T0344658

Antibodies
for Infectious Diseases

Antibodies
for Infectious Diseases

Edited by

James E. Crowe, Jr.
Vanderbilt University Medical Center
Nashville, Tennessee

Diana Boraschi
National Research Council
Napoli, Italy

AND

Rino Rappuoli
Novartis Vaccines
Siena, Italy

ASM
PRESS

Washington, DC

Library of Congress Cataloging-in-Publication Data

Antibodies for infectious diseases / edited by James E. Crowe, Jr., Vanderbilt University Medical Center, Nashville, Tennessee, Diana Boraschi, National Research Council, Napoli, Italy, and Rino Rappuoli, Novartis Vaccines, Siena, Italy.
   pages cm
   Includes bibliographical references and index.
   ISBN 978-1-55581-735-0 (alk. paper)
   1. Immunoglobulins. 2. Communicable diseases--Immunological aspects. I. Crowe, James E., Jr., editor. II. Boraschi, D. (Diana), editor. III. Rappuoli, Rino, editor.
   QR186.7.A534 2015
   616.07'98--dc23
   2015009356
   eISBN: 978-1-55581-741-1
   doi:10.1128/9781555817411
   10 9 8 7 6 5 4 3 2 1

All Rights Reserved
Printed in the United States of America

Address editorial correspondence to ASM Press, 1752 N St., N.W.,
Washington, DC 20036-2904, USA
Send orders to ASM Press, P.O. Box 605, Herndon, VA 20172, USA
Phone: 800-546-2416; 703-661-1593
Fax: 703-661-1501
E-mail: books@asmusa.org
Online: http://estore.asm.org

Cover image: Cancer cell with high details (source: 123RF)

Contents

ALTERNATE SYSTEMS FOR EXPRESSION

Contributors

Edith Acquaye-Seedah
Department of Biochemistry
University of Texas at Austin
Austin, TX 78712

Ramesh Akkina
Department of Microbiology, Immunology, and Pathology
Colorado State University
1619 Campus Delivery
Fort Collins, CO 80523

Shanta P. Boddapati
Department of Biomedical Engineering
Oregon Health and Science University
3181 SW Sam Jackson Park Road
Portland, OR 97239

Scott D. Boyd
Department of Pathology
Stanford University
Stanford, CA 94305

Arturo Casadevall
Departments of Microbiology and Immunology, and Medicine
Albert Einstein College of Medicine of Yeshiva University
1695A Eastchester Road
Bronx, NY 10461

Davide Corti
Humabs BioMed SA
via Mirasole 1
Bellinzona, 6500
Switzerland

James E. Crowe, Jr.
School of Medicine
Vanderbilt University
Nashville, TN 37232

Ekaterina (Kate) Dadachova
Departments of Radiology, Microbiology and Immunology
Albert Einstein College of Medicine of Yeshiva University
1695A Eastchester Road
Bronx, NY 10461

Donald N. Forthal
Department of Infectious Diseases
3044 Hewitt Hall
University of California, Irvine
Irvine, CA 92617

Manuel A. Franco
Facultad de Ciencias y MedicinaPontificia
Universidad Javeriana
Oficina 306, Edificio 50
Carrera 7 # 40-62
Bogotá
Colombia

Bettina C. Fries
Department of Medicine/Infectious Diseases and
Department of Microbiology and Immunology
Albert Einstein College of Medicine
Bronx, NY 10461

Zachary P. Frye
Department of Chemical Engineering
University of Texas at Austin
Austin, TX 78712

Amy E. Gilbert
Cutaneous Medicine and Immunotherapy Unit
St. John's Institute of Dermatology
Division of Genetics and Molecular Medicine & NIHR
Biomedical Research Centre at Guy's and St. Thomas's Hospitals and
King's College London School of Medicine
Guy's Hospital
London SE1 9RT
United Kingdom

Hannah J. Gould
Randall Division of Cell and Molecular Biophysics
Division of Asthma, Allergy and Lung Biology
MRC and Asthma UK Centre for Allergic Mechanisms of Asthma
King's College London
New Hunt's House
Guy's Campus
London SE1 1UL
United Kingdom

Harry B. Greenberg
Departments of Medicine and Microbiology and Immunology
Stanford University
School of Medicine and the VAPAHCS
Palo Alto, CA 94305

Scott B. Halstead
Department of Preventive Medicine and Biometrics
Uniformed Services University of the Health Sciences
Bethesda, MD 20814

Shen Y. Helvig
Department of Pharmacy
Center for Pharmaceutical Nanotechnology and Nanotoxicology
Faculty of Health and Medical Sciences
University of Copenhagen
Copenhagen, DK-2100
Denmark

Adam Hey
Preclinical Safety, Biologics
Novartis AG
Basel
Switzerland

Andrew Hiatt
Mapp Biopharmaceutical, Inc.
6160 Lusk Blvd. #C105
San Diego, CA 92121

Björn Hock
Department of Protein Engineering and Antibody Technologies
Merck Serono, Merck KgaA
Frankfurter Str. 250
D-64293 Darmstadt
Germany

Kelly Huang
Department of Infectious Disease
MedImmune, LLC
One MedImmune Way
Gaithersburg, MD 20878

Philip R. Johnson
The Children's Hospital of Philadelphia
Abramson Research Center
Philadelphia, PA 19104

Debra H. Josephs
Cutaneous Medicine and Immunotherapy Unit
St. John's Institute of Dermatology
Division of Genetics and Molecular Medicine & NIHR
Biomedical Research Centre at Guy's and St. Thomas's Hospitals
King's College London School of Medicine
Guy's Hospital
London SE1 9RT
United Kingdom

Shilpa A. Joshi
Department of Pathology
Stanford University
Stanford, CA 94305

Sophia N. Karagiannis
Cutaneous Medicine and Immunotherapy Unit
St. John's Institute of Dermatology
Division of Genetics and Molecular Medicine & NIHR Biomedical Research
Centre at Guy's and
St. Thomas's Hospitals
King's College London School of Medicine
Guy's Hospital
London SE1 9RT
United Kingdom

Panagiotis Karagiannis
Cutaneous Medicine and Immunotherapy Unit
St. John's Institute of Dermatology
Division of Genetics and Molecular Medicine & NIHR Biomedical Research
Centre at Guy's and
St. Thomas's Hospitals
King's College London School of Medicine
Guy's Hospital
London SE1 9RT
United Kingdom

Jens C. Krause
Children's Hospital
University of Freiburg Medical Center
79106 Freiberg
Germany

Antonio Lanzavecchia
Institute for Research in Biomedicine
via Vincenzo Vela 6
Bellinzona, 6500
Switzerland

Marie-Paule Lefranc
Laboratoire d'ImmunoGénétique Moléculaire LIGM
IMGT®, the international ImMunoGeneTics information system®
Institut de Génétique Humaine IGH
Université Montpellier 2
UPR CNRS 1142
Montpellier, 34396
cedex 5, 40202
France

Olivier Leger
Department of Protein Engineering and Antibody Technologies
Merck Serono S.A.--Geneva
9, chemin des Mines
1202 Geneva
Switzerland

Kin-Ming Lo
Department of Protein Engineering and Antibody Technologies
EMD Serono Research Institute
45A Middlesex Turnpike
Billerica, MA 01821

Wayne A. Marasco
Department of Cancer Immunology and AIDS
Dana-Farber Cancer Institute
Harvard Medical School
Boston, MA 02215

Jennifer A. Maynard
Department of Chemical Engineering
University of Texas at Austin
Austin, TX 78712

Luzia M. Mayr
INSERM U1109
Université de Strasbourg
3 Rue Koeberlé
67000 Strasbourg
France

Jens Meiler
Department of Chemistry and Center for Structural Biology
Vanderbilt University
Nashville, TN 37212

S. Moein Moghimi
Department of Pharmacy
Center for Pharmaceutical Nanotechnology and Nanotoxicology
Faculty of Health and Medical Sciences
University of Copenhagen
Copenhagen, DK-2100
Denmark

Susan Zolla-Pazner
New York University School of Medicine
550 First Avenue
New York, NY 10016

Louise Saul
Cutaneous Medicine and Immunotherapy Unit
St. John's Institute of Dermatology
Division of Genetics and Molecular Medicine & NIHR Biomedical Research
Centre at Guy's and
St. Thomas's Hospitals
King's College London School of Medicine
Guy's Hospital
London SE1 9RT
United Kingdom

Bruce C. Schnepp
The Children's Hospital of Philadelphia
Abramson Research Center
Philadelphia, PA 19104

Jennifer E. Schuster
Department of Pediatrics
Children's Mercy Hospital
Kansas City, MO 64108-4619

Alexander M. Sevy
Department of Chemistry and Center for Structural Biology
Vanderbilt University
Nashville, TN 37212

Jared Sheehan
Department of Cancer Immunology and AIDS
Dana-Farber Cancer Institute
Harvard Medical School
Boston, MA 02215

Michael R. Sierks
Department of Chemical Engineering
Arizona State University
Tempe, AZ 85287-6006

Scott A. Smith
The Vanderbilt Vaccine Center and the Department of Medicine
Vanderbilt University Medical Center
Nashville, TN 37232

Robyn L. Stanfield
Department of Molecular Biology
The Scripps Research Institute
10550 North Torrey Pines Road
La Jolla, CA 92037

Nadine Upton
Randall Division of Cell and Molecular Biophysics
Division of Asthma, Allergy and Lung Biology
MRC and Asthma UK Centre for Allergic Mechanisms of Asthma
King's College London
New Hunt's House
Guy's Campus
London SE1 1UL
United Kingdom

Avanish K. Varshney
Department of Medicine/Infectious Diseases and
Department of Microbiology and Immunology
Albert Einstein College of Medicine
Bronx, NY 10461

Stefanie N. Velgos
Mayo Clinic Arizona
5777 East Mayo Boulevard
Phoenix, AZ 85054

Kevin J. Whaley
Mapp Biopharmaceutical, Inc.
6160 Lusk Blvd. #C105
San Diego, CA 92121

Peter P. Wibroe
Centre for Pharmaceutical Nanotechnology and Nanotoxicology
Department of Pharmacy
Faculty of Health and Medical Sciences
University of Copenhagen
Copenhagen, DK-2100
Denmark

John V. Williams
Department of Pediatrics
School of Medicine
Vanderbilt University
Nashville, TN 37232-2581

Ian A. Wilson
Department of Molecular Biology and Skaggs Institute for Chemical Biology
The Scripps Research Institute
10550 North Torrey Pines Road
La Jolla, CA 92037

Herren Wu
Department of Antibody Discovery and Protein Engineering
MedImmune, LLC
One MedImmune Way
Gaithersburg, MD 20879

Guocheng Yang
Department of Chemical Engineering
Arizona State University
Tempe, AZ 85287-6006

Larry Zeitlin
Mapp Biopharmaceutical, Inc.
6160 Lusk Blvd. #C105
San Diego, CA 92121

Preface

Antibodies form the principal foundation for modern intervention against infectious diseases. Emil Adolf von Behring was awarded the first Nobel Prize in Physiology or Medicine in 1901 *"for his work on serum therapy, especially its application against diphtheria, by which he has opened a new road in the domain of medical science and thereby placed in the hands of the physician a victorious weapon against illness and deaths."* Antibodies now provide the focus for understanding mechanisms of immunity to most infectious diseases, and they play a central role in passive immunotherapy and active vaccination as mechanisms or correlates of immunity. For most of the 20th century, immunotherapy was based on passive transfer of polyclonal hyperimmune animal serum, immune human serum, or even hyperimmune human serum. Georges J.F. Köhler and César Milstein reported the generation of monoclonal antibodies in 1979, for which they shared the 1984 Nobel Prize in Physiology or Medicine *"for . . .the discovery of the principle for production of monoclonal antibodies."* Since that time, entire fields related to antibodies for infectious diseases, including antibody gene cloning, engineering, and expression; antibody libraries; and high-throughput antibody gene repertoire sequence analysis have extended our capabilities to explore the diversity of antibody specificity and function with unprecedented depth and breadth.

This book provides a broad survey of many of the most important aspects of the field of antibodies for infectious diseases. The book begins with a general introduction, followed by chapters 2 through 5 on general features pertaining to structure, function, isotype, and the role of complement in antibody function. Chapters 6 through 10 review contemporary approaches for antibody discovery using phage and yeast display, plasma cell and memory B cell cloning, human hybridomas, humanized mice, and computational methods. Chapters 11 through 18 review in depth the biology of antibodies specific for particular pathogens, including viruses and bacterial toxins, to illustrate the role of antibodies in antimicrobial immunity with specific targets. These chapters reveal that attempts to raise effective antibody responses to each of these pathogens faces unique and pathogen-specific challenges. Chapters 19 to 23 cover major technical advances pertaining to antibody engineering, repertoire sequencing and analysis, and new methods for study or therapeutic use of antibodies, including radiotherapy. Finally, chapters 24 and 25 cover new methods for expression of monoclonal antibodies, in plants or by transfer of antibody genes for *in vivo* expression in treated subjects.

Recent literature is exploding with new antibody-related techniques and reports of antimicrobial antibodies with unprecedented potency, breadth of activity, and therapeutic potential. We hope that this timely compilation of state-of-the-art reviews of major aspects of this field will be of interest to both antibody cognoscenti and those new to this exciting field. We thank the authors for their dedication in producing definitive reviews of the topics at hand.

James E. Crowe, Jr.
Diana Boraschi
Rino Rappuoli

INTRODUCTION

History and Practice:
Antibodies in Infectious Diseases

ADAM HEY[1]

Antibodies in Infectious Diseases aims to inform, update, and inspire students, teachers, researchers, pharmaceutical developers, and health care professionals on the status of the development of antibody-based therapies for treating infectious diseases and the potential for these in times of growing antibiotic resistance to provide alternative treatment solutions to the currently used antibiotics and new treatments for infectious diseases where no proper treatments are available.

This introductory article will provide a historical perspective on the use of antibody-based therapies, followed by a high-level overview of what makes antibodies attractive tools for this purpose. This will include the pros and cons of such therapies compared to the use of antibiotics and the practical and strategic considerations involved in selecting the best format and development path for new antibody-based therapies targeting specific infectious agents. Then, examples of antibody-based therapies in the development of treatments for infectious diseases will be presented, and finally a look into the future will summarize the different aspects that will influence what the future might bring for this type of treatments for infectious diseases.

[1]Preclinical Safety, Biologics, Novartis AG, Basel, Switzerland.
Antibodies for Infectious Diseases
Edited by James E. Crowe, Jr., Diana Boraschi, and Rino Rappuoli
© 2015 American Society for Microbiology, Washington, DC
doi:10.1128/microbiolspec.AID-0026-2014

HISTORICAL PERSPECTIVE

Antibodies and the use of passive antibody therapy in the treatment of infectious diseases is the story of a treatment concept which dates back more than 120 years, to the late 19th century, and which originally, by the use of serum from immunized animals, provided the first effective treatment options against severe bacterial infections (1, 2). By immunizing horses with bacterial toxins from *Clostridium tetani* and *Corynebacterium diphtheriae*, Emil A. Von Behring and Shibasaburo Kitasato (3) generated serum containing antibodies capable of neutralizing the effects of the toxins produced by these bacteria and successfully provided treatment for these serious diseases where the pathogenesis is driven by the effects of the bacterial toxins. For his work on providing treatment for diphtheria, Behring received the Nobel Prize in Physiology or Medicine in 1901. These radical treatment results quickly prompted development of multiple additional serum therapies for the treatment of infectious diseases caused by, e.g., *Neisseria meningitidis, Haemophilus influenza*, and group A *Streptococcus*. Since serum therapy involved administration of large amounts of crude mixtures of animal proteins including antibodies, they were associated with side effects in the form of hypersensitivity and serum sickness (2).

Due to the crude and unpurified nature of these products, side effects were seen even when administering human serum preparations. Side effects were observed in up to 50% of patients and were considered to be caused by immune complex formations that resulted in symptoms such as rash, itching, joint pain, fever, and in serious cases hypotension and shock. However, due to the lack of alternative options, these treatments were, despite their side effects, widely used. Serum was normally administered by intravenous infusion in patients after a test for hypersensitivity where a small amount of serum was injected subcutaniously (1). As described

above, serum therapy applied in these early days (late 19th century and early 20th century) involved preparations of serum from rabbits and horses immunized with the infectious agent or in live and/or neutralized versions or toxins from these (1). The costs of keeping the immunized animals and the production and potency testing of the materials made this a relatively expensive treatment. In 1891, data from Klemperer (4) showed serum therapy to protect rabbits from *Streptococcus pneumoniae* infection and paved the way for this type of treatment and for development of similar serum-based treatments of streptococcal infections in humans. When treating humans, early administration of serum could reduce mortality significantly down to around 5% compared to when administered 4 to 5 days after onset of symptoms, when serum treatment was largely without effect. This strongly indicated the need for quick diagnosis and quick treatment to control the infection before it got out of control. Consequently, in the absence of a specific diagnosis, mixtures of serum from immunizations with different serotypes were used to circumvent this need for early treatment without having a serotype-specific diagnosis. The understanding that different serotypes existed for pneumococci and that efficient treatment relied on using serotype-specific serum was being built up during the 1920s and 1930s through experience from extensive clinical trials.

By the end of the 1930s serum therapy was the standard of care for treatment of pneumococcal pneumonia. At that time, the efficacy and potency of the derived sera were assessed in mice, in "the mouse protection test" by testing survival after a concomitant intraperitoneal injection of a lethal dose of pneumococci and the serum to be tested. Due to the inherent variation in this test, efficacy and survival in two thirds of the animals was the acceptance criteria, and 10 times the lowest dose providing this was used for defining a unit of the serum. This allowed for large batch-to-batch variation, and the use of different strains of bacteria for immunization probably explains part of the missing responses observed (1). In the early 20th century a pandemic of meningitis in Europe and the United States, with mortality rates up to 80%, spurred the development of serum therapy treatment options. Although in the 1930s this became the recommended treatment in children assumed to be suffering from meningitis, failure to reduce mortality in several meningitis epidemics during that time raised doubts about the general applicability of serum treatment. In those days serum therapy often involved quite extensive procedures and infusion of large volumes of serum. The following example clearly illustrates this. Data from Flexner and Jobling (5) from treating meningitis in monkeys resulted in the development of sera from immunized horses for treatment in humans. The treatment protocol included lumbar puncture and withdrawal of more than 30 ml of spinal fluid representing an amount slightly larger than the expected amount of horse serum to be injected subsequently. This treatment involved such daily slow infusions of up to 30 ml of serum until the patient's condition improved. This treatment was used in outbreaks in New York in 1905 and 1906 and did markedly decrease mortality.

After the discovery of penicillin by Fleming in 1928, and the subsequent introduction of antibiotics in the 1930s, serum therapy was largely abandoned over a period of 10 years due to the availability of these new, more broadly effective and cheaper treatment options, which also had fewer side effects. Although improvements in the purification of antibodies had resulted in preparations with better safety and side effect profiles, high manufacturing costs and narrow specificity resulted in antibody therapy being mostly restricted to a smaller number of selected treatments for snake venoms, bacterial toxins, and some viral infections (1, 2). Currently, antibody administration is used for treatment and prevention of hepatitis B virus, rabies virus, respiratory syncytial virus (RSV), *Clostridium tetani, Clostridium botulinum*, vaccinia virus, echovirus, and enterovirus. For the most part, these treatments consist of pooled immunoglobulin, also known as IVIG (intravenous immunoglobulin), from several postexposure donors. This results in both batch-to-batch variation, in the need for relatively large amounts of serum due to low specificity and to restricted supplies due to reliance on exposed donors.

However, several challenges have resulted in the need for new tools in the treatment and prevention of infectious diseases. The broad and general use of antibiotics in human and veterinary medicine for many years has resulted in the development of multi-resistant strains of bacteria with limited to no response to existing treatments such as methicillin-resistant *Staphylococcus aureus* (MRSA), vancomycin-resistant *S. aureus*, and others. This has resulted in patients needing screening and treatment with several antibacterial agents and longer treatment time, causing extra strain on patients and health care providers (6; http://www.cdc.gov/drugresistance/threat-report-2013/index.html). According to the WHO and CDC more than 25,000 people in European Union countries and similar numbers in the United States die every year as a result of antibiotic-resistant infections. This together with the emergence of new pathogens (e.g., severe acute respiratory syndrome, Middle East respiratory syndrome), the re-emergence/epidemics of old/known pathogens (e.g., Ebola), and the difficulties in treating infections in immune-deficient patients (e.g., HIV patients) has highlighted the need for new solutions. The 2014 Ebola epidemic in West Africa (Liberia, Sierra Leone, Guinea, Nigeria, and Senegal) has further highlighted this. No treatment or prophylactic vaccine is available to treat or prevent the spread of Ebola infections, which have an average mortality of >50%. Local health authorities in the affected countries are struggling to contain and handle the disease, which is threatening to go out of control and spread more widely. Various products, mainly antibody cocktails from previously recovered patients, are being used despite a lack of clinical data on their safety and efficacy, and those are the only sporadically available treatment options and only in small amounts and for a few patients.

Ebola is an example of a disease which normally affects only a small number of individuals and which normally burns out when disease outbreaks are contained. Therefore, given the small number of potential patients affected by previous Ebola infections to date, there was no incentive for big pharma companies to do research and development of drugs for Ebola. With the increasing number of infected (13,567) and a death toll of 4,951 (7) and the lack of the ability to contain the epidemic, it will be interesting to follow the aftermath of this outbreak and see whether there will be requests for new ways to ensure that vaccines and treatment options are available for Ebola and similar high-mortality and potential bio-warfare infections that have no available treatments or procedures to for mass-production upon the first signs/reports of active infections. Although both the CDC and the WHO have special programs focusing on these types of infections, the Ebola outbreak in 2014 clearly shows that more financial support for research and development of new diagnostics and treatments is needed. This is one example where antibody-based treatments would have the potential to play a major role. To put this in the right perspective, one should, however, not forget that other infectious diseases such as tuberculosis, influenza, and malaria kill hundreds of thousands each year. There is therefore plenty of room for improvement in developing treatments for these diseases as well, but the high attention drawn to, e.g., the Ebola outbreak creates a special niche and opportunity where antibody treatments could gain extraordinary development funding and support and prove their value and treatment potential.

That antibody-based therapies could take this role is supported by the revolution in technologies for the development, selection, generation, and purification of fully human antibodies described in more detail later in the section "Methods and Platforms for Generating Antibodies". Antibody-based programs currently at different stages of development include investigations into the potential use of single antibody preparations, combinations of antibodies (to avoid survival of escape mutants), fragments of antibodies, and antibodies carrying radioactive isotopes or cytotoxic drugs or antibody-like frameworks (e.g., fibronectin) either alone, as a first-line treatment, or as an adjunct to existing treatments. This multitude of possible formats, the ability to raise antibodies to almost any target and the ability to engineer both size, effector functions, and half-life are now considered by many to provide very valuable tools for designing specific antibody-based treatments to eradicate specific targeted infectious agents. However, although several antibody-based therapies have been approved for oncology and anti-inflammatory indications (see Table 1), only one monoclonal antibody (mAb) is approved against an infectious disease agent—Synagis (palivizumab, MedImmune) for the prevention and treatment of respiratory syncytical virus (RSV) in high-risk children. Economic obstacles such as the high cost of mAb therapies and relatively small markets have resulted in less interest from pharmaceutical companies in developing these. Also highlighting the challenges in developing these types of antibody-based treatments are the difficulties encountered in developing a follow-up higher-affinity candidate to Synagis. Poor translatability of data obtained in the available animal disease models for RSV in cotton rats has resulted in non-approval due to inferiority relative to Synagis. In other viral diseases such as cytomegalovirus (CMV) the high species specificity of the strains of CMV makes it impossible to test human antibody therapies *in vivo*. Therefore, any real data on the efficacy of treatments for CMV will not be obtained until testing in clinical trials. As described later in this article several new antibody-based therapies for infectious diseases are in development, and hopefully this will gradually open the field and result in better treatment options and outcomes for patients.

TABLE 1 Approved and pending antibody-based therapies

Name: antibody	Target: antibody type	Indication	Company	Approval date
OKT3[a]: Muronomab-CD3	CD3: murine, IgG2a	Autoimmune	Johnson & Johnson	1986 (U.S.)
ReoPro: abciximab	PIIb/IIIa: chimeric, IgG1, Fab	Homeostasis	Johnson & Johnson	1984 (U.S.)
Rituxan: rituximab	CD20: chimeric, IgG1	Cancer	Genentech	1997 (U.S.) 1998 (E.U.)
Zenapax[a]: daclizumab	CD25: humanized, IgG1	Autoimmune	Roche	1997 (U.S.) 1999 (E.U.)
Simulect: basiliximab	CD25: chimeric, IgG1	Autoimmune	Novartis	1998 (U.S., E.U.)
Synagis: palivizumab	RSV: humanized, IgG1	Infections	MedImmune	1998 (U.S.) 1999 (E.U.)
Remicade: infliximab	TNFα: chimeric, IgG1	Autoimmune	Johnson & Johnson	1998 (U.S.) 1999 (E.U.)
Herceptin: trastuzumab	HER2: humanized, IgG1	Cancer	Genentech/ Roche	1998 (U.S.) 2000 (E.U.)
Mylotarg[a]: gemtuzumab ozogamicin	CD33: humanized, IgG4, immunotoxin	Cancer	Wyeth/Pfizer	2000 (U.S.)
Campath: alemtuzumab	CD52: humanized, IgG1	Cancer	Genzyme	2001 (U.S.) 2001 (E.U.)
Zevalin: ibritumomab tiuxetan	CD20: murine, IgG1, radiolabeled (yttrium 90)	Cancer	Biogen Idec	2002 (U.S.) 2004 (E.U.)
Humira: adalimumab	TNFα: human, IgG1	Autoimmune	Abbott	2002 (U.S.) 2003 (E.U.)
Xolair: omalizumab	IgE: humanized, IgG1	Autoimmune	Genentech/ Roche	2003 (U.S.)
Bexxar: tositumomab-I-131	CD20: murine, IgG2a, radiolabeled (iodine 131)	Cancer	Corixa/GSK	2003 (U.S.)
Raptiva[a]: falizumab	CD11a: humanized, IgG1	Autoimmune	Genentech/ Roche	2003 (U.S.) 2004 (E.U.)
Erbitux: cetuximab	EGFR: chimeric, IgG1	Cancer	Imclone/Lilly	2004 (U.S.) 2004 (E.U.)
Avastin: bevacizumab	VEGF: humanized, IgG1	Cancer	Genentech/ Roche	2004 (U.S.) 2005 (E.U.)
Tysabri: natalizumab	α4-Intergrin: humanized, IgG4	Autoimmune	Biogen Idec	2004 (U.S.)
Actemra: tocilizumab	Anti-IL-6R: humanized, IgG1	Autoimmune	Chugai/ Roche	2005 (Japan) 2010 (U.S.)
Vectibix: panitumumab	EGFR: human, IgG2	Cancer	Amgen	2006 (U.S.)
Lucentis: ranibizumab	VEGF: humanized IgG1 Fab	Macular degeneration	Genentech/ Roche	2006 (U.S.)
Soliris: eculizumab	C5: humanized IgG2/4	Blood disorders	Alexion	2007 (U.S.)
Cimzia: certolizumab pegol	TNFα: humanized, pegylated Fab	Autoimmune	UCB	2008 (US)
Simponi: golimumab	TNFα: human IgG1	Autoimmune	Johnson & Johnson	2009 (U.S., E.U., Canada)
Ilaris: canakinumab	IL1b: human IgG1	Infalmmatory	Novartis	2009 (U.S., E.U.)
Stelara: ustekinumab	IL-12/23: human IgG1	Autoimmune	Johnson & Johnson	2008 (E.U.) 2009 (U.S.)
Arzerra: ofatumumab	CD20: human IgG1	Cancer	Genmab	2009 (E.U.)
Prolia: denosumab	RANK ligand: human IgG2	Bone loss	Amgen	2010 (U.S.)
Numax: motavizumab	RSV: humanized IgG1	Anti-infective	MedImmune	Pending
ABthrax: Raxibacumab	*B. anthrasis* PA: human IgG1	Anti-infection	GSK	2012 (U.S.)
Benlysta: belimumab	BLyS: human IgG1	Autoimmune	HGS	2011 (U.S.)
Yervoy: ipilimumab	CTLA-4: human IgG1	Cancer	BMS	2011 (U.S.)
Adcetris: brentuximab vedotin	CD30: chimeric, IgG1, drug- conjugate	Cancer	Seattle Genetics	2011 (U.S.)

(Continued on next page)

TABLE 1 Approved and pending antibody-based therapies *(Continued)*

Name: antibody	Target: antibody type	Indication	Company	Approval date
Perjeta: pertuzumab	Her2: humanized, IgG1	Cancer	Genentech/ Roche	2012 (U.S.)
Kadcyla: ado-trastuzumab emtansine	Her2: humanized, IgG1, Drug-conjugate	Cancer	Genentech/ Roche	2013 (U.S.)
Raxibacumab	Anti-B anthrasis PA: human IgG1	Anthrax infection	Not approved	2012
Entyvio: vedolizumab	Integrin $\alpha_4\beta_7$: humanized IgG1	Crohn's disease, ulcerative colitis	Takeda	2014 (U.S.)
Cyramza: ramuciruumab	Anti-VEGFR2: Human IgG1	Gastric cancer	Lilly	2014 (U.S.)
Gazyva: obinutuzumab	Anti-CD20: humanized IgG1 glucoengineered	Cancer/CLL[b]	Genentech/ Roche	2014 (U.S.)
Sylvant: situximab	Anti IL-6: chimeric IgG1	Castleman disease	Janssen	2014 (U.S.), 2014 (E.U.)
Cosentyx: sekukinumab	Anti IL-17a: human IgG1	Psoriasis	Novartis	2015 (U.S.), 2015 (E.U.)
Nivolumab	Anti PD-1: human IgG4	Melanoma	BMS	Not approved
Keytruda: pembrolizuumab	Anti-PD-1: humanized IgG4	Melanoma	Merck	2014 (U.S.)

[a]Antibodies approved but later withdrawn.
[b]CLL, chronic lymphocytic leukemia.

INTRODUCTION TO ANTIBODIES

Antibodies, also called immunoglobulins based on their combined structure and function in immune responses, are produced by B cells of the immune system. They are part of the adaptive immune response and are specially designed for neutralizing and eliminating the infectious agents and toxins produced by these. Antibodies are present in blood, plasma, and extracellular fluids, and since these fluids were formerly known as humors, they were said to be part of the humoral immune response. Antibodies are Y-shaped structures consisting of two main parts: the upper arms of the Y, which contain two identical variable-region antigen binding sites, and the lower region, called the constant region, which is responsible for the initiation of effector functions that lead to the removal and destruction of the pathogen or cells harboring the pathogen (see Fig. 1). The antigen-binding sites on an antibody can by themselves bind to and neutralize bacterial toxins and viruses, thereby preventing them from binding to their target cells or receptors causing toxic effects or spread of the infection.

Antibodies consist of two pairs of heavy and light chains which, as described above, are held together in a Y-shaped arrangement. Each of the heavy and light chains in these pairs is separated into constant and variable chains. The upper arms of the Y each contain a variable and a constant section of the light and the heavy chain, where the upper variable parts of the heavy and light chains contain the antigen-binding site, and the constant parts are connected via disulfide bonds. The lower part of the Y, called the constant part, consists of two or three constant segments (immunoglobulin domains) from each of the two heavy chains interacting and also linked via disulfide bonds. The sections of the heavy chains connecting the constant part of the upper arms to the constant parts of the constant region contain special hinge regions that provide flexibility to the different sections of the antibody to bind to antigens and effector cells. The constant regions of the heavy chain also contain attached oligosaccharide moieties which provide functional specialization to the antibodies (8).

The variable domains of the heavy and light chains form the antigen-binding sites and

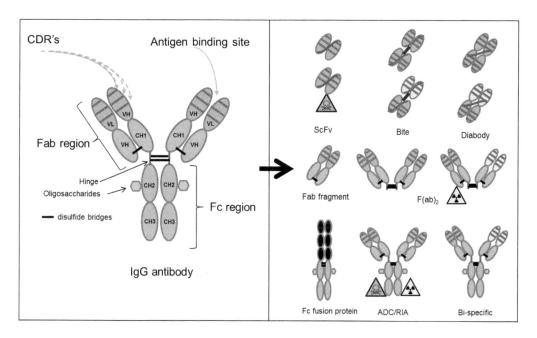

FIGURE 1 (Left panel) Model of antibody structure exemplified by IgG. On top the antigen-binding sites in orange each contain one variable light and variable heavy domain with the three complementarity determining regions (CDRs) that are responsible for the specific binding of the antibody to its target. For each arm of the antibody, an additional set of variable heavy and light domains, together with the CDR-containing domains, represent the two fragment antigen binding (Fab) regions. The two Fabs are held together via two disulfide bridges. Below the Fabs is the Fc region, which contains four constant heavy domains. On the upper pair of these domains are binding sites for oligosaccharides, which have major importance for the ability of the antibody Fc part to trigger effector functions when the Fc portion is bound to Fc gamma receptors on natural killer cells, neutrophil granulocytes, monocytes/macrophages, dendritic cells, and B cells. (Right panel) Examples of some of the antibody-derived alternative formats used to exploit the specific features of the CDRs, the Fabs, and the Fc parts of the antibodies. ScFv: The single chain fragment variable consists of the variable domains of the heavy and light chains held together by a flexible linker. This can also be used as a carrier of a cytotoxic drug in a so-called antibody drug complex (ADC) where the specificity of the ScFv is used to target the cytotoxic drug to, e.g., a tumor. Bite (bi-specific T cell engager): Fusion proteins consisting of two ScFvs, one directed against the target on a tumor cell and the other against the T cell receptor (CD3). Diabody: ScFv dimers where short linker peptides (five amino acids) ensure dimerization, and not folding, of the ScFvs. Fab and F(ab)$_2$ fragments: Single Fab fragments or fragments containing two Fabs linked via disulfide bridges. This is used where effector functions related to the Fc part of the antibody are unwanted and where a smaller size is desired to obtain better tissue penetration in, e.g., tumors. Due to the lack of the FcRn binding via the Fc part, Fab and F(ab)$_2$ fragments have much shorter half-lives (hours or days) than full-size antibodies (weeks). These can also be used as carriers of cytotoxic payloads or cytotoxic radioactive isotopes and for the F(ab)$_2$ fragments can be constructed as bi-specifics which can cross-link immune cells and target cells. Fc fusion protein: Fusion protein containing the Fc domain of an immunoglobulin bound to a peptide. The peptide can be a ligand for a specific receptor on a target cell or a blocking peptide for a soluble ligand. The Fc part provides a longer half-life to the construct and the potential to bind to and engage effector functions in the killing of, e.g., tumor cells or infected cells. ADCs/RIAs and bi-specifics: Full-size IgG antibodies carrying either a cytotoxic chemical or radioactive payload, which may also carry different CDRs, enabling cross-linking of effector and target cells for increased killing. doi:10.1128/microbiolspec.AID-0026-2014.f1

contain special hyper-variable segments called complementarity-determining regions (CDRs), which allow the B cells, via genetic recombination, to generate antibodies to all the different antigens specific to amino acid sequences or three-dimensional structural motifs (polysaccharides, DNA, and RNA) found on pathogens.

Based on the structure of their heavy chain constant regions, antibodies, or immunoglobulins, are separated into five classes—IgM, IgG, IgE, IgD, and IgA. Differences in the sequences of the constant regions provide distinct characteristics to these different classes. These characteristics include the number of heavy chain constant segments, the number and location of interconnecting disulfide bridges, the length of the hinge region, and the number and location of oligosaccharide moieties. For IgG, four heavy chain versions exist, creating IgG1, 2, 3, and 4 isotypes, each with different characteristics in their serum half-lives and ability to trigger different effector functions. Because of the combined advantage from ability to trigger effector mechanisms, long [21 days] half-life, their ability to be transported over the placenta, and their stability in the production process, antibodies of the IgG class and of the IgG1 isotype are preferred as the basis for new antibody-based therapies. The effector functions are triggered by the Fc part of an antibody when the variable parts of the antibody are bound directly to an infectious agent or to proteins from an infectious agent expressed on an infected cell. This binding leaves the Fc part free to interact with Fc receptors on phagocytic cells and neutrophils, eosinophils, and natural killer cells capable of inducing phagocytosis or lysis of infectious agents or infected cells. These effector functions include (i) the ability to activate the complement system for lysis (complement-dependent cellular cytotoxicity); (ii) triggering of uptake and destruction by phagocytic cells such as macrophages and neutrophils via interaction with Fc receptors on these cells; (iii) activation of macrophages, eosinophils, neutrophils, and natural killer cells to kill infected cells via binding to Fc receptors on these cells and antibody-dependent cellular cytotoxicity; and (iv) neutralization of bacterial toxins and blocking of binding and uptake of bacteria or viruses to target cells (see Fig. 2) (9).

The Fc part of IgG antibodies also contains a region that interacts with the neonatal Fc receptor (FcRn) expressed on most immunocompetent cells and in many other cells such as endothelial cells in kidney, liver, placenta, lung, and breast (10), which protects antibodies from degradation by phagocytotic/exocytotic cycling into FcRn-expressing cells, thereby prolonging their half-life. This results in half-lives of 20 to 21 days for most IgG1, 2, and 4 antibodies, whereas half-lives are 10, 6, and 2 days, respectively, for IgM, IgA, and IgE. The highly specific binding sites on the variable regions of the upper arms of the antibody allow for several important features of antibodies–binding to and neutralization of, e.g., bacterial toxins, binding to pathogens and blocking their binding to or interaction with target cells (e.g., cyncytia formation of CMV-infected cells); or blocking of binding and interactions of infectious agents with target cells via blocking receptors on the target cells.

METHODS AND PLATFORMS FOR GENERATING ANTIBODIES

As described above, the early use of passive antibody transfer as a therapy in infectious diseases involved the use of immune serum from immunized sheep and horses. These preparations were crude and contained a broad mixture of neutralizing and non-neutralizing antibodies and both the foreign nature of the antibodies and the numerous host serum proteins. This resulted in less specific and thus less efficient therapies due to a high variability in efficacy between batches derived from different animals immunized with different strains of bacteria in different laboratories and resulted in multiple unwanted side effects related to hypersensitivity and

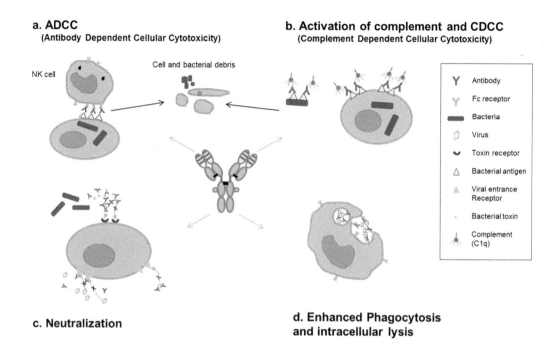

a. ADCC
(Antibody Dependent Cellular Cytotoxicity)

b. Activation of complement and CDCC
(Complement Dependent Cellular Cytotoxicity)

NK cell

Cell and bacterial debris

Y	Antibody
Y	Fc receptor
▬	Bacteria
	Virus
	Toxin receptor
△	Bacterial antigen
▲	Viral entrance Receptor
-	Bacterial toxin
	Complement (C1q)

c. Neutralization

d. Enhanced Phagocytosis and intracellular lysis

FIGURE 2 **Effector functions of antibodies. (a) Antibodies bind to pathogen-derived or endogenous antigens expressed on the surface of an infected cell, which triggers binding to Fc receptors on natural killer cells and lysis of the infected cell by antibody-dependent cellular cytotoxicity. (b) Antibodies bind to pathogen-derived or endogenous antigens expressed on the surface of infected cells, which triggers activation of complement through binding of complement factor C1q. (c) Neutralization. Top: Bacterial toxin neutralized by bound antigen. Bottom: Antibody bound to either receptor for the virus or to the virus itself, which blocks virus binding and entry into the cell. (d) Antibody bound to viral surface proteins binds to Fc receptors on phagocytic cells, e.g., macrophages, and triggers endocytosis and destruction of virus in endolysosome. doi:10.1128/microbiolspec.AID-0026-2014.f2**

anaphylactic reactions to foreign proteins. These days, antibodies being developed for treatment of diseases in humans are highly purified and are mostly fully human monoclonal antibodies. The term monoclonal antibody refers to that cell cultures used for generating these antibodies each originates from a single cell and thus produces only one specific antibody. Development of fully human monoclonal antibodies happened in stages over a time span of more than 15 years. First stage in this process was generation of monoclonal murine IgG antibodies (e.g., OKT3 [muronomab-CD3, Johnson and Johnson] approved in 1986). Next stage was generation of so called chimeric antibodies consisting of human heavy and light chain constant sections but with murine variable sections (e.g.,

Rituxan [rituximab, Genentech]). Next stage was then the humanized antibodies where the only remaining murine part of the antibody is the antigen-binding CDR (e.g., Xolair [omalizumab, Novartis/Genentech]). Both the first chimeric and humanized antibodies were approved in the late 1990s. Then finally 16 years later, the first fully human antibody Humira (adalimumab, Abbott) was approved in 2002. Since the time of the crude and low-scale manufacturing of the original antibody serum products, much has changed, and therapeutic antibodies are now produced by fermentation in 5,000 liter scale using highly controlled and documented yeast or mammalian cell lines that are genetically engineered to express a single specific antibody. This has resulted in a pure and highly specific antibody product, and thanks to great improvements in cell line design and fermentation efficiency, monoclonal antibody therapeutics can now be produced at more reasonable, although still high, costs.

The price of antibody-based therapies is, however, still much higher than chemically synthesized antibiotics. Although they do provide very welcome and needed treatment options, the cost of antibody-based treatments approved for cancer and inflammatory diseases is creating major economic challenges for health care systems and health care providers around the world. Targeted immune therapy in, e.g., colorectal cancer with 8 weeks of treatment with a monoclonal antibody like Erbitux (cetuximab, Imclone/ Lilly) cost up to $31,790 in the 1990s. In comparison, $63 for an 8-week treatment with fluorouracil, which was the standard treatment until the mid-1990s, puts the cost of antibody treatments in perspective.

Highly specific antibodies monoclonal antibodies (each produced by culture of cells all derived from the same single cell), can be selected for and generated from immunized humans or animals in several different ways: (i) phage display of a human variable light segment library from several donors and B cells, followed by cycles of panning against target antigen, selection of phages with the desired target specificity, and subsequent cloning and expression in a cell line for expression; (ii) the use of transgenic mice carrying the genes for human IgG and immortalization of the mouse B cells by fusing them with myeloma cells (the hybridoma technology); and (iii) isolation of memory B cells or activated memory B cells (plasmablasts) from patients that have been or are exposed to the infectious agent. After isolation the memory B cells are then first screened for reaction to the relevant antigen and positive cells are then immortalized by transformation with Epstein Barr virus transformation in the presence of a oligodeoxynucleotide (CpG) and irradiated peripheral blood mononuclear cells (11, 12). Finally the cell cultures are subjected to several steps of "limiting dilution" where the concentration of cells in the subsequent seeding cultures are less than one. This is done to ensure that each cell culture is derived from one cell only (monoclonal) and that only identical antibodies from a single clone is harvested from each of the cell cultures.

An essential technological step on the way to the current antibody products was the method to produce monoclonal antibodies by immortalizing B cells, which is the basis for the "hybridoma technology" (13). This allowed the production of large amounts of homogenous antibodies with defined specificity and a single Ig class and isotype (14). This was quickly adapted for clinical use, and in the 1980s the OKT3 anti-CD3 monoclonal murine IgG2 antibody was the first one in the class approved for prevention of organ transplant rejection (14). The ability to generate monoclonal antibodies in unlimited amounts and against almost any target protein provided extremely valuable tools for detecting, locating, inhibiting, and blocking specific markers and pathways in general biological and medical research and in setting up analyses for numerous markers via enzyme-linked immunosorbent assay or immunohistochemistry. It also played a major role in basic research into the mechanisms of antibody action.

STRATEGIC CONSIDERATIONS IN DEVELOPING ANTIBODY-BASED THERAPIES FOR INFECTIOUS DISEASES

As mentioned above, the past 10 to 15 years saw a revolution in development and approvals of monoclonal antibody-based therapies for inflammatory and neoplastic diseases. This revolution, however, did not include treatments for infectious diseases. As can be seen in Table 1, more than 40 antibody-based treatments have been approved or are under final evaluation. Although many products for infectious diseases are in different stages of development, still only one monoclonal antibody-based product, Synagis, is currently approved for use in infectious diseases. The main reason for this is the availability of the much cheaper, easier to administer, and more broadly acting anti-microbials or antibiotics. However, the increasing development of resistant strains of bacteria (e.g., MRSA) and viruses has opened the door for a re-emergence of antibody-based therapies. Several features of monoclonal antibodies are, however, working against them when comparing with antimicrobial therapies. First, and most importantly, is the very high cost of production already mentioned above. In addition, since antibodies are proteins, they need to be treated carefully, kept refrigerated, and they are administered by intravenous or subcutaneous injection. In contrast, antibiotics usually come in the form of tablets that can be taken orally and can be kept in a bag or in a closet at room temperature. Antibiotics normally target general mechanisms, e.g., cell wall formation in bacteria, and can act against, e.g., a broad spectrum of bacteria, whereas antibodies are very specific to a single virus, bacteria, or bacterial subtype, and a clear diagnosis should be made before initiating treatment with a monoclonal antibody. This highlights the need for improving or developing diagnostics in parallel with developing antibody therapies. The specificity also has an economical angle since it results in a smaller market compared to broad-spectrum antibiotics, making antibody-based therapies less attractive for pharmaceutical companies to develop.

The specificity is, however, also a strength in the sense that the antibody works only on a specific infectious agent, and although mutations in that agent can render the antibody ineffective, this does not affect other similar agents and thus does not cause the spread of resistance. The specificity also results in very low off-target binding and therefore very few side effects, including the gastrointestinal effects often observed with antibiotics due to broad effects on bacterial flora in the gut. The balance between antibody therapies and antibiotics with respect to costs and ease of use in the clinic should, however, be seen in a broad and more realistic context, including the current situation around the development of resistance, which has resulted in antibiotic

therapy in the United Kingdom not working in one in seven patients (15). In the United States this situation has resulted in multiple cases with the need for dosing up to 10 different antibiotics before proper control of infection can be obtained. Table 2 lists the pros and cons of antibody-based therapies and antibiotics.

To make antibody therapeutics more efficacious and more convenient for patients and treating physicians, several approaches have been and are being taken.

Strategy To Avoid Escape Mutants

Although antibody treatments do not induce resistance in nontarget bacteria or viruses, both bacteria and viruses have the ability to escape the host immune system and specific antibody treatments via mutations that change their surface proteins or structure, creating so-called escape mutants that are no longer neutralized by the specific antibody. The best way to circumvent this is by using a combination of antibodies directed at different viral targets. The use of cocktails of two or more antibodies was shown to provide synergism or additive effects in neutralizing, e.g., hepatitis B virus (HBV) and RSV infections (16). Combinations of antibodies have also been used in HIV, targeting GP41 and GP120 viral proteins (17), and rabies (18) and are part of the strategy in most pharmaceutical companies that are developing antiviral antibodies. Therefore, part of the early preclinical development of such antibody combinations consists of serial passage of virally infected cells (>20 generations) to ensure continued efficacy and the absence of escape mutants. This is combined with testing against known patient isolates, when available. Cocktails of antibodies would also be an interesting approach to target groups of infectious agents often seen in parallel in, e.g., burn wounds.

Antibody Engineering

Another strategy to increase efficacy, increase the ability of the treatment to reach the intended target, and avoid unwanted side

TABLE 2 Pros and cons of antibody based therapies related to serum therapy and antibiotics

Parameter	Serum therapy	Antibiotics	mAbs	Comments
Source	Animals Humans	Chemical synthesis Fermentation	Tissue culture Bioreactor Fermentation	
Lot variation	High	Low	Low	
Specificity	Narrow	Broad	Narrow	Narrow specificity prevents development of resistance in non-target species but results in the requirement for a specific diagnosis before treatment. Restricts treatment to single species.
Toxicity	High	Low	Low	Original crude antibodies from animals had poor tolerability, but current human- and animal-derived immunoglobulins have been proven safe
Ease of administration	Difficult (intravenous [i.v.], intramuscular [i.m.], subcutaneous [s.c.])	Easy/difficult (oral/i.v.)	Easy (i.v., i.m., s.c.)	Many antibiotics can be administered orally, whereas serum or mAbs are given by i.v or s.c injection
Pharmacokinetics	Variable	Consistent	Consistent	
Cost/dose	High (in the hundreds)	Very high (in the thousands)	Low (in the single digits)	

effects resulting from the killing of nontarget cells is antibody engineering—more precisely, genetic manipulation of the Fc domain (mainly in the CH2 domain) or changes to the glucosylation pattern of the N-linked oligosaccharide moieties attached at antibody N297 in the Fc part of the heavy chain. For generating antibodies with enhanced effector functions, different mutations have been identified that have increased affinity to the FcγIIIa receptor and a significant enhanced cellular cytotoxicity (S239D/A330L/I332E, also known as 3M [19, 20], F243L [21], and G236A). These antibodies either directly or indirectly enhance binding of Fc receptors and thus significantly enhance cellular cytotoxicity. Enhanced effector function can also be achieved by modulating the oligosaccharide moieties. Removal of fucose from the A297 linked oligosaccharide moietites, which creates so-called afucosylated Fc domains, has been shown to greatly increase the potency for inducing antibody-dependent cel-

lular cytotoxicity (22). This is achieved by manufacturing the antibodies in cell lines lacking the enzyme fucosyl transferase, which renders them unable to add fucose to the oligosaccharide moieties (22).

Similarly, ways to reduce or ablate the ability of antibodies to trigger effector functions have been described and are being used broadly in cases where the aim is to block specific membrane-bound receptors/targets and where killing of the cell harboring the target is not desired. Again, mutations in the Fc part, e.g., the mutations L234A and L235A, also called the LALA mutation, greatly reduce but do not completely remove effector functions by removing amino acids important for the C1q factor of complement (23, 24). Modulation of the glucosylation pattern, in this case creating completely aglucosylated antibodies, has also been shown to remove the ability to properly bind Fc receptors on effector cells and trigger effector functions. One alternative approach used especially when developing immuno-modulatory agonistic antibodies is the use of antibodies of the IgG4 isotype, which does not trigger effector functions. Finally, mutations in the Fc part that increase the affinity to the FcRn receptor have also been used to create antibodies with an increased half-life. Introduction of three mutations in the Fc domain (M252Y, S254T, and T2556E, also called the YTE) has been shown to provide a half-life extension of 3- to 4-fold (25). From a convenience point of view, a long half-life is obviously attractive, but it can be a down-side in the case of severe adverse effects due to the long duration of action.

Creating "Magic Bullets"

In oncology, to enhance the efficacy of therapeutic antibodies, the tactic of using the specific binding capacity of the antibody to deliver a cargo in the form of a cell toxin or a radioactive isotope to kill tumor cells has long been recognized. The first treatments using radiolabeled antibodies were the anti-CD20 antibodies Zevalin (ibritumomab tioxetan; yttrium 90 labeled) and Bexxar (tositumumab; iodine 131 labeled), which were approved in the United States in 2002 and 2003, respectively. These demonstrated the potential for developing such antibodies. However, they are not widely used in cancer therapy. Successful generation of labeled antibodies against fungal infections with *Cryptococcus neoformans* and *Histoplasma capsulatum* and bacterial infections with *S. pneumoniae* was reported by Saylor et al. (26), and efficacy was shown *in vitro* and in animal models. However, clinical efficacy still needs to be demonstrated. One opportunity with this approach is that these antibodies can be directed at infected cells and not the pathogen itself, killing the infected cells and thereby potentially removing reservoirs of infected cells (26). The challenges in selecting the right isotopes, achieving distribution and uptake into tumors and tissues, and minimizing exposure of non-target tissues have slowed the pace of development of these types of antibody

treatments. Difficulties in handling and disposing of such products have also contributed to this.

With a similar approach but with antibodies aimed at delivering cytotoxic drugs via antibodies also known as antibody-drug complexes (ADCs) there is currently great enthusiasm and activity, especially in oncology. The first antibody of this kind, Myoltarg (gemtuzumab ozogamicin), was approved by the FDA in 2000 but was later withdrawn due to major toxicities in patients, caused by instability and heterogenicity. Two other ADC antibodies have been approved for the treatment of cancer: Adcetris (brentuximab vedotin) and Kadcyla (ado-trastuzumab emtansine), which were approved in 2011 and 2013, respectively. The ADC field is expanding, and many products are in development in cancer and inflammatory diseases, but has not resulted in any approvals for products in infectious diseases. A major challenge in this approach is the selection of the right linker to create a stable complex, as well as ensuring minimal off-target exposure and, most importantly, achieving internalization and release in the proper compartment of the target cells. The antibody CDRs should ensure specific binding and delivery of the cytotoxic drugs, but in animal studies using a specific ADC and an ADC without target but labeled with same toxin, the same broad pattern of toxicity was observed with both products. This indicates that the desired specific targeting to mainly affect target cells or tissues is currently not achievable. So far, this concept is used only in cancer treatment; for any successful development of such treatments in infectious diseases, a critical case-by-case risk/benefit evaluation combined with considerations of availability of other effective drugs will be needed.

Antibody Formats

In the era of antibody-based therapies, full-size antibodies were and are still the main format. There is, however, an increase in companies offering/researching into new variants of antibodies or new combinations of antibody-derived structures. Examples of these can be seen in Fig. 1 and include both bispecific full-size antibodies with antigen-binding sites with different targets, Fab or F(ab)$_2$ fragments, single-chain variable fragments (ScFv), pairs of ScFvs linked in different ways (diabodies and bites), fusion-proteins containing, e.g., a receptor fused to an antibody Fc part, and many others not shown. Much creativity has been demonstrated in this field of research, and every imaginable variation and combination of antibody structures is being created and tested. This is done to test how these different formats and the attributes of the different parts of antibodies potentially can overcome the challenges facing the development of antibody-based therapies. These challenges include the high costs of production and finding optimal combinations of size, stability, half-life, efficacy, and very importantly, safety. These new formats also introduces new structures foreign to the immune system and thus immunogenicity is likely going to be a major factor in these developments with the potential risk of loss of efficacy, loss of exposure, potential hypersensitivity reactions, and potential cross-reactivity to endogenous receptors or immunoglobulins. As described above, a lot of work was put into reducing immunogenicity and immune reactions to the animal-derived or chimeric antibodies by turning them into more and more fully human antibodies. It is therefore a paradox that with the introduction of these new formats (e.g., new scaffolds with fibrinogen carrying antigen-binding sites), the risk of immunogenicity and immune reactions is being reintroduced. Time will show whether the safety and efficacy of these new formats will actually support their registration and use in patients with infectious diseases.

EXAMPLES OF ANTIBODIES THAT ARE OR WERE IN DEVELOPMENT FOR INFECTIOUS DISEASES

When searching for antibody-based treatments in different stages of development, it becomes obvious that the vast majority of these focus on viral and some on bacteriological infections. Around 70% of these focus on five main pathogens: hepatitis C virus (HCV), HIV, *Bacillus anthracis*, *Escherichia coli*, and *S. aureus*. The following section describes examples of projects targeting infections with these and a few additional treatments divided into antibacterials, antivirals, and antifungals.

Antibacterials

Due to their ability to cause a multitude of serious infections and due to their high propensity for developing resistance, MRSA infections are a major problem in hospitals and in local community settings. However, despite several clinical trials with antibodies targeting the clumping factor A, e.g., Aurexis (tefibazumab, Inhibitex) (27) and Aurograb (Novartis), a single-chain variable fragment (ScFv) targeting an *S. aureus* surface protease has failed to show efficacy of any of these treatments (28). Some hope has arisen from the work on pagibaximab (Biosynexus), which is an antibody for the prevention of staphylococcal sepsis in premature infants with low birth weight. Clinical phase I and II trials have shown good safety and no cases of treatment related adverse events when doses of 90 mg/kg were given. A phase III study is ongoing (29).

Research into mAbs targeting the adhesins SA I and II from *Streptococcus mutans*, which aims at recolonizing the bacterial flora in the oral cavity to prevent caries, did not show the expected effects in the first human trials, and further development work was stopped (30).

Some optimism has been generated in finding an antibody-based treatment of *Pseudomonas aeruginosa*. Two antibody-based treatments are in development for the prevention and treatment of infections with *Pseudomonas* in ventilated patients: a full-size antibody, panobacumab (Kenta Biotech), directed against LPS 011, and a pegylated Fab product targeting the type 3 secretion system. Both of these have shown good tolerability and efficacy in patients, and phase II studies are ongoing (31, 32).

B. anthracis causes highly lethal pulmonary infections and is recognized as a potential biological warfare weapon. Four antibodies, raxibacumab (ABthrax, Human Genome Sciences), Valortim (PharmAthene/Medarex), Thravixa (Emergent Biosolutions), and Anthim (Elusys Therapeutics), are human antibodies directed against the protective antigen which interacts with the toxin's lethal factor and edema factor to facilitate their toxic action. All are undergoing clinical trials for tolerability, but raxibacumab was approved in 2012 for treatment of inhalation anthrax. It was, however, not a traditional approval based on phase II and III clinical trials showing efficacy but was the first treatment approved under the so-called animal rule, where the efficacy, for good reasons, is approved based on animal studies.

For treatment of infections with *Clostridium difficile* a cocktail of two antibodies, CDA-1 and CDB-1 MK3415A (Merck), for neutralization of toxins A and B are in phase II development (33). Clinical trial data with MK3415A given on top of a standard of care showed a lower recurrence rate compared to the standard of care alone. This was an example of positive data where a therapeutic antibody treatment was given as an adjunct to standard of care antibiotics.

Another cocktail of two antibodies (caStx1, caStx2; Shigamabs [LFB Biotechnologies/Thallion Pharmaceutics]) is being developed to treat infections with strains of *E. coli* producing Shiga toxin. There is currently no treatment for the hemolytic uremic syndrome caused by infections with these strains of *E. coli* which affects around 300,000 people every year. Phase I trials showed the cocktail to be well tolerated in healthy volunteers, and a phase II study is looking at pharmacokinetics and efficacy of treatment (34).

Antivirals

Synagis (palivizumab, MedImmune), for the prevention of RSV infection in infants, is currently the only approved monoclonal anti-body treatment for infectious diseases. An affinity maturation and half-life extended third-generation monoclonal, Numax (motavizumab, AstraZeneca/MedImmune), is currently in clinical development but due to safety issues and an inability to demonstrate superiority has so far not been approved by the FDA. This is an interesting example of a case where a back-up for antibody, despite higher affinity and potency, fails to show improved efficacy in clinical trials (35).

A number of antibodies against HCV are in development. One of these (MBL-HCV-1) is directed against an envelope protein on the virus (36). The others are directed against host cell proteins, and one of these, bavituximab (Peregrine Pharmaceuticals) (37), is directed against phosphatidylserine, which normally is expressed only on the inner surface of the cell membrane but which in cancer- and virus-infected cells flips out and gets expressed on the external part of the membrane, allowing its use as a target for mAbs. Another approach adopted from cancer treatment is immuno-modulation. Another example of a mAb being tested in HCV is the two anti-PD-1 receptor antibodies, CTZ-11 and BMS-936558, where blocking the inhibitory receptor PD-1 on CD8 T cells restores the ability of these cells to lyse HCV-infected cells.

Shifting the focus to HIV, a number of mAbs which targeted the GP120 envelope protein were being tested but suffered from escape mutants causing a rebound of viral loads. A different strategy targeting conserved receptors such as CCR5 or CXCR4, which serve coreceptors for the virus on target CD4 T cells, has had some success in reducing viral loads (38, 39). Two such antibody therapies, Ibalizumab (WuXi Pharma Tech) and PRO140 (CytoDyn), are in late-stage clinical development and have caused some modest optimism.

In rabies the current treatment practice after potential exposure is vaccination and administration of immunoglobulin from vaccinated humans (human rabies immunoglobulin [HRIG]) or from horses. In Asia >50,000 people annually die from rabies (35), and a shortage of specific immunoglobulins has resulted in the testing of a polyclonal antibody product (CL-184, foravirumab, Sanofi/Crucell); virus-neutralizing effects similar to what is observed with immunoglobulin treatment in dosed humans has been observed (40).

Antifungal

Fungal infections with yeasts such as *Candida albicans* and *C. neoformans* cause morbidity and mortality in immunocompromised individuals. For candidiasis one antibody, efungumab (Mycograb, Novartis), which targets heat-shock protein 90 (HSP90), was in late-stage clinical development for treatment on top of antifungal therapy. However, safety concerns and lack of proven efficacy compared to antifungal treatment alone resulted in discontinuation of the program. For *Cryptococcus* a murine antibody, MAb18b7, which targets capsular glucuronoxylomannan and acts through complement activation, was tested in HIV patients, but due to generation of anti-mouse antibodies, this program was halted (41).

FUTURE PERSPECTIVES FOR ANTIBODY TREATMENTS IN INFECTIOUS DISEASES

There is no questioning the fact that new treatment options are needed in infectious diseases. Increasing multidrug resistance, inability to treat immunocompromised patients, risk of bioterrorism, and new emerging diseases call for alternatives to the current armament. For that purpose, antibodies and antibody-derived treatments offer very attractive tools and attributes to kill or neutralize infectious agents, lyse infected cells, or modulate the immune system to enable effector cells to escape immunosuppressed conditions and contribute to the elimination of infections. The ability to raise antibodies to any target, and the ability to modulate effector functions, half-life, and size of the treatment units makes antibodies ideal for tailoring treatments for specific infectious agents.

Antibody-based treatments have been going through a time of great excitement and development in generating treatments for cancer and inflammatory diseases, and many new antibody-based products are now approved for clinical use (Table 1). This development passed by the field of infectious diseases, and despite multiple programs in multiple diseases only one treatment, the anti-RSV antibody Synagis, has been approved. Inherent challenges such as high cost, the need for parallel development of specific diagnostics, and ease of storage and dosing have been difficult to overcome in a field where cheap and functioning antibiotics are available. For cancer and inflammatory disease there is usually no alternative treatment, which increases the need and demand for a proper treatment and acceptance of, e.g., high costs of treatment. Furthermore, in many programs a lack of predictive animal models has resulted in many disappointments in translating apparent efficacy in animals to humans. In addition, in diseases with large potential markets the vaccine and antibiotic development approach will generally be used. It is therefore time to take a new and revised look into the future to find appropriate niches in infectious diseases where new antibody-based treatments could prove their value and make a major difference. In this, the ability to provide treatments for infections in immunocompromised subjects such as HIV patients or very young or elderly people, as well as treatments for some of the severe potential bioterror infections such as Ebola, could open the eyes of health care providers, researchers, and pharmaceutical developers and provide stepping stones for broader acceptance of the potential for these treatments.

In addition, the general approach to the format and use of these treatments should be reconsidered. The use of cocktails of multiple antibodies more and more seems to be required to avoid escape mutations and to more efficiently neutralize several toxins or target infection with different mechanisms. Regulatory pathways for developing such cocktails now seem to be in place where mostly only the actual cocktail is tested and only limited additional clinical data demonstrating the contribution from each element is needed. What is also clear is that to generate efficacious antibody treatments, further research into specific mechanisms of pathogenesis is needed, which will assist in choosing the right target antigens. In this respect the vast flexibility that can be achieved by modulating format, effector functions, half-life, and other features provides many opportunities but also challenges in conducting the necessary testing to enable selection of the product with the optimal combination of these features.

Another consideration for the future is to focus more on developing treatments that are adjunct to existing ones, e.g., antibiotic treatment instead of a stand-alone treatment. This might provide that extra efficacy in patients with failing immune response and potentially also compensate for and reduce the development of resistance, thereby ensuring available efficacious treatment options. On the cost side, research into the use of the smaller and cheaper antibody-based fragments could contribute to making antibody-based treatments more attractive and more efficient, and cheaper ways of manufacturing antibodies would contribute to this. In summary, there is no doubt that antibody-based treatments, through their great flexibility to be designed for specific targets on infectious agents or the host immune cells, will and should play a major role in designing new treatments for infectious diseases in the future. Hopefully, several of the programs currently in development will show clinical efficacy and through their approval provide the basis and enthusiasm for this process.

ACKNOWLEDGMENT

Conflicts of interest: I declare no conflicts.

CITATION

Hey A. 2015. History and practice: antibodies in infectious diseases. Microbiol Spectrum 3(1):AID-0026-2014.

REFERENCES

1. **Casadevall A, Sharff MD.** 1994. Serum therapy revisited: animal models of infection and development of passive antibody therapy. *Antimicrob Agents Chemother* **38:**1695–1702.
2. **Casadevall A.** 1996. Antibody-based therapies for emerging infectious diseases. *Emerg Infect Dis* **2:**200–208.
3. **Behring EA, Kitasato S.** 1890. Ueber das zustandekommen der diptherie-immunität und der tetanus-immunität bei thieren. *Deutch Med Woch* **49:**1113–1114.
4. **Klemperer G, Klemperer F.** 1891. Versuche uber immunisirung und heilung bei der pneumokokkeninfection. *Berlin Klin Wochenschr* **28:**833–835.
5. **Flexner S, Jobling JW.** 1908. Serum treatment of epidemic cerebro-spinal meningitis. *J Exp Med* **10:**141–195.
6. **Rosington B.** 2013. The drugs won't work: top doctor warns of "apocalypse" in 20 years as bugs become resistant to antibiotics. *Daily Mirror*, January 24.
7. **WHO.** 2014. *Ebola response roadmap update report.* http://www.who.int/csr/resources/publications/ebola/response-roadmap/en/.
8. **Chan CEZ, Chan AHY, Hanson BJ, Ooi EE.** 2009. The use of antibodies in the treatment of infectious diseases. *Singapore Med J* **50:**663–672.
9. **Berry JD, Gaudet RG.** 2011. Antibodies in infectious diseases: polyclonals, monoclonals and niche biotechnology. *New Biotechnol* **28:**489–501.
10. **Cauza K, Hinterhuber G, Dingelmaier-Hovorka R, Brugger K, Klosner G, Horvat R, Wolff K, Foedinger D.** 2005. Expression of FcRn, the MHC class I-related receptor for IgG, in human keratinocytes. *J Invest Dermatol* **124:**132–139.
11. **Marasco WA, Sui J.** 2007. The growth and potential of human antiviral monoclonal antibody therapeutics. *Nat Biotechnol* **25:**1421–1434.
12. **Wrammert J, Koutsonanos D, Li G-M, Edupganti S, Sui J, Morrissey M, McCausland M, Skountzou I, Hornig M, Lipkin WI, Metha A, Razave B, DelRio C, Zheng N-Y, Lee J-H, Huang M, All Z, Kaur K, Andrews S, Amara RR,**

Wang Y, Das SR, O'Donnel CD, Yewdell JW, Subbarao K, Marasco WA, Mulligan M, Compans R, Ahmed R, Wilson PC. 2011. Broadly cross-reactive antibodies dominate the human B cell response against 2009 pandemic H1N1 influenza virus infection. *J Exp Med* **208**:181–193.

13. Köhler G, Milstein C. 1975. Continuous cultures of fused cells secreting antibody of predefined specificity. *Nature* **256**:495–497.

14. Casadevall A, Dadachova E, Pirofski LA. 2004. Passive antibody therapy for infectious diseases. *Nat Rev Microbiol* **2**:695–703.

15. Triggle N. Antibiotic treatments from GPs "fail 15% of the time". *BBC News, Health*, September 25.

16. Bregenholt S, Jensen A, Lantto J, Hyldig S, Haurum J. 2006. Recombinant human polyclonal antibodies: a new class of therapeutic antibodies against viral infections. *Curr Pharm Des* **12**:2007–2015.

17. Flego M, Ascione A, Cianfriglia M, Vella S. 2013. Clinical development of monoclonal antibody-based therapy drugs in HIV and HCV diseases. *BMC Med* **11**:1–17.

18. de Kruif J, Bakker ABH, Marissen WE, Arjen Kramer R, Throsby M, Rupprecht CE, Goudsmit J. 2007. A human monoclonal antibody cocktail as a novel component of rabies post-exposure prophylaxis. *Annu Rev Med* **50**: 359–368.

19. Lazar GA, Dang W, Karki S, Vafa OPeng JS, Hyun L, Chan C, Chung HS, Eivazi A, Yoder SC. 2006. Engineered antibody Fc variants with enhanced effector function. *Proc Natl Acad Sci USA* **103**:4005–4010.

20. Shields RL, Namenuk AK, Hong K, Meng YG, Rae J, Briggs J, Xie D, Lai J, Stadlen A, Li B. 2001. High resolution mapping of the binding site on human IgG1 for FcγRI, FcγRII, FcγRIII, and FcRn and design of IgG1 variants with improved binding to the FcγR. *J Biol Chem* **276**:6591–6604.

21. Stewart R, Thom G, Levens M, Güler-Gane G, Holgate R, Rudd PM, Webster C, Jermutus L, Lund J. 2011. A variant human IgG1-Fc mediates improved ADCC. *Protein Eng Des Sel* **24**:671–678.

22. Niwa R, Hatanaka S, Shoji-Hosaka E, Sakurada M, Kobayashi Y, Uehara A, Yokoi H, Nakamura K, Shitara K. 2004. Enhancement of the antibody-dependent cellular cytotoxicity of low-fucose IgG1 is independent of Fc-q gammaRIIIa functional polymorphism. *Clin Cancer Res* **10**:6248–6255.

23. Hezareh M, Hessell AJ, Jensen RC, van de Winkel JGJ, Parren PWHI. 2001. Effector function activities of a panel of mutants of a broadly neutralizing antibody against human immunodeficiency virus type 1. *J Virol* **75**: 12161–12168.

24. Hessell AJ, Hangartner L, Hunter M, Havenith CD, Beursken FJ, Bakker JM, Lanigan CM, Landucci G, Forthal DN, Parren PW, Marx PA, Burton DR. 2007. Fc receptor but not complement binding is important in antibody protection against HIV. *Nature* **449**(7158):101–104.

25. Dall'Acqua WF, Kiener PA, Wu H. 2006. Properties of human IgG1s engineered for enhanced binding to the neonatal Fc receptor (FcRn). *J Biol Chem* **281**:23514–23524.

26. Saylor C, Dadachova E, Casadevall A. 2009. Monoclonal antibody-based therapies for microbial diseases. *Vaccine* **275**:G38–G46.

27. Hall AE, Domanski PJ, Vernachio JH, Syrbeys PJ, Gorovits EL, Johnson MA, Ross JM, Patti JM. 2003. Characterization of a protective monoclonal antibody recognizing *Staphylococcus aureus* MSCRAMM protein clumping factor A. *Infect Immun* **71**:6864–6870.

28. Bebbington C, Yarranton G. 2008. Antibodies for the treatment of bacterial infections: current experience and future prospects. *Curr Opin Biotechnol* **19**:613–619.

29. Weisman LE, Thackray HM, Steinhorn RH, Walsh WF, Lassiter HA, Dhanireddy R, Brozanski BS, Palmer KG, Trautman MS, Escobedo M, Meissner HC, Sasidharan P, Fretz J, Kokai-Kun JF, Mond JJ. 2011. A randomized study of a monoclonal antibody (pagibaximab) to prevent staphylococcal sepsis. *Pediatrics* **128**:271–279.

30. Weintraub JA, Hilton JF, White JM, Hoover CI, Wycoff KL, Yu L, Larrick JW, Featherstone JD. 2005. Clinical trial of a plant-derived antibody on recolonization of mutans streptococci. *Caries Res* **19**:241–250.

31. Baer M, Sawa T, Flynn P. 2009. An engineered human antibody Fab fragment specific for *Pseudomonas aeruginosa* PcrV antigen has potent antibacterial activity. *Infect Immun* **77**:1083–1090.

32. Secher T, Fauconnier L, Szade A. 2011. Antipseudomonas aeruginosa serotype 011 LPS immunoglobulin M monoclonal antibody panobacumab (KBPA101) confers protection in a murine model of acute lung infection. *J Antimicrob Chemother* **66**:1100–1109.

33. Migone T, Subramanian GM, Bolmer SD. 2009. Raxibacumab for the treatment of inhalational anthrax. *N Engl J Med* **361**:135–144.

34. Lowy I, Molrine DC, Leav BA. 2010. Treatment with monoclonal antibodies against *Clostridium\ difficile* toxins. *N Engl J Med* **362**:197–205.

35. **Ter Meulen J.** 2011. Monoclonal antibodies in infectious diseases: clinical pipeline in 2011. *Infect Dis Clin N Am* **25:**798–802.

36. **Broering TJ, Garrity KA, Boatright NK.** 2009. Identification and characterization of broadly neutralizing human monoclonal antibodies directed against the E2 envelope glycoprotein of hepatitis C virus. *J Virol* **83:**12473–12482.

37. **Soares MM, King SW, Thorpe PE.** 2008. Targeting inside-out phosphatidylserine as a therapeutic strategy for viral diseases. *Nat Med* **14:**1357–1362.

38. **Bruno BJ, Jacobson JM.** 2010. Ibalizumab: an anti-CD4 monoclonal antibody for the treatment of HIV-1 infection. *J Antimicrob Chemother* **65:**1839–1841.

39. **Li L, Sun T, Yang K.** 2010. Monoclonal CCR5 antibody for treatment of people with HIV infection (review). *Cochrane Database Syst Rev* 8:CD008439.

40. **Quiambao B, Bakker A, Bermal NN.** 2009. Evaluation of the safety and neutralizing activity of CL184, a monoclonal antibody cocktail against rabies, in a phase II study in healthy adolescents and children. Quebec, Canada: Presentation at RITA XX, Rabies in the Americas.

41. **Larsen RA, Pappas PG, Perfect J, Aberg JA, Casadevall A, Cloud GA.** 2005. Phase I evaluation of the safety and pharmacokinetics of murine-derived anticryptococcal antibody 18b7 in subjects with treated cryptococcal meningitis. *Antimicrob Agents Chemother* **49:**952–958.

GENERAL FEATURES OF IMMUNOGLOBULINS

Functions of Antibodies

2

DONALD N. FORTHAL[1]

INTRODUCTION

In the setting of infectious diseases, antibody function refers to the biological effect that an antibody has on a pathogen or its toxin. Thus, assays that measure antibody function are differentiated from those that strictly measure the ability of an antibody to bind to its cognate antigen. Examples of antibody functions include neutralization of infectivity, phagocytosis, antibody-dependent cellular cytotoxicity (ADCC), and complement-mediated lysis of pathogens or of infected cells.

Antibodies can impact pathogens in the presence or in the absence of effector cells or effector molecules such as complement, and experiments can often sort out with precision the mechanisms by which an antibody inhibits a pathogen *in vitro*. In addition, *in vivo* models, particularly those engineered to knock in or knock out effector cells or effector molecules are excellent tools for understanding antibody functions. However, it is highly likely that multiple antibody functions occur simultaneously or sequentially in the presence of an infecting organism *in vivo*.

The most critical incentive for measuring antibody functions is to provide a basis for vaccine development and for the development of therapeutic antibodies.

[1]Department of Infectious Diseases, University of California, Irvine, Irvine, CA 92617.
Antibodies for Infectious Diseases
Edited by James E. Crowe, Jr., Diana Boraschi, and Rino Rappuoli
© 2015 American Society for Microbiology, Washington, DC
doi:10.1128/microbiolspec.AID-0019-2014

In this respect, some functions, such as virus neutralization, serve to inhibit the acquisition of a pathogen or limit its pathogenesis. However, an antibody can also enhance replication or contribute to pathogenesis. This review will emphasize those functions of the antibody that are potentially beneficial to the host; a separate article is devoted to a discussion of antibody-dependent enhancement of infection. In addition, this article will focus on the effects of antibodies on the organisms themselves, rather than on the toxins the organisms may produce. Finally, the role of antibody in modulating T-cell immunity is not discussed in detail.

ANTIBODY FUNCTIONS INDEPENDENT OF EFFECTOR CELLS OR EFFECTOR MOLECULES

Antibodies are capable of having an impact on organisms in the absence of effector cells or effector molecules such as complement. For the most part, the impact of antibodies by themselves can be measured *in vitro* as neutralization of organism infectivity. Neutralization is herein referred to as the ability of the antibody by itself to inhibit the infection of susceptible cells or, in the case of some extracellular organisms, to inhibit an initial pathogenic step. Importantly, as described below, neutralization involves many potential mechanisms. Furthermore, it should be emphasized that other antibody functions in addition to neutralization may ultimately be involved in the prevention or clearance of infection, even by antibodies that neutralize the relevant organism *in vitro* (1).

Neutralization of Infectivity

In vitro, antibodies are capable of blocking the infectivity or pathogenesis of viruses, bacteria, parasites, and fungi. Neutralization generally occurs as a result of interfering with an organism's attachment to host tissues. However, it is now clear that several mechanisms account for neutralization and that a single antibody or antibodies with different speci-

ficities can neutralize a given organism, at least *in vitro*, through multiple mechanisms.

Preattachment Neutralization

Some antibodies have been shown to inhibit infectivity by binding to organisms and causing them to aggregate. Aggregation or agglutination by immunoglobulin A (IgA) may allow more efficient entrapment of bacteria in mucus and subsequent clearance by peristalsis (2, 3). Although aggregation is more likely to occur with polymeric IgA and IgM, some neutralizing IgG antibodies can aggregate poliovirus; the aggregation results in less infectivity, probably by reducing the number of encounters between virus and host cells (4, 5).

Antibodies have also been shown to immobilize or "paralyze" organisms, such as the channel catfish pathogen *Ichthyophthirius multifiliis* (6). The IgA monoclonal antibody (mAb) Sal4 can render *Salmonella enterica* serovar Typhimurium immobile, independently of agglutination, although Sal4 also specifically interferes with uptake into epithelial cells. Antibodies directed against *Pseudomonas aeruginosa* flagella inhibit motility of that organism (7). Polyclonal antibodies, induced by immunizing mice with *Vibrio cholerae* outer membrane vesicles, protect suckling mice from oral *V. cholerae* challenge, likely by inhibiting the motility of the organism (8). Antibody may slow the random movement of human immunodeficiency virus type 1 (HIV-1) in vaginal mucus, presumably reducing the number of times the virus can make contact with the epithelial surface; this antibody function appears to rely in part on Fc interactions with components of the mucus (9).

Some antibodies appear to destabilize organisms, rendering them noninfectious. For example, the anti-foot-and-mouth-disease virus mAb 4C9 disrupts virion capsids, possibly by mimicking the virus' cell receptor (10). A neutralizing antibody against the E1 glycoprotein of Sindbis virus also induces conformational changes (11). Binding of HIV-1 gp120 can result in the shedding of gp120, leaving the transmembrane glycoprotein on the surface. However, the overall effect of such shedding on neutralization sensitivity is unclear (12).

mAbs binding to a surface protein of *Borrelia* can kill the organism by inducing pores in the outer membrane (13). A mAb directed against fungal heat shock protein 90, a component of yeast cell walls, directly inhibits the growth of *Candida* (14, 15) and works in synergy with antifungal drugs to inhibit *Cryptococcus neoformans* (16). IgG1 and IgM mAbs that bind to the *C. neoformans* capsule affect gene expression, lipid biosynthesis, cellular metabolism, and protein phosphorylation or susceptibility to amphotericin B (17). Other mechanisms by which antibody inhibits bacterial and fungal infections directly and prior to attachment have been described (18, 19, 20).

Interference with Pathogen Attachment

Antibodies that bind to pathogen ligands essential for attachment of the pathogen to its host receptor have been described for many pathogens. In the case of viruses, such antibodies generally inhibit infectivity without altering their cognate antigen, thus strictly inhibiting by virtue of steric interference. This mechanism of virus inhibition has been described for many enveloped and non-enveloped antibodies. Well-studied example are antibodies against HIV-1 gp120 that interfere with binding of gp120 to CD4 (21). In addition, antibodies that neutralize, among others, flaviviruses (22), Newcastle disease virus (23), papillomavirus (24), and rotavirus (25) may do so by interfering with attachment. Some antibodies that block virus attachment do not bind directly to the site on the virus involved with attachment. For example, an antibody against human rhinovirus type 14 binds to surrounding viral structures but nonetheless sterically hinders interactions between the virus and its intercellular adhesion molecule-1 host receptor (26).

The stoichiometry of antibody-antigen interactions required for neutralization has been studied for many viruses, and evidence supports a "multiple hit" phenomenon in which neutral-

ization requires the engagement of more than one antibody on the virion (27). Both antibody affinity and the accessibility of epitopes on the organism are the critical factors in determining whether antibody binding will exceed the threshold required for neutralization. Thus, for example, one cannot necessarily predict neutralizing potency by measuring antibody affinity alone or on the basis of epitope specificity. Antibody Fab or F(ab′)2 fragments are often capable of providing sufficient blockade of attachment to inhibit neutralization. These and other details regarding virus neutralization, including kinetics and requirements for steric hindrance can be found elsewhere (12, 28, 29).

Adhesion of bacteria to the surface of host cells or tissue allows targeting of the organism to a specific cell type and allows the bacteria to resist physical removal by hydrodynamic shear forces (30). Thus, adhesion is a first step in bacterial pathogenesis. The molecules responsible for bacterial adhesion are known as adhesins and are generally incorporated into pili or fimbriae (30, 31). These adhesins are targets for antibodies that, in a manner somewhat analogous to virus neutralization, can inhibit attachment (32, 33, 34). Thus, vaccines have been developed in order to elicit antibodies directed against adhesions. In most cases, this strategy has failed because of sequence variation in the structural proteins of fimbriae. Nonetheless, vaccination with FimH was able to reduce bladder infection of mice and monkeys with uropathogenic *Escherichia coli* (35, 36, 37). The use of this vaccination strategy in humans is made difficult by a shared epitope between FimH and human LAMP-2 and thus a fear of autoimmunity (38). Another example of adherence inhibition was described by Manjarrez-Hernanadez et al., who found that secretory IgA (sIgA) in breast milk was able to inhibit the adherence of enteropathogenic *E. coli* to cells (39). An mAb against lipoarabinomannan, a surface lipoglycan of *Mycobacterium tuberculosis*, is able to prevent adherence of *M. tuberculosis* to human monocyte-derived macrophages (40). Antibodies can also inhibit the attachment of bacteria to abiotic surfaces (41).

Antibodies to merozoite surface protein 1 (MSP1) on *Plasmodium* spp. can protect rodents against infection (42). One mechanism that might account for this is inhibition of the attachment of the parasite to red blood cells (43, 44). *Plasmodium*-infected red blood cells express *Plasmodium falciparum* erythrocyte membrane protein 1 (PfEMP1), which mediates binding to host endothelia and placenta. Antibodies have been elicited that can inhibit the interaction between infected erythrocytes and chondroitin sulfate proteoglycan, their ligand on placenta (45). Inhibition of binding in this manner would not impact infection *per se*, but might influence pathogenesis.

As with other organisms, binding of fungi to host-cell surfaces is a first step in infection. mAb 2G8, directed against β1,3-glucan, can inhibit binding of *Candida albicans* to human epithelial cells (49). It should be noted that mAb 2G8 also directly inhibits fungal growth and facilitates antifungal activity of human polymorphonuclear neutrophils (49, 50). Other antibodies can also inhibit adhesion of *C. albicans* to HEC cells (51) and of *C. neoformans* to a human lung epithelial cell line (52). As with bacteria, antibodies can inhibit *C. albicans* adherence to abiotic surfaces (53).

In the case of several parasites that infect the gastrointestinal tract, the mechanisms by which Ig, and, in particular, IgA, may function are unclear, but it is likely that the inhibition of attachment plays a role (46). For example, mucosal anti-*Giardia* IgA antibodies may prevent infection by inhibiting attachment of the organism to the intestinal epithelium (47). Intestinal IgE antibodies might contribute to the elimination of *Trichinella spiralis* in rats, possibly by blockade of the attachment to intestinal epithelium (48), and immune serum can block the attachment of *Cryptosporidium parvum* to epithelial cells (49).

Finally, antibodies generated against the host receptors themselves can also block infection of a number of different organisms (50, 51, 52, 53, 54, 55, 56, 57).

Postattachment Neutralization

Inhibition of fusion/entry

Intracellular pathogens can be neutralized by antibodies at postattachment steps in their life cycle. In the case of viruses, several studies have identified antibodies that inhibit fusion of viral and host membranes or entry into susceptible target cells. For enveloped viruses, antibodies can block an interaction between a viral protein necessary for fusion and its cellular receptor (58). mAb 2F5, an HIV-1-neutralizing antibody, may block fusion of HIV-1 by obstructing the juxtaposition of viral and cellular membranes (29, 59). 4E10, another HIV-1-neutralizing mAb, may interfere with the formation of fusion-competent complexes of gp41 (60). In the case of West Nile virus, a neutralizing monoclonal antibody likely sterically constrains low-pH-mediated rearrangements of E proteins (61, 62). Similarly, anti-influenza virus hemagglutinin (HA) antibodies can hinder the low pH-induced structural changes necessary for fusion of viral and endosomal membranes (63, 64). It is possible that anti-influenza HA antibodies can inhibit both attachment and postattachment steps (65).

An interesting twist on fusion inhibition was described for an mAb against influenza virus HA. The mAb becomes internalized at acid pH through the Fc neonatal receptor (FcRn) and reduces viral replication following apical exposure of Madin-Darby canine kidney cells to influenza virus. As virus, mAb, and FcRn colocalize within endosomes, it is possible that inhibition of infectivity occurs by interfering with fusion of viral envelope and endosomal membranes (66).

Nonenveloped viruses generally enter cells by endocytosis, and escape from the endocytic vesicle is mediated by capsid protein. Antibodies against polio virus may stabilize the capsid and prevent the structural rearrangements necessary for vesicle escape (29, 67, 68).

Inhibition of other steps in organism life cycles

A number of studies have revealed the ability of antibodies to inhibit organisms once they have successfully entered cells. In order for intracellular neutralization to be accomplished, antibodies must be internalized by host cells. Internalization of antibodies can occur as a result of coating of the organism, in which case, the coated organism must be capable of cell entry, or through Fc receptors. In addition, cells have been engineered to express intracellular antibodies (intrabodies) for potential therapeutic purposes (69). Intracellular neutralization can potentially interrupt an organism's life cycle by interfering with the release, replication, or expression of genomic material. As an example, adenovirus type 5 antihexon mAb (9C12) allows viral attachment, cell entry, and intracellular transport of the virus to the nuclear periphery (70). Nonetheless, 9C12 neutralizes virus infectivity, likely by interfering with capsid uncoating and the release of viral genome (70). A rabbit anti-HPV16 L2 serum was able to neutralize HPV16 pseudoviruses through a mechanism that appeared to involve, at least in part, blocking the transport of viral genome to the nucleus (71).

IgA directed against surface proteins or glycoproteins can mediate neutralization of Sendai virus, influenza virus, and measles virus within susceptible target cells (72, 73, 74). In addition, IgA directed against measles virus M and N proteins, which are internal to the membrane, can inhibit measles virus replication within Vero cells (73, 75). Polymeric IgA or sIgM can intracellularly block the transcytosis of HIV-1 through epithelial cells. Although the epithelial cells are not thought to be a target of HIV-1 infection and replication, such blocking of transcytosis could block access *in vivo* to subepithelial CD4+ cells (76). Similarly, IgA inhibits transcytosis of rotavirus through polarized Caco-2 cells (77). IgA can also introduce a conformational change in the rotavirus VP6 trimer, which is exposed after internalization of virus. The

structural change results in transcriptionally incompetent particles (78, 79).

A novel mechanism of intracellular virus inhibition was described by Mallery et al., wherein antibody bound to adenovirus interacted with cytosolic TRIM21; this interaction resulted in the antibody-bound virus being targeted to the proteasome for degradation (80). This mechanism of inhibition would not be expected to work with enveloped virus, since the antibody would be shed along with the envelope prior to internalization within the cytoplasm.

An interesting example of intracellular antibody function in a bacterial infection was described by Wang et al., who showed that a mAb against *Anaplasma phagocytophilum* inhibits morulae formation within HL-60 cells (a human promyelocytic leukemia cell line) (81). A mAb against listeriolysin O, the pore-forming toxin of *Listeria monocytogenes*, blocks *L. monocytogenes* infection within macrophages. Inhibition likely occurs as a result of intracellular neutralization of a secreted *Listeria* virulence factor (82).

With respect to parasites, IgA is reported to inhibit the replication of *Toxoplasma gondii* in enterocytes (83). In addition, a mouse monoclonal IgG2b antibody, which enters host fibroblasts upon invasion of the antibody-treated organism, inhibits the intracellular growth of *T. gondii* (84).

INHIBITION OF LATER STEPS

Antibodies are capable of binding to nascent viruses and inhibiting their liberation from infected cells. This function has been described for antibodies directed against the neuraminidase of influenza A virus (85). It has also been suggested that the antibody directed against influenza A virus M2 protein influences the efficiency of virus budding (86). An mAb against rubella virus E1 glycoprotein was reported to delay the release of virus, perhaps by affecting virion assembly (87).

ANTIBODY FUNCTIONS DEPENDENT ON COMPLEMENT

Activation of the complement cascade by antibody can result in the lysis of organisms or of infected cells (88). In addition, organisms bound by complement can be internalized by phagocytic cells, with resultant clearance of the organism. Internalization through complement receptors on antigen-presenting cells can also result in the processing of antigen for presentation to T lymphocytes. The details of complement activation have been reviewed elsewhere (88). It is important to note that antibodies that bind and activate complement may also directly inhibit pathogens in the absence of complement. Complement activation may also have an indirect effect on pathogens by recruiting and activating leukocytes to sites of infection (89, 90). Similarly, complement-activating antibodies may engage Fc receptors (see below). The Ig subtype and IgG subclass of antibody are major determinants of complement activation (91). For the most part, in this review, we limit the discussion to antibodies that affect pathogens in the presence of complement but that, in the absence of complement, either have no or reduced antimicrobial activity.

A role for IgM and complement in limiting West Nile virus infection in mice has been suggested (92). More recently, Vogt et al. determined that a nonneutralizing mouse IgG1 mAb decreased West Nile virus load in mice in a manner that required C1q as well as phagocytic cells and FcγRIII (93). C1q, as well as FcγRs, contributed to the enhancement of CD4+ T-cell responses mediated by nonneutralizing anti-respiratory syncytial virus (RSV) antibody during RSV infection (94).

Antibodies that both neutralize and mediate complement-dependent lysis of influenza virus-infected cells may provide broader strain cross-reactivity than antibodies that only neutralize (95). Furthermore, the addition of complement has long been known to increase the infectivity-inhibiting activity of neutralizing antibodies against several viruses, including influenza viruses (96), Newcastle disease virus (97), herpes simplex virus (98), and Japanese encephalitis virus (99). Paramyxoviruses represent an interesting case in terms of the role of complement, since one study has shown that antibody can neutralize human parainfluenza virus type 2 with little contribution by complement, whereas neutralization of mumps virus and simian virus 5 was dependent on complement (100).

In a mouse model of respiratory syncytial virus, passive immunization of a nonneutralizing mAb was shown to protect animals from intranasal challenge. The mAb lost protective activity as a Fab, and decomplementation of mice reduced the degree of protection (101). Similarly, protective mAbs against Semliki Forest virus lose some effect in complement-depleted mice (102).

HIV-1 Env-specific antibodies are capable of lysing HIV-1-infected cells or virus in the presence of complement. However, such complement-mediated effects are inhibited by the presence of regulators of complement activation found on infected cells or on the virus itself (103, 104). Recently, complement-mediated phagocytosis of apoptotic, HIV-1-infected T cells by polyreactive antibodies has been reported (105). Another study has found that antibody from human immunodeficiency virus type 2 (HIV-2)-infected subjects is more potent than that from HIV-1-infected subjects in complement-mediated inactivation of the respective virus. Given the multiple potential consequences of complement, either directly or indirectly, its role in human immunodeficiency virus (HIV) infection *in vivo* remains unsettled (106, 107, 108).

Natural antibodies, generally of the IgM subtype, activate complement and can neutralize influenza virus (109). Moreover, natural IgM recognizing influenza virus or a surface protein of *Leishmania* may be involved in regulating CD4+ or CD8+ T cells through complement (110, 111).

A unique function of antibody is to initiate the clearance of pathogens via complement activation and binding to erythrocyte complement receptor 1 (CR1); the result of such binding sequesters the pathogen from invading susceptible tissue and may facilitate the destruction of the organisms by tissue macrophages (112). This phenomenon was first noted for bacteria by Nelson in 1953 (113).

Bacterial pathogens have developed strategies to evade the effects of complement. However, in the presence of specific antibody, effective activation of complement can result in the death or clearance of organisms such as *Neisseria meningitidis, Neisseria gonorrhoeae,* and *Haemophilus influenzae* (114). Individuals with complement deficiencies are at higher risk of infection with these organisms, and, in the case of *N. meningitidis* and *H. influenzae,* vaccine-induced antibody may protect through complement-mediated bacterial killing (115, 116). However, even with late complement component deficiencies, C3b deposition allows antibodies to kill the organisms by complement-mediated phagocytosis (115, 116, 117, 118, 119).

Antibody-mediated complement lysis of *Legionella pneumophila* is ineffective; however, organisms opsonized with both antibody and complement are phagocytosed by polymorphonuclear leukocytes (PMNs), although killing of ingested bacteria is limited (120). Vaccination of humans with an oral typhoid vaccine, M01ZH09, results in antibodies that are bactericidal to *S. enterica* serovar Typhi in the presence of complement; the antibodies also promote phagocytosis of *S. enterica* serovar Typhi by macrophages in a complement-independent manner (121).

Antibody and complement augment proinflammatory cytokine production of human peripheral blood mononuclear cells stimulated with *C. albicans,* which could be a factor in host defense against *C. albicans* infection (122). Han et al. found that protective IgM or IgG3 mAbs more efficiently bind C3 to the yeast cell than does a nonprotective mAb and that protection is likely associated with enhanced phagocytosis and killing (123). In *C. neoformans,* immune serum or an IgG1 mAb localize C3 at the edge of the organism's capsule, allowing phagocytosis

through complement receptors (124). IgM also promotes complement deposition and PMN phagocytosis of *C. neoformans* (125). Interestingly, IgM, IgA, and IgG1 can promote the phagocytosis of *C. neoformans* through complement receptors in the absence of complement; this occurs because of an antibody-mediated change in the organism's capsule that allows an interaction with complement receptors (126).

Nonspecific autologous antibodies can opsonize *P. falciparum*-parasitized erythrocytes, activate complement, and clear the infected cells through phagocytosis (127). Interestingly, antibody and complement deposition and phagocytosis are increased with erythrocytes from individuals with glucose-6-phosphate dehydrogenase deficiency, sickle trait, and β-thalassemia; it has been proposed that this antibody-mediated phenomenon underlies the protection against falciparum malaria in individuals with certain genetic disorders of red blood cells (127, 128, 129, 130). Antibody and complement can promote the killing of *P. falciparum* blood forms by THP-1 cells (a myelomonocytic cell line) and neutrophils (131, 132). In addition, antibody-dependent complement-mediated lysis of schizonts results in growth inhibition of *P. falciparum* (133). Antibodies to *P. falciparum* gametes can abolish infectivity of the gametes to mosquitoes; the gametes are lysed in the presence of complement and antibody, and antibody that binds to gametes but does not lyse them does not abolish mosquito infectivity (134, 135, 136, 137). Antibody has also been shown to clear experimental *Trypanosoma brucei* infection in a manner dependent on C3 and associated with uptake of organisms in the liver (138). Moreover, clearance of African trypanosomes by IgM, which is a major factor in controlling parasitemia, is mediated by complement and CR3 (139). Complement may also be involved in the pathogenesis of severe malaria (140, 141).

Finally, it is important to note that antibodies that neutralize *in vitro* only in the presence of complement may protect *in vivo* through other means (142).

ANTIBODY FUNCTIONS DEPENDENT ON Fc-Fc RECEPTOR INTERACTIONS

Much of the biological activity of antibody is mediated through interactions between Fc and Fc receptors found on a number of cells important for host defense. The engagement of Fc receptors by immune complexes (ICs) results in several downstream effects, depending on the Fc receptor-bearing cell, the form of the IC, the cytokine milieu, and the presence of complement. Fc receptor-mediated antibody activity can impact virus, bacteria, fungi, and parasites and can have beneficial or adverse consequences to the host.

Fc receptors have been identified for IgG (FcγR), IgE (FcεR), and IgA (FcαR), and for both IgA and IgM (FcRα/μ). Five FcγRs have been identified in humans: FcγRI, FcγRIIa, FcγRIIb, FcγRIIIa, and FcγRIIIb that differ from one another in their cellular distribution, function, and binding to IgG Fc (143, 144). There are two known forms of FcεR and one expressed form each of FcRα and FcRα/μ (144). FcγRIIa, FcγRIIIa, and FcγRIIIb are each encoded by polymorphic genes that result in phenotypically different receptors with respect to binding to different IgG subclasses (145, 146, 147, 148, 149). As a rule, IgG1 and IgG3 bind best to FcγRs, whereas IgG2 and IgG4 bind less well (150). Despite the similar magnitude of IgG1 and IgG3 binding to FcγRs, it has been reported that IgG3 mAbs are less able to mediate phagocytosis of antibody-coated red blood cells than are IgG1 mAbs, whereas ADCC activity of IgG3 is greater than that of IgG1 (151). In addition, glycosylation of the Fc segment of antibody can impact binding to FcRs (152, 153, 154, 155).

Interactions between Fc and FcRs can result in the death of pathogens or of cells infected with pathogens by a process known as antibody-dependent cellular cytotoxicity (156, 157, 158). Fc-FcR interactions are also important for phagocytosis of pathogens or of infected cells, although phagocytosis can occur in the absence of antibody or in the presence of antibody through other receptors (including complement receptors) (144). Engagement of FcRs can also inhibit intracellular pathogens without apparently killing the host cell (159). Modulation of inflammation is another FcR-mediated antibody function that can impact several pathogens (160, 161, 162, 163, 164). Finally, studies have documented the impact of FcR engagement on assays used to measure the neutralizing activity of antibodies (165, 166, 167, 168).

Antibody-Dependent Cellular Cytotoxicity

ADCC occurs when antibody forms a bridge between an infected target cell (or directly with some pathogens) and an FcR-bearing effector cell. The result of this three-way interaction is the death of the target cell, either by lysis or apoptosis. ADCC is likely to play an important role in the clinical effects of antitumor mAbs, such as rituximab and trastuzumab, but its role in infections is less clear and complicated by the multiple functions of antibody (169, 170, 171).

ADCC, first described against virus-infected cells by Shore et al. for HSV-1 (172), becomes most interesting with regard to antibodies that protect animals but that poorly neutralize the pathogen *in vitro*. Nonneutralizing mAbs directed against HSV-2 glycoproteins can protect mice after a footpad injection of a lethal dose of HSV-2. The mAbs are equally efficient in protection in complement-sufficient and complement-deficient mice (173). More recently, Gorander et al. found that vaccination of mice with glycoprotein G of HSV-2 plus CpG could protect animals from vaginal challenge with HSV-2. The protective vaccine was associated with CD4+ T-cell interferon-γ responses. In addition, the vaccine resulted in nonneutralizing antibodies that mediated ADCC and might have been involved in protection (174). Chu et al. found that passive infusion of IgG antibodies decreased symptoms and mortality and decreased vaginal viral quantity in normal mice infected with HSV-2; although the antibody had neutralizing activity, protection was significantly diminished in mice lacking FcγR expression (175). Influenza A virus M2 vaccination results in partial protection of mice from influenza A infection that is mediated by nonneutralizing antibodies; ADCC is likely involved, since protection is not dependent on complement, whereas NK cells depletion reduces the protective effect (176).

The role of ADCC in HIV-1 and other lentivirus infections has been reviewed recently (156, 177). A great deal of correlative evidence in monkeys, as well as in humans, suggests a role for ADCC or other FcγR-mediated antibody activities in preventing or modulating lentivirus infections. A more definitive study has demonstrated that mutations in the Fc segment of antibody that abrogate FcγR binding render a neutralizing mAb (IgG1b12) less protective *in vivo* against vaginal SHIV challenge than the unmutated mAb (1). However, whether the decreased protection is due to a lack of ADCC or to some other FcγR-mediated activity remains unknown.

There is scant literature on the role of ADCC in bacterial infections. However, complement-independent killing of bacteria *in vitro* in the presence of "killer" lymphocytes has been described for *N. meningitidis* and *Shigella flexneri* (178, 179). IgA, as well as IgG, in combination with lymphocytes from murine gut-associated lymphoid tissue, is reported to mediate ADCC against *S. flexneri* and *Salmonella* spp. (180, 181). Similarly, the same group found antibacterial activity against *Streptococcus pneumoniae* by mouse lung lymphocytes in conjunction with IgA (182). ADCC has also been described for *Ehrlichia risticii* and *Coxiella burnetii*-infected cells and for *Brucella abortus*, although, as with other bacteria, the role, if any, of ADCC in these infections *in vivo* is unknown (183, 184, 185). In the case of *C. burnetii*, passive antibody treatment can protect mice from *C. burnetii* infection in common γ-chain knockout mice, suggesting that Fc-FcγR interactions were not required for protection (186).

ADCC has been documented *in vitro* for a number of parasites. IgG opsonized *T. spiralis* larvae are susceptible to ADCC by eosinophils, neutrophils, and monocytes (187, 188). Schistosomula are killed by eosinophils, macrophages, or platelets in the presence of specific antibody, including IgE and IgG (189, 190, 191, 192). *In vivo* protection of rats from *Schistosoma mansoni* infection is likely the result of such IgE-mediated ADCC (193). Antibodies that bind poorly to FcRs, such as IgM, IgG2, and IgG4, can inhibit ADCC against schistosomula and have been epidemiologically linked to increased susceptibility of infection in humans (194, 195, 196). ADCC mediated by IgG or IgE and by macrophages, eosinophils, or neutrophil effector cells has also been shown *in vitro* to kill larval or adult filaria (197, 198, 199, 200, 201, 202). *In vivo*, clearance of *Brugia malayi* microfilaria is very likely mediated through ADCC (203). ADCC activity against trypanosomes and other parasites has also been documented (204, 205, 206, 207, 208, 209, 210).

It is important to note that many of the effector cells mediating ADCC against parasites are capable of antibody-mediated phagocytosis as well. In both ADCC and phagocytosis, organisms are killed and radioisotopes or dyes are released, and distinguishing between these two antibody functions requires careful consideration (204, 205).

Finally, antibodies may also inhibit infections in a manner that requires the components of ADCC (i.e., infected target cells, antibody, and FcR-bearing effector cells) but does not necessarily rely on target cell lysis. Thus, antibody-dependent cell-mediated inhibition of *P. falciparum* has been described, where the development of intracellular parasites is blocked in a manner dependent on blood monocytes and antibody; triggering of both FcγRIIa and FcγRIIIa may be required, but erythrocyte target cells do not appear to be killed (159, 211, 212). Forthal et al. have described antibody-dependent cell-mediated virus inhibition (ADCVI) with measles virus

HIV, simian immunodeficiency virus (SIV) and simian-human immunodeficiency virus (SHIV) (1, 160, 213, 214). ADCVI is a measure of virus inhibition occurring as a result of antibody-FcR interactions and is likely dependent on combinations of ADCC, phagocytosis, and chemokine/cytokine production.

Phagocytosis

The internalization and degradation of antibody-coated pathogens by phagocytes via FcRs has been well described for a number of organisms and is likely a critical antibody function for clearance of pathogens *in vivo*. Since phagocytosis and ADCC often require the same components (antibody and effector cells), it may be difficult to definitively and specifically demonstrate a role for phagocytosis in preventing or modulating infections in animals or humans.

With respect to viruses, passive infusion of antibodies results in the rapid elimination of cell-free organisms from the blood of animals (215, 216). This is consistent with information indicating that the rate of clearance of antigens by the reticuloendothelial system is greatly increased in the presence of specific antibodies (217, 218).

A recent example comes close to demonstrating a key role for phagocytosis in preventing a viral infection (93). In that study, a poorly neutralizing antibody against the West Nile virus envelope could reduce viremia in mice via an FcγRIII- and C1q-dependent mechanism that required phagocytic cells. Since NK cells did not seem to be involved, it is less likely that ADCC played a significant role in protection. However, it remains possible that the lysis of infected cells mediated by the phagocytes, in addition to or instead of phagocytosis of antibody-coated virus, was involved in protection. A possible role for phagocytosis in clearing influenza virus from the lungs of mice was suggested by Fujisawa (219). In that study, both PMNs and the passive infusion of neutralizing antibody were required for maximum viral clearance and survival. A particularly interesting point about this study was the need for PMNs despite the high neutralizing titer of the infused immune serum; this finding is consistent with that of Hessell et al. where maximal protection against SHIV was afforded by a neutralizing antibody that engaged Fc receptors (1). Huber et al., using passive antibody transfer in FcRγ$^{-/-}$ mice, also concluded that phagocytosis is important in the clearance of influenza virus (220). In all of these studies, however, it is not possible to precisely define the antibody function responsible for protection, because phagocytosis, ADCC, or soluble factors could have contributed.

An interesting phenomenon related to phagocytosis was described by Chan et al. (221) who showed that inhibition of dengue virus phagocytosis, by aggregating virus and cross-linking of FcγRIIb, resulted in neutralization of virus infectivity.

Phagocytosis of antibody-coated infected cells, in addition to phagocytosis of immune complexed cell-free virus, could be a contributor to protection, although virus-infected cells can be phagocytosed in the absence of antibody (222, 223). Surprisingly, two studies indicated that neither human monocytes nor human neutrophils were able to phagocytose IgA or IgG immune complexes formed with influenza virus *in vitro* (224, 225).

FcγR-mediated phagocytosis and clearance of *Bordetella pertussis* has been demonstrated *in vitro* and in a mouse model (226). Similarly, natural and vaccine-induced antibodies mediate phagocytosis of *S. pneumoniae*, and such FcγR-mediated phagocytosis may play a role in protection (227). In FcγRIIb-deficient mice, phagocytosis and survival after *S. pneumoniae* challenge are both improved relative to control mice, although the survival advantage is reversed after immunization followed by challenge with a high dose of bacteria (227). In the later case, it is likely that inflammatory cytokines triggered by interactions between antipneumococcal antibody and activating FcγRs—in the absence of the inhibitory FcγRIIb—were responsible for the higher mortality. Other studies in mice have found that antibody-mediated protection from *S. pneumoniae* does not depend on FcγRs (228). In humans, IgG2, a relatively inefficient activator of complement, is thought to be important in protection against *S. pneumoniae*. Although IgG2 is also relatively poor at engaging FcγRs, it binds best to the H isoform of FcγRIIa and to the V isoform of FcγRIIIa (150). Consistent with a role for FcγR-mediated phagocytosis, there appears to be an association between homozygosity for the R isoform of FcγRIIa and severe or invasive pneumococcal disease (229, 230). Moreover, PMNs from FcγRIIa HH homozygous donors have higher phagocytic activity against antibody-opsonized *S. pneumoniae* (231). In the case of *N. meningitidis*, complement-mediated clearance or bactericidal activity appears to be more important than FcγR-mediated phagocytosis (see above). However, FcγR-mediated phagocytosis can be demonstrated *in vitro* (232, 233). Furthermore, some studies, but not all, have found associations between FcγRIIa genotypes and susceptibility to or severity of meningococcal infection (233, 234, 235, 236, 237, 238). Finally, γδT cells capable of phagocytosing antibody-opsonized *E. coli* via FcγRIIIa have been described (239).

Opsonization and phagocytosis by IgG subclass-switched mouse mAbs has been described for *C. neoformans* (240). Passive infusion of the mAbs had some effect on clearing yeast from mice, but the phagocytic activity *in vitro* did not correlate well with clearing of organisms *in vivo* (241). A study of *C. neoformans* phagocytosis has suggested a specific receptor for IgG3 in mice different from the known FcγRs (242). A recent study using X-linked immunodeficient mice indicated that IgM promotes containment of *C. neoformans* in the lungs by augmenting phagocytosis (243).

In many cases, parasites may be too large for phagocytosis: lysosomal and parasitic membranes fuse after Fc-FcR (γ, α, or ε) interactions, resulting in the lysis of parasites extracellularly (244). However, IgG from individuals living in malaria-endemic areas can mediate the phagocytosis of *P. falciparum*-infected erythrocytes by monocytes (245). In addition, the PfEMP1 is the major target of antibodies that mediate phagocytosis, and anti-PfEMP1 antibodies are associated with a reduced risk of developing symptomatic malaria (246).

OTHER ANTIBODY FUNCTIONS

Apart from specific effects on organisms, antibodies may modulate inflammation and thereby indirectly affect pathogenesis. Such immune modulation is well described for FcγR triggering by immune complexes, which results in the generation, secretion, or repression of various pro- or anti-inflammatory substances (247, 248, 249, 250, 251, 252, 253, 254, 255, 256). In addition to modulation of cytokines by FcRs themselves, internalization of immune complexes via FcRs can result in the engagement of toll-like receptors, adding a further layer of complexity and control over inflammation (255, 257, 258, 259, 260).

An example of the role of FcγRs in inflammation was the demonstration that soluble FcγRII, by competing with IC binding to cellular FcγRs, can limit the inflammation due to the IC (i.e., the Arthus reaction) (261). Soon thereafter, it was established that the Arthus reaction was markedly attenuated in FcRγ-chain knockout mice (262). These types of studies have important implications for autoimmune diseases (263).

Engagement of FcγRIIb by IgG immune complexes serve to regulate B-cell activity and survival and may serve as a means of maintaining peripheral tolerance for B cells (264, 265, 266). Immune complex binding and internalization via FcγRs also result in dendritic cell maturation and in efficient major histocompatibility complex class I-restricted presentation of the exogenous peptides making up the immune-complexed antigen (267).

Another important mechanism of immune modulation by antibodies is through the activation of complement components, which can then serve as chemotactic agents (268). Moreover, C5a anaphylatoxin is involved in immune complex-mediated injury in part because it results in a shifting of the balance between activating and inhibitory FcγRs toward a more inflammatory phenotype (269). Activation of C3bi on immune complexes can result in blunting of the inflammatory response by diverting interactions of the IC away from FcγRs and toward CR3 (270).

CONCLUSIONS

The inhibitory effects of antibodies on pathogenic organisms have been documented since the late 1800s (271). Since that time, much has been learned regarding the mechanisms that underlie the antimicrobial activity of antibodies. However, antibodies often have multiple functions *in vitro* and *in vivo*, either directly or through interactions with FcRs or complement. Modern tools, such as knockout mice or antibodies engineered to abrogate or enhance functions have proven useful for more precise explorations of antibody function. Nonetheless, major questions regarding the way in which an antibody functions *in vivo* remain, and multiple activities are likely to contribute to the antimicrobial effect.

ACKNOWLEDGMENTS

I received financial support from the U.S. Public Health Service (grants AI084136, AI0797775, and AI102715).

I acknowledge the editorial assistance of Gabriel J. A. Forthal.

Conflicts of interest: I declare no conflicts.

CITATION

Forthal DN. Functions of antibodies. 2014. Microbiol Spectrum 2(4):AID-0019-2014.

REFERENCES

1. **Hessell AJ, Hangartner L, Hunter M, Havenith CE, Beurskens FJ, Bakker JM, Lanigan CM, Landucci G, Forthal DN, Parren PW, Marx PA, Burton DR.** 2007. Fc receptor but not complement binding is important in antibody protection against HIV. *Nature* 449:101–104.
2. **Brandtzaeg P.** 2007. Induction of secretory immunity and memory at mucosal surfaces. *Vaccine* 25:5467–5484.
3. **Phalipon A, Cardona A, Kraehenbuhl JP, Edelman L, Sansonetti PJ, Corthesy B.** 2002. Secretory component: a new role in secretory IgA-mediated immune exclusion in vivo. *Immunity* 17:107–115.
4. **Brioen P, Dekegel D, Boeye A.** 1983. Neutralization of poliovirus by antibody-mediated polymerization. *Virology* 127:463–468.
5. **Thomas AA, Vrijsen R, Boeye A.** 1986. Relationship between poliovirus neutralization and aggregation. *J Virol* 59:479–485.
6. **Lin TL, Clark TG, Dickerson H.** 1996. Passive immunization of channel catfish (Ictalurus punctatus) against the ciliated protozoan parasite Ichthyophthirius multifiliis by use of murine monoclonal antibodies. *Infect Immun* 64:4085–4090.
7. **Campodonico VL, Llosa NJ, Grout M, Doring G, Maira-Litran T, Pier GB.** 2010. Evaluation of flagella and flagellin of *Pseudomonas aeruginosa* as vaccines. *Infect Immun* 78:746–755.
8. **Bishop AL, Schild S, Patimalla B, Klein B, Camilli A.** 2010. Mucosal immunization with Vibrio cholerae outer membrane vesicles provides maternal protection mediated by antilipopolysaccharide antibodies that inhibit bacterial motility. *Infect Immun* 78:4402–4420.
9. **Hope T.** 2010. Defining the interaction of HIV with the mucosal barriers to gain insights into the mechanisms of sexual transmission. Abstr. AIDS Vaccine Conference 2010, Atlanta, GA.
10. **McCullough KC, Smale CJ, Carpenter WC, Crowther JR, Brocchi E, De Simone F.** 1987. Conformational alteration in foot-and-mouth disease virus virion capsid structure after complexing with monospecific antibody. *Immunology* 60:75–82.
11. **Hernandez R, Paredes A, Brown DT.** 2008. Sindbis virus conformational changes induced by a neutralizing anti-E1 monoclonal antibody. *J Virol* 82:5750–5760.
12. **Klasse PJ, Sattentau QJ.** 2002. Occupancy and mechanism in antibody-mediated neutralization of animal viruses. *J Gen Virol* 83:2091–2108.

13. **LaRocca TJ, Holthausen DJ, Hsieh C, Renken C, Mannella CA, Benach JL.** 2009. The bactericidal effect of a complement-independent antibody is osmolytic and specific to Borrelia. *Proc Natl Acad Sci USA* **106:**10752–10757.

14. **Matthews RC, Rigg G, Hodgetts S, Carter T, Chapman C, Gregory C, Illidge C, Burnie J.** 2003. Preclinical assessment of the efficacy of mycograb, a human recombinant antibody against fungal HSP90. *Antimicrob Agents Chemother* **47:**2208–2216.

15. **Pachl J, Svoboda P, Jacobs F, Vandewoude K, van der Hoven B, Spronk P, Masterson G, Malbrain M, Aoun M, Garbino J, Takala J, Drgona L, Burnie J, Matthews R.** 2006. A randomized, blinded, multicenter trial of lipid-associated amphotericin B alone versus in combination with an antibody-based inhibitor of heat shock protein 90 in patients with invasive candidiasis. *Clin Infect Dis* **42:**1404–1413.

16. **Nooney L, Matthews RC, Burnie JP.** 2005. Evaluation of Mycograb, amphotericin B, caspofungin, and fluconazole in combination against *Cryptococcus neoformans* by checkerboard and time-kill methodologies. *Diagn Microbiol Infect Dis* **51:**19–29.

17. **McClelland EE, Nicola AM, Prados-Rosales R, Casadevall A.** 2010. Ab binding alters gene expression in *Cryptococcus neoformans* and directly modulates fungal metabolism. *J Clin Invest* **120:**1355–1361.

18. **Watanabe M, Blobel G.** 1989. Site-specific antibodies against the PrlA (secY) protein of Escherichia coli inhibit protein export by interfering with plasma membrane binding of preproteins. *Proc Natl Acad Sci USA* **86:**1895–1899.

19. **Gregory RL, Michalek SM, Shechmeister IL, McGhee JR.** 1984. Function of anti-*Streptococcus mutans* antibodies: anti-ribosomal antibodies inhibit acid production, growth, and glucose phosphotransferase activity. *Infect Immun* **45:**286–289.

20. **Casadevall A, Pirofski LA.** 2012. Immunoglobulins in defense, pathogenesis, and therapy of fungal diseases. *Cell Host Microbe* **11:**447–456.

21. **Klasse PJ, Sanders RW, Cerutti A, Moore JP.** 2012. How can HIV-type-1-Env immunogenicity be improved to facilitate antibody-based vaccine development? *AIDS Res Hum Retroviruses* **28:**1–15.

22. **He RT, Innis BL, Nisalak A, Usawattanakul W, Wang S, Kalayanarooj S, Anderson R.** 1995. Antibodies that block virus attachment to Vero cells are a major component of the human neutralizing antibody response against dengue virus type 2. *J Med Virol* **45:**451–461.

23. **Iorio RM, Glickman RL, Riel AM, Sheehan JP, Bratt MA.** 1989. Functional and neutralization profile of seven overlapping antigenic sites on the HN glycoprotein of Newcastle disease virus: monoclonal antibodies to some sites prevent viral attachment. *Virus Res* **13:**245–261.

24. **Booy FP, Roden RB, Greenstone HL, Schiller JT, Trus BL.** 1998. Two antibodies that neutralize papillomavirus by different mechanisms show distinct binding patterns at 13 A resolution. *J Mol Biol* **281:**95–106.

25. **Ruggeri FM, Greenberg HB.** 1991. Antibodies to the trypsin cleavage peptide VP8 neutralize rotavirus by inhibiting binding of virions to target cells in culture. *J Virol* **65:**2211–2219.

26. **Smith TJ, Olson NH, Cheng RH, Liu H, Chase ES, Lee WM, Leippe DM, Mosser AG, Rueckert RR, Baker TS.** 1993. Structure of human rhinovirus complexed with Fab fragments from a neutralizing antibody. *J Virol* **67:**1148–1158.

27. **Della-Porta AJ, Westaway EG.** 1978. A multi-hit model for the neutralization of animal viruses. *J Gen Virol* **38:**1–19.

28. **Platt EJ, Gomes MM, Kabat D.** 2012. Kinetic mechanism for HIV-1 neutralization by antibody 2G12 entails reversible glycan binding that slows cell entry. *Proc Natl Acad Sci USA* **109:**7829–7834.

29. **Reading SA, Dimmock NJ.** 2007. Neutralization of animal virus infectivity by antibody. *Arch Virol* **152:**1047–1059.

30. **Klemm P, Vejborg RM, Hancock V.** 2010. Prevention of bacterial adhesion. *Appl Microbiol Biotechnol* **88:**451–459.

31. **Cegelski L, Marshall GR, Eldridge GR, Hultgren SJ.** 2008. The biology and future prospects of antivirulence therapies. *Nat Rev Microbiol* **6:**17–27.

32. **Smani Y, McConnell MJ, Pachón J.** 2012. Role of fibronectin in the adhesion of *Acinetobacter baumannii* to host cells. *PLoS One* **7:**e33073. doi:10.1371/journal.pone.0033073.

33. **Tsang TM, Annis DS, Kronshage M, Fenno JT, Usselman LD, Mosher DF, Krukonis ES.** 2012. Ail protein binds ninth type III fibronectin repeat (9FNIII) within central 120-kDa region of fibronectin to facilitate cell binding by *Yersinia pestis.* *J Biol Chem* **287:**16759–16767.

34. **Khan MN, Pichichero ME.** 2012. Vaccine candidates PhtD and PhtE of *Streptococcus pneumoniae* are adhesins that elicit functional antibodies in humans. *Vaccine* **30:**2900–2907.

35. **Langermann S, Ballou WR.** 2003. Development of a recombinant FimCH vaccine for urinary tract infections. *Adv Exp Med Biol* **539:**635–648.

36. **Langermann S, Palaszynski S, Barnhart M, Auguste G, Pinkner JS, Burlein J, Barren P, Koenig S, Leath S, Jones CH, Hultgren SJ.** 1997. Prevention of mucosal *Escherichia coli* infection by FimH-adhesin-based systemic vaccination. *Science* **276:**607–611.

37. **Langermann S, Mollby R, Burlein JE, Palaszynski SR, Auguste CG, DeFusco A, Strouse R, Schenerman MA, Hultgren SJ, Pinkner JS, Winberg J, Guldevall L, Soderhall M, Ishikawa K, Normark S, Koenig S.** 2000. Vaccination with FimH adhesin protects cynomolgus monkeys from colonization and infection by uropathogenic *Escherichia coli*. *J Infect Dis* **181:**774–778.

38. **Kain R, Exner M, Brandes R, Ziebermayr R, Cunningham D, Alderson CA, Davidovits A, Raab I, Jahn R, Ashour O, Spitzauer S, Sunder-Plassmann G, Fukuda M, Klemm P, Rees AJ, Kerjaschki D.** 2008. Molecular mimicry in pauci-immune focal necrotizing glomerulonephritis. *Nat Med* **14:**1088–1096.

39. **Manjarrez-Hernandez HA, Gavilanes-Parra S, Chavez-Berrocal E, Navarro-Ocana A, Cravioto A.** 2000. Antigen detection in enteropathogenic *Escherichia coli* using secretory immunoglobulin A antibodies isolated from human breast milk. *Infect Immun* **68:**5030–5036.

40. **Schlesinger LS, Hull SR, Kaufman TM.** 1994. Binding of the terminal mannosyl units of lipoarabinomannan from a virulent strain of Mycobacterium tuberculosis to human macrophages. *J Immunol* **152:**4070–4079.

41. **Kornspan JD, Tarshis M, Rottem S.** 2011. Adhesion and biofilm formation of Mycoplasma pneumoniae on an abiotic surface. *Arch Microbiol* **193:**833–836.

42. **Holder AA, Freeman RR.** 1981. Immunization against blood-stage rodent malaria using purified parasite antigens. *Nature* **294:**361–364.

43. **Perkins ME, Rocco LJ.** 1988. Sialic acid-dependent binding of *Plasmodium falciparum* merozoite surface antigen, Pf200, to human erythrocytes. *J Immunol* **141:**3190–3196.

44. **Bolad A, Berzins K.** 2000. Antigenic diversity of *Plasmodium falciparum* and antibody-mediated parasite neutralization. *Scand J Immunol* **52:**233–239.

45. **Clausen TM, Christoffersen S, Dahlback M, Langkilde AE, Jensen KE, Resende M, Agerbaek MO, Andersen D, Berisha B, Ditlev SB, Pinto VV, Nielsen MA, Theander TG, Larsen S, Salanti A.** 2012. Structural and functional insight into how the Plasmodium falciparum VAR2CSA protein mediates binding to chondroitin sulfate A in placental malaria. *J Biol Chem* **287:**23332–23345.

46. **Yun CH, Lillehoj HS, Lillehoj EP.** 2000. Intestinal immune responses to coccidiosis. *Dev Comp Immunol* **24:**303–324.

47. **Eckmann L.** 2003. Mucosal defences against Giardia. *Parasite Immunol* **25:**259–270.

48. **Negrao-Correa D.** 2001. Importance of immunoglobulin E (IgE) in the protective mechanism against gastrointestinal nematode infection: looking at the intestinal mucosae. *Rev Inst Med Trop Sao Paulo* **43:**291–299.

49. **Cevallos AM, Zhang X, Waldor MK, Jaison S, Zhou X, Tzipori S, Neutra MR, Ward HD.** 2000. Molecular cloning and expression of a gene encoding *Cryptosporidium parvum* glycoproteins gp40 and gp15. *Infect Immun* **68:**4108–4116.

50. **Lopalco L, Barassi C, Pastori C, Longhi R, Burastero SE, Tambussi G, Mazzotta F, Lazzarin A, Clerici M, Siccardi AG.** 2000. CCR5-reactive antibodies in seronegative partners of HIV-seropositive individuals down-modulate surface CCR5 in vivo and neutralize the infectivity of R5 strains of HIV-1 In vitro. *J Immunol* **164:**3426–3433.

51. **Barassi C, Soprana E, Pastori C, Longhi R, Buratti E, Lillo F, Marenzi C, Lazzarin A, Siccardi AG, Lopalco L.** 2005. Induction of murine mucosal CCR5-reactive antibodies as an anti-human immunodeficiency virus strategy. *J Virol* **79:**6848–6858.

52. **Wintachai P, Wikan N, Kuadkitkan A, Jaimipuk T, Ubol S, Pulmanausahakul R, Auewarakul P, Kasinrerk W, Weng WY, Panyasrivanit M, Paemanee A, Kittisenachai S, Roytrakul S, Smith DR.** 2012. Identification of prohibitin as a Chikungunya virus receptor protein. *J Med Virol* **84:**1757–1770.

53. **Kondratowicz AS, Lennemann NJ, Sinn PL, Davey RA, Hunt CL, Moller-Tank S, Meyerholz DK, Rennert P, Mullins RF, Brindley M, Sandersfeld LM, Quinn K, Weller M, McCray PB Jr, Chiorini J, Maury W.** 2011. T-cell immunoglobulin and mucin domain 1 (TIM-1) is a receptor for Zaire Ebolavirus and Lake Victoria Marburgvirus. *Proc Natl Acad Sci USA* **108:**8426–8431.

54. **Bruno CJ, Jacobson JM.** 2010. Ibalizumab: an anti-CD4 monoclonal antibody for the treatment of HIV-1 infection. *J Antimicrob Chemother* **65:**1839–1841.

55. **Meuleman P, Hesselgesser J, Paulson M, Vanwolleghem T, Desombere I, Reiser H, Leroux-Roels G.** 2008. Anti-CD81 antibodies can prevent a hepatitis C virus infection in vivo. *Hepatology* **48:**1761–1768.

56. **Silvie O, Rubinstein E, Franetich JF, Prenant M, Belnoue E, Renia L, Hannoun L, Eling W, Levy**

S, Boucheix C, Mazier D. 2003. Hepatocyte CD81 is required for *Plasmodium falciparum* and *Plasmodium yoelii* sporozoite infectivity. *Nat Med* **9:**93–96.

57. Schubert A, Zakikhany K, Pietrocola G, Meinke A, Speziale P, Eikmanns BJ, Reinscheid DJ. 2004. The fibrinogen receptor FbsA promotes adherence of Streptococcus agalactiae to human epithelial cells. *Infect Immun* **72:**6197–6205.

58. Edwards MJ, Dimmock NJ. 2001. Hemagglutinin 1-specific immunoglobulin G and Fab molecules mediate postattachment neutralization of influenza A virus by inhibition of an early fusion event. *J Virol* **75:**10208–10218.

59. de Rosny E, Vassell R, Jiang S, Kunert R, Weiss CD. 2004. Binding of the 2F5 monoclonal antibody to native and fusion-intermediate forms of human immunodeficiency virus type 1 gp41: implications for fusion-inducing conformational changes. *J Virol* **78:**2627–2631.

60. Lorizate M, Cruz A, Huarte N, Kunert R, Perez-Gil J, Nieva JL. 2006. Recognition and blocking of HIV-1 gp41 pre-transmembrane sequence by monoclonal 4E10 antibody in a Raft-like membrane environment. *J Biol Chem* **281:**39598–39606.

61. Kaufmann B, Nybakken GE, Chipman PR, Zhang W, Diamond MS, Fremont DH, Kuhn RJ, Rossmann MG. 2006. West Nile virus in complex with the Fab fragment of a neutralizing monoclonal antibody. *Proc Natl Acad Sci USA* **103:**12400–12404.

62. Pierson TC, Diamond MS. 2008. Molecular mechanisms of antibody-mediated neutralisation of flavivirus infection. *Expert Rev Mol Med* **10:**e12. doi:10.1017/S1462399408000665.

63. Barbey-Martin C, Gigant B, Bizebard T, Calder LJ, Wharton SA, Skehel JJ, Knossow M. 2002. An antibody that prevents the hemagglutinin low pH fusogenic transition. *Virology* **294:**70–74.

64. Ekiert DC, Bhabha G, Elsliger MA, Friesen RH, Jongeneelen M, Throsby M, Goudsmit J, Wilson IA. 2009. Antibody recognition of a highly conserved influenza virus epitope. *Science* **324:**246–251.

65. Cao Z, Meng J, Li X, Wu R, Huang Y, He Y. 2012. The epitope and neutralization mechanism of AVFluIgG01, a broad-reactive human monoclonal antibody against H5N1 influenza virus. *PLoS One* **7:**e38126. doi:10.1371/journal.pone.0038126.

66. Bai Y, Ye L, Tesar DB, Song H, Zhao D, Bjorkman PJ, Roopenian DC, Zhu X. 2011. Intracellular neutralization of viral infection in polarized epithelial cells by neonatal Fc receptor (FcRn)-mediated IgG transport. *Proc Natl Acad Sci USA* **108:**18406–18411.

67. Stewart PL, Nemerow GR. 1997. Recent structural solutions for antibody neutralization of viruses. *Trends Microbiol* **5:**229–233.

68. Wien MW, Filman DJ, Stura EA, Guillot S, Delpeyroux F, Crainic R, Hogle JM. 1995. Structure of the complex between the Fab fragment of a neutralizing antibody for type 1 poliovirus and its viral epitope. *Nat Struct Biol* **2:**232–243.

69. Maciejewski JP, Weichold FF, Young NS, Cara A, Zella D, Reitz MS Jr, Gallo RC. 1995. Intracellular expression of antibody fragments directed against HIV reverse transcriptase prevents HIV infection in vitro. *Nat Med* **1:**667–673.

70. Varghese R, Mikyas Y, Stewart PL, Ralston R. 2004. Postentry neutralization of adenovirus type 5 by an antihexon antibody. *J Virol* **78:**12320–12332.

71. Ishii Y, Tanaka K, Kondo K, Takeuchi T, Mori S, Kanda T. 2010. Inhibition of nuclear entry of HPV16 pseudovirus-packaged DNA by an anti-HPV16 L2 neutralizing antibody. *Virology* **406:**181–188.

72. Mazanec MB, Kaetzel CS, Lamm ME, Fletcher D, Nedrud JG. 1992. Intracellular neutralization of virus by immunoglobulin A antibodies. *Proc Natl Acad Sci USA* **89:**6901–6905.

73. Yan H, Lamm ME, Bjorling E, Huang YT. 2002. Multiple functions of immunoglobulin A in mucosal defense against viruses: an in vitro measles virus model. *J Virol* **76:**10972–10979.

74. Mazanec MB, Coudret CL, Fletcher DR. 1995. Intracellular neutralization of influenza virus by immunoglobulin A anti-hemagglutinin monoclonal antibodies. *J Virol* **69:**1339–1343.

75. Zhou D, Zhang Y, Li Q, Chen Y, He B, Yang J, Tu H, Lei L, Yan H. 2011. Matrix protein-specific IgA antibody inhibits measles virus replication by intracellular neutralization. *J Virol* **85:**11090–11097.

76. Bomsel M, Heyman M, Hocini H, Lagaye S, Belec L, Dupont C, Desgranges C. 1998. Intracellular neutralization of HIV transcytosis across tight epithelial barriers by anti-HIV envelope protein dIgA or IgM. *Immunity* **9:**277–287.

77. Corthesy B, Benureau Y, Perrier C, Fourgeux C, Parez N, Greenberg H, Schwartz-Cornil I. 2006. Rotavirus anti-VP6 secretory immunoglobulin A contributes to protection via intracellular neutralization but not via immune exclusion. *J Virol* **80:**10692–10699.

78. Feng N, Lawton JA, Gilbert J, Kuklin N, Vo P, Prasad BV, Greenberg HB. 2002. Inhibition of rotavirus replication by a non-neutralizing,

rotavirus VP6-specific IgA mAb. *J Clin Invest* **109:**1203–1213.

79. **Thouvenin E, Schoehn G, Rey F, Petitpas I, Mathieu M, Vaney MC, Cohen J, Kohli E, Pothier P, Hewat E.** 2001. Antibody inhibition of the transcriptase activity of the rotavirus DLP: a structural view. *J Mol Biol* **307:**161–172.

80. **Mallery DL, McEwan WA, Bidgood SR, Towers GJ, Johnson CM, James LC.** 2010. Antibodies mediate intracellular immunity through tripartite motif-containing 21 (TRIM21). *Proc Natl Acad Sci USA* **107:**19985–19990.

81. **Wang X, Kikuchi T, Rikihisa Y.** 2006. Two monoclonal antibodies with defined epitopes of P44 major surface proteins neutralize *Anaplasma phagocytophilum* by distinct mechanisms. *Infect Immun* **74:**1873–1882.

82. **Edelson BT, Unanue ER.** 2001. Intracellular antibody neutralizes Listeria growth. *Immunity* **14:**503–512.

83. **Bout D, Moretto M, Dimier-Poisson I, Gatel DB.** 1999. Interaction between *Toxoplasma gondii* and enterocyte. *Immunobiology* **201:** 225–228.

84. **Mineo JR, Khan IA, Kasper LH.** 1994. *Toxoplasma gondii*: a monoclonal antibody that inhibits intracellular replication. *Exp Parasitol* **79:**351–361.

85. **Webster RG, Laver WG.** 1967. Preparation and properties of antibody directed specifically against the neuraminidase of influenza virus. *J Immunol* **99:**49–55.

86. **Hughey PG, Roberts PC, Holsinger LJ, Zebedee SL, Lamb RA, Compans RW.** 1995. Effects of antibody to the influenza A virus M2 protein on M2 surface expression and virus assembly. *Virology* **212:**411–421.

87. **Corboba P, Grutadauria S, Cuffini C, Zapata M.** 2000. Neutralizing monoclonal antibody to the E1 glycoprotein epitope of rubella virus mediates virus arrest in VERO cells. *Viral Immunol* **13:**83–92.

88. **Murphy K, Travers P, Walport M.** 2008. The complement system and innate immunity, p 61–80. *Janeway's Immunobiology*, 7th ed. Garland Science, New York, NY.

89. **DiScipio RG, Schraufstatter IU.** 2007. The role of the complement anaphylatoxins in the recruitment of eosinophils. *Int Immunopharmacol* **7:**1909–1923.

90. **Walport MJ.** 2001. Complement. First of two parts. *N Engl J Med* **344:**1058–1066.

91. **Prodinger WM, Wurzner R, Stoiber H, Dierich MP.** 2003. Complement, p 1077–1103. *In* Paul W (ed), *Fundamental Immunology*, 5th ed. Lippincott Williams & Wilkins, Philadelphia, PA.

92. **Diamond MS, Shrestha B, Mehlhop E, Sitati E, Engle M.** 2003. Innate and adaptive immune responses determine protection against disseminated infection by West Nile encephalitis virus. *Viral Immunol* **16:**259–278.

93. **Vogt MR, Dowd KA, Engle M, Tesh RB, Johnson S, Pierson TC, Diamond MS.** 2011. Poorly neutralizing cross-reactive antibodies against the fusion loop of West Nile virus envelope protein protect in vivo via Fcgamma receptor and complement-dependent effector mechanisms. *J Virol* **85:**11567–11580.

94. **Kruijsen D, Bakkers MJ, van Uden NO, Viveen MC, van der Sluis TC, Kimpen JL, Leusen JH, Coenjaerts FE, van Bleek GM.** 2010. Serum antibodies critically affect virus-specific CD4+/CD8+ T cell balance during respiratory syncytial virus infections. *J Immunol* **185:**6489–6498.

95. **Terajima M, Cruz J, Co MD, Lee JH, Kaur K, Wrammert J, Wilson PC, Ennis FA.** 2011. Complement-dependent lysis of influenza a virus-infected cells by broadly cross-reactive human monoclonal antibodies. *J Virol* **85:** 13463–13467.

96. **Frank AL, Puck J, Hughes BJ, Cate TR.** 1980. Microneutralization test for influenza A and B and parainfluenza 1 and 2 viruses that uses continuous cell lines and fresh serum enhancement. *J Clin Microbiol* **12:**426–432.

97. **Linscott WD, Levinson WE.** 1969. Complement components required for virus neutralization by early immunoglobulin antibody. *Proc Natl Acad Sci USA* **64:**520–527.

98. **Yoshino K, Taniguchi S.** 1965. Studies on the neutralization of herpes simplex virus. I. Appearance of neutralizing antibodies having different grades of complement requirement. *Virology* **26:**44–53.

99. **Ozaki Y, Tabeyi K.** 1967. Studies on the neutralization of Japanese encephalitis virus. I. Application of kinetic neutralization to the measurement of the neutralizing potency of antiserum. *J Immunol* **98:**1218–1223.

100. **Johnson JB, Capraro GA, Parks GD.** 2008. Differential mechanisms of complement-mediated neutralization of the closely related paramyxoviruses simian virus 5 and mumps virus. *Virology* **376:**112–123.

101. **Corbeil S, Seguin C, Trudel M.** 1996. Involvement of the complement system in the protection of mice from challenge with respiratory syncytial virus Long strain following passive immunization with monoclonal antibody 18A2B2. *Vaccine* **14:**521–525.

102. **Boere WA, Benaissa-Trouw BJ, Harmsen T, Erich T, Kraaijeveld CA, Snippe H.** 1986. The

role of complement in monoclonal antibody-mediated protection against virulent Semliki Forest virus. *Immunology* **58**:553–559.

103. **Saifuddin M, Parker CJ, Peeples ME, Gorny MK, Zolla-Pazner S, Ghassemi M, Rooney IA, Atkinson JP, Spear GT.** 1995. Role of virion-associated glycosylphosphatidylinositol-linked proteins CD55 and CD59 in complement resistance of cell line-derived and primary isolates of HIV-1. *J Exp Med* **182**:501–509.

104. **Schmitz J, Zimmer JP, Kluxen B, Aries S, Bogel M, Gigli I, Schmitz H.** 1995. Antibody-dependent complement-mediated cytotoxicity in sera from patients with HIV-1 infection is controlled by CD55 and CD59. *J Clin Invest* **96**:1520–1526.

105. **Zhou ZH, Wild T, Xiong Y, Sylvers P, Zhang Y, Zhang L, Wahl L, Wahl SM, Kozlowski S, Notkins AL.** 2013. Polyreactive Antibodies Plus Complement Enhance the Phagocytosis of Cells Made Apoptotic by UV-Light or HIV. *Sci Rep* **3**:2271. doi:10.1038/srep02271.

106. **Willey S, Aasa-Chapman MM, O'Farrell S, Pellegrino P, Williams I, Weiss RA, Neil SJ.** 2011. Extensive complement-dependent enhancement of HIV-1 by autologous non-neutralising antibodies at early stages of infection. *Retrovirology* **8**:16. doi:10.1186/1742-4690-8-16.

107. **Stoiber H, Banki Z, Wilflingseder D, Dierich MP.** 2008. Complement-HIV interactions during all steps of viral pathogenesis. *Vaccine* **26**:3046–3054.

108. **Huber G, Banki Z, Lengauer S, Stoiber H.** 2011. Emerging role for complement in HIV infection. *Curr Opin HIV AIDS* **6**:419–426.

109. **Jayasekera JP, Moseman EA, Carroll MC.** 2007. Natural antibody and complement mediate neutralization of influenza virus in the absence of prior immunity. *J Virol* **81**:3487–3494.

110. **Carroll MC.** 2004. The complement system in regulation of adaptive immunity. *Nat Immunol* **5**:981–986.

111. **Stager S, Alexander J, Kirby AC, Botto M, Rooijen NV, Smith DF, Brombacher F, Kaye PM.** 2003. Natural antibodies and complement are endogenous adjuvants for vaccine-induced CD8+ T-cell responses. *Nat Med* **9**:1287–1292.

112. **Lindorfer MA, Hahn CS, Foley PL, Taylor RP.** 2001. Heteropolymer-mediated clearance of immune complexes via erythrocyte CR1: mechanisms and applications. *Immunol Rev* **183**:10–24.

113. **Nelson RA Jr.** 1953. The immune-adherence phenomenon; an immunologically specific reaction between microorganisms and erythrocytes leading to enhanced phagocytosis. *Science* **118**:733–737.

114. **Ram S, Lewis LA, Rice PA.** 2010. Infections of people with complement deficiencies and patients who have undergone splenectomy. *Clin Microbiol Rev* **23**:740–780.

115. **Amir J, Scott MG, Nahm MH, Granoff DM.** 1990. Bactericidal and opsonic activity of IgG1 and IgG2 anticapsular antibodies to *Haemophilus influenzae* type b. *J Infect Dis* **162**:163–171.

116. **Frasch CE, Borrow R, Donnelly J.** 2009. Bactericidal antibody is the immunologic surrogate of protection against meningococcal disease. *Vaccine* **27**(Suppl 2):B112–B116.

117. **Welsch JA, Moe GR, Rossi R, Adu-Bobie J, Rappuoli R, Granoff DM.** 2003. Antibody to genome-derived neisserial antigen 2132, a Neisseria meningitidis candidate vaccine, confers protection against bacteremia in the absence of complement-mediated bactericidal activity. *J Infect Dis* **188**:1730–1740.

118. **Plested JS, Welsch JA, Granoff DM.** 2009. Ex vivo model of meningococcal bacteremia using human blood for measuring vaccine-induced serum passive protective activity. *Clin Vaccine Immunol* **16**:785–791.

119. **Granoff DM.** 2009. Relative importance of complement-mediated bactericidal and opsonic activity for protection against meningococcal disease. *Vaccine* **27**(Suppl 2):B117–B125.

120. **Horwitz MA, Silverstein SC.** 1981. Interaction of the Legionnaires' disease bacterium (Legionella pneumophila) with human phagocytes. I. *L. pneumophila* resists killing by polymorphonuclear leukocytes, antibody, and complement. *J Exp Med* **153**:386–397.

121. **Lindow JC, Fimlaid KA, Bunn JY, Kirkpatrick BD.** 2011. Antibodies in action: role of human opsonins in killing *Salmonella enterica* serovar Typhi. *Infect Immun* **79**:3188–3194.

122. **Cheng SC, Sprong T, Joosten LA, van der Meer JW, Kullberg BJ, Hube B, Schejbel L, Garred P, van Deuren M, Netea MG.** 2012. Complement plays a central role in *Candida albicans*-induced cytokine production by human PBMCs. *Eur J Immunol* **42**:993–1004.

123. **Han Y, Kozel TR, Zhang MX, MacGill RS, Carroll MC, Cutler JE.** 2001. Complement is essential for protection by an IgM and an IgG3 monoclonal antibody against experimental, hematogenously disseminated candidiasis. *J Immunol* **167**:1550–1557.

124. **Zaragoza O, Casadevall A.** 2006. Monoclonal antibodies can affect complement deposition on the capsule of the pathogenic fungus *Cryptococcus neoformans* by both classical pathway activation and steric hindrance. *Cell Microbiol* **8**:1862–1876.

125. **Zhong Z, Pirofski LA.** 1998. Antifungal activity of a human antiglucuronoxylomannan antibody. *Clin Diagn Lab Immunol* **5:**58–64.

126. **Taborda CP, Casadevall A.** 2002. CR3 (CD11b/CD18) and CR4 (CD11c/CD18) are involved in complement-independent antibody-mediated phagocytosis of *Cryptococcus neoformans. Immunity* **16:**791–802.

127. **Ayi K, Turrini F, Piga A, Arese P.** 2004. Enhanced phagocytosis of ring-parasitized mutant erythrocytes: a common mechanism that may explain protection against falciparum malaria in sickle trait and beta-thalassemia trait. *Blood* **104:**3364–3371.

128. **Luzzi GA, Merry AH, Newbold CI, Marsh K, Pasvol G.** 1991. Protection by alpha-thalassaemia against *Plasmodium falciparum* malaria: modified surface antigen expression rather than impaired growth or cytoadherence. *Immunol Lett* **30:**233–240.

129. **Yuthavong Y, Bunyaratvej A, Kamchonwongpaisan S.** 1990. Increased susceptibility of malaria-infected variant erythrocytes to the mononuclear phagocyte system. *Blood Cells* **16:**591–597.

130. **Cappadoro M, Giribaldi G, O'Brien E, Turrini F, Mannu F, Ulliers D, Simula G, Luzzatto L, Arese P.** 1998. Early phagocytosis of glucose-6-phosphate dehydrogenase (G6PD)-deficient erythrocytes parasitized by *Plasmodium falciparum* may explain malaria protection in G6PD deficiency. *Blood* **92:**2527–2534.

131. **Kumaratilake LM, Ferrante A, Jaeger T, Morris-Jones SD.** 1997. The role of complement, antibody, and tumor necrosis factor alpha in the killing of *Plasmodium falciparum* by the monocytic cell line THP-1. *Infect Immun* **65:**5342–5345.

132. **Salmon D, Vilde JL, Andrieu B, Simonovic R, Lebras J.** 1986. Role of immune serum and complement in stimulation of the metabolic burst of human neutrophils by *Plasmodium falciparum. Infect Immun* **51:**801–806.

133. **Pang XL, Horii T.** 1998. Complement-mediated killing of *Plasmodium falciparum* erythrocytic schizont with antibodies to the recombinant serine repeat antigen (SERA). *Vaccine* **16:**1299–1305.

134. **Healer J, McGuinness D, Hopcroft P, Haley S, Carter R, Riley E.** 1997. Complement-mediated lysis of *Plasmodium falciparum* gametes by malaria-immune human sera is associated with antibodies to the gamete surface antigen Pfs230. *Infect Immun* **65:**3017–3023.

135. **Read D, Lensen AH, Begarnie S, Haley S, Raza A, Carter R.** 1994. Transmission-blocking antibodies against multiple, non-variant target epitopes of the *Plasmodium falciparum* gamete surface antigen Pfs230 are all complement-fixing. *Parasite Immunol* **16:**511–519.

136. **Rener J, Graves PM, Carter R, Williams JL, Burkot TR.** 1983. Target antigens of transmission-blocking immunity on gametes of *Plasmodium falciparum. J Exp Med* **158:**976–981.

137. **Roeffen W, Geeraedts F, Eling W, Beckers P, Wizel B, Kumar N, Lensen T, Sauerwein R.** 1995. Transmission blockade of *Plasmodium falciparum* malaria by anti-Pfs230-specific antibodies is isotype dependent. *Infect Immun* **63:**467–471.

138. **Macaskill JA, Holmes PH, Whitelaw DD, McConnell I, Jennings FW, Urquhart GM.** 1980. Immunological clearance of 75Se-labelled Trypanosoma brucei in mice. II. Mechanisms in immune animals. *Immunology* **40:**629–635.

139. **Pan W, Ogunremi O, Wei G, Shi M, Tabel H.** 2006. CR3 (CD11b/CD18) is the major macrophage receptor for IgM antibody-mediated phagocytosis of African trypanosomes: diverse effect on subsequent synthesis of tumor necrosis factor alpha and nitric oxide. *Microbes Infect* **8:**1209–1218.

140. **Owuor BO, Odhiambo CO, Otieno WO, Adhiambo C, Makawiti DW, Stoute JA.** 2008. Reduced immune complex binding capacity and increased complement susceptibility of red cells from children with severe malaria-associated anemia. *Mol Med* **14:**89–97.

141. **Patel SN, Berghout J, Lovegrove FE, Ayi K, Conroy A, Serghides L, Min-oo G, Gowda DC, Sarma JV, Rittirsch D, Ward PA, Liles WC, Gros P, Kain KC.** 2008. C5 deficiency and C5a or C5aR blockade protects against cerebral malaria. *J Exp Med* **205:**1133–1143.

142. **Farrell HE, Shellam GR.** 1991. Protection against murine cytomegalovirus infection by passive transfer of neutralizing and non-neutralizing monoclonal antibodies. *J Gen Virol* **72**(Pt 1):149–156.

143. **Horton RE, Vidarsson G.** 2013. Antibodies and their receptors: different potential roles in mucosal defense. *Front Immunol* **4:**200. doi:10.3389/fimmu.2013.00200.

144. **Takai T.** 2002. Roles of Fc receptors in autoimmunity. *Nat Rev Immunol* **2:**580–592.

145. **Clark MR, Clarkson SB, Ory PA, Stollman N, Goldstein IM.** 1989. Molecular basis for a polymorphism involving Fc receptor II on human monocytes. *J Immunol* **143:**1731–1734.

146. **Warmerdam PA, van de Winkel JG, Vlug A, Westerdaal NA, Capel PJ.** 1991. A single amino acid in the second Ig-like domain of the human

Fc gamma receptor II is critical for human IgG2 binding. *J Immunol* **147:**1338–1343.

147. **Ravetch JV, Perussia B.** 1989. Alternative membrane forms of Fc gamma RIII(CD16) on human natural killer cells and neutrophils. Cell type-specific expression of two genes that differ in single nucleotide substitutions. *J Exp Med* **170:**481–497.

148. **Ory PA, Goldstein IM, Kwoh EE, Clarkson SB.** 1989. Characterization of polymorphic forms of Fc receptor III on human neutrophils. *J Clin Invest* **83:**1676–1681.

149. **Ory PA, Clark MR, Kwoh EE, Clarkson SB, Goldstein IM.** 1989. Sequences of complementary DNAs that encode the NA1 and NA2 forms of Fc receptor III on human neutrophils. *J Clin Invest* **84:**1688–1691.

150. **Bruhns P, Iannascoli B, England P, Mancardi DA, Fernandez N, Jorieux S, Daeron M.** 2009. Specificity and affinity of human Fcgamma receptors and their polymorphic variants for human IgG subclasses. *Blood* **113:**3716–3725.

151. **Wiener E, Jolliffe VM, Scott HC, Kumpel BM, Thompson KM, Melamed MD, Hughes-Jones NC.** 1988. Differences between the activities of human monoclonal IgG1 and IgG3 anti-D antibodies of the Rh blood group system in their abilities to mediate effector functions of monocytes. *Immunology* **65:**159–163.

152. **Shields RL, Lai J, Keck R, O'Connell LY, Hong K, Meng YG, Weikert SH, Presta LG.** 2002. Lack of fucose on human IgG1 N-linked oligosaccharide improves binding to human Fcgamma RIII and antibody-dependent cellular toxicity. *J Biol Chem* **277:**26733–26740.

153. **Forthal DN, Gach JS, Landucci G, Jez J, Strasser R, Kunert R, Steinkellner H.** 2010. Fc-glycosylation influences Fcgamma receptor binding and cell-mediated anti-HIV activity of monoclonal antibody 2G12. *J Immunol* **185:**6876–6882.

154. **Lux A, Nimmerjahn F.** 2011. Impact of differential glycosylation on IgG activity. *Adv Exp Med Biol* **780:**113–124.

155. **Moldt B, Shibata-Koyama M, Rakasz EG, Schultz N, Kanda Y, Dunlop DC, Finstad SL, Jin C, Landucci G, Alpert MD, Dugast AS, Parren PW, Nimmerjahn F, Evans DT, Alter G, Forthal DN, Schmitz JE, Iida S, Poignard P, Watkins DI, Hessell AJ, Burton DR.** 2012. A nonfucosylated variant of the anti-HIV-1 monoclonal antibody b12 has enhanced FcgammaRIIIa-mediated antiviral activity in vitro but does not improve protection against mucosal SHIV challenge in macaques. *J Virol* **86:**6189–6196.

156. **Forthal DN, Moog C.** 2009. Fc receptor-mediated antiviral antibodies. *Curr Opin HIV AIDS* **4:**388–393.

157. **Lyerly HK, Reed DL, Matthews TJ, Langlois AJ, Ahearne PA, Petteway SR Jr, Weinhold KJ.** 1987. Anti-GP 120 antibodies from HIV seropositive individuals mediate broadly reactive anti-HIV ADCC. *AIDS Res Hum Retroviruses* **3:**409–422.

158. **Torben W, Ahmad G, Zhang W, Nash S, Le L, Karmakar S, Siddiqui AA.** 2012. Role of antibody dependent cell mediated cytotoxicity (ADCC) in Sm-p80-mediated protection against Schistosoma mansoni. *Vaccine* **30:**6753–6758.

159. **Bouharoun-Tayoun H, Oeuvray C, Lunel F, Druilhe P.** 1995. Mechanisms underlying the monocyte-mediated antibody-dependent killing of *Plasmodium falciparum* asexual blood stages. *J Exp Med* **182:**409–418.

160. **Forthal DN, Landucci G, Daar ES.** 2001. Antibody from patients with acute human immunodeficiency virus (HIV) infection inhibits primary strains of HIV type 1 in the presence of natural-killer effector cells. *J Virol* **75:**6953–6961.

161. **Weber S, Tian H, van Rooijen N, Pirofski LA.** 2012. A serotype 3 pneumococcal capsular polysaccharide-specific monoclonal antibody requires Fcgamma receptor III and macrophages to mediate protection against pneumococcal pneumonia in mice. *Infect Immun* **80:**1314–1322.

162. **Sun D, Raisley B, Langer M, Iyer JK, Vedham V, Ballard JL, James JA, Metcalf J, Coggeshall KM.** 2012. Anti-peptidoglycan antibodies and Fcgamma receptors are the key mediators of inflammation in Gram-positive sepsis. *J Immunol* **189:**2423–2431.

163. **Song X, Tanaka S, Cox D, Lee SC.** 2004. Fcgamma receptor signaling in primary human microglia: differential roles of PI-3K and Ras/ERK MAPK pathways in phagocytosis and chemokine induction. *J Leukoc Biol* **75:**1147–1155.

164. **Porcherie A, Mathieu C, Peronet R, Schneider E, Claver J, Commere PH, Kiefer-Biasizzo H, Karasuyama H, Milon G, Dy M, Kinet JP, Louis J, Blank U, Mecheri S.** 2011. Critical role of the neutrophil-associated high-affinity receptor for IgE in the pathogenesis of experimental cerebral malaria. *J Exp Med* **208:**2225–2236.

165. **Forthal DN, Landucci G, Phan TB, Becerra J.** 2005. Interactions between natural killer cells and antibody Fc result in enhanced antibody neutralization of human immunodeficiency virus type 1. *J Virol* **79:**2042–2049.

166. **Brown BK, Wieczorek L, Kijak G, Lombardi K, Currier J, Wesberry M, Kappes JC, Ngauy V, Marovich M, Michael N, Ochsenbauer C, Montefiori DC, Polonis VR.** 2012. The role of

natural killer (NK) cells and NK cell receptor polymorphisms in the assessment of HIV-1 neutralization. *PLoS One* **7:**e29454. doi:10.1371/journal.pone.0029454.

167. **Holl V, Peressin M, Decoville T, Schmidt S, Zolla-Pazner S, Aubertin AM, Moog C.** 2006. Nonneutralizing antibodies are able to inhibit human immunodeficiency virus type 1 replication in macrophages and immature dendritic cells. *J Virol* **80:**6177–6181.

168. **Holl V, Hemmerter S, Burrer R, Schmidt S, Bohbot A, Aubertin AM, Moog C.** 2004. Involvement of Fc gamma RI (CD64) in the mechanism of HIV-1 inhibition by polyclonal IgG purified from infected patients in cultured monocyte-derived macrophages. *J Immunol* **173:**6274–6283.

169. **Anderson DR, Grillo-Lopez A, Varns C, Chambers KS, Hanna N.** 1997. Targeted anticancer therapy using rituximab, a chimaeric anti-CD20 antibody (IDEC-C2B8) in the treatment of non-Hodgkin's B-cell lymphoma. *Biochem Soc Trans* **25:**705–708.

170. **Sliwkowski MX, Lofgren JA, Lewis GD, Hotaling TE, Fendly BM, Fox JA.** 1999. Nonclinical studies addressing the mechanism of action of trastuzumab (Herceptin). *Semin Oncol* **26:**60–70.

171. **Clynes RA, Towers TL, Presta LG, Ravetch JV.** 2000. Inhibitory Fc receptors modulate in vivo cytotoxicity against tumor targets. *Nat Med* **6:**443–446.

172. **Shore SL, Nahmias AJ, Starr SE, Wood PA, McFarlin DE.** 1974. Detection of cell-dependent cytotoxic antibody to cells infected with herpes simplex virus. *Nature* **251:**350–352.

173. **Balachandran N, Bacchetti S, Rawls WE.** 1982. Protection against lethal challenge of BALB/c mice by passive transfer of monoclonal antibodies to five glycoproteins of herpes simplex virus type 2. *Infect Immun* **37:**1132–1137.

174. **Gorander S, Harandi AM, Lindqvist M, Bergstrom T, Liljeqvist JA.** 2012. Glycoprotein G of herpes simplex virus 2 as a novel vaccine antigen for immunity to genital and neurological disease. *J Virol* **86:**7544–7553.

175. **Chu CF, Meador MG, Young CG, Strasser JE, Bourne N, Milligan GN.** 2008. Antibody-mediated protection against genital herpes simplex virus type 2 disease in mice by Fc gamma receptor-dependent and -independent mechanisms. *J Reprod Immunol* **78:**58–67.

176. **Jegerlehner A, Schmitz N, Storni T, Bachmann MF.** 2004. Influenza A vaccine based on the extracellular domain of M2: weak protection mediated via antibody-dependent NK cell activity. *J Immunol* **172:**5598–5605.

177. **Forthal D, Hope TJ, Alter G.** 2013. New paradigms for functional HIV-specific non-neutralizing antibodies. *Curr Opin HIV AIDS* **8:**392–400.

178. **Lowell GH, Smith LF, Artenstein MS, Nash GS, MacDermott RP Jr.** 1979. Antibody-dependent cell-mediated antibacterial activity of human mononuclear cells. I. K lymphocytes and monocytes are effective against meningococci in cooperation with human imune sera. *J Exp Med* **150:**127–137.

179. **Lowell GH, MacDermott RP, Summers PL, Reeder AA, Bertovich MJ, Formal SB.** 1980. Antibody-dependent cell-mediated antibacterial activity: K lymphocytes, monocytes, and granulocytes are effective against shigella. *J Immunol* **125:**2778–2784.

180. **Tagliabue A, Nencioni L, Villa L, Keren DF, Lowell GH, Boraschi D.** 1983. Antibody-dependent cell-mediated antibacterial activity of intestinal lymphocytes with secretory IgA. *Nature* **306:**184–186.

181. **Tagliabue A, Boraschi D, Villa L, Keren DF, Lowell GH, Rappuoli R, Nencioni L.** 1984. IgA-dependent cell-mediated activity against enteropathogenic bacteria: distribution, specificity, and characterization of the effector cells. *J Immunol* **133:**988–992.

182. **Sestini P, Nencioni L, Villa L, Boraschi D, Tagliabue A.** 1988. IgA-driven antibacterial activity against Streptococcus pneumoniae by mouse lung lymphocytes. *Am Rev Respir Dis* **137:**138–143.

183. **Messick JB, Rikihisa Y.** 1992. Presence of parasite antigen on the surface of P388D1 cells infected with *Ehrlichia risticii*. *Infect Immun* **60:**3079–3086.

184. **Koster FT, Kirkpatrick TL, Rowatt JD, Baca OG.** 1984. Antibody-dependent cellular cytotoxicity of Coxiella burnetii-infected J774 macrophage target cells. *Infect Immun* **43:**253–256.

185. **Galdiero F, Romano Carratelli C, Nuzzo I, Folgore A.** 1985. Cytotoxic antibody dependent cells in mice experimentally infected with *Brucella abortus*. *Microbiologica* **8:**217–224.

186. **Shannon JG, Cockrell DC, Takahashi K, Stahl GL, Heinzen RA.** 2009. Antibody-mediated immunity to the obligate intracellular bacterial pathogen Coxiella burnetii is Fc receptor- and complement-independent. *BMC Immunol* **10:**26. doi:10.1186/1471-2172-10-26.

187. **Kazura JW.** 1981. Host defense mechanisms against nematode parasites: destruction of newborn *Trichinella spiralis* larvae by human antibodies and granulocytes. *J Infect Dis* **143:**712–718.

188. Venturiello SM, Giambartolomei GH, Costantino SN. 1993. Immune killing of newborn Trichinella larvae by human leucocytes. *Parasite Immunol* **15**:559–564.

189. Gounni AS, Lamkhioued B, Ochiai K, Tanaka Y, Delaporte E, Capron A, Kinet JP, Capron M. 1994. High-affinity IgE receptor on eosinophils is involved in defence against parasites. *Nature* **367**:183–186.

190. Capron M, Capron A. 1994. Immunoglobulin E and effector cells in schistosomiasis. *Science* **264**:1876–1877.

191. Zhou S, Liu S, Song G, Xu Y, Sun W. 2000. Protective immunity induced by the full-length cDNA encoding paramyosin of Chinese *Schistosoma japonicum*. *Vaccine* **18**:3196–3204.

192. Capron A. 1998. Schistosomiasis: forty years' war on the worm. *Parasitol Today* **14**:379–384.

193. Joseph M, Auriault C, Capron A, Vorng H, Viens P. 1983. A new function for platelets: IgE-dependent killing of schistosomes. *Nature* **303**:810–812.

194. Khalife J, Capron M, Capron A, Grzych JM, Butterworth AE, Dunne DW, Ouma JH. 1986. Immunity in human schistosomiasis mansoni. Regulation of protective immune mechanisms by IgM blocking antibodies. *J Exp Med* **164**:1626–1640.

195. Auriault C, Gras-Masse H, Pierce RJ, Butterworth AE, Wolowczuk I, Capron M, Ouma JH, Balloul JM, Khalife J, Neyrinck JL. 1990. Antibody response of *Schistosoma mansoni*-infected human subjects to the recombinant P28 glutathione-S-transferase and to synthetic peptides. *J Clin Microbiol* **28**:1918–1924.

196. Demeure CE, Rihet P, Abel L, Ouattara M, Bourgois A, Dessein AJ. 1993. Resistance to *Schistosoma mansoni* in humans: influence of the IgE/IgG4 balance and IgG2 in immunity to reinfection after chemotherapy. *J Infect Dis* **168**:1000–1008.

197. Lawrence RA. 2001. Immunity to filarial nematodes. *Vet Parasitol* **100**:33–44.

198. Haque A, Joseph M, Ouaissi MA, Capron M, Capron A. 1980. IgE antibody-mediated cytotoxicity of rat macrophages against microfilaria of *Dipetalonema citeae* in vitro. *Clin Exp Immunol* **40**:487–495.

199. Weiss N, Tanner M. 1979. Studies on *Dipetalonema viteae* (*Filarioidea*) 3. Antibody-dependent cell-mediated destruction of microfilariae in vivo. *Tropenmed Parasitol* **30**:73–80.

200. Mehta K, Sindhu RK, Subrahmanyam D, Hopper K, Nelson DS, Rao CK. 1981. Antibody-dependent cell-mediated effects in bancroftian filariasis. *Immunology* **43**:117–123.

201. Sim BK, Kwa BH, Mak JW. 1982. Immune responses in human *Brugia malayi* infections:

202. Parab PB, Rajasekariah GR, Chandrashekar R, Alkan SS, Braun DG, Subrahmanyam D. 1988. Characterization of a monoclonal antibody against infective larvae of *Brugia malayi*. *Immunology* **64**:169–174.

203. Gray CA, Lawrence RA. 2002. A role for antibody and Fc receptor in the clearance of *Brugia malayi* microfilariae. *Eur J Immunol* **32**:1114–1120.

204. Albright JW, Stewart MJ, Latham PS, Albright JF. 1994. Antibody-facilitated macrophage killing of *Trypanosoma musculi* is an extracellular process as studied in several variations of an in vitro analytical system. *J Leukoc Biol* **56**:636–643.

205. Townsend J, Duffus WP. 1982. *Trypanosoma theileri*: antibody-dependent killing by purified populations of bovine leucocytes. *Clin Exp Immunol* **48**:289–299.

206. Kierszenbaum F, Hayes MM. 1980. Mechanisms of resistance against experimental *Trypanosoma cruzi* infection. Requirements for cellular destruction of circulating forms of T. cruzi in human and murine in vitro systems. *Immunology* **40**:61–66.

207. Piedrafita D, Parsons JC, Sandeman RM, Wood PR, Estuningsih SE, Partoutomo S, Spithill TW. 2001. Antibody-dependent cell-mediated cytotoxicity to newly excysted juvenile *Fasciola hepatica* in vitro is mediated by reactive nitrogen intermediates. *Parasite Immunol* **23**:473–482.

208. Nolan TJ, Rotman HL, Bhopale VM, Schad GA, Abraham D. 1995. Immunity to a challenge infection of Strongyloides stercoralis third-stage larvae in the jird. *Parasite Immunol* **17**:599–604.

209. Bekhti K, Kazanji M, Pery P. 1992. In vitro interactions between murine neutrophils and *Eimeria falciformis* sporozoites. *Res Immunol* **143**:909–917.

210. Smith PD, Keister DB, Elson CO. 1983. Human host response to Giardia lamblia. II. Antibody-dependent killing in vitro. *Cell Immunol* **82**:308–315.

211. Khusmith S, Druilhe P. 1983. Cooperation between antibodies and monocytes that inhibit in vitro proliferation of *Plasmodium falciparum*. *Infect Immun* **41**:219–223.

212. Jafarshad A, Dziegiel MH, Lundquist R, Nielsen LK, Singh S, Druilhe PL. 2007. A novel antibody-dependent cellular cytotoxicity mechanism involved in defense against malaria requires costimulation of monocytes FcgammaRII and FcgammaRIII. *J Immunol* **178**:3099–3106.

serum dependent cell-mediated destruction of infective larvae in vitro. *Trans R Soc Trop Med Hyg* **76**:362–370.

213. **Forthal DN, Landucci G.** 1998. In vitro reduction of virus infectivity by antibody-dependent cell-mediated immunity. *J Immunol Methods* **220:**129–138.

214. **Forthal DN, Landucci G, Cole KS, Marthas M, Becerra JC, Van Rompay K.** 2006. Rhesus macaque polyclonal and monoclonal antibodies inhibit simian immunodeficiency virus in the presence of human or autologous rhesus effector cells. *J Virol* **80:**9217–9225.

215. **Brunner KT, Hurez D, Mc CR, Benacerraf B.** 1960. Blood clearance of P32-labeled vesicular stomatitis and Newcastle disease viruses by the reticuloendothelial system in mice. *J Immunol* **85:**99–105.

216. **Igarashi T, Brown C, Azadegan A, Haigwood N, Dimitrov D, Martin MA, Shibata R.** 1999. Human immunodeficiency virus type 1 neutralizing antibodies accelerate clearance of cell-free virions from blood plasma. *Nat Med* **5:**211–216.

217. **Kim YB, Bradley SG, Watson DW.** 1967. Ontogeny of the immune response. IV. The role of antigen elimination in the true primary immune response in germ-free, colostrum-deprived piglets. *J Immunol* **99:**320–326.

218. **Glenny AT, Hopkins BE.** 1923. Duration of passive immunity. *J Hyg (Lond)* **22:**208–221.

219. **Fujisawa H.** 2008. Neutrophils play an essential role in cooperation with antibody in both protection against and recovery from pulmonary infection with influenza virus in mice. *J Virol* **82:**2772–2783.

220. **Huber VC, Lynch JM, Bucher DJ, Le J, Metzger DW.** 2001. Fc receptor-mediated phagocytosis makes a significant contribution to clearance of influenza virus infections. *J Immunol* **166:**7381–7388.

221. **Chan KR, Zhang SL, Tan HC, Chan YK, Chow A, Lim AP, Vasudevan SG, Hanson BJ, Ooi EE.** 2011. Ligation of Fc gamma receptor IIB inhibits antibody-dependent enhancement of dengue virus infection. *Proc Natl Acad Sci USA* **108:**12479–12484.

222. **Chung KM, Thompson BS, Fremont DH, Diamond MS.** 2007. Antibody recognition of cell surface-associated NS1 triggers Fc-gamma receptor-mediated phagocytosis and clearance of West Nile Virus-infected cells. *J Virol* **81:**9551–9555.

223. **Hashimoto Y, Moki T, Takizawa T, Shiratsuchi A, Nakanishi Y.** 2007. Evidence for phagocytosis of influenza virus-infected, apoptotic cells by neutrophils and macrophages in mice. *J Immunol* **178:**2448–2457.

224. **Ratcliffe DR, Michl J, Cramer EB.** 1993. Neutrophils do not bind to or phagocytize human immune complexes formed with influenza virus. *Blood* **82:**1639–1646.

225. **Scott CB, Ratcliffe DR, Cramer EB.** 1996. Human monocytes are unable to bind to or phagocytize IgA and IgG immune complexes formed with influenza virus in vitro. *J Immunol* **157:**351–359.

226. **Hellwig SM, van Oirschot HF, Hazenbos WL, van Spriel AB, Mooi FR, van De Winkel JG.** 2001. Targeting to Fcgamma receptors, but not CR3 (CD11b/CD18), increases clearance of *Bordetella pertussis*. *J Infect Dis* **183:**871–879.

227. **Clatworthy MR, Smith KG.** 2004. FcgammaRIIb balances efficient pathogen clearance and the cytokine-mediated consequences of sepsis. *J Exp Med* **199:**717–723.

228. **Mold C, Rodic-Polic B, Du Clos TW.** 2002. Protection from *Streptococcus pneumoniae* infection by C-reactive protein and natural antibody requires complement but not Fc gamma receptors. *J Immunol* **168:**6375–6381.

229. **Yee AM, Phan HM, Zuniga R, Salmon JE, Musher DM.** 2000. Association between FcgammaRIIa-R131 allotype and bacteremic pneumococcal pneumonia. *Clin Infect Dis* **30:**25–28.

230. **Yuan FF, Wong M, Pererva N, Keating J, Davis AR, Bryant JA, Sullivan JS.** 2003. FcgammaRIIA polymorphisms in Streptococcus pneumoniae infection. *Immunol Cell Biol* **81:**192–195.

231. **Rodriguez ME, van der Pol WL, Sanders LA, van de Winkel JG.** 1999. Crucial role of FcgammaRIIa (CD32) in assessment of functional anti-Streptococcus pneumoniae antibody activity in human sera. *J Infect Dis* **179:**423–433.

232. **Bredius RG, Fijen CA, De Haas M, Kuijper EJ, Weening RS, Van de Winkel JG, Out TA.** 1994. Role of neutrophil Fc gamma RIIa (CD32) and Fc gamma RIIIb (CD16) polymorphic forms in phagocytosis of human IgG1- and IgG3-opsonized bacteria and erythrocytes. *Immunology* **83:**624–630.

233. **Fijen CA, Bredius RG, Kuijper EJ, Out TA, De Haas M, De Wit AP, Daha MR, De Winkel JG.** 2000. The role of Fcgamma receptor polymorphisms and C3 in the immune defence against *Neisseria meningitidis* in complement-deficient individuals. *Clin Exp Immunol* **120:**338–345.

234. **Bredius RG, Derkx BH, Fijen CA, de Wit TP, de Haas M, Weening RS, van de Winkel JG, Out TA.** 1994. Fc gamma receptor IIa (CD32) polymorphism in fulminant meningococcal septic shock in children. *J Infect Dis* **170:**848–853.

235. **Platonov AE, Shipulin GA, Vershinina IV, Dankert J, van de Winkel JG, Kuijper EJ.**

1998. Association of human Fc gamma RIIa (CD32) polymorphism with susceptibility to and severity of meningococcal disease. *Clin Infect Dis* **27**:746–750.

236. **Domingo P, Muniz-Diaz E, Baraldes MA, Arilla M, Barquet N, Pericas R, Juarez C, Madoz P, Vazquez G.** 2002. Associations between Fc gamma receptor IIA polymorphisms and the risk and prognosis of meningococcal disease. *Am J Med* **112**:19–25.

237. **Domingo P, Muniz-Diaz E, Baraldes MA, Arilla M, Barquet N, Pericas R, Juarez C, Madoz P, Vazquez G.** 2004. Relevance of genetically determined host factors to the prognosis of meningococcal disease. *Eur J Clin Microbiol Infect Dis* **23**:634–637.

238. **Smith I, Vedeler C, Halstensen A.** 2003. FcgammaRIIa and FcgammaRIIIb polymorphisms were not associated with meningococcal disease in Western Norway. *Epidemiol Infect* **130**:193–199.

239. **Wu Y, Wu W, Wong WM, Ward E, Thrasher AJ, Goldblatt D, Osman M, Digard P, Canaday DH, Gustafsson K.** 2009. Human gamma delta T cells: a lymphoid lineage cell capable of professional phagocytosis. *J Immunol* **183**:5622–5629.

240. **Schlageter AM, Kozel TR.** 1990. Opsonization of *Cryptococcus neoformans* by a family of isotype-switch variant antibodies specific for the capsular polysaccharide. *Infect Immun* **58**:1914–1918.

241. **Sanford JE, Lupan DM, Schlageter AM, Kozel TR.** 1990. Passive immunization against *Cryptococcus neoformans* with an isotype-switch family of monoclonal antibodies reactive with cryptococcal polysaccharide. *Infect Immun* **58**:1919–1923.

242. **Saylor CA, Dadachova E, Casadevall A.** 2010. Murine IgG1 and IgG3 isotype switch variants promote phagocytosis of *Cryptococcus neoformans* through different receptors. *J Immunol* **184**:336–343.

243. **Szymczak WA, Davis MJ, Lundy SK, Dufaud C, Olszewski M, Pirofski LA.** 2013. X-linked immunodeficient mice exhibit enhanced susceptibility to *Cryptococcus neoformans* Infection. *MBio* **4**. doi:10.1128/mBio.00265-13.

244. **Murphy K, Travers P, Walport M.** 2008. The destruction of antibody-coated pathogens via Fc receptors. *In Janeway's Immunobiology*, 7th ed. Garland Science, New York

245. **Celada A, Cruchaud A, Perrin LH.** 1982. Opsonic activity of human immune serum on in vitro phagocytosis of *Plasmodium falciparum* infected red blood cells by monocytes. *Clin Exp Immunol* **47**:635–644.

246. **Chan JA, Howell KB, Reiling L, Ataide R, Mackintosh CL, Fowkes FJ, Petter M, Chesson JM, Langer C, Warimwe GM, Duffy MF, Rogerson SJ, Bull PC, Cowman AF, Marsh K, Beeson JG.** 2012. Targets of antibodies against Plasmodium falciparum-infected erythrocytes in malaria immunity. *J Clin Invest* **122**:3227–3238.

247. **Tsuboi N, Asano K, Lauterbach M, Mayadas TN.** 2008. Human neutrophil Fcgamma receptors initiate and play specialized nonredundant roles in antibody-mediated inflammatory diseases. *Immunity* **28**:833–846.

248. **Lendvai N, Qu XW, Hsueh W, Casadevall A.** 2000. Mechanism for the isotype dependence of antibody-mediated toxicity in *Cryptococcus neoformans*-infected mice. *J Immunol* **164**:4367–4374.

249. **Alonso A, Bayon Y, Crespo MS.** 1996. The expression of cytokine-induced neutrophil chemoattractants (CINC-1 and CINC-2) in rat peritoneal macrophages is triggered by Fc gamma receptor activation: study of the signaling mechanism. *Eur J Immunol* **26**:2165–2171.

250. **Fernandez N, Renedo M, Sanchez Crespo M.** 2002. FcgammaR receptors activate MAP kinase and up-regulate the cyclooxygenase pathway without increasing arachidonic acid release in monocytic cells. *Eur J Immunol* **32**:383–392.

251. **Abrahams VM, Cambridge G, Lydyard PM, Edwards JC.** 2000. Induction of tumor necrosis factor alpha production by adhered human monocytes: a key role for Fcgamma receptor type IIIa in rheumatoid arthritis. *Arthritis Rheum* **43**:608–616.

252. **Fernandez N, Renedo M, Garcia-Rodriguez C, Sanchez Crespo M.** 2002. Activation of monocytic cells through Fc gamma receptors induces the expression of macrophage-inflammatory protein (MIP)-1 alpha, MIP-1 beta, and RANTES. *J Immunol* **169**:3321–3328.

253. **Zhang Y, Zhou Y, Yang Q, Mu C, Duan E, Chen J, Yang M, Xia P, Cui B.** 2012. Ligation of Fc gamma receptor IIB enhances levels of antiviral cytokine in response to PRRSV infection in vitro. *Vet Microbiol* **160**:473–480.

254. **Gallo P, Goncalves R, Mosser DM.** 2010. The influence of IgG density and macrophage Fc (gamma) receptor cross-linking on phagocytosis and IL-10 production. *Immunol Lett* **133**:70–77.

255. **Parcina M, Wendt C, Goet F, Zawatzky R, Zahringer U, Heeg K, Bekeredjian-Ding I.** 2008. *Staphylococcus aureus*-induced plasmacytoid dendritic cell activation is based on an IgG-mediated memory response. *J Immunol* **181**:3823–3833.

256. **Jancar S, Sanchez Crespo M.** 2005. Immune complex-mediated tissue injury: a multistep paradigm. *Trends Immunol* **26**:48–55.

257. Bunk S, Sigel S, Metzdorf D, Sharif O, Triantafilou K, Triantafilou M, Hartung T, Knapp S, von Aulock S. 2010. Internalization and coreceptor expression are critical for TLR2-mediated recognition of lipoteichoic acid in human peripheral blood. *J Immunol* **185:**3708–3717.

258. Lovgren T, Eloranta ML, Kastner B, Wahren-Herlenius M, Alm GV, Ronnblom L. 2006. Induction of interferon-alpha by immune complexes or liposomes containing systemic lupus erythematosus autoantigen- and Sjogren's syndrome autoantigen-associated RNA. *Arthritis Rheum* **54:**1917–1927.

259. Boule MW, Broughton C, Mackay F, Akira S, Marshak-Rothstein A, Rifkin IR. 2004. Toll-like receptor 9-dependent and -independent dendritic cell activation by chromatin-immunoglobulin G complexes. *J Exp Med* **199:**1631–1640.

260. Means TK, Latz E, Hayashi F, Murali MR, Golenbock DT, Luster AD. 2005. Human lupus autoantibody-DNA complexes activate DCs through cooperation of CD32 and TLR9. *J Clin Invest* **115:**407–417.

261. Ierino FL, Powell MS, McKenzie IF, Hogarth PM. 1993. Recombinant soluble human Fc gamma RII: production, characterization, and inhibition of the Arthus reaction. *J Exp Med* **178:**1617–1628.

262. Sylvestre DL, Ravetch JV. 1994. Fc receptors initiate the Arthus reaction: redefining the inflammatory cascade. *Science* **265:**1095–1098.

263. Hogarth PM, Pietersz GA. 2012. Fc receptor-targeted therapies for the treatment of inflammation, cancer and beyond. *Nat Rev Drug Discov* **11:**311–331.

264. Ravetch JV, Lanier LL. 2000. Immune inhibitory receptors. *Science* **290:**84–89.

265. Pearse RN, Kawabe T, Bolland S, Guinamard R, Kurosaki T, Ravetch JV. 1999. SHIP recruitment attenuates Fc gamma RIIB-induced B cell apoptosis. *Immunity* **10:**753–760.

266. Nimmerjahn F, Ravetch JV. 2008. Fcgamma receptors as regulators of immune responses. *Nat Rev Immunol* **8:**34–47.

267. Regnault A, Lankar D, Lacabanne V, Rodriguez A, Thery C, Rescigno M, Saito T, Verbeek S, Bonnerot C, Ricciardi-Castagnoli P, Amigorena S. 1999. Fcgamma receptor-mediated induction of dendritic cell maturation and major histocompatibility complex class I-restricted antigen presentation after immune complex internalization. *J Exp Med* **189:**371–380.

268. DiScipio RG, Daffern PJ, Jagels MA, Broide DH, Sriramarao P. 1999. A comparison of C3a and C5a-mediated stable adhesion of rolling eosinophils in postcapillary venules and transendothelial migration in vitro and in vivo. *J Immunol* **162:**1127–1136.

269. Godau J, Heller T, Hawlisch H, Trappe M, Howells E, Best J, Zwirner J, Verbeek JS, Hogarth PM, Gerard C, Van Rooijen N, Klos A, Gessner JE, Kohl J. 2004. C5a initiates the inflammatory cascade in immune complex peritonitis. *J Immunol* **173:**3437–3445.

270. Fernandez N, Renedo M, Alonso S, Crespo MS. 2003. Release of arachidonic acid by stimulation of opsonic receptors in human monocytes: the FcgammaR and the complement receptor 3 pathways. *J Biol Chem* **278:** 52179–52187.

271. Casadevall A, Scharff MD. 1994. Serum therapy revisited: animal models of infection and development of passive antibody therapy. *Antimicrob Agents Chemother* **38:**1695–1702.

Antibody Structure

3

ROBYN L. STANFIELD[1] and IAN A. WILSON[1,2]

Currently, well over 1,000 antibody Fab or Fab variable (Fv) structures have been determined and deposited in the Protein Data Bank (www.rcsb.org). Many of these antibodies target proteins found on or secreted by infectious agents, such as viruses or bacteria. At first glance, one antibody Fab fragment may look just like another, but closer inspection shows that these workhorses of the adaptive immune system can capitalize on novel structural features to tailor their binding sites to accommodate targets of diverse shapes, sizes, and properties. Recent crystallographic and electron microscopy studies of human antibodies against human immunodeficiency virus type 1 (HIV-1) and influenza viruses have revealed some unusual structural features and modes of antigen recognition that enable these antibodies to effectively and broadly neutralize their rapidly evolving targets. We will focus here on immunoglobulin G (IgG) antibodies, as these are the best characterized from a structural perspective.

[1]Department of Integrative Structural and Computational Biology, The Scripps Research Institute, La Jolla, CA 92037; [2]Skaggs Institute for Chemical Biology, The Scripps Research Institute, La Jolla, CA 92037.

Antibodies for Infectious Diseases
Edited by James E. Crowe, Jr., Diana Boraschi, and Rino Rappuoli
© 2015 American Society for Microbiology, Washington, DC
doi:10.1128/microbiolspec.AID-0012-2013

BASICS OF ANTIBODY STRUCTURE

A typical mammalian IgG antibody has two copies each of two protein chains: the light chain (~24 kDa) and the heavy chain (~55 kDa). These chains pair in such a way as to create three structural domains, two Fabs and one Fc, that are linked by a flexible "hinge" region and can be readily cleaved into Fab and Fc fragments by proteases. The Fc fragment is a heavy chain dimer of the constant heavy 2 (C_H2) and constant heavy 3 (C_H3) segments, and the Fab fragment is a mixed light-heavy chain dimer of variable light (V_L)-constant light (C_L) paired with variable heavy (V_H)-constant heavy 1 (C_H1) segments. Each of the eight component units of an IgG adopts an immunoglobulin protein fold. The variable regions of the heavy and light chains are created by a genetic recombination event called V(D)J (heavy chain) or VJ (light chain) recombination, where all possible combinations of numerous different V, D, and J gene segments can theoretically lead to around one million different antibody sequence combinations. In fact, this number is much, much larger, as nucleotide additions and deletions at the V-D, D-J, and V-J junctions can create extensive diversity in length and sequence, and somatic mutations in response to antigen challenge can further alter the sequence and structure of each antibody. Further diversity can arise from posttranslational modifications, such as glycosylation and tyrosine sulfation. The Fab fragment recognizes antigen using some or all of its six complementarity-determining region (CDR) loops (three from each light and heavy chain), which extend out from the structurally conserved framework region and make the vast majority of contacts to antigen. Of these six CDRs (L1, L2, L3, H1, H2, and H3), CDR H3 is the most variable in length, sequence, and structure. This loop is formed at the V-D-J junction, and extra nucleotides inserted or deleted between V-D and D-J account for its extremely high level of variability. Recent 454 deep sequencing studies have shown that a single adult has anywhere from 3 to 9 million unique CDR H3 sequences in circulation (1).

Since the first X-ray crystal structures of Fab fragments were determined in the early 1970s (2, 3), over a thousand structures of intact IgGs, Fabs, and Fvs have been determined and deposited in the Protein Data Bank (4). Early studies of the different antibody structures noted many common features. For example, CDR loops L1, L2, L3, H1, and H2 usually are found in a "canonical" conformation, which can be predicted from conserved sequence motifs (5, 6, 7, 8). Other analyses of antibody-antigen complexes showed that, while some antibodies use all six CDR loops to recognize antigen, CDRs H3, H2, and L3 usually make the largest contributions to the interface with antigen and CDR L2 usually makes the smallest (9). In fact, CDR L2 often makes no contact with small ligands, although there are of course a few exceptions to these generalizations. As would be expected, Fabs recognizing large protein antigens normally have the largest combining sites (around 700 to 900 Å^2 of buried surface on the Fab) and often, but not always, use all 6 CDR loops, while Fabs interacting with small haptens or peptides have smaller combining sites (~160 to 300 Å^2 for haptens and 470 to 560 Å^2 for peptides) and are more likely to use a smaller number of CDR loops (10). Antigen size also correlates with trends in the shape of the combining site. For example, large antigens, such as proteins, often interact with a largely flat, undulating combining site, while peptides and small antigens usually bind into grooves or pocket-shaped combining sites (10, 11). Analyses of Fab and Fv fragments in their unliganded and antigen-bound forms have shown that, while some antibody combining sites are "preformed" and do not undergo conformational changes upon binding antigen, others show varying degrees of flexibility, ranging from small shifts in CDR position, to large conformational rearrangements of the CDR loops, to shifts in the relative positions and orientations of the V_L and V_H domains, and sometimes combinations of all of these (12, 13). However, as phage-display technology (14, 15), interrogation of memory B cells (16, 17), and improved hybridoma techniques (18) have been developed to allow for the isolation and structure determination of a large number of interesting antibodies, some unusual structural features have been revealed, especially in human antibodies against viruses, such as HIV-1 and influenza.

CDR H3: SIZE AND SUBTERFUGE

It has long been known that CDR H3 is the most variable of all the CDR loops in length, sequence, and structure. However, for many years, the majority of antibody structures determined were from mice, whose antibodies have inherently shorter CDR H3 regions than those of humans (19), with an average H3 length (H3 defined with IMGT [international ImMunoGeneTics information system, http://www.imgt.org] boundaries and Kabat numbering H93 to H102; insertions can occur after H100) of around 11 to 12 and observed lengths of 1 to 21. In contrast, human CDR H3 regions have an average length of about 15 residues, and range from 1 to 35 amino acids in length (19). Recent structures of anti-HIV-1 antibodies derived from infected donors have revealed several antibodies with extremely long CDR H3 regions. Two such antibodies are the clonally related PG16 and PG9, which are potent and broadly neutralizing anti-HIV-1 antibodies that recognize the V1/V2 region in gp120 of the trimeric viral envelope protein. PG16 and PG9 differ at just 9 amino acid positions within their 28/30-residue CDR H3 (in the text and in Table 1, we list the H3 length as defined by both Kabat and IMGT boundaries [Kabat/IMGT], with the IMGT length always 2 amino acids longer). In the unliganded PG16 structure, the large CDR H3 hovers above the other CDR loops in a hydrogen-bond-stabilized

subdomain termed a "hammerhead" that has a two-headed, bifurcated loop structure (20, 21) (Fig. 1). The loop conformation is maintained when PG9 is bound to a scaffold-supported gp120 V1/V2 domain (22) (Fig. 1), where the large CDR H3 binds to a V2 β-strand at the base of a crevice formed by two glycan moieties from gp120. The glycan linked to Asn160 is critical for the interaction, and a second glycan at either Asn156 or Asn173 contributes to the binding interface. Another potent and broadly neutralizing HIV-1 antibody that also targets the V1/V2 region is PGT145. This Fab has been structurally characterized in its unliganded form, and its 31/33-residue CDR H3 loop adopts an extremely long β-hairpin finger capped by a type I β-turn that extends about 25 Å above the platform formed by the tips of the other CDR loops (Fig. 1). Keeping in mind that a typical Fab measures about 65 Å along its long axis, this CDR H3 is almost 40% as long as the main body of the Fab itself. It has been noted that long CDR H3 loops are often found in antiviral antibodies (23) and perhaps are necessary to access recessed regions on the viral proteins. This perceived requirement for long CDR H3 regions has long concerned antiviral vaccine developers, but recently, a 454 deep-sequencing study (24) has shown that antibodies with these extremely long H3 CDR loops are found in the naive repertoire, albeit infrequently, with long ($\geq 22/24$) and very long ($\geq 26/28$) H3 loops found in 3.5% and 0.43% of the naive population, respectively. Thus, long CDR H3s are generated during the original V(D)J recombination event, often using the longest D and J genes, in combination with nucleotide additions at the joining junctions (24). Thus, although long CDR H3s could also be created through extensive somatic mutation, antibodies with these loops are likely available for activation in the naive repertoire.

PG9, PG16, and PGT145 also share the unusual posttranslational modification of tyrosine sulfation in their CDR H3 regions (22), with up to 2, 1, and 2 tyrosine residues sulfated in PG9, PG16, and PGT145, respectively. The CDRs are all highly negatively charged, and, in

TABLE 1 CDR lengths and posttranslational modifications of unusual human antibodies

Antibody	Epitope	Length of CDR (residues)[a]:							Modification(s)
		L1 (24–34)	L2 (50–56)	L3 (89–97)	H1 (31–35x)	H2 (50–65)	H3 (95–102; Kabat)	H3 (93–102; IMGT)	
PG9	HIV-1 V1/V2	14	7	10	5	17	28	30	Long H3, tyrosine sulfation
PG16	HIV-1 V1/V2	14	7	10	5	17	28	30	Long H3, tyrosine sulfation, N-linked glycan
PGT128	HIV-1 V3 glycans	9	7	10	7	22	19	21	Long H2, short L1
PGT145	HIV-1 V1/V2	16	7	9	5	19	31	33	Long H3, tyrosine sulfation
2G12	HIV-1 glycan shield	11	7	9	5	17	14	16	Domain-swapped Fab
2D1	Influenza head	13	7	12	7	18	14	16	Unusual 3-residue insert after residue H62; only physically lengthens CDR by 1 residue
CR6261	Influenza HA[b] stem	13	7	12	5	17	12	14	Heavy-chain-only binding
C05	Influenza HA receptor binding site	11	7	9	10	17	24	26	Long H3 dominates binding, long H1 due to unusual 5-residue insert at H27 not accounted for in Kabat CDR definition

[a]CDR lengths are defined using the Kabat boundaries, except for H3, which is defined using both Kabat and IMGT boundaries. Note that C05 has a long H1 due to an unusual insert at H27; the length in the table reflects that insertion.
[b]HA, hemagglutinin.

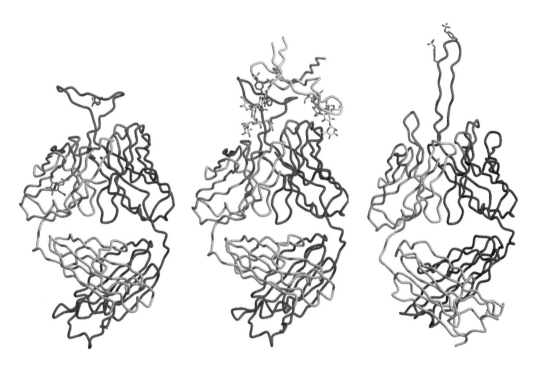

FIGURE 1 Extremely long CDR H3 loops in human anti-HIV-1 antibodies targeting the V1/V2 region of gp120 in the Env trimer. Fab PG16 (left, PDB 3mug) has a large (28/30 residue), structured "hammerhead" CDR H3 (red) with posttranslational modifications of one sulfated tyrosine and one N-linked glycan. PG9 (middle, PDB 3u4e) in complex with the V1/V2 domain (yellow) from HIV-1 gp120 (CAP45 isolate) uses its large CDR H3 to bisect two glycans (shown in yellow ball-and-stick representation) and form a parallel β-sheet interaction with one strand from V1/V2. PG9 has two sulfated tyrosine residues at its tip. Fab PGT145 (right, PDB 3u1s) has the longest CDR H3 (31/33 residues) yet seen in human antibodies. This CDR also has two sulfated tyrosine residues at its tip. For the Cα trace of both Fabs, the CDR loops are colored orange (L1), magenta (L2), green (L3), blue (H1), pink (H2), and red (H3), with light chains in light gray and heavy chains in dark gray. All figures were made with MOLSCRIPT (56) and rendered with Raster3D (57). doi:10.1128/microbiolspec.AID-0012-2013.f1

PG9, the sulfated tyrosines have been shown to specifically interact with residues in its cationic β-strand binding site located in the gp120 V2 region (22). Two other antibodies that target the V1/V2 region, 2909 and CHO4, also have sulfated tyrosines within their highly anionic CDR H3 loops (22, 25, 26). Sulfated tyrosines have also been found in several other HIV-1 neutralizing antibodies (27, 28) against a CD4 receptor-induced epitope, which overlaps the coreceptor binding site. When HIV-1 enters cells, it does so by interacting with two receptors, first CD4 and then a coreceptor that is usually the G protein-coupled receptor CCR5. The CCR5 N terminus contains a number of sulfated tyrosine residues that are thought to interact with gp120, so antibodies with this same posttranslational modification are thought to bind to regions on gp120 that interact with CCR5. Some antibodies to other viral and nonviral targets also contain sulfated tyrosines that arise from cellular processing of tyrosines embedded in a sea of acidic residues (27).

HEAVY CHAIN DOMINATION AND FRAMEWORK CONTACTS

We have discussed the important role CDR H3 can play in antibody-antigen interactions, and it is interesting that jawless vertebrates (the most primitive animals to possess immunoglobulin-based antibodies) have as part of their repertoire heavy-chain-only antibodies called "new antigen receptors" that bind antigen with only a single V_H domain that contains only two CDR loops (H1 and H3) (29, 30). Camels, llamas, and alpacas also have functional heavy-chain-only antibodies that originated from a mutation resulting in loss of the C_H1 domain. The resulting V_H-C_H2-C_H3 heavy chain dimerizes, forming a normal Fc region, but does not associate with the light chain (31, 32, 33). The camelid and shark heavy chain variable regions have structurally converged to have very long CDR H3 regions that often contain noncanonical disulfide bonds that can link H3 to other CDRs or to different parts of the V_H framework region, and several structures have shown that the loop (~H72 to H75) analogous to HV4 in a T-cell receptor can also be used to contact antigen (34, 35). These camelid and shark heavy-chain-only antibodies have inspired extensive research into single domain (V_HH) antibody fragments that are currently in use as drugs and reagents (36).

Since these shark and camel antibodies work perfectly well with only a single V_H domain, it is perhaps not surprising that the epitopes of some conventional light-heavy chain Fabs have a larger contribution from V_H than from V_L. Heavy chain domination of the antibody-antigen interaction is not uncommon with small antigens or peptides; however, it is more unusual with protein antigens, where all six CDR loops are usually used to contact antigen. Recently, some Fabs have been found that use only their V_H domain to contact large, protein antigens. Antibody C05 (37) is a broadly neutralizing influenza antibody that uses its long CDR H3 (24/26 residues) to access the very small, but highly conserved, receptor binding site on the hemagglutinin surface glycoprotein, with minor additional contacts from an unusually long CDR H1, which has a 5-amino-acid insertion at position H27 (rather than the more common 0- or 2-residue insertion at residue H31) (Fig. 2). By using mainly one loop for recognition, the large Fab mimics the mechanism, but not the specific interaction, of the small sialic acid receptors of influenza virus. Two other interesting anti-influenza antibodies, Fab CR6261 (38) and scFv F10 (39), also use only their heavy chain and bind to closely overlapping epitopes on the conserved stalk region of the trimeric hemagglutinin (Fig. 2) in nearly identical fashions, using primarily the H2 CDR loop and contributions from CDR H3, as well as residues from the framework V_H72–75 loop (HV4), in the case of CR6261. These antibodies neutralize virus by preventing a conformational rearrangement necessary for viral fusion. Interestingly, CR6261, F10, and some other related anti-influenza antibodies (40) all use the V_H1–69 germ line gene (41). This germ line gene codes for a CDR H2 with a hydrophobic tip that is used by these antibodies to bind into hydrophobic pockets. Other anti-HIV and anti-influenza antibodies derived from V_H1–69 include at least 9 different CD4-induced anti-HIV-1 antibodies (42) that all have protruding hydrophobic residues at the tip of CDR H2 and anti-HIV antibody D5 that targets a gp41 fusion intermediate (43) and also contacts a hydrophobic pocket on gp41 with its hydrophobic H2 residues.

DISULFIDES IN THE CDRS

While noncanonical disulfide bonds in the CDRs of camels and sharks are common, disulfide bonds within or between human or murine antibody CDR loops are not. Cysteine is coded in one human germ line DH gene, and 1.2% of all human CDR H3 residues have been found to be cysteine (19). With no homologous germ line gene in mice, cysteines in H3 are rarer in that system. Within complete human CDR H3 regions, 3.35% of the CDRs were found to have one cysteine and 5.98% contained two

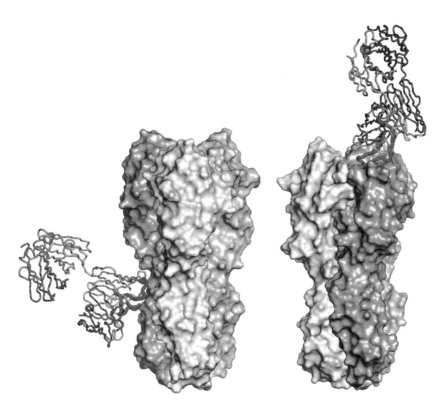

FIGURE 2 Broadly neutralizing Fab CR6261 (left) uses only its heavy chain (dark gray, with blue, pink, and red CDR loops) to recognize the stem region of a hemagglutinin trimer. Fab C05 (right) binds to a conserved region near the receptor binding site, using mainly its large CDR H3 (red), with minor contact from CDR H1 (blue). doi:10.1128/microbiolspec.AID-0012-2013.f2

cysteine residues. One of the earliest antibodies to have its Fab crystal structure determined, human KOL (2), has a disulfide within its CDR H3, between residues H100a and H100f. Crystal structures for other antibodies containing H3 disulfides exist for human Fab 8F9 (44) to human cytomegalovirus (disulfide between H98 and H100c), human Fab CB3S (45) that recognizes BLyS receptor 3 (disulfide between H97 and H100d), and a human anti-influenza Fab F045-092 (P. Lee, personal communication) (disulfide between H100c and H100f). Anti-HIV Fab PGT128 (46) has a disulfide bond linking CDR H1 to CDR H2 (residues H32 and H52B), and murine anti-HIV Fab 59.1 against the gp120 V3 region (47) also has a disulfide bond linking these two CDRs (residues H35 and H52). In some

of the ligand-bound structures, such as PGT128 and F045-092, the Fab contacts with the antigen include the disulfide, so these are important for the antigen recognition process. The disulfides may also be of importance in stabilizing a particular CDR conformation or position.

SELF-CARBOHYDRATE RECOGNITION: PENETRATING THE GLYCAN SHIELD

The envelope proteins on viruses, such as HIV-1, are extensively glycosylated using host-derived enzymes, so the viral glycans contain only human carbohydrate moieties. Thus, one would expect that antibodies would not target such glycosylated regions in viral proteins. In fact, the dense coat of carbohydrates covering most of the outside of the gp120 envelope protein has long been termed the "glycan shield" or "silent" face (48) because it was thought to make the protein invisible to the immune system. However, several anti-HIV-1 antibodies have now been discovered whose primary targets are these same self glycans. It is thought that the extremely high density of high-mannose glycans on gp120 is unusual among human proteins and, thus, is responsible for the surprising immunogenicity. The first such antibody, 2G12, that was found to target the HIV-1 glycan shield is among the most unusual antibodies found to date because the two Fab fragments on the IgG are domain-swapped through their V_H domains so that the two Fab fragments are intimately interlocked in a side-by-side arrangement (Fig. 3). 2G12 is extensively mutated in comparison to its putative germ line sequence, with 38 and 16 somatic mutations in the heavy and light chains, respectively. However, just 5 to 7 of these mutations are enough to cause the germ line Fab to become significantly domain exchanged (49), with four being especially important: Ala at H14, Glu at H75, Ile at H19, and Pro at H113. Structures of 2G12 in complex with $Man_9GlcNAc_2$ carbohydrates and other, smaller, components of high-mannose sugars (50, 51), show that each antigen-combining site of the dimeric Fab binds to the D1 arm of one $Man_9GlcNAc_2$ sugar, closely contacting the two terminal mannose sugars. In addition, sugar groups from a crystallographic symmetry-related D2 arm bind in the cleft between the two closely spaced V_H domains, suggesting

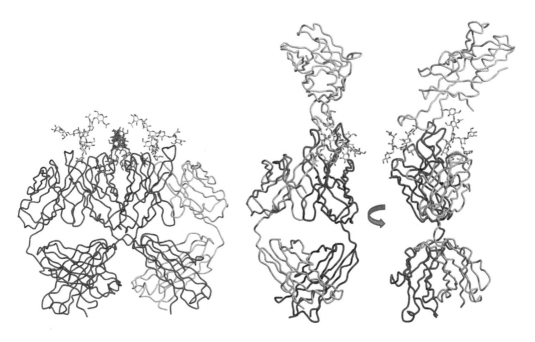

FIGURE 3 **Self-carbohydrate recognition by HIV-1 antibodies. (Left) Dimeric, domain-swapped 2G12 binds the D1 arms of $GlcNAc_2Man_9$ (yellow) via two closely spaced primary combining sites. A third potential binding site, located between the closely spaced V_H and V_H' domains, binds symmetry-related sugars (orange). (Middle and right) PGT128 also binds to two sugar moieties and inserts its CDR H3 (red) and long H2 (magenta) between two high-mannose sugars to contact the protein surface. The Fab-antigen complex is shown from two different sides to illustrate the interaction. 2G12, PGT128, and PG9 (Fig. 1) bind two high-mannose sugars, either with two separate binding sites, as in 2G12, or by wedging long CDR loops between two carbohydrates, as in PGT128 and PG9 recognition. doi:10.1128/ microbiolspec.AID-0012-2013.f3**

a possible secondary binding site. Antibody affinity for carbohydrates is usually weak (micro- to millimolar range); however, multivalent binding of the dimeric 2G12 Fab increases avidity to the nanomolar range, which increases the effectiveness of 2G12 in viral neutralization.

More recently, several extremely broad and potent neutralizing antibodies have been discovered that also bind to high-mannose glycans on gp120 without the use of 2G12-like domain exchange. Already mentioned above are PG9 and PG16, which use their large "hammerhead" CDR H3 to bind in a cleft between two sugars on the gp120 V1/V2 region, with one sugar on each side of the large CDR H3, and backbone-backbone hydrogen bonds from the β-strand-like top of H3 to a β-strand of the V1/V2 region (22). PGT128 is another broad and potent antibody that binds to a carbohydrate-containing epitope at the base of the gp120 V3 loop (Fig. 3). A glycan at gp120 residue Asn332 binds into the primary combining site of PGT128, contacting residues in H2, H3, L3, and framework region 2, while the Asn301 glycan contacts residues in CDR H1, framework region 3, and the disulfide bond linking CDR H1 to CDR H2. Contact is also made from Fab to several backbone atoms of the gp120 in another β-strand-like interaction. PGT128 has a moderately long CDR H3 loop (19/21 amino acids), the longest H2 CDR loop yet seen, with a 6-amino-acid insert after residue H52 (insertions here are usually 1 or 3 amino acids in length), and a very short CDR L1 (residues 28 and 29 are missing). These insertions and deletions combine to make the heavy chain component of the Fab paratope much more elevated than the light chain part (Fig. 3), and most of the interactions between PGT128 and gp120 are with the heavy chain.

PGT128, PG9, and PG16 all bind to carbohydrates so that they contact multiple mannose and/or GlcNAc sugar moieties, as opposed to merely contacting the distal tips of the $Man_9GlcNAc_2$ residues, as with 2G12. Thus, 2G12, PG9, PG16, and PGT128 have all devised ways to create multiple or large binding sites for carbohydrate to increase the avidity of an otherwise weak interaction. The heavy chain regions of PG9, PG16, PGT128, and PGT145 also give rise to uniquely shaped, convex paratopes that can penetrate the glycan shield. These paratope topologies differ from the more traditional flat and undulating, or concave pocket or groove shapes (10, 11) (Fig. 4). In addition, the 2G12 paratope is very broad, extending from one Fab binding site to another, in which up to four potential binding pockets for carbohydrate are located.

UNUSUAL INDELS

Some recently isolated influenza and HIV-1 antibodies have highly unusual insertion mutations. We have already described the long H1 insert in Fab C05 and the long H2 insert in Fab PGT128. In both of these cases, the inserted residues cause the CDR loop to become longer but do not alter any of the Fab framework structure (Fig. 5). Antibody 2D1 is an influenza antibody with a 3-amino-acid insertion on the C-terminal side of CDR H2 at position H62 (52). This insertion causes a register shift, lengthening the CDR H2 by one residue and, surprisingly, extending the H65-H66 loop (which faces toward the Fab Fc region) (Fig. 5). The bulge at the tip of H2 also causes distortion of the neighboring H1 CDR. This is the first insertion that we are aware of that has not simply resulted in extension of a CDR loop. Removal of the inserted residues in 2D1 results in canonical structures for the H1 and H2 CDRs but reduced affinity for hemagglutinin and reduced viral neutralization.

MECHANISMS OF ANTIBODY NEUTRALIZATION

Working in concert with the novel antiviral antibody structural features are some equally novel mechanisms of neutralization. The classic model for antibody neutralization of virus is the binding of antibody to virus and

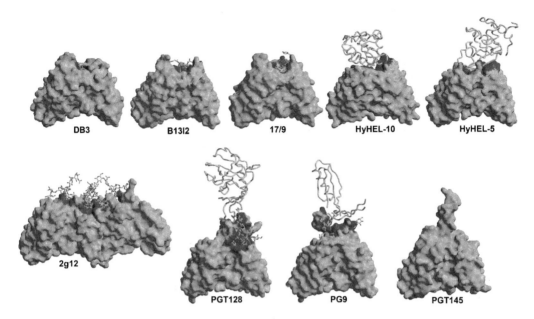

FIGURE 4 **Diversity in the shape of antibody combining sites. Fab domain swapping and extremely long CDR H3 loops result in unusually shaped paratopes. (Top) Fv molecular surfaces are shown in gray, with paratopes (if known) colored in magenta and antigens shown in yellow. Classic antibody binding sites are usually pockets for small haptens (DB3, progesterone), grooves for peptides (B13I2, myohemerythrin peptide; 17/9, influenza peptide), or flat, undulating surfaces for proteins (HyHEL-10, lysozyme; HyHEL-5, lysozyme). (Bottom) In contrast, domain-swapped 2G12 has created a paratope consisting of 4 different binding pockets, and PGT128 and PG9 have protruding, convex paratopes that can be inserted between two large carbohydrate moieties. A structure of PGT145 with its antigen has not yet been determined, but its very long CDR H3 can be clearly visualized. doi:10.1128/microbiolspec.AID-0012-2013.f4**

the subsequent blocking by the bulky IgG of virus attachment to a host cell receptor. However, some recent work has uncovered other mechanisms. The anti-influenza antibodies CR6261, F10, and CR9114 (53) all bind to the hemagglutinin trimer stem and have been shown to block conformational changes that must take place in the hemagglutinin to bring about membrane fusion. Two other anti-influenza antibodies, CR8033 and CR8071 (53), bind to two different epitopes on the hemagglutinin head and, while they do not prevent viral entry or genomic replication, they do prevent the virus from propagating. In the presence of these antibodies, newly created viruses are not released from the infected cell, similar to what is seen with the neuraminidase inhibitor zanamivir. The anti-HIV antibody PGT128 has been shown to neutralize virus much more

potently as an IgG than as an Fab, although the binding affinities for Fab and IgG to isolated gp120 trimers are very similar. Thus, the IgG is postulated to cross-link different gp120 trimers on the viral surface. The PGT128 also reduces the lifetime of viral infectivity more than comparable antibodies, so the cross-linking may be causing conformational changes in the gp120 trimers that interfere with their functionality (46).

SUMMARY

Recent advances in the isolation, identification, and production of potent and broadly neutralizing human, antiviral antibodies have resulted in many exciting new crystal structures for these antibodies in complex with their antigens. While the ultimate goal

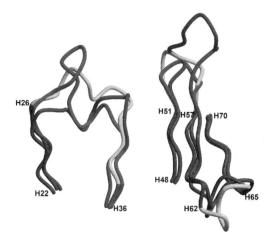

FIGURE 5 Unusual insertions in CDRs H1 and H2 from Fabs C05 (red), 2D1 (yellow), and PGT128 (blue). (Left) In these H1 CDRs, the colored areas cover residues H26 to H35b. C05 has an unusually long 5-residue insertion in H1, while PGT128 and 2D1 have more common 2-residue insertions in H1. The 2D1 H1 CDR has shifted away its canonical conformation due to a clash with its long H2 loop. (Right) H2 CDRs from the same Fabs, with the same coloring from positions H51 to H57. C05 has a normal H2 CDR with a 1-residue insertion after residue 52. PGT128 has a very rare 6-residue insertion in this CDR, which is reflected in its unusually long H2 CDR loop. 2D1 has a 3-residue insertion in the CDR that extends the physical CDR length by 1 residue, but the other inserted residues are accommodated in the loop around H63–H64 that faces the C$_H$1 domain. doi:10.1128/microbiolspec.AID-0012-2013.f5

of producing effective vaccines to prevent viral infection has been advanced by the identification of novel epitope regions on viral antigens, many structural features of the antibodies themselves have proven to be surprising. Almost 30 years have passed since the first Fab structure was determined at atomic resolution, yet new insights into how these immune receptors can adapt to any pathogen are constantly being revealed. A plethora of mouse antibody structures, from the few that trickled out in the 1970s to increasing numbers in the 1980s and 1990s, led one to believe that everything was known about antibody structure and function. Structures of camel and shark antibodies

altered the landscape, and human antibodies have now completely changed our view of the range of structural features and mechanisms that can be used to target the universe of potential antigens. The last few years have been very exhilarating and suggest that the next 30 years of antibody structural studies will prove just as exciting, as more novel human antibodies are discovered, as well as those from other species such as cows, whose extravagantly long and cysteine-rich CDR H3s far exceed anything seen so far (54, 55). More importantly, these studies will no doubt prove helpful in the design of new vaccines and antibody therapeutics to prevent human disease.

ACKNOWLEDGMENT

Conflicts of interest: I declare no conflicts.

CITATION

Stanfield RL, Wilson IA. 2014. Antibody structure. Microbiol Spectrum 2(2):AID-0012-2013.

REFERENCES

1. **Arnaout R, Lee W, Cahill P, Honan T, Sparrow T, Weiand M, Nusbaum C, Rajewsky K, Koralov SB.** 2011. High-resolution description of antibody heavy-chain repertoires in humans. *PLoS One* **6:** e22365.
2. **Palm W.** 1974. The physico-chemical characterization and crystallization of immunoglobulins and their fragmentation products: a contribution to the elucidation of the three-dimensional structure of antibodies. II. Human immunoglobulin Kol: a myeloma protein of the class IgG, gamma2 kappa2. *Hoppe Seylers Z Physiol Chem* **355:**877–880.
3. **Amzel LM, Poljak RJ, Saul F, Varga JM, Richards FF.** 1974. The three dimensional structure of a combining region-ligand complex of immunoglobulin NEW at 3.5-Å resolution. *Proc Natl Acad Sci USA* **71:**1427–1430.
4. **Berman H, Henrick K, Nakamura H.** 2003. Announcing the worldwide Protein Data Bank. *Nat Struct Biol* **10:**980.
5. **Chothia C, Lesk AM.** 1987. Canonical structures for the hypervariable regions of immunoglobulins. *J Mol Biol* **196:**901–917.

6. **Al-Lazikani B, Lesk AM, Chothia C.** 1997. Standard conformations for the canonical structures of immunoglobulins. *J Mol Biol* **273:**927–948.

7. **Martin AC, Thornton JM.** 1996. Structural families in loops of homologous proteins: automatic classification, modelling and application to antibodies. *J Mol Biol* **263:**800–815.

8. **North B, Lehmann A, Dunbrack RL Jr.** 2011. A new clustering of antibody CDR loop conformations. *J Mol Biol* **406:**228–256.

9. **Wilson IA, Stanfield RL.** 1994. Antibody-antigen interactions: new structures and new conformational changes. *Curr Opin Struct Biol* **4:**857–867.

10. **Wilson IA, Stanfield RL.** 1993. Antibody-antigen interactions. *Curr Opin Struct Biol* **3:**113–118.

11. **MacCallum RM, Martin AC, Thornton JM.** 1996. Antibody-antigen interactions: contact analysis and binding site topography. *J Mol Biol* **262:**732–745.

12. **Stanfield RL, Takimoto-Kamimura M, Rini JM, Profy AT, Wilson IA.** 1993. Major antigen-induced domain rearrangements in an antibody. *Structure* **1:**83–93.

13. **Stanfield RL, Wilson IA.** 1994. Antigen-induced conformational changes in antibodies: a problem for structural prediction and design. *Trends Biotechnol* **12:**275–279.

14. **Kang AS, Barbas CF, Janda KD, Benkovic SJ, Lerner RA.** 1991. Linkage of recognition and replication functions by assembling combinatorial antibody Fab libraries along phage surfaces. *Proc Natl Acad Sci USA* **88:**4363–4366.

15. **Clackson T, Hoogenboom HR, Griffiths AD, Winter G.** 1991. Making antibody fragments using phage display libraries. *Nature* **352:**624–628.

16. **Scheid JF, Mouquet H, Feldhahn N, Walker BD, Pereyra F, Cutrell E, Seaman MS, Mascola JR, Wyatt RT, Wardemann H, Nussenzweig MC.** 2009. A method for identification of HIV gp140 binding memory B cells in human blood. *J Immunol Methods* **343:**65–67.

17. **Walker LM, Phogat SK, Chan-Hui PY, Wagner D, Phung P, Goss JL, Wrin T, Simek MD, Fling S, Mitcham JL, Lehrman JK, Priddy FH, Olsen OA, Frey SM, Hammond PW, Kaminsky S, Zamb T, Moyle M, Koff WC, Poignard P, Burton DR.** 2009. Broad and potent neutralizing antibodies from an African donor reveal a new HIV-1 vaccine target. *Science* **326:**285–289.

18. **Zhang C.** 2012. Hybridoma technology for the generation of monoclonal antibodies. *Methods Mol Biol* **901:**117–135.

19. **Zemlin M, Klinger M, Link J, Zemlin C, Bauer K, Engler JA, Schroeder HW Jr, Kirkham PM.** 2003. Expressed murine and human CDR-H3 intervals of equal length exhibit distinct repertoires that differ in their amino acid composition and predicted range of structures. *J Mol Biol* **334:**733–749.

20. **Pejchal R, Walker LM, Stanfield RL, Phogat SK, Koff WC, Poignard P, Burton DR, Wilson IA.** 2010. Structure and function of broadly reactive antibody PG16 reveal an H3 subdomain that mediates potent neutralization of HIV-1. *Proc Natl Acad Sci USA* **107:**11483–11488.

21. **Pancera M, McLellan JS, Wu X, Zhu J, Changela A, Schmidt SD, Yang Y, Zhou T, Phogat S, Mascola JR, Kwong PD.** 2010. Crystal structure of PG16 and chimeric dissection with somatically related PG9: structure-function analysis of two quaternary-specific antibodies that effectively neutralize HIV-1. *J Virol* **84:**8098–8110.

22. **McLellan JS, Pancera M, Carrico C, Gorman J, Julien JP, Khayat R, Louder R, Pejchal R, Sastry M, Dai K, O'Dell S, Patel N, Shahzadul-Hussan S, Yang Y, Zhang B, Zhou T, Zhu J, Boyington JC, Chuang GY, Diwanji D, Georgiev I, Kwon YD, Lee D, Louder MK, Moquin S, Schmidt SD, Yang ZY, Bonsignori M, Crump JA, Kapiga SH, Sam NE, Haynes BF, Burton DR, Koff WC, Walker LM, Phogat S, Wyatt R, Orwenyo J, Wang LX, Arthos J, Bewley CA, Mascola JR, Nabel GJ, Schief WR, Ward AB, Wilson IA, Kwong PD.** 2011. Structure of HIV-1 gp120 V1/V2 domain with broadly neutralizing antibody PG9. *Nature* **480:**336–343.

23. **Collis AV, Brouwer AP, Martin AC.** 2003. Analysis of the antigen combining site: correlations between length and sequence composition of the hypervariable loops and the nature of the antigen. *J Mol Biol* **325:**337–354.

24. **Briney BS, Willis JR, Crowe JE Jr.** 2012. Human peripheral blood antibodies with long HCDR3s are established primarily at original recombination using a limited subset of germline genes. *PLoS One* **7:**e36750.

25. **Changela A, Wu X, Yang Y, Zhang B, Zhu J, Nardone GA, O'Dell S, Pancera M, Gorny MK, Phogat S, Robinson JE, Stamatatos L, Zolla-Pazner S, Mascola JR, Kwong PD.** 2011. Crystal structure of human antibody 2909 reveals conserved features of quaternary structure-specific antibodies that potently neutralize HIV-1. *J Virol* **85:**2524–2535.

26. **Spurrier B, Sampson JM, Totrov M, Li H, O'Neal T, Williams C, Robinson J, Gorny MK, Zolla-Pazner S, Kong XP.** 2011. Structural analysis of human and macaque mAbs 2909 and 2.5B: implications for the configuration of the

quaternary neutralizing epitope of HIV-1 gp120. *Structure* **19**:691–699.

27. **Choe H, Li W, Wright PL, Vasilieva N, Venturi M, Huang CC, Grundner C, Dorfman T, Zwick MB, Wang L, Rosenberg ES, Kwong PD, Burton DR, Robinson JE, Sodroski JG, Farzan M.** 2003. Tyrosine sulfation of human antibodies contributes to recognition of the CCR5 binding region of HIV-1 gp120. *Cell* **114**:161–170.

28. **Huang CC, Lam SN, Acharya P, Tang M, Xiang SH, Hussan SS, Stanfield RL, Robinson J, Sodroski J, Wilson IA, Wyatt R, Bewley CA, Kwong PD.** 2007. Structures of the CCR5 N terminus and of a tyrosine-sulfated antibody with HIV-1 gp120 and CD4. *Science* **317**:1930–1934.

29. **Stanfield RL, Dooley H, Flajnik MF, Wilson IA.** 2004. Crystal structure of a shark single-domain antibody V region in complex with lysozyme. *Science* **305**:1770–1773.

30. **Nuttall SD.** 2012. Overview and discovery of IgNARs and generation of VNARs. *Methods Mol Biol* **911**:27–36.

31. **Muyldermans S, Atarhouch T, Saldanha J, Barbosa JA, Hamers R.** 1994. Sequence and structure of VH domain from naturally occurring camel heavy chain immunoglobulins lacking light chains. *Protein Eng* **7**:1129–1135.

32. **Spinelli S, Frenken L, Bourgeois D, de Ron L, Bos W, Verrips T, Anguille C, Cambillau C, Tegoni M.** 1996. The crystal structure of a llama heavy chain variable domain. *Nat Struct Biol* **3**:752–757.

33. **Muyldermans S, Cambillau C, Wyns L.** 2001. Recognition of antigens by single-domain antibody fragments: the superfluous luxury of paired domains. *Trends Biochem Sci* **26**:230–235.

34. **Stanfield RL, Dooley H, Verdino P, Flajnik MF, Wilson IA.** 2007. Maturation of shark single-domain (IgNAR) antibodies: evidence for induced-fit binding. *J Mol Biol* **367**:358–372.

35. **Fanning SW, Horn JR.** 2011. An anti-hapten camelid antibody reveals a cryptic binding site with significant energetic contributions from a nonhypervariable loop. *Protein Sci* **20**:1196–1207.

36. **Vanlandschoot P, Stortelers C, Beirnaert E, Ibanez LI, Schepens B, Depla E, Saelens X.** 2011. Nanobodies(R): new ammunition to battle viruses. *Antiviral Res* **92**:389–407.

37. **Ekiert DC, Kashyap AK, Steel J, Rubrum A, Bhabha G, Khayat R, Lee JH, Dillon MA, O'Neil RE, Faynboym AM, Horowitz M, Horowitz L, Ward AB, Palese P, Webby R, Lerner RA, Bhatt RR, Wilson IA.** 2012. Cross-neutralization of influenza A viruses mediated by a single antibody loop. *Nature* **489**:526–532.

38. **Ekiert DC, Bhabha G, Elsliger MA, Friesen RH, Jongeneelen M, Throsby M, Goudsmit J, Wilson IA.** 2009. Antibody recognition of a highly conserved influenza virus epitope. *Science* **324**:246–251.

39. **Sui J, Hwang WC, Perez S, Wei G, Aird D, Chen LM, Santelli E, Stec B, Cadwell G, Ali M, Wan H, Murakami A, Yammanuru A, Han T, Cox NJ, Bankston LA, Donis RO, Liddington RC, Marasco WA.** 2009. Structural and functional bases for broad-spectrum neutralization of avian and human influenza A viruses. *Nat Struct Mol Biol* **16**:265–273.

40. **Kashyap AK, Steel J, Oner AF, Dillon MA, Swale RE, Wall KM, Perry KJ, Faynboym A, Ilhan M, Horowitz M, Horowitz L, Palese P, Bhatt RR, Lerner RA.** 2008. Combinatorial antibody libraries from survivors of the Turkish H5N1 avian influenza outbreak reveal virus neutralization strategies. *Proc Natl Acad Sci USA* **105**:5986–5991.

41. **Throsby M, van den Brink E, Jongeneelen M, Poon LL, Alard P, Cornelissen L, Bakker A, Cox F, van Deventer E, Guan Y, Cinatl J, ter Meulen J, Lasters I, Carsetti R, Peiris M, de Kruif J, Goudsmit J.** 2008. Heterosubtypic neutralizing monoclonal antibodies cross-protective against H5N1 and H1N1 recovered from human IgM+ memory B cells. *PLoS One* **3**:e3942.

42. **Huang CC, Venturi M, Majeed S, Moore MJ, Phogat S, Zhang MY, Dimitrov DS, Hendrickson WA, Robinson J, Sodroski J, Wyatt R, Choe H, Farzan M, Kwong PD.** 2004. Structural basis of tyrosine sulfation and VH-gene usage in antibodies that recognize the HIV type 1 coreceptor-binding site on gp120. *Proc Natl Acad Sci USA* **101**:2706–2711.

43. **Luftig MA, Mattu M, Di Giovine P, Geleziunas R, Hrin R, Barbato G, Bianchi E, Miller MD, Pessi A, Carfi A.** 2006. Structural basis for HIV-1 neutralization by a gp41 fusion intermediate-directed antibody. *Nat Struct Mol Biol* **13**:740–747.

44. **Thomson CA, Bryson S, McLean GR, Creagh AL, Pai EF, Schrader JW.** 2008. Germline V-genes sculpt the binding site of a family of antibodies neutralizing human cytomegalovirus. *EMBO J* **27**:2592–2602.

45. **Lee CV, Hymowitz SG, Wallweber HJ, Gordon NC, Billeci KL, Tsai SP, Compaan DM, Yin J, Gong Q, Kelley RF, DeForge LE, Martin F, Starovasnik MA, Fuh G.** 2006. Synthetic anti-BR3 antibodies that mimic BAFF binding and target both human and murine B cells. *Blood* **108**:3103–3111.

46. **Pejchal R, Doores KJ, Walker LM, Khayat R, Huang PS, Wang SK, Stanfield RL, Julien JP, Ramos A, Crispin M, Depetris R, Katpally U, Marozsan A, Cupo A, Maloveste S, Liu Y, McBride R, Ito Y, Sanders RW, Ogohara C, Paulson JC, Feizi T, Scanlan CN, Wong CH, Moore JP, Olson WC, Ward AB, Poignard P, Schief WR, Burton DR, Wilson IA.** 2011. A potent and broad neutralizing antibody recognizes and penetrates the HIV glycan shield. *Science* **334:**1097–1103.

47. **Ghiara JB, Stura EA, Stanfield RL, Profy AT, Wilson IA.** 1994. Crystal structure of the principal neutralization site of HIV-1. *Science* **264:**82–85.

48. **Wyatt R, Kwong PD, Desjardins E, Sweet RW, Robinson J, Hendrickson WA, Sodroski JG.** 1998. The antigenic structure of the HIV gp120 envelope glycoprotein. *Nature* **393:**705–711.

49. **Huber M, Le KM, Doores KJ, Fulton Z, Stanfield RL, Wilson IA, Burton DR.** 2010. Very few substitutions in a germ line antibody are required to initiate significant domain exchange. *J Virol* **84:**10700–10707.

50. **Calarese DA, Scanlan CN, Zwick MB, Deechongkit S, Mimura Y, Kunert R, Zhu P, Wormald MR, Stanfield RL, Roux KH, Kelly JW, Rudd PM, Dwek RA, Katinger H, Burton DR, Wilson IA.** 2003. Antibody domain exchange is an immunological solution to carbohydrate cluster recognition. *Science* **300:**2065–2071.

51. **Calarese DA, Lee HK, Huang CY, Best MD, Astronomo RD, Stanfield RL, Katinger H,** Burton DR, Wong CH, Wilson IA. 2005. Dissection of the carbohydrate specificity of the broadly neutralizing anti-HIV-1 antibody 2G12. *Proc Natl Acad Sci USA* **102:**13372–13377.

52. **Krause JC, Ekiert DC, Tumpey TM, Smith PB, Wilson IA, Crowe JE Jr.** 2011. An insertion mutation that distorts antibody binding site architecture enhances function of a human antibody. *MBio* **2:**e00345–e00310.

53. **Dreyfus C, Laursen NS, Kwaks T, Zuijdgeest D, Khayat R, Ekiert DC, Lee JH, Metlagel Z, Bujny MV, Jongeneelen M, van der Vlugt R, Lamrani M, Korse HJ, Geelen E, Sahin O, Sieuwerts M, Brakenhoff JP, Vogels R, Li OT, Poon LL, Peiris M, Koudstaal W, Ward AB, Wilson IA, Goudsmit J, Friesen RH.** 2012. Highly conserved protective epitopes on influenza B viruses. *Science* **337:**1343–1348.

54. **Saini SS, Allore B, Jacobs RM, Kaushik A.** 1999. Exceptionally long CDR3H region with multiple cysteine residues in functional bovine IgM antibodies. *Eur J Immunol* **29:**2420–2426.

55. **Wang F, Ekiert DC, Ahmad I, Yu W, Zhang Y, Bazirgan O, Torkamani A, Raudsepp T, Mwangi W, Criscitiello MF, Wilson IA, Schultz PG, Smider VV.** 2013. Reshaping antibody diversity. *Cell* **153:**1379–1393.

56. **Kraulis PJ.** 1991. MOLSCRIPT: a program to produce both detailed and schematic plots of protein structures. *J Appl Crystallogr* **24:**946–950.

57. **Merritt EA, Bacon DJ.** 1997. Raster3D: photorealistic molecular graphics. *Methods Enzymol* **277:**505–524.

The Role of Complement in Antibody Therapy for Infectious Diseases

4

PETER P. WIBROE,[1] SHEN Y. HELVIG,[1] and S. MOEIN MOGHIMI[1]

INTRODUCTION

The complement system is an integral and evolutionarily ancient component of the innate immune system, serving as the first line of defense against common pathogens (Fig. 1) (1). The prime functions of complement in innate host defense are accomplished through three effector pathways. These include lysis, inflammation, and opsonization (Fig. 2). The latter is central to microbial recognition and clearance by phagocytic cells. Complement further cooperates with Toll-like receptors in response to microbial structure and infection, in which immune responses are determined through both synergistic and antagonistic manners (1). Complement is also a functional bridge between innate and adaptive immunity, orchestrating an integrated host defense response to pathogenic challenges. For instance, complement can modulate adaptive immunity by providing signals that reinforce humoral responses to antigens by priming and regulating T cells and lowering the B-cell activation threshold (2, 3). It is also an important integral point for cross talk with other biological cascades to ensure homeostasis is maintained. One example is the interplay between the complement and coagulation cascades,

[1]Centre for Pharmaceutical Nanotechnology and Nanotoxicology, Department of Pharmacy, Faculty of Health and Medical Sciences, University of Copenhagen, DK-2100 Copenhagen Ø, Denmark.

Antibodies for Infectious Diseases
Edited by James E. Crowe, Jr., Diana Boraschi, and Rino Rappuoli
© 2015 American Society for Microbiology, Washington, DC
doi:10.1128/microbiolspec.AID-0015-2014

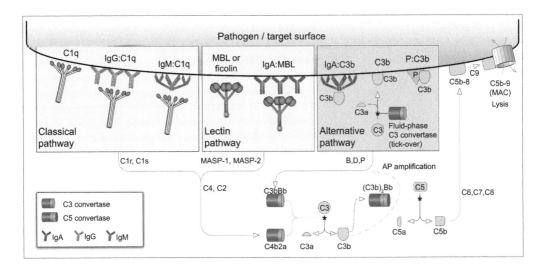

FIGURE 1 Schematic representation of complement activation by pathogens. The diagram shows the role of surface-bound antibodies and other complement-sensing molecules in complement triggering. Serum IgA is monomeric, but IgA in secretions is dimeric. IgM is pentameric. P, properdin; AP, alternative pathway. doi:10.1128/microbiolspec.AID-0015-2014.f1

whereby the complement system can amplify coagulation by enhancing local clotting and, as a result, preventing microbial spread through the systemic circulation. Likewise, the activated clotting factor XII can activate the classical complement pathway and thrombin can directly cleave the third and fifth complement components (C3 and C5, respectively) (4, 5).

In addition to effector functions, complement also plays a vital role in the maintenance of homeostasis by aiding in the removal of cell debris and aging cells from the host in a noninflammatory manner. The safe removal of endogenous debris is tactful, whereby apoptotic cells are opsonized without downstream amplification that would result in inflammation, thus ensuring cell integrity and

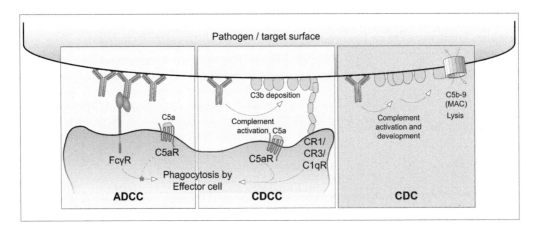

FIGURE 2 Antibody-mediated pathogen attack and elimination mechanisms. doi:10.1128/microbiolspec. AID-0015-2014.f2

maintenance of homeostasis (6). Complement also plays regulatory roles in organ regeneration, neuroprotection, and the mobilization of hematopoietic stem progenitor cells from the bone marrow (6).

On account of its potency, selectivity, and rapid amplifying nature, complement plays a central role in the field of antibody (Ab) therapy. A promising future has been forecast for Abs in the treatment of many pathologies, including cancer and infectious diseases, owing to their targeting properties and efficient use of inherent elimination procedures. However, there are only a few drugs on the market and in clinical trials for the treatment of infectious diseases, mainly due to competition pressure from cheaper broad-spectrum antibiotics (7) and the crucial need for correct early diagnosis. Consequently, Ab therapy is unlikely to outcompete treatments for diseases where cheaper and efficient treatments are widely accessible. Nevertheless, emerging antimicrobial drug resistance affirms the need for more targeted treatments, as in methicillin-resistant *Staphylococcus aureus* (8), where Ab treatments could have potential.

Anti-infectious Ab therapy targets either the pathogen or its toxins. Currently, there is only one approved anti-infectious monoclonal antibody (MAb) on the market (palivizumab) for the treatment and prevention of respiratory syncytial virus infection in infants (9). A further few are currently in clinical trials (7). The highly complex nature of Ab binding in affinity and effector functions is another challenge in the development of new and more-efficient therapeutic Abs. This was the case for motavizumab, an intended new and improved version of palivizumab. However, clinical trials were disappointing both in the lack of efficacy and in initiating adverse reactions in some patients (7).

Abs mediate pathogen elimination through different effector mechanisms (Fig. 2). Surface neutralization is one approach, where bound Abs form a barrier that passivates the invading pathogen independent of Fc isotype (10). Moreover, bound Abs can directly recruit

effector cells to the site of interest. This may result in pathogen engulfment via Fc receptors (FcRs), complement receptors (CRs), and/or cytokine release. The latter process is known as Ab-dependent cell cytotoxicity (ADCC) and may involve natural killer cells, macrophages, neutrophils, and eosinophils. Finally, bound Abs recruit the complement components that kill the cell either directly by complement-dependent lysis (complement-dependent cytotoxicity [CDC]) or through C1q and/or C3b/iC3b opsonization processes that activate leukocytes (complement-dependent cell cytotoxicity [CDCC]).

The advantage of Ab therapy is in its targeting properties. A preparation of MAbs consisting of a single purified Ab with only one epitope may target specific infectious agents and leave host resident flora cells undisturbed. The response development from Ab binding to pathogen killing or elimination is, however, complex. Accordingly, important considerations on the effector mechanisms must be made to achieve the full potential of the formulation, where complement plays a central role.

COMPLEMENT ACTIVATION

The complement system consists of more than 30 circulating and cell-bound proteins (11). This array of proteins is organized into a hierarchy of proteolytic cascades operating through three major distinct pathways: the classical, lectin, and alternative pathways (Fig. 1). These pathways all converge at the step where C3 is cleaved by C3 convertases, thereby amplifying complement response and propagating the cascade.

Classical Pathway

The classical pathway is primarily Ab dependent and is initiated by antigen-Ab complexes. Only immunoglobulin G (IgG) clusters and IgM are capable of initiating the classical pathway (4), as discussed below. Complement component C1q can also act as a pattern recognition molecule that can recognize and bind to microbial and apoptotic cells without the aid of Abs, thus activating the classical pathway directly (12). C1q has a hexameric structure, which is formed by six globular heads that are held together by a collagen-like tail. Together with two other proteins, C1r and C1s, they form the C1 complex. Upon binding of more than one globular head of the C1q to the constant regions of IgG/IgM or directly to a pathogen surface, C1q undergoes a conformational change that can activate zymogens C1r and C1s, forming an enzymatically active C1 complex that cleaves the C2 and C4 proteins to form the classical pathway C3 convertase, C4b2a.

Lectin Pathway

The lectin pathway is triggered when mannose-binding lectin (MBL) and ficolins bind to a surface. These species recognize repeating carbohydrate patterns (e.g., mannose and N-acetylated sugars) on invading pathogens. Host cells also display carbohydrate units, but these are protected by sialic acid, which prevents the binding of MBL (13). The binding of MBL or ficolin to a surface triggers activation of their associated serine protease zymogens (mannose-activating serine protease 1 [MASP-1], MASP-2, and MASP-3). Activated MASP-2 cleaves C4, which in turn results in C2 cleavage and formation of a C3 convertase identical to that of the classical pathway.

Alternative Pathway

The alternative pathway is spontaneously activated at a low but constant rate (tick over). This is also a mechanism that provides an ongoing probing of the surrounding cells. There are abundant amounts of circulating C3 in the host, which is spontaneously hydrolyzed to $C3b_{H2O}$. This exposes a binding site for factor B. Upon binding, factor B is cleaved by factor D, forming the alternative pathway fluid-phase C3 convertase C3bBb. The resulting soluble convertase cleaves C3 to give C3a and C3b. The latter can attach to pathogen or host cells, where covalently bound C3b binds factor B, which in turn is rapidly cleaved by factor D, forming surface-bound C3bBb and aiding deposition of many molecules of C3b on the surface. Properdin, a positive complement regulator, stabilizes the C3bBb convertase, extending its half-life severalfold (14). On host cells, complement regulatory proteins such as CR1 and decay-accelerating factor can displace Bb from C3b. Factor H is also recruited and accelerates Bb displacement from C3b. In addition to these processes, CR1, membrane cofactor of proteolysis, and factor H catalyze the cleavage of bound C3b by recruiting the plasma protease factor I to produce inactive C3b.

C3 convertases from all three pathways can cleave C3 into C3b and C3a components, with the deposits of C3b quickly forming new C3 convertases in the presence of factor B and D through the alternative pathway. This positive reinforcement turns into a large amplification loop, responsible for 80 to 90% of complement response, independent of the original pathway (6).

AB-MEDIATED COMPLEMENT ACTIVATION

The three Ab subtypes, IgA, IgG, and IgM, have shown complement-activating properties (Fig. 1). Collectively, they are able to activate all three complement pathways, with IgG-mediated classical pathway activation standing as the most essential. Common to all isotypes is the requirement of a tight interaction between the Ab and a surface (e. g., a cell membrane, allograft, or drug carrier surface). This binding induces a conformational change in the Fc/Fab hinge regions or associates the Abs into a spatial orientation that allows the complement proteins (e.g., C1q, C3b) to become both bound and activated. The conformational change is vital for complement activation. For example, IgG can bind to some particulate materials (e.g., SiO_2 particles), but the binding may not be strong enough to accomplish the conformational change necessary for efficient complement activation (15). IgMs also require specific conformations for activation, as they have been shown to bind equally well on different-sized dextran nanoparticles but only induce complement activation when a distinct curvature criteria is fulfilled (16).

IgG

IgG is the most abundant immunoglobulin isotype and is believed to be the most important in complement activation. It is responsible for the linkage between the diversification of the adaptive system and the rapid response of complement, as IgG can bind to epitopes on nonself surfaces, resulting in recruitment and activation of C1q via the classical pathway. The active conformation of C1q is achieved by the binding of more than one C1q head group to Fcγ domains of surface-bound IgGs. Multiple IgGs must therefore be bound to a surface in a proper intermolecular distance to be able to initiate a complement response.

There are four subtypes of IgG (IgG1 to IgG4), each with different biological activities (C1q and FcR affinity) and pharmacokinetic profiles (half-life and protease susceptibility) (17). IgG1 is the isotype used in the majority of MAbs because of its ability to strongly associate with both C1q and FcγR while possessing good circulation half-lives and stability. IgG3 has a similar biological activity, only with a reduced half-life, which is most likely due to a longer hinge region that renders the Ab susceptible to proteolysis. Despite the lack of biological activity from IgG2 and IgG4, these isotypes have shown superior bactericidal function against *Cryptococcus neoformans* infections in mice (18). This finding highlights the complex effector function in Ab therapies in general and suggests specific demands for different infections. It further questions the general role of complement in Ab therapies and is discussed below.

IgM

Another activator of the classical pathway is the IgM Ab, which possesses an activation mechanism similar to that of IgG. Secreted IgMs circulate in its inactive, planar pentameric conformation. When efficiently bound to a target surface, the pentamer adopts a staple conformation by kinking its Fab regions relative to the Fc plane. This change in conformation exposes binding sites for C1q and initiates a complement response. The fact that a single pentamer is sufficient to initiate complement further removes the requirement for specific Ab densities. Accordingly, IgM species could make promising candidates in MAb therapies, provided that the production of stable expression of the native pentameric form can be achieved on a large scale (19).

IgA

The role of IgA in complement activation is less studied, though IgA can activate complement through different pathways. It activates the lectin pathway mainly by acting as a ligand for MBL (20). Furthermore, it is also believed to increase the alternative pathway turnover (21, 22). Its complement-activating properties largely depend on its multimeric state and its extent of glycosylation, with the most potent activators being the polymeric and heavily glycosylated species. Polymeric IgA is also a ligand for the FcαR present on phagocytes and has thereby shown, in concert with its complement-activating properties, to mediate phagocytosis of *Streptococcus pneumoniae* (21). This elimination mechanism is highly similar to the IgG-mediated activation through FcγR affinity. However, where IgG can induce phagocytosis directly through FcγR in the absence of complement activation, IgA-mediated killing is dependent on phagocyte preactivation by C5a or tumor necrosis factor alpha (21). Its relatively passive inflammatory nature is convenient, given the high abundance of IgA at mucosal sites, where a continuous exposure to microorganisms and foreign molecules would otherwise cause host cell damage.

After response initiation and coating by active complement complexes on the Fc region, the IgA1 isotype has been reported to be able to detach from the antigenic surface while retaining its binding properties toward new antigens. This phenomenon is termed complement-coated Ab transfer and is believed to be an efficient mechanism for transferring activated complement compounds to nearby antigens without the need to initialize a new response (23).

Coadministration of IgA and IgG has been shown to induce tumor cell killing by polymorphonuclear cells by activating their respective Fc receptors simultaneously (24). On the other hand, IgA's affinity to bacterial capsular polysaccharides has (paradoxically) been reported to sterically block IgG binding and the following inflammatory functions (25, 26), thus questioning the robustness of the IgA/IgG synergistic effects.

EFFECTOR RESPONSES AND THEIR ROLE IN MAB TREATMENTS

Following the detection of a pathogenic surface and initiation of one of the three pathways, there are three main effector functions that contribute to pathogen removal. These functions and their effect on MAb treatments are outlined below.

MAC and CDC

As the complement activation amplifies and propagates, the density of C3b increases dramatically, which leads to the binding of C3b to already formed C3 convertases, producing the C5 convertase [C4b2a3b, $(C3b)_2Bb$]. This permits complement activation to enter the terminal phase, where all three pathways converge. C5 convertase cleaves C5 into C5a and C5b. C5a is a potent soluble anaphylatoxin, whereas C5b quickly

associates with C6 and C7 components and partitions into a lipid bilayer membrane. Subsequently, C8 binds to the complex, which then induces the binding and polymerization of 10 to 16 C9 components, producing a channel-like structure that penetrates the cellular membrane, known as the membrane attack complex (MAC). Water, electrolytes, and even enzymes can freely pass the channel, which leads to a disruption of cell homeostasis and cell lysis (12).

MAbs engineered to target specific pathogens can direct a complement activation leading to the development of the MAC, thereby lysing the targeted cells by taking advantage of the body's own defense system. This action forms the basic mechanism of CDC and is believed to play a major role in Ab-based therapy of certain hematological malignancies and solid tumors (27, 28) and a less-defined role in elimination of pathogens, especially bacterial toxins and viruses (7).

Opsonization

The large amounts of opsonins, in particular C3b produced from the amplification loop, efficiently coat the surface of the pathogen, tagging it for recognition by neutrophils, NK cells, and monocytes carrying the CRs and C1q receptors. But as opposed to Ab-mediated cell activation through FcRs, CRs do not internalize particles unless they are costimulated by external factors like tumor necrosis factor alpha, colony-stimulating factors, or the complement anaphylatoxins C3a and C5a. Furthermore, CR-mediated phagocytosis does not release inflammatory mediators like reactive oxygen intermediates and arachidonic acid metabolites (29). This may be a reason why CDCC is believed to have limited influence in clinically available immunotherapies (30).

The polysaccharide β-glucan can enhance CR3-dependent cellular cytotoxicity, sometimes referred to as CR3-DCC (31). It is naturally present on cell walls of yeasts and fungi, but its coadministration in MAb therapy targeting surfaces inherently absent of the molecule has been shown to induce cytotoxicity (32). Activation of complement also facilitates the adaptive immune system via the binding of opsonized antigens to CR2 on B cells, which activates specific Ab production and the differentiation of B memory cells. Thus, complement does not only become activated by Abs, but may direct Ab production against C3b-bound surfaces. Clearly C3b is a key molecule in translating complement activation into effector responses (14).

Inflammatory Responses

The potent anaphylatoxins C3a and C5a are capable of inducing an inflammatory state by degranulation of mast cells and basophil granulocytes, giving rise to vasodilation and capillary leakage (14). Furthermore, they are strong chemoattractants that guide the migration of circulating neutrophils, monocytes, and macrophages to the site of complement activation, exerting an important role in indirectly facilitating the interaction between opsonins and phagocytes (4). These powerful bioactive fragments are quickly cleaved by carboxypeptidases to give C5a-desArg and C3a-desArg. C5a-desArg retains up to 10% of the C5a inflammatory properties, while C3a-desArg is devoid of proinflammatory functions (33).

Though not directly responsible for pathogen clearance, the complement anaphylatoxins with their effector cell-activating and chemoattractive properties are important mediators in any cell-mediated immune response, including Ab-mediated FcR activation (i.e., ADCC). An activated complement response thereby has the potential to act synergistically with ADCC, especially by the C5a-dependent upregulation of activating FcγRIII on macrophages (34, 35).

MANIPULATING AB-MEDIATED COMPLEMENT RESPONSES

Many of the MAbs already in clinical use do not seem to exploit the full potential of complement. However, since most of the applied Abs are of the IgG1 isotype that has the potential to activate complement, and has been shown to do so in vitro, their clinical efficiency may be improved by providing the proper conditions for a complement response development, as suggested before (31). The substantial amount of experience within CDC and complement initiation should provide approaches to strategically manipulate the complement system to improve the efficacy of immunotherapies, either by improving CDC or by providing synergistic effects between CDC and ADCC. Different approaches can be applied, as briefly outlined below.

Increasing Complement Response

Since Ab density is an important parameter for proper complement activation, choosing the right conserved epitope or introducing a cocktail of MAbs with different epitope specificities may not only avoid escape variants of the targeted pathogen but also result in improved complement effector functions in addition to potential effects of neutralizing properties (19, 36). In general, simulating a controlled pool of polyclonal Abs is believed to have several beneficial roles in terms of broader specificity, potency, and robustness and may target groups of infectious agents that are common for specific diseases or exposures (19, 36). The prevalence of infectious diseases is commonly increased in the case of a dysfunctional or immature immune system, and the effector functions expected to accompany Ab therapies are similarly compromised. Immune function assessment and coadministration of complement sources or adjuvants could therefore be necessary to achieve expected drug effects (7).

A central property of the complement system is its fast-acting nature. Due to its efficient amplification, a response rapidly develops and exerts its function. Within a relatively short period, the plasma becomes drained for native complement proteins, and the constant activity of the nonconsumed regulatory proteins ensures down-regulation of the response. Indeed, in the case of rituximab infusions against chronic lymphocytic leukemia (CLL), the least-abundant complement plasma protein, C2, is rapidly consumed and is the limiting factor of rituximab cell-killing efficiency (37). The same group demonstrated that boosting the rituximab-initiated complement response by administering a secondary Ab toward cell-bound C3b and its breakdown products greatly enhanced C3b coating (38). Based on these findings, it was recently shown that the effect of rituximab on five patients with CLL was markedly improved when coadministered with fresh plasma as a source of uncleaved complement proteins (39). It should be noted that CLL is well associated with low levels of complement proteins, especially classical pathway components and properdin. However, since long, repetitive infusions are not uncommon, consumption of complement proteins is likely to occur, resulting in a reduced therapeutic efficiency and increased risk of infectious diseases. Furthermore, most MAb therapies target extravascular spaces, where complement protein levels may be reduced or unevenly distributed compared to plasma. This may explain why many in vitro experiments performed in serum show high complement contributions, whereas in vivo data are less convincing. If target cells are located in extravascular spaces, it is therefore imperative to evaluate the availability of complement proteins and potentially consider coadministration of a complement protein source at the target site (37, 40).

Reducing Negative Effects from Complement

The mechanism of action of MAb therapies is likely to be a combination of ADCC, CDC, and CDCC (Fig. 2). However, the exact nature of their interaction, i.e., whether it is synergistic, additive, or antagonistic, remains uncertain (27, 41). Activated complement components would be expected to have positive effects of the recruitment and activation of phagocytes necessary for ADCC, but recent studies with cancer MAb therapies have questioned the positive contributions from complement. In an in vitro study (42), the activation of complement was found to inhibit NK cell-mediated cytotoxicity brought on by ADCC. This inhibition was due to a C3b-dependent interference of the binding of NK cells to rituximab, thus preventing the activation of NK cells. In the same study, the depletion of C3b components in an in vivo model was able to enhance the ability of rituximab-coated target cells to activate human NK cells and improve the efficacy of the MAb. Yet another study showed that the presence of C5a in the tumor microenvironment could suppress the antitumor CD8$^+$ T-cell-mediated response, which would normally recruit myeloid-derived suppressor cells into tumors and augment T-cell-directed suppressive abilities (43). The same study showed that deficiency of complement in mice was coupled with a hindered tumor growth, a suppression that was comparable to pharmacologically blocking C5a receptors (C5aRs). The inhibition of C5aR signaling was also associated with enhanced CD8$^+$ T cell antitumor response (43). Since CDC depends on late-stage complement development, attempts that block complement activation or deficiency of complement proteins in specific target tissues or in some individuals is likely to reduce ADCC without gaining any effect from CDC. Accordingly, complete blocking of complement may not be a plausible approach in antimicrobial therapies with Abs.

COMPLEMENT EVASIVE PROPERTIES OF PATHOGENS

Pathogens generally lack complement regulatory proteins and are susceptible to opsonization and complement attack. However, millions of years of evolution have allowed pathogenic microorganisms to develop sophisticated strategies to dampen or even overcome complement activity (1, 44, 45, 46). Some have successfully employed surface strategies to mask or camouflage antigenic components on their surfaces, while others can express surface proteins to bind to, recruit, or mimic host complement regulators (44). It is not unusual for pathogens to apply several defense strategies, exploiting complement cascades at different stages (47). *Staphylococcus aureus* is an excellent example of a pathogen that can evade several different points of a complement attack by preventing activation, degrading opsonin C3b, and inhibiting C3 convertase, thereby preventing downstream complement effector responses (44). This pathogen also expresses staphylococcal protein A (SpA) with the ability to bind to the Fc fragments of IgGs, thereby reducing the FcR-mediated phagocytosis (48). Other mechanisms include the expression of adhesins by pathogens to anchor to host cell surfaces or to present invasin to mediate uptake into host cells (49).

All surface strategies serve the purpose of avoiding recognition, opsonization, and clearance by host complement response, which lead to the survival of pathogens in an otherwise immunocompetent host (4, 49). Over and above, mutating or new merging pathogenic microorganisms persist to accomplish new ways to counterstrike complement defense, presenting a real challenge for the host and the application for MAb treatments against certain infectious diseases (5).

Persisting malignant cells have the inherent ability to express high levels of endogenous membrane-bound complement regulators, including CD46, decay-accelerating factor, and CD59, which efficiently prevent complement amplification and MAC formation. They can further block complement activation by recruiting fluid-phase complement regulators, contributing to the evasion of complement surveillance that leads to progression in malignant growth (4). However, considering the success of CDC-dependent MAb treatments against malignant cells with upregulated complement regulators, it is plausible to speculate that a well-targeted complement activation may overcome the pathogen's immune evasive properties.

CONCLUSIONS AND FUTURE PERSPECTIVE

The complement system protects the host from pathogenic invaders in a very effective manner. Although defined as a part of the innate immune system, there is a large overlap area shared with the adaptive effector functions. Complement is able to induce inflammation responses that permit the functions of the adaptive system as well as stimulate B-cell-specific Ab production and differentiation of memory B cells. Likewise, target-bound Abs can act as pattern recognition molecules and activate complement. Further, it interacts dynamically with multiple systems, which highlights the complexity of both the biological system and the complement system. The poor understanding of this complexity has led to past failures in the pharmaceutical development in the field. A particular challenge lies in the in vitro/in vivo correlation, in which theory obtained from the linear and often well-controlled experimental environments fails to apply to in vivo performances, where multiple systems are at play. For example, it might be difficult to predict the biological response in tissues where certain effector proteins are dysregulated or in immunocompromised patients.

Our immune system is in constant battle with invading and opportunist pathogens. A lowering of this guard, for example, in immune-compromised individuals, could have consequences that might require pharmaceutical interventions. However, the present anti-infectious development is not advancing at the same pace as the rapid emerging strategies of pathogens to counterstrike both the immune system and the current broad-spectrum antibiotic treatments. On the other hand, particulate nanoparticles are receiving increasing attention to enhance the immunogenicity of subunit vaccines through both antigen protection and targeting to antigen-presenting cells as well as immunostimulation (50). The latter may involve the complement system (for instance, some complement activation products can induce B cell activation) or direct activation of the NALP3 inflammasome complex (apoptosis-associated speck-like protein and caspase 1 protease), which in turn cleave and activate the immunostimulatory cytokine interleukin 1β (51).

Ab treatment holds the potential to open a new approach to fight infectious diseases. Properties like direct targeting and selectivity, even for mutant strains, should be taken advantage of. However, issues such as efficiency and precision of diagnosis, cost of drug discovery, and the lack of comprehensive understanding of the mode of action of development candidates signify that much more attention is needed to succeed in building this new platform. When their potentials are fully explored, they would definitely provide a promising future for complement in Ab treatments.

ACKNOWLEDGMENTS

Financial support from the Danish Agency for Science, Technology, and Innovation (Det Strategiske Forskningsråd), reference 09-065746, is gratefully acknowledged.

Conflicts of interest: We declare no conflicts.

CITATION

Wibroe PP, Helvig SY, Moghimi SM. 2014. The role of complement in antibody therapy for infectious diseases. Microbiol Spectrum 2(2):AID-0015-2014.

REFERENCES

1. **Ricklin D, Hajishengallis G, Yang K, Lambris JD.** 2010. Complement: a key system for immune surveillance and homeostasis. *Nat Immunol* **11:**785–797.
2. **Carroll MC.** 2004. The complement system in regulation of adaptive immunity. *Nat Immunol* **5:**981–986.
3. **Mastellos D, Germenis AE, Lambris JD.** 2005. Complement: an inflammatory pathway fulfilling multiple roles at the interface of innate immunity and development. *Curr Drug Targets Inflamm Allergy* **4:**125–127.
4. **Markiewski MM, Nilsson B, Nilsson-Ekdahl K, Mollnes TE, Lambris JD.** 2007. Complement and coagulation: strangers or partners in crime? *Trends Immunol* **28:**184–192.
5. **Rittirsch D, Flierl MA, Ward PA.** 2008. Harmful molecular mechanisms in sepsis. *Nat Rev Immunol* **8:**776–787.
6. **Zipfel PF, Skerka C.** 2009. Complement regulators and inhibitory proteins. *Nat Rev Immunol* **9:**729–740.
7. **ter Meulen J.** 2011. Monoclonal antibodies in infectious diseases: clinical pipeline in 2011. *Infect Dis Clin N Am* **25:**789–802.
8. **Saylor C, Dadachova E, Casadevall A.** 2009. Monoclonal antibody-based therapies for microbial diseases. *Vaccine* **27**(Suppl 6):G38–G46.
9. **Krilov LR.** 2011. Respiratory syncytial virus disease: update on treatment and prevention. *Expert Rev Anti Infect Ther* **9:**27–32.
10. **Martínez I, Melero JA.** 1998. Enhanced neutralization of human respiratory syncytial virus by mixtures of monoclonal antibodies to the attachment (G) glycoprotein. *J Gen Virol* **79:**2215–2220.
11. **Moghimi SM, Hamad I.** 2008. Liposome-mediated triggering of complement cascade. *J Liposome Res* **18:**195–209.
12. **Murphy K, Travers P, Walport M.** 2008. *Janeway's Immunobiology*, 7th ed. Garland Science, New York, NY.
13. **Favoreel HW, Van de Walle GR, Nauwynck HJ, Pensaert MB.** 2003. Virus complement evasion strategies. *J Gen Virol* **84:**1–15.
14. **Ehrnthaller C, Ignatius A, Gebhard F, Huber-Lang M.** 2011. New insights of an old defense system: structure, function, and clinical relevance of the complement system. *Mol Med* **17:**317–329.
15. **Sellborn A, Andersson M, Hedlund J, Andersson J, Berglin M, Elwing H.** 2005. Immune complement activation on polystyrene and silicon dioxide surfaces. Impact of reversible IgG adsorption. *Mol Immunol* **42:**569–574.
16. **Pedersen MB, Zhou XF, Larsen EKU, Sorensen US, Kjems J, Nygaard JV, Nyengaard JR, Meyer RL, Boesen T, Vorup-Jensen T.** 2010. Curvature of synthetic and natural surfaces is an important target feature in classical pathway complement activation. *J Immunol* **184:**1931–1945.
17. **Salfeld JG.** 2007. Isotype selection in antibody engineering. *Nat Biotechnol* **25:**1369–1372.
18. **Beenhouwer DO, Yoo EM, Lai C-W, Rocha MA, Morrison SL.** 2007. Human immunoglobulin G2 (IgG2) and IgG4, but not IgG1 or IgG3,

protect mice against *Cryptococcus neoformans* infection. *Infect Immun* **75**:1424–1435.

19. **Berry JD, Gaudet RG.** 2011. Antibodies in infectious diseases: polyclonals, monoclonals and niche biotechnology. *Nat Biotechnol* **28**:489–501.

20. **Roos A, Bouwman LH, van Gijlswijk-Janssen DJ, Faber-Krol MC, Stahl GL, Daha MR.** 2001. Human IgA activates the complement system via the mannan-binding lectin pathway. *J Immunol* **167**:2861–2868.

21. **Janoff EN, Fasching C, Orenstein JM, Rubins JB, Opstad NL, Dalmasso AP.** 1999. Killing of *Streptococcus pneumoniae* by capsular polysaccharide-specific polymeric IgA, complement, and phagocytes. *J Clin Investig* **104**:1139–1147.

22. **Hiemstra PS, Gorter A, Stuurman ME, Van Es LA, Daha MR.** 1987. Activation of the alternative pathway of complement by human serum IgA. *Eur J Immunol* **17**:321–326.

23. **Boackle RJ, Nguyen QL, Leite RS, Yang X, Vesely J.** 2006. Complement-coated antibody-transfer (CCAT); serum IgA1 antibodies intercept and transport C4 and C3 fragments and preserve IgG1 deployment (PGD). *Mol Immunol* **43**:236–245.

24. **van Egmond M, van Spriel AB, Vermeulen H, Huls G, van Garderen E, van de Winkel JG.** 2001. Enhancement of polymorphonuclear cell-mediated tumor cell killing on simultaneous engagement of fcgammaRI (CD64) and fcalphaRI (CD89). *Cancer Res* **61**:4055–4060.

25. **Jarvis GA, Griffiss JM.** 1991. Human IgA1 blockade of IgG-initiated lysis of *Neisseria meningitidis* is a function of antigen-binding fragment binding to the polysaccharide capsule. *J Immunol* **147**:1962–1967.

26. **Griffiss JM.** 1975. Bactericidal activity of meningococcal antisera. Blocking by IgA of lytic antibody in human convalescent sera. *J Immunol* **114**:1779–1784.

27. **Weiner LM, Surana R, Wang S.** 2010. Monoclonal antibodies: versatile platforms for cancer immunotherapy. *Nat Rev Immunol* **10**:317–327.

28. **Scott AM, Wolchok JD, Old LJ.** 2012. Antibody therapy of cancer. *Nat Rev Cancer* **12**:278–287.

29. **Wright SD, Silverstein SC.** 1983. Receptors for C3b and C3bi promote phagocytosis but not the release of toxic oxygen from human phagocytes. *J Exp Med* **158**:2016–2023.

30. **Zhou X, Hu W, Qin X.** 2008. The role of complement in the mechanism of action of rituximab for B-cell lymphoma: implications for therapy. *Oncologist* **13**:954–966.

31. **Gelderman KA, Tomlinson S, Ross GD, Gorter A.** 2004. Complement function in mAb-mediated cancer immunotherapy. *Trends Immunol* **25**:158–164.

32. **Vetvicka V, Thornton BP, Ross GD.** 1996. Soluble beta-glucan polysaccharide binding to the lectin site of neutrophil or natural killer cell complement receptor type 3 (CD11b/CD18) generates a primed state of the receptor capable of mediating cytotoxicity of iC3b-opsonized target cells. *J Clin Investig* **98**:50–61.

33. **Klos A, Tenner AJ, Johswich KO, Ager RR, Reis ES, Kohl J.** 2009. The role of the anaphylatoxins in health and disease. *Mol Immunol* **46**:2753–2766.

34. **Shushakova N, Skokowa J, Schulman J, Baumann U, Zwirner J, Schmidt RE, Gessner JE.** 2002. C5a anaphylatoxin is a major regulator of activating versus inhibitory FcgammaRs in immune complex-induced lung disease. *J Clin Investig* **110**:1823–1830.

35. **Schmidt RE, Gessner JE.** 2005. Fc receptors and their interaction with complement in autoimmunity. *Immunol Lett* **100**:56–67.

36. **Logtenberg T.** 2007. Antibody cocktails: next-generation biopharmaceuticals with improved potency. *Trends Biotechnol* **25**:390–394.

37. **Kennedy AD, Beum PV, Solga MD, DiLillo DJ, Lindorfer MA, Hess CE, Densmore JJ, Williams ME, Taylor RP.** 2004. Rituximab infusion promotes rapid complement depletion and acute CD20 loss in chronic lymphocytic leukemia. *J Immunol* **172**:3280–3288.

38. **Kennedy AD, Solga MD, Schuman TA, Chi AW, Lindorfer MA, Sutherland WM, Foley PL, Taylor RP.** 2003. An anti-C3b(i) mAb enhances complement activation, C3b(i) deposition, and killing of CD20+ cells by rituximab. *Blood* **101**:1071–1079.

39. **Klepfish A, Gilles L, Ioannis K, Rachmilewitz EA, Eliezer R, Schattner A, Ami S.** 2009. Enhancing the action of rituximab in chronic lymphocytic leukemia by adding fresh frozen plasma: complement/rituximab interactions and clinical results in refractory CLL. *Ann N Y Acad Sci* **1173**:865–873.

40. **Wang S-Y, Veeramani S, Racila E, Cagley J, Fritzinger DC, Vogel C-W, St John W, Weiner GJ.** 2009. Depletion of the C3 component of complement enhances the ability of rituximab-coated target cells to activate human NK cells and improves the efficacy of monoclonal antibody therapy in an in vivo model. *Blood* **114**: 5322–5330.

41. **Wang S-Y, Weiner G.** 2008. Complement and cellular cytotoxicity in antibody therapy of cancer. *Expert Opin Biol Ther* **8**:759–768.

42. **Wang SY, Veeramani S, Racila E, Cagley J, Fritzinger DC, Vogel CW, St John W, Weiner GJ.** 2009. Depletion of the C3 component of complement enhances the ability of rituximab-coated target cells to activate human NK cells and

improves the efficacy of monoclonal antibody therapy in an in vivo model. *Blood* **114:**5322–5330.

43. **Markiewski MM, DeAngelis RA, Benencia F, Ricklin-Lichtsteiner SK, Koutoulaki A, Gerard C, Coukos G, Lambris JD.** 2008. Modulation of the antitumor immune response by complement. *Nat Immunol* **9:**1225–1235.

44. **Sarma JV, Ward PA.** 2011. The complement system. *Cell Tissue Res* **343:**227–235.

45. **Rooijakkers SH, van Strijp JA.** 2007. Bacterial complement evasion. *Mol Immunol* **44:**23–32.

46. **Lambris JD, Ricklin D, Geisbrecht BV.** 2008. Complement evasion by human pathogens. *Nat Rev Microbiol* **6:**132–142.

47. **Szebeni J.** 2004. *The Complement System.* Kluwer Academic Publisher, Boston, MA.

48. **Peterson PK, Verhoef J, Sabath LD, Quie PG.** 1977. Effect of protein A on staphylococcal opsonization. *Infect Immun* **15:**760–764.

49. **Finlay BB, McFadden G.** 2006. Anti-immunology: evasion of the host immune system by bacterial and viral pathogens. *Cell* **124:**767–782.

50. **Moghimi SM.** 2009. The innate immune responses, adjuvants and delivery systems, p 113–127. *In* Jorgensen L, Nielsen HM (ed), *Delivery Technologies for Biopharmaceuticals. Peptides, Proteins, Nucleic Acids and Vaccines.* Wiley, Chichester, United Kingdom.

51. **Li H, Willingham SB, Ting JP, Re F.** 2008. Cutting edge: inflammasome activation by alum and alum's adjuvant effects are mediated by NLRP3. *J Immunol* **181:**17–21.

Immunoglobulin E and Allergy: Antibodies in Immune Inflammation and Treatment

5

SOPHIA N. KARAGIANNIS,[1] PANAGIOTIS KARAGIANNIS,[1]
DEBRA H. JOSEPHS,[1] LOUISE SAUL,[1] AMY E. GILBERT,[1] NADINE UPTON,[2]
and HANNAH J. GOULD[2]

IMMUNOLOGICAL MECHANISMS OF ALLERGIC DISEASES AND THE ROLE OF IGE ANTIBODIES

Clinical Perspective on Allergic Inflammation

Allergic inflammation, caused by development of an allergen-induced immune response, is largely driven via immunoglobulin E (IgE)-dependent mechanisms. It manifests clinically as asthma, rhinoconjunctivitis (more commonly known as hay fever), allergic skin inflammation (the main example of which is atopic dermatitis), food allergy, urticaria, and/or anaphylaxis, with several known disease variants caused by different underlying cellular and molecular mechanisms (1). Increased levels of circulating IgE, allergen-specific IgE reactivity profiles measured with radioallergosorbent tests and positive skin prick tests for specific allergens,

[1]Cutaneous Medicine and Immunotherapy Unit, St. John's Institute of Dermatology, Division of Genetics and Molecular Medicine & NIHR Biomedical Research Centre at Guy's and St. Thomas's Hospitals and King's College London, King's College London School of Medicine, Guy's Hospital, King's College London, London SE1 9RT, United Kingdom; [2]Randall Division of Cell and Molecular Biophysics, Division of Asthma, Allergy, and Lung Biology, MRC and Asthma UK Centre for Allergic Mechanisms of Asthma, King's College London, New Hunt's House, Guy's Campus, London SE1 1UL, United Kingdom.

Antibodies for Infectious Diseases
Edited by James E. Crowe, Jr., Diana Boraschi, and Rino Rappuoli
© 2015 American Society for Microbiology, Washington, DC
doi:10.1128/microbiolspec.AID-0006-2012

together with auxiliary ex vivo and in vitro mast cell and basophil activation functional readouts, support the importance of IgE antibodies in the clinical manifestation of allergies (2, 3). Allergic inflammation can be local (that is, within the target organ), as is the case for allergic rhinoconjunctivitis and allergic asthma, or systemic, as is the case for anaphylaxis. The etiology of allergic immune responses has been shown to be influenced by several factors, including genetic susceptibility (4), route of exposure, dose of the allergen, and in some cases, structural characteristics of the allergen (5).

The allergic inflammatory cascade is thought to have evolved from the natural immune defenses to parasite and worm infections. This response can provide swift protection against these organisms but also participates in wound healing following tissue damage accrued as a result of the infection or accumulation of toxins. The same inflammatory cascades, originally evolved to neutralize invading parasites, are activated in response to innocuous antigens such as house dust mite and pollen proteins in the context of allergic diseases, triggering mast cell degranulation and eosinophil inflammation to the sites of allergen challenge. Furthermore, acute protective immune responses to infection evolve into chronic inflammatory cascades with long and persistent exposure to allergens. The consequences are persistent inflammation, tissue remodeling, and undesirable pathologies (6).

IgE Antibodies Activate Immune Responses in the Presence of Allergens

The discovery and characterization of IgE, culminating in the independent descriptions of this class of antibody by Ishizaka et al. and Johansson and Bennich, arguably represents the most crucial advance in our understanding of the immunological basis of allergic disorders (7, 8). Allergic inflammation is characterized by IgE-dependent activation of mast cells and an infiltration of inflammatory cells to sites of allergen challenge, orchestrated by increased numbers of activated CD4$^+$ T helper type 2 (Th2) lymphocytes.

Production of allergen-specific IgE requires that allergens are taken up by dendritic cells (DCs), monocytes, B cells, or other antigen presenting cells (APCs), which, in the presence of cytokines such as interleukin-4 (IL-4) or IL-13 present the processed antigens to cognate naive T cells that then acquire a Th2 cell phenotype (9). Th2 cells then engage cognate B cells through both B cell major histocompatibility complex class II and costimulatory molecules and secrete IL-4 and IL-13, inducing B cells to undergo class-switch recombination, resulting in the variable, diverse, and joining segments that were initially linked to another constant (C) region in the immunoglobulin heavy chain locus to instead be linked to the Cε region (10). Class-switch recombination can also be induced by IL-4 and/or IL-13 derived from cells other than Th2 cells, which may include mast cells and basophils (11). Allergen sensitization was previously thought to occur primarily in lymphoid germinal centers; however, IgE-producing B cells that undergo clonal selection and affinity maturation can also be generated locally at sites of antigen challenge such as the respiratory mucosa, gastrointestinal tract, and lymph nodes of individuals with food allergy, seasonal or perennial allergic rhinitis, or atopic or nonatopic asthma (11).

A Glance at IgE Receptors

IgE antibodies have two known cell surface receptors, FcεRI (the high-affinity receptor) and CD23 (otherwise known as FcεRII, the low-affinity receptor) (10). Each Fcε receptor recognizes a distinct epitope located on opposite sites of the Cε3 domain of the IgE constant region, and binding of one receptor to this domain prevents binding of the other to IgE (12). IgE antibodies also recognize the IgE- and FcεRI-binding protein galectin-3 (10).

FcεRI, which has affinity for IgE in the nanomolar range (K_a = 10^8 to 10^{10} M^{-1}) is expressed on basophils and mast cells as an αβγ2 tetramer and on Langerhans cells, myeloid DCs, plasmacytoid DCs, monocytes, and eosinophils as an αγ2 trimer (13). The α subunit has two extracellular immunoglobulin domains, which form the binding site of IgE to the receptor, and regulates movement of the receptor from the endoplasmic reticulum, where the subunits of the receptor are assembled to the cell surface membrane via an immunoreceptor tyrosine-based activation motif. The γ chain which is shared with FcγRs is necessary for receptor assembly and cell surface expression, while the β subunit is thought to enhance receptor functions and to also be responsible for enhanced receptor (αβγ2 tetramer) expression on the surface of mast cells and basophils. The downstream signaling events that culminate in degranulation in mast cells and basophils are mediated by the associated β and γ subunits.

The low-affinity receptor, CD23, can be induced on a broad range of immune cells, such as activated B cells, activated monocytes and macrophages, eosinophils, natural killer T cells, T cells, follicular DCs, and platelets, and also on nonimmune cells, such as airway epithelial cells and smooth muscle cells (10, 14, 15). Unlike the high-affinity receptor, the low-affinity receptor, CD23, displays a micromolar affinity ($K_a = 10^7$ to 10^8 M^{-1}) for IgE as a monomer, but trimeric fragments are released from the cell membrane by metalloproteases and bind with 10 nM avidity (16). The CD23a splice variant is exclusively expressed on B cells activated by antigen, and it plays a key role in antigen endocytosis, processing, and presentation and in the regulation of IgE synthesis. Expression of the CD23b form can be triggered by IL-4 on a variety of effector cells, including B cells and macrophages. Engagement of CD23 by IgE-antigen complexes is thought to induce nitric oxide synthase and the release of cytokines such as tumor necrosis factor alpha (TNF-α) by macrophages, and these events have been reported to participate in phagocytosis and killing of parasites (17, 18).

Galectin-3, the beta-galactoside-binding lectin which recognizes both IgE Fc and FcεRI, exists in a secreted form and is also stored intracellularly. Its expression is associated with activated IgE immune cells such as monocytes/macrophages, DCs, mast cells, and eosinophils and also with B cells following stimulation by IL-4 and CD40-CD40L engagement (19).

IgE Effector Cells and Their Roles in IgE Responses

Mast Cells: Hallmarks of IgE-Driven Allergic Response

The hallmark of an acute allergic response, mediated by allergen-IgE-FcεRI complexes cross-linking FcεRI on the surface of mast cells, is immediate (type I) hypersensitivity. Cross-linking can occur when the targeted antigen is multivalent, as two or more receptors need to be engaged to activate the ensuing signaling cascade, although the presence of cytokinergic IgEs capable of activating mast cells in the absence of multivalent antigen have been reported (20). Cross-linking of IgE-FcεRI complexes on the mast cell surface by allergens leads, within minutes, to the so-called "early phase" of the allergic response, involving mast cell degranulation and the rapid release of preformed vasoactive amines (mainly histamine), lipid mediators (such as prostaglandin D, platelet-activating factor, leukotriene C4 [LTC4], LTD4, and LTE4), chemokines (CXC-chemokine ligand 8, CXC-chemokine ligand 10, CC-chemokine ligand 2 [CCL2], CCL4, and CCL5), and cytokines (such as IL-4, IL-5, and IL-13). Mast cell activation plays a key role in generating the symptoms of allergy; the cytokines and chemokines liberated in this early phase initiate the "late phase," which peaks some hours later and involves the recruitment and activation of inflammatory cells (neutrophils, followed by eosinophils, monocytes, and lymphocytes) at sites sensitive to allergen. Similarly, but without overt symptoms, allergens activate the IgE-sensitized APCs, which in turn promote de novo immunoglobulin production by B cells, thereby maintaining mast cell and APC sensitization (10).

APCs Trigger Th2 Responses and IgE Inflammation

Th2 cells are recruited and activated at the sites of allergic inflammation. A key research focus aims to understand the mechanisms by which allergens regulate Th2 cells through antigen presentation by professional APCs such as DCs. It has been proposed that allergic inflammation is initiated following allergen-epithelial cell contact, leading to the promotion of Th2 immunity via the production of a number of cytokines. Of key importance among these is epithelial cell-derived thymic stromal lymphopoietin, which conditions DCs to favor Th2 induction (21), while other epithelial cell-derived cytokines, namely IL-25 and IL-33, are also capable of inducing and maintaining Th2 immunity (22, 23). In addition, by secreting the chemokines CCL17 and CCL22, DCs possess definitive roles in the recruitment and activation of Th2 cells, while other cells secrete IL-4 which is necessary for Th2 cell differentiation (24). There is increasing evidence that basophils express FcεRI, major histocompatibility complex class II, and costimulatory molecules CD80/CD86, may participate in antigen recognition and processing, and can induce Th2 cell differentiation through the release of IL-4 (25, 26, 27). Other cells may also possess antigen presentation properties and can also secrete Th2 cytokines when activated by IL-25 and IL-33; these include mast cells, macrophages, eosinophils, and natural helper cells (28).

B Cells and CD23 Participate in Antigen Presentation

Allergen-IgE complexes bound to CD23 expressed by allergen-activated B cells can facilitate antigen presentation to T cells. The process of antigen presentation by way of CD23 is termed facilitated antigen presentation (FAP). The association between CD23 and HLA-DR in the cell membrane is involved in the trafficking of allergen-IgE-CD23 complexes to endosomes, where the allergen-derived peptides are loaded onto the HLA-DR molecules for presentation at the B-cell surface (29). An antigen-activated B cell expressing CD23 can simultaneously process unrelated antigens through FcRs and cause epitope spreading to other antigens. Indeed, CD23-mediated FAP is known to be as efficient as FcR-mediated antigen presentation by DCs (30), orders of magnitude more efficient than B-cell internalization via surface immunoglobulin (the BCR).

B cells in draining lymph nodes participate in allergic inflammation through IgE synthesis. However, they are also present in the respiratory mucosa, and their capacity to produce IgE locally in tissues has been demonstrated (31). Following exposure to allergens, production of IgE is triggered by key Th2 cytokines IL-4 and IL-13, with IL-9 participating by enhancing IgE synthesis in situ (32, 33). Regulatory functions have also been attributed to B cells through secretion of IL-10, but the role of different subsets of B cells in allergic diseases remains to be determined (6).

Monocytes and Eosinophils Mediate IgE Effector Functions and Tissue Remodeling

Monocytes and eosinophils are among the IgE effector cell types that are drawn to sites of allergic inflammation. IgE upregulates the expression of FcεRI, whereas IL-4 and IL-13 can stimulate the expression of CD23 by these cells. This in turn arms the cells for functions such as clearance of antigen-IgE complexes, and killing and phagocytosis of pathogens (for example, helminth parasites) and tumor cells that bear "foreign" antigens (34, 35). In carrying out their functions, monocytes and eosinophils inevitably also inflict some damage on bystander cells in the tissue. This side effect may ultimately contribute to tissue remodeling and exacerbates the symptoms of chronic asthma. The IgE-binding protein galectin-3, which is expressed by monocytes, has both IgE-dependent and IgE-independent proinflammatory activities in the allergic response. Its expression is elevated in peribronchial monocytes, and it is released into the extracellular space. It contributes to cell survival and activation and to the retention of cells in the extracellular matrix in allergic inflammation (10). Galectin-3 also enhances the hypersensitivity of mast cells and the phagocytic activity of monocytes, perhaps by cross-linking additional IgE and FcεRI molecules on these cells when they have engaged their specific targets. The pentameric molecule galectin-3 may by itself contribute through FcεRI to airway smooth muscle cell contractile responses and thus to airway hyperresponsiveness and remodeling in asthma.

Interactions Between Allergens, IgE, and FcεRI Trigger Hypersensitivity Responses

The high-affinity IgE receptor, FcεRI, is of primary interest to researchers investigating allergy, since its activation through engagement of IgE-multimeric antigen complexes mediates allergic reactions and could in some instances trigger anaphylactoid responses (36). Disrupting IgE-FcεRI interactions is expected to reduce IgE-mediated allergic responses and may result in loss of allergic inflammatory cascades, including anaphylactic functions. Mice lacking FcεRI showed normal development and differentiation of mast cells, B cells, and T cells, as well as a normal level of expression of the low-affinity IgE receptor, CD23 (37). However, these mice were resistant to systemic and cutaneous anaphylaxis induced by intravenous and subcutaneous injection of allergen-specific IgE and the allergen shortly afterwards. These data demonstrated that the interaction between IgE and the FcεRI could be interrupted to prevent escalation of the allergic response.

Upon multivalent antigen-IgE complex binding to the receptor, cross-linked FcεRI is mobilized in lipid rafts, where downstream signaling events potentiated by the associated β and γ chains activate phosphorylation by Src kinases (38), leading to degranulation, release of proinflammatory mediators, and the onset of allergic responses. In mast cells, these events are mediated through activation of RhoGTPases and mitogen-activated protein kinase pathways (39, 40). As well as the activation of signaling cascades to promote degranulation, the receptor also has sequences which interact with the actin cytoskeleton and microtubules, initiating signaling cascades that are calcium dependent and calcium independent, respectively (41, 42).

The central role of FcεRI signaling in triggering mast cell activation renders this receptor an attractive target for therapeutic approaches, which include neutralizing monoclonal antibodies.

Allergen-Specific IgG Antibodies Can Trigger Hypersensitivity Responses in Murine Models

IgE antibodies can mediate allergies and anaphylactic reactions, and several cell types have been described to be involved in these processes; among them are mast cells, basophils, and macrophages, which express Fcε receptors, and also neutrophils, which do not express Fcε receptors. Interestingly, studies with mice have demonstrated that effector cells are not exclusively activated by the combination of IgE, its high-affinity receptor, and antigens and that IgG antibodies can trigger cell activation and degranulation which can lead to anaphylactoid responses. It has been reported that active systemic anaphylaxis (ASA) can be induced through activation of FcγRs in vivo via IgE-independent effector mechanisms in mice (43, 44). Human neutrophils transferred into mice that lack active IgG Fc receptors on mouse immune cells were described to restore ASA. FcγRIIA and FcγRIIIB are expressed on human neutrophils, but only FcγRIIA can bind mouse IgG, indicating that this receptor was responsible for restored ASA after human neutrophil transfer into mice (45, 46). In support of the role of FcγRIIA in anaphylactic reactions, a recent study using an FcγRIIA transgenic mouse model demonstrated that induction of FcγRIIA engagement and signaling was sufficient to trigger active and passive anaphylaxis as well as airway inflammation. Additionally, blocking FcγRIIA in the absence of IgE abolished the reactions induced by IgG antibodies in vivo (47). Further investigations revealed that IgG1 induced passive systemic anaphylaxis by activating basophils, whereas IgG2 induced passive systemic anaphylaxis via neutrophils, while ASA depended on monocytes/macrophages or neutrophils and not on mast cells and basophils (47, 48).

Thus, emerging evidence in murine models suggests that IgG and FcγR complexes contribute to allergic and anaphylactoid processes, although the precise requirements and pathways involved need to be elucidated.

IGE ANTIBODIES IN INFECTIOUS DISEASES

IgE Mechanisms of Protection in Parasitic Infections

Besides their critical role in allergy, IgE antibodies play a key physiological role in immunity against multicellular parasitic infections by a number of different mechanisms and via a number of IgE receptor-expressing cell types (49). The first in vivo evidence that IgE antibodies could be an essential component of the protective immunity against parasites was provided by passive transfer of monoclonal IgE antibodies directed against schistosomes (50). In this study, a rat monoclonal IgE antibody raised against *Schistosoma mansoni* afforded a significant level of protection against a challenge infection with *S. mansoni* when passively transferred into naive recipient rats. Furthermore, in another study, induction of resistance to infection by adoptive transfer of eosinophils or platelets bearing IgE indicated that the presence of IgE on these effector cells was crucial (51).

Subsequently, support for a role of IgE in parasite immunity was found when it was demonstrated that human eosinophils, platelets, and macrophages could harness IgE in vitro to mediate cytotoxicity and phagocytosis of *Schistosoma mansoni* or *Leishmania major* via FcεRI and CD23, respectively (17, 18, 52). These observations were subsequently established to be relevant to human immunity when epidemiological studies with *Schistosoma haematobium* provided evidence that host protection against reinfection in *S. haematobium*-infected populations was associated with high levels of parasite-specific IgE (53), and subsequently, IgE antibodies against *Schistosoma mansoni* were shown to positively predict resistance against reinfection with this blood fluke (54).

More recently, studies have demonstrated evidence that IgE antibodies are capable of activating a different cell type, namely mast cells to induce elimination of parasites via the release of toxic granules (55). *Trichinella spiralis* infection induces intestinal mastocytosis and heightened IgE responses, and elimination of this parasite requires expulsion of the adult worms from the gut and destruction of the larval cysts deposited in the muscles (56). In IgE-sufficient animals, intense deposition of IgE around the necrotic larval cysts was demonstrated with associated accelerated removal of worms from the intestine and a reduction in the viability of larval parasites in muscle (56). Indeed, *T. spiralis* infection drove a marked splenic mastocytosis and elevated serum levels of mouse mast cell protease-1 (MMCP-1), consistent with a systemic expansion of mast cells driven by the parasite. This mast cell increase was dramatically attenuated in IgE$^{-/-}$ mice, implicating IgE antibodies in this mast cell protection from parasitic infections. Furthermore, protective roles for mast cells during *T. spiralis* infection have also been observed using mast cell-deficient mice and by antibody inhibition of the mast cell marker, c-Kit (56).

Hyper-IgE Syndrome and Sensitivity to Infections

Elevated serum IgE is a major hallmark of hyper-IgE syndrome (HIES), a rare primary immunodeficiency disease. Common clinical manifestations include eczema and skin abscesses, often described as "cold boils" (57). HIES is clinically subdivided into autosomal dominant HIES (AD-HIES) and autosomal recessive HIES (AR-HIES). AD-HIES is associated with additional somatic abnormalities of the vascular, connective tissue, and skeletal systems, whereas AR-HIES is limited to skin conditions, including eczema, and is frequently more severe (58). HIES is further classified according to underlying mutations in key proteins involved in intracellular signaling networks, namely STAT3 and DOCK8. Dominant negative mutations in STAT3 are more frequent in AD-HIES (59) and DOCK8 mutations are more frequent in AR-HIES (60, 61), which may be directly related to the clinical and underlying immunological differences observed. In terms of allergy, patients with DOCK8 mutations frequently suffer from symptoms of atopic disease such as asthma (62). It has been suggested that despite elevated serum IgE being a feature of both forms of HIES, differences in mechanisms of IgE regulation may be apparent. Xiong et al. suggested that affinity maturation pathways of IgE-producing cells may differ between atopic and nonatopic HIES patients, and such investigation would be very informative (63).

Recurrent *Staphylococcus aureus* infections in the lungs and skin is common in HIES and, to a lesser degree, *Haemophilus influenzae* and *Streptococcus pneumoniae* infections (58). It has been suggested that increased susceptibility to infection in AD-HIES is a direct consequence of STAT3 mutations (59, 64). STAT3 regulates multiple families of cytokines, including IL-6, IL-21, IL-22, and IL-23, which are involved in the generation of Th17 cells (65, 66). Th17 cells are essential for clearance of bacterial and fungal infections via induction and expansion of neutrophilic and antimicrobial responses (67). Impaired Th17 immune responses are a likely explanation for recurrent infection in AD-HIES (68).

The precise role, if any, of IgE in recurrent infections in HIES is unknown. It is likely that elevated serum IgE in nonatopic HIES patients is simply a marker of deregulated immune responses, with a dominating Th2 lineage driving the generation of IgE cells. In addition, impaired STAT3 induction of IL-21, a critical negative regulator of IgE class switching and B-cell death, is evident in animal models of AD-HIES (69) and may largely contribute to the associated high serum IgE levels observed in patients with HIES. As allergy and asthma are common in patients with DOCK8 mutations, the role of allergen-specific IgE may be more prominent in both the underlying pathogenesis of AR-HIES and its role in recurrent infections. Recent reports demonstrate that in nasal polyps from patients with chronic rhinosinusitis, which are frequently associated with *Staphylococcus aureus* infections, ongoing local receptor revision and class switching to IgE occurs (70). It is possible that such events occur during *Staphylococcus aureus* infection in AR-HIES, which could suggest a mechanism of interplay between infection and allergy in AR-HIES.

Current strategies to prevent recurrent *Staphylococcus aureus* infection in HIES involve administration of antibiotics and regular steroid treatment (58). Treatment of a patient with HIES with omalizumab, an anti-IgE antibody that blocks binding of circulating IgE to its Fc receptors on effector cells, resulted in significant clinical improvement (71). This report indicates that targeting IgE in AR-HIES may prove to be a beneficial alternative to current treatment strategies.

Virus-Induced IgE Antibodies

Multiple reports demonstrate that viral infection can induce IgE production. Infection of human tonsil B cells with measles virus induced germ line epsilon expression (72), which suggests that direct viral infection triggers IgE class switch recombination. It has been suggested that virus-induced activation of B-cell antiviral protein kinase R drives virus-induced class switching to IgE, via cellular detection of viral double-stranded RNA (73).

In allergic disease, viral infection may increase production of allergen-specific IgE antibodies and so increase susceptibility to allergen-induced IgE reactions such as mast cell degranulation. In atopic asthma, respiratory viral infections induce over 80% of asthma exacerbations, and 60% of these are strains of rhinovirus (74, 75), also known as the "common cold virus." The risk of hospitalization is greatest in asthmatics infected with rhinovirus who are both sensitized and have been exposed to allergen (76, 77), indicating an additive effect of viral infection on underlying allergic inflammatory reactions. In addition, serum levels of total IgE (78) and dust mite IgE (79) are elevated during rhinovirus infection in atopic asthmatics, which suggests that rhinovirus infection increases susceptibility to IgE-mediated reactions. The precise mechanisms for how in vivo rhinovirus infection increases production of IgE are unknown; however, an advanced understanding of rhinovirus-induced inflammation has generated logical hypotheses. Both in vitro and in vivo rhinovirus infection enhance Th2-mediated airway inflammation in asthma (80, 81, 83). It is possible that rhinovirus-induced inflammation drives germinal center reactions within the bronchial mucosa. Local germinal center reactions could generate B cells within the lungs to class switch to IgE and induce differentiation into IgE-secreting plasma cells. It is possible that this excessive local production of IgE during rhinovirus infection could spill over into the circulation, giving rise to the detected increase in serum IgE during infection in asthma. In 1998, Rager et al. demonstrated that infection of Ramos B cell line with rhinovirus 14 and 16 strains (RV14 and RV16) induced germ line epsilon expression (73). Whether in vivo rhinovirus infection induces IgE class switching or B-cell proliferation and differentiation into IgE plasma cells would be informative.

The role of respiratory syncytial virus (RSV) in the development of asthma and allergies in children has been well established (84). Children with recurrent RSV infections developed high titers of serum IgE and tested positive with allergen skin prick tests (85). The risk of developing asthma was significantly greater in these children, highlighting RSV as a major risk factor for the development of allergic asthma. RSV has been shown to induce production of RSV-specific IgE (86). Dakhama et al. demonstrated a positive correlation between RSV-IgE production and severity of airway hyperresponsiveness in mice (86).

Investigation into mechanisms of virus-induced IgE antibodies in allergic disease will prove very informative and could aid the development of novel preventative therapies for both virus-induced asthma exacerbations and the development of asthma.

ANTIBODIES IN THE TREATMENT OF ALLERGIES

Recombinant Antibodies Targeting IgE Interactions with Fcε Receptors

Designing therapeutic antibodies targeting IgE represents an approach for the treatment of patients with allergies. The primary aim of anti-IgE therapy is to reduce the amount of circulating IgE in patients and to neutralize the interactions between free IgE and immune cells responsible for mediating allergic reactions (87). One approach entails blocking free IgE from binding to its Fc receptors expressed on immune effector cells, such as basophils and mast cells, to prevent the release of inflammatory mediators, such as histamines and tryptases, from these cells which lead to hypersensitivity. Another would be to downregulate the production of IgE by B cells.

IgE-Blocking Antibodies for Passive Immunotherapy: Omalizumab

There have been numerous anti-IgE antibodies in preclinical and clinical development, with omalizumab (Xolair) being the first licensed anti-IgE therapy approved for the treatment of allergic bronchial asthma in 2003 (88). Omalizumab represents an important breakthrough in the development of antibodies for anti-IgE immunotherapy in allergy. Omalizumab is a humanized IgG1 monoclonal antibody that recognizes an epitope in the Cϵ3 region of IgE, the IgE Fc region which contains the binding sites for both the high- and low-affinity IgE Fc receptors (10, 89). This anti-IgE antibody can block the binding of circulating IgE to both of its Fc receptors, which are expressed on the surfaces of various effector cells, thus preventing IgE-mediated allergic immune responses (Fig. 1).

Treatment with omalizumab also has been shown to result in downregulating the expression of FcϵRI on immune cells (Table 1) (90, 91, 92). Notably, omalizumab is not able to bind to IgE in the complex with its receptors, possibly due to allosteric inhibition. It was recently shown that engagement of IgE with omalizumab triggers a lower degree of bending in IgE compared to that adopted through recognition of FcϵRI, inducing a conformational change that is incompatible with FcϵRI recognition (93). Due to these properties, the antibody is not capable of cross-linking IgE already bound to receptors on the surfaces of mast cells and basophils, and therefore, any unwanted immune cell activation and release of inflammatory mediators is avoided (94). Examination of cross-linking is essential in the design of IgE immunotherapy to ameliorate the risk of any acute allergic reactions such as type 1 hypersensitivity in patients (Table 1).

Anti-IgE therapy has widespread applicability in asthma. Currently, omalizumab is being evaluated for the treatment of many other IgE-mediated allergic diseases, including atopic dermatitis, seasonal allergic rhinitis, food allergy, and urticaria (Table 2). Although discontinued for clinical development, due to partnership agreements rather than clinical utility, the anti-IgE antibody talizumab (TNX-901) demonstrated the ability to increase the sensitivity threshold to peanuts, supporting the use of anti-IgE therapy for some food allergies to prevent mast cell/basophil degranulation (95). Talizumab can also inhibit the presentation of allergens, since it was shown to block allergen-CD23 complex formation on the surface of B cells, and can prevent proliferation of allergen-specific T cells (96).

Antibodies Blocking CD23 Functions and B Cells

Another approach centers on targeting CD23 with the aim of regulating IgE production through blocking the functions of the low-affinity IgE receptor, CD23, on B cells. A prominent agent featuring this approach is primatized anti-CD23 macaque/human chimeric antibody, lumiliximab (IDEC-152), which was designed to modulate antigen presentation, reduce activation of Th2 responses, and hinder IgE production by B cells (97). This agent reached clinical evaluations for the treatment of allergic asthma, but it is now evaluated for use in hematological oncology indications such as chronic lymphocytic leukemia.

New anti-IgE antibodies are undergoing preclinical evaluations and development and include agents aimed at downregulating the production of IgE by B cells. One emerging strategy is the engineering of an antibody (8D6) which, like omalizumab, prevents the binding of free IgE to cell surface FcϵRI but additionally interacts with CD23-bound IgE

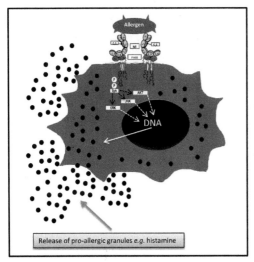 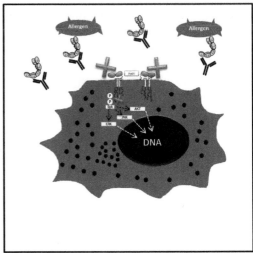

 IgE antibody

 Omalizumab

FIGURE 1 Omalizumab blocks IgE-mediated mast cell activation. The allergic response mediated by multivalent allergen-IgE-FcεRI complex formation on the surface of mast cells triggers cross-linking of FcεRI, leading to downstream signaling events potentiated by the β and γ chains (left). These entail phosphorylation (P) by Src kinases and cellular activation through RhoGTPases and mitogen-activated protein kinase pathways, leading to mast cell degranulation and the rapid release of a range of vasoactive amines (e.g., histamine), prostaglandins, leukotrienes, cytokines, and chemokines, inducing and maintaining allergic inflammatory responses. Omalizumab, a humanized IgG1 monoclonal antibody that recognizes an epitope in the Cε3 region of IgE, can block the binding of circulating IgE to FcεRI, sequestering free and allergen-bound IgE (right). These interactions prevent allergen-IgE-FcεRI complex formation on the surface of mast cells and interfere with the signaling cascades that trigger degranulation and the onset of IgE-mediated allergic inflammatory cascades. Syk, spleen tyrosine kinase; AKT, Ak strain thymoma serine/threonine-specific protein kinase; ERK, extracellular signal-regulated kinase; JNK, Jun N-terminal protein kinase; P, phosphorylation. doi:10.1128/microbiolspec. AID-0006-2012.f1

with the aim of also inhibiting IgE production on B cells, thereby controlling circulating IgE levels (98). Another approach encompasses an anti-IgE antibody, XmAb7195, with modified IgG Fc domains that feature increased affinity to the inhibitory FcγRIIB expressed on B cells and also the ability to suppress B-cell activation. Like omalizumab, this agent was recently reported to target the Cε3 domains of free IgE but to also cointeract with IgE in the complex with FcγRIIB on the surface of IgE-expressing B cells (99). This antibody was shown to suppress B-cell signaling and prevent maturation of B cells into IgE⁺ plasma cells, reducing

total IgE in circulation in vivo while neutralizing IgE in a manner similar to omalizumab. The two complementary properties resulted in prolonged efficacy for XmAb7195 compared to antibodies exerting only one of the two mechanisms.

Another strategy involved use of the anti-CD20 chimeric antibody rituximab, which has been approved for the B-cell malignancy non-Hodgkin lymphoma and has also demonstrated efficacy in some autoimmune disorders (100). The antibody was examined as a potential tool to eliminate B cells and therefore remove allergen-induced B-cell

TABLE 1 Interactions of omalizumab with IgE, the resulting mechanisms of action, and clinical effects of treatment in patients with allergies

Monoclonal antibody property	Mechanism	Biological function	Immunological effects	Clinical impact
Binds to the Cε3 region of free circulating IgE	Sequesters free IgE	Reduction of IgE titers in human sera and reduced levels of cell-bound IgE	Reduced mast cell and basophil activation, reduced antigen presentation	Reduced allergic symptoms/efficacy
	Prevents IgE-FcεRI interactions on cell surfaces	Decreased FcεRI density on circulating basophils	Decreased basophil/mast cell responsiveness upon challenge with IgE-allergen complexes	Reduced allergic symptoms/efficacy
		Decreased FcεRI density on APCs (e.g., DCs)	Inhibition of antigen processing and presentation to T cells, reduced Th2 cellular and cytokine responses	Reduced allergic inflammation/efficacy
	Prevents IgE-FcεRII interactions on cell surfaces	Inhibition of allergen-IgE-FcεRII complex formation	Decreased antigen presentation to T cells	Reduced chronic allergic responses/efficacy
		Cross-linking and IgE-mediated endocytosis	Decreased de novo synthesis of IgE	
Does not interfere with variable regions of IgE	Circulating IgEs of any specificity sequestered Blocks cell surface interactions of FcεRs with any IgEs	Blocks IgE-FcεR-IgE functions mediated by any allergen	Inhibition of allergic responses irrespective of allergen specificity	Broad applicability in allergic diseases
Binds to a Cε3 epitope in proximity to both binding sites recognized by FcεRI and FcεRII	Does not recognize IgE bound to cell surface IgE-FcεRs	Addition of antibody could not trigger FcεRI cross-linking and mast cell/basophil degranulation	Reduced potential for type 1 hypersensitivity responses that may lead to onset of anaphylaxis	Improved safety profile
High specificity for IgE Fc	Sequesters free IgE only	Reduction of IgE titers but no reduction of IgG	Normal immunity is unaffected	No off-target effects/safety

TABLE 2 **Active phase II, III, and IV interventional clinical studies for antibody immunotherapies of allergic diseases in 2012**[a]

Trial title	Intervention	Target	Phase	Indication	Primary endpoint(s)	Sponsor	Status
Oral immunotherapy combined with humanized monoclonal anti-IgE antibody Xolair (omalizumab) in the treatment of cow's milk allergy	MAb + OIT[b]: omalizumab + milk OIT	IgE	II	Milk allergy	Efficacy: percentage of subjects developing clinical tolerance to milk	National Institute of Allergy and Infectious Diseases (NIAID)	Recruiting
Peanut oral immunotherapy and anti-IgE for peanut allergy	MAb + OIT: omalizumab + peanut OIT	IgE	I/II	Peanut hypersensitivity	Efficacy: percentage of subjects developing clinical tolerance to peanuts	University of North Carolina (collaborator, Genentech)	Active, not recruiting
Effect of KB003 in subjects with asthma inadequately controlled by corticosteroids	MAb: KB003-04	GM-CSF[c]	II	Moderate-to-severe asthma	Safety, tolerability, and efficacy: effects on lung function measured by FEV1[d]	KaloBios Pharmaceuticals	Recruiting
A phase 2b, randomized, double-blind study to evaluate the efficacy of tralokinumab in adults with asthma	MAb: tralokinumab	IL-13	IIb	Asthma	Efficacy: asthma exacerbation rate	MedImmune LLC	Recruiting
Dose ranging pharmacokinetics and pharmacodynamics study with mepolizumab in asthma patients with elevated eosinophils	MAb: mepolizumab (SB-240563)	IL-5	II	Asthma	Pharmacokinetics, pharmacodynamics, immunogenicity analysis; effects on blood eosinophil levels, drug plasma levels	GlaxoSmithKline	Recruiting

Study	MAb[b]	Target	Phase	Condition	Efficacy outcome	Sponsor	Status
Omalizumab in patients with moderate to severe persistent allergic asthma not adequately controlled despite GINA (2009) step 4 therapy	MAb: omalizumab	IgE	III	Persistent allergic asthma	Efficacy: change from baseline in mean morning PEF[e]	Novartis Pharmaceuticals (collaborator, Genentech)	Recruiting
A study of lebrikizumab in patients whose asthma is uncontrolled with inhaled corticosteroids and a second controller medication (LUTE)	MAb: lebrikizumab	IL-13	III	Asthma	Efficacy: rate of asthma exacerbations	Genentech	Recruiting
A study of lebrikizumab in patients with uncontrolled asthma who are on inhaled corticosteroids and a second controller medication (VERSE)	MAb: lebrikizumab	IL-13	III	Asthma	Efficacy: rate of asthma exacerbations	Genentech	Recruiting
Effect of Xolair on airway hyperresponsiveness	MAb: omalizumab	IgE	IV	Allergic asthma	Efficacy: reduction in abnormal increase in limitation to airflow in patients with asthma; decrease the amount of inflammation in the lungs	Creighton University (collaborator, Genentech)	Active, not recruiting

[a]Source: ClinicalTrials.gov; U.S. National Institutes of Health.
[b]MAb, monoclonal antibody; OIT, oral immunotherapy.
[c]GM-CSF, granulocyte-macrophage colony-stimulating factor.
[d]FEV1, forced expiratory volume in 1 s.
[e]PEF, peak expiratory flow.

class switching and synthesis of IgE and also IgG autoantibodies, for applications in atopic dermatitis and urticaria, and anecdotal successes for individual patients treated with this agent have been reported (101, 102).

As demonstrated by the success of omalizumab and the other anti-IgE therapies undergoing preclinical and clinical evaluations, monoclonal antibodies targeting IgE are emerging as important therapeutic modalities for the treatment of allergic diseases, while new approaches are being examined which aim to improve the efficacy of omalizumab. Other strategies with indirect effects on IgE production, such as those aimed at neutralizing B cells and targeting CD23, have been less successful to date.

Antibodies Targeting Key Cytokines, Chemokines, and Their Receptors

Th2-type cytokines (e.g., IL-4, IL-5, IL-9, and IL-13) are produced by mast cells, basophils, Th2 lymphocytes, and eosinophils but also by nonimmune cells such as lung airway epithelial cells. They play key roles in triggering and maintaining allergic inflammation and contribute to the resulting pathologies. Targeting cytokines associated with allergies with antibodies has been explored as a treatment option, and various strategies are being examined in preclinical studies and in clinical trials, with asthma being a major therapeutic indication for these efforts.

Production of IL-4 by basophils, mast cells, NK cells, or eosinophils and subsequently also by Th2 lymphocytes is linked to a number of processes in allergic inflammation, such as upregulation of FcεRI and CD23 on the surface of effector cells and class switching from IgM to IgE by B lymphocytes. Therefore, neutralizing IL-4 would be expected to inhibit IgE synthesis, formation of Th2-type T cells, and upregulation of IgE receptors. Preclinical studies in a murine model of asthma demonstrated that an anti-IL-4 antibody could inhibit IgE production, but this agent did not abrogate

allergic inflammatory cascades in animal lungs (103). Phase I and II clinical studies in patients with asthma using a humanized antibody (pascolizumab, SB-240683) which blocks IL-4– IL-4 receptor interactions did not result in clinical improvements in patients (104).

By sharing a receptor with IL-4 in the form of IL-4R subunit α, IL-13 is thought to be involved in class switching to IgE but also has functions distinct from IL-4, such as regulation of epithelial cell maturation, muscle contractility, production of extracellular matrix proteins, and recruitment of monocytes, T cells, and eosinophils. Targeting IL-13 is presently an area of translational and clinical activity. Tralokinumab (CAT-354), a human IgG4 antibody which can neutralize IL-13, was associated with improved lung function when tested in patients with asthma, although results from phase IIb clinical studies are pending (Table 2) (105). Another agent presently undergoing clinical evaluations in phase III clinical trials is the IgG4 humanized anti-IL-13 antibody, lebrikizumab. Small improvements in lung functions were observed when this antibody was administered in asthmatics with inhaled glucocorticoid-resistant disease, and clinical responses were associated with increased levels of serum periostin, suggesting the merits of utilizing biomarkers to select patients most likely to respond (106).

Eosinophilia comprises an important component of the inflammatory infiltrate in asthmatic lungs, and increased levels of eosinophils are found in the blood of allergic subjects. Because of its role in potentiating activation and proliferation of eosinophils and their terminal differentiation in tissues, IL-5 constitutes an attractive therapeutic target for allergic conditions characterized by eosinophilia (107). Three humanized antibodies targeting IL-5 are in clinical trials for the treatment of eosinophilia-associated allergic conditions. Clinical studies of patients with hypereosinophilic conditions reported that treatment with mepolizumab (SB-240563) resulted in increased titers of serum IL-5 and IL-5 receptor, while reduced eosinophil activation and lower blood eosinophil levels were observed (108). One study demonstrated disease management with lower doses of corticosteroid treatment and reduced bronchial mucosal eosinophilia in asthmatic subjects receiving this antibody. Others reported reduced exacerbation of symptoms in asthmatics, with further clinical trials with this agent presently in progress (Table 2) (109, 110). Two other humanized antibodies, the anti-IL-5 antibody reslizumab (CTx55700) and the anti-IL-5 receptor-specific antibody benralizumab (MEDI-563), have demonstrated favorable safety profiles and reductions in eosinophil counts in patients. So far, clinical utility has not been proven for anti-IL-5 therapies, although clinical studies are still underway (111, 112, 113).

Studies of murine models of asthma demonstrated that IL-9 provides activatory and proliferative signals to mast cells, contributing to airway hyperresponsiveness and airway fibrosis. Targeting this cytokine with an antibody reduced these allergen-induced inflammatory symptoms, and antibody treatment was associated with reduced levels of known profibrotic cytokines transforming growth factor β, vascular endothelial growth factor, and fibroblast growth factor 2 (114). A humanized antibody targeting IL-9 (MEDI-528) has been tested in clinical trials in healthy individuals and patients with asthma with some encouraging clinical responses (115).

Expressed by macrophages and mast cells following activation with different stimuli, including IgE-FcεRI associations, TNF-α triggers infiltration of immune effector cells in tissues and has a role in inflammatory processes, including those associated with asthma (116). Anti-TNF-α antibodies tested in the clinic include the chimeric infliximab, the humanized certolizumab pegol, the human antibodies adalimumab and golimumab, and the soluble TNF-α receptor 2-Fc fusion protein, etanercept. All of these agents are expected to neutralize TNF-α. However, any moderate clinical responses observed have been overshadowed with reports of induction of opportunistic infections and cancer, which

may reflect the importance of considering the complex balance between mounting natural protective immune functions and reducing allergic inflammatory environments when designing therapeutics for allergic diseases (117).

Active Allergen Immunotherapy Induces Neutralizing Antibody Responses in Patients

An attractive therapeutic direction entails strategies to interrupt IgE binding to allergens to reduce IgE-mediated responses in patients with allergies. For known allergens, it is possible to produce a vaccine that would reduce the inflammatory response of antigen-bound IgE binding to mast cells by disrupting the binding of the Fab region of IgE to allergenic epitopes, and this has formed the focus of recombinant allergen immunotherapy. This therapy has been examined now for decades; the availability of allergen sequences has led to the expression of recombinant allergens and production of synthetic allergenic peptides, and there now exists a database where these sequences have been deposited for comparison (118). Immunization with recombinant allergen induces the production of allergen-specific IgGs, which compete with IgEs for binding to the allergen, thus blocking downstream IgE cross-linking and suppressing allergic responses (119).

There are a number of subclasses of these recombinant and synthetic allergens. Of particular interest to those who study the allergic response stimulated by the cross-linking of IgE are the wild-type hypoallergens. These are designed to be allergen mimics and may consist of a fragment of the allergen, a mutant of the allergen, or the whole recombinant allergen. The net result of this subclass is reduced IgE activity in patients. The first clinical trial of the wild-type hypoallergen was with the Birch pollen allergen, Bet v 1, with patients who showed an allergic response to the crude extract. Application of rBet v 1, as well as fragments of the Bet v 1, showed efficacy in reducing histamine release in basophils, an important step in the progression of an allergic response (120). The same trial also showed that there was an increased production of allergen-specific IgG1 and IgG4 with both the full-length allergenic recombinant and smaller fragments, suggesting that a few allergenic residues are all that are required to induce a clinical regression of symptoms in patients. Not only was there a notable lack of histamine reaction to the use of recombinant therapies but there were also no T-cell-mediated toxic effects noted.

The efficacy of recombinantly expressed allergen has been characterized and shown to be capable of inducing desensitization to specific allergens. The Der p 2 allergen is the major allergen responsible for dust mite allergies, and there are a number of allergenic isoforms. One of these isoforms was selected and expressed in the yeast strain *Pichia pastoris* and as inclusion bodies in *Escherichia coli*, where they were refolded to a stable tertiary structure. The secondary structures of these recombinant products were compared to the native allergen, obtained from dust mites by circular dichroism, and showed that different structures were obtained for each of the products. However, in a mouse model, both of the recombinant products were capable of inducing desensitization to the Der p 2 allergen, despite differential structural properties. These findings suggest that potentially linear epitopes may be sufficient for allergenic vaccine therapy (121).

Based upon the success of recombinant allergens, rational design of allergenic epitopes was the next logical step, since, as far back as 1970, allergens were being chemically modified to reduce IgE binding capacity while retaining the ability to prompt the production of antigen-specific IgGs (122, 123). More recently, the use of recombinant technology yielded new tools with which to mutate specific residues that alter the activity of the allergen. An example of this approach was the use of mutated forms of the mouse allergen Mus m 1. The high resolution crystal structure of a domain of the allergen

highlighted a potentially important residue (124). When this residue was mutated, in two single-point mutant forms of the allergen, it resulted in very different circular dichroism spectra, suggesting a change in conformation of the allergen based on altering this site. Both of the mutants had reduced ability to bind IgE and activate basophils but could be recognized by allergen-specific T cells. These findings suggest that site-directed mutagenesis retains the immunogenicity of these allergens while counteracting initiation of an allergic response.

In 2011, there were 11 clinical trials running in the United Kingdom using recombinant allergens to combat allergic diseases, with 4 of these being in phase III (125). The relative success of this therapy suggests that targeting the interaction of the antibody with the allergen may be an effective therapeutic alternative to or complementary to the use of anti-IgE antibodies.

Triggering Protective Immunity with Immunotherapy—the Role of IgG4

Specific immunotherapy (SIT) involves the administration of allergens to achieve clinical tolerance, with the aim of easing the symptoms in patients with allergic conditions. Long-term clinical benefits of SIT persist even after discontinuation of therapy, indicating the involvement of a cellular memory component to therapy. The mechanism behind the therapy has extensively been studied but still remains a matter of research and debate.

Research on SIT has to date focused on altered T-lymphocyte responses and induction of allergen-specific IgG4 antibodies. Two individual patterns of change, which may occur sequentially, have been described. The first event is induced within 1 to 4 weeks and entails the generation of regulatory T cells secreting IL-10 and transforming growth factor β, accompanied by suppression of allergen-induced late cutaneous responses. Subsequently, around week 10 postchallenge, elevated serum titers of allergen-specific IgG4 and IgA are observed. Although these titers appeared proportional to the dose of administered antigen rather than to clinical improvements, recent studies reported that the functional capacity of IgG4 antibodies to block IgE functions correlates with clinical responses (126, 127). These events coincide with a decrease of allergen-specific IgE antibodies and a shift in the allergen-specific T-cell response from predominantly Th2 to Th1 (126).

Serum obtained from patients following SIT has been shown to inhibit allergen-IgE binding to B cells, an effect mediated largely by IgG4 antibodies in patient sera. This in vitro system introduced the idea that SIT triggers production of "blocking antibodies" that inhibit IgE functions, such as IgE-FAP on B cells. Similarly, basophil histamine release assays or basophil activation assays have demonstrated the functional ability of IgG4 to inhibit IgE-dependent activation and mediator release, either by competing with IgE for the antigen and/or by stimulating cell surface IgG-inhibitory receptors present on basophils and mast cells (127, 128). Interestingly, IgA antibodies could not block allergen-IgE binding to B cells. The contribution of IgA in the responses to SIT may lie in engagement of surface IgA receptors and release of the inhibitory cytokine IL-10, which may participate in the induction of immune tolerance to allergens (129).

The mechanisms triggering elevated IgE-neutralizing antibodies following SIT are not completely understood, although it is known that prolonged exposure to antigenic stimuli can direct production of IgG4 by B cells. B cells can switch from IgG4 to IgE but not vice versa, as these sections of the gene are spliced out during class switching. Thus, IgG4 must be produced by switching from IgM, IgG1–3, or IgA1 or by proliferation of preexisting IgG4$^+$ B cells during SIT. It has been suggested that Th2 cytokine environments with elevated levels of IL-10 can drive the differentiation of IgG4-switched B cells to IgG4-secreting plasma cells (130). In addition to IL-10, the immunoregulatory cytokine, IL-21, has been found to increase IgG4 production in vitro (131).

The IgE-neutralizing and -tolerogenic properties of IgG4 may be partly due to competing with allergen-specific IgE for antigen specificity. This would interrupt IgE-FcεRI-multivalent allergen complex formation on the surface of immune effector cells, preventing downstream signaling and effector cell activation (Fig. 2). However, since only a fraction of IgG4 antibodies are allergen specific after immunotherapy, other mechanisms may also be involved. van der Neut Kolfschoten and colleagues used recombinant IgG4 antibodies against grass and cat allergens, which when coinjected in a mouse graft, became bispecific in a process termed Fab-arm exchange. Although this process was not observed when antibodies were combined in vitro, these findings raise the possibility that IgG4 antibodies may also operate by Fab-arm exchange (132). If this is true in patients receiving allergen immunotherapy, IgE/IgG4 bispecific antibody formation may reduce the affinity of IgE antibodies for allergens and interrupt IgE-FcεRI-multivalent allergen complex formation on the surface of immune effector cells. These properties would therefore moderate IgE-mediated inflammatory cascades. This latter possible mechanism by which IgG4 antibodies may function would be consistent with the observations that IgE effector cells such as eosinophils, mast cells, or basophils are reduced after SIT against house dust mite and grass pollen (133). An additional mechanism by which SIT can tolerize allergic immune responses lies with the ineffective Fc-mediated functions of IgG4 in lacking complement activator properties and mediating ineffective FcR signals, reducing the capacity of this antibody class to trigger cytotoxicity or phagocytosis.

Additionally, involvement of IgG4 and also IgA antibodies in natural induction of tolerance is supported by reports of increased allergen-specific IgG4 serum levels in patients who spontaneously become tolerant to cow's milk and from findings that these serum levels are maintained and remain higher than those measured from individuals with diagnosed active cow's milk allergies (134, 135). Finally,

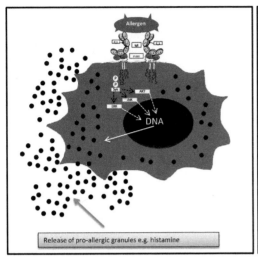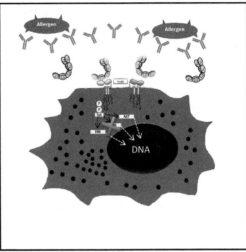

 IgE antibody

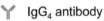 IgG₄ antibody

FIGURE 2 IgG4 antibodies induced by allergen immunotherapies modulate IgE-mediated activation of effector cells. The allergic response mediated by multivalent allergen-IgE FcεRI complex assembly and downstream signaling events leading to release of inflammatory mediators (left) may be blocked by adaptive immune responses triggered in response to SIT with recombinant antigens. IgG4 antibodies, induced following SIT, could compete with IgE for binding to allergens and prevent the formation of allergen-IgE-FcεRI complexes on the surface of effector cells, blocking effector functions such as degranulation (right). Syk, spleen tyrosine kinase; AKT, Ak strain thymoma serine/threonine-specific protein kinase; ERK, extracellular signal-regulated kinase; JNK, Jun N-terminal protein kinase; P, phosphorylation. doi:10.1128/microbiolspec.AID-0006-2012.f2

favored production of IgG4 antibodies was recently demonstrated in patients with melanomas and extrahepatic cholangiocarcinomas, suggesting the association of IgG4 antibodies with immune tolerance favored by IL-10-rich environments such as those in tumors (136, 137).

THE OPPOSITE SIDE OF THE COIN: HARNESSING THE ALLERGIC RESPONSE AGAINST CANCER AND THE EMERGENCE OF ANTIBODIES OF THE IGE CLASS FOR CANCER THERAPY

Monoclonal antibodies of the IgG class have emerged as an important therapeutic modality over the last 20 years, and a number of these agents are in clinical use for the treatment of cancer. There have been many efforts to enhance the efficacy of these antibodies by engineering Fc regions with enhanced affinity to Fc receptors to create antibodies with desirable pharmacokinetic properties and improved cellular immune functions. Our group's approach has been to enhance antibody Fc-mediated functions by engineering therapeutic antitumoral antibodies with Fc regions of the IgE class (138). Employing this strategy, therapeutic antibodies of the IgE class may confer several advantages over antibodies of the IgG class, particularly with respect to the treatment of solid tumors. The advantages of IgE would include (i) high affinity of IgE to its Fcε receptors; (ii) lack of IgE inhibitory Fc receptors; (iii) natural immune activatory functions in tissues; (iv) presence of IgE effector cells in tumors; (v) the activation of

Fc receptors (i.e., FcεRI and FcεRII) other than Fcγ receptors on a set of effector cells (e.g., mast cells, eosinophils, and monocytes/macrophages) different from those bearing IgG receptors; and (vi) desirable pharmacokinetic properties such as fast clearance from circulation, reducing the chance of antibody-neutralizing antibody responses (35, 139, 140, 141).

Exploiting IgE as a novel class of therapeutic antibodies may prove successful in harnessing a potent allergic response against tumor cells. The multimerization of therapeutic IgE antibodies bound to multimeric antigens or multivalent antigens expressed on tumor cells can result in the cross-linking of antibody receptors on immune cells, high-avidity binding and cell activation, and the release of inflammatory mediators such as histamines, leukotrienes, tryptases, inflammatory cytokines, and cytotoxic granules which would result in tumor cell death. We have demonstrated that IgE antibodies targeting the tumor antigens folate receptor alpha (FRα) and the human epidermal growth factor receptor 2 (HER2/neu) are capable of mediating effective cytotoxicity against tumor cells through IgE Fc-mediated interactions with Fcε receptors present on frequently tumor-resident immune cells such as monocytes, mast cells, and eosinophils (34, 35, 139, 140, 142). Furthermore, in a number of animal models of ovarian carcinoma, the administration of MOv18 IgE antibodies, which target the tumor antigen FRα, resulted in increased survival and restriction of tumor growth compared to dosing with the IgG1 counterparts (35, 139, 140). Thus, IgE antibodies targeting tumor antigens are capable of mediating allergic responses in solid tumors by the activation of immune cells generally involved in allergic responses, and such a strategy resulted in the redirection of the cytotoxic effects of these immune cells against tumor cells (141).

We envisage that a successful clinical utility setting for therapeutic IgE antibodies includes the selection of appropriate disease settings such as those of solid tumor types, with immune cell infiltrates bearing Fcε receptors capable of mediating potent cytotoxic effects. The systemic administration of IgE therapeutic antibodies also warrants immunological monitoring of patients, to ensure allergic responses are primarily harnessed in solid tumors and do not lead to potentially harmful type 1 hypersensitivity responses in patient circulation. Here, since only soluble multimeric antigens at high concentrations in blood would have the potential to cross-link IgE-FcεRI complexes that may give rise to type 1 hypersensitivity, the design of antibodies to antigenic targets known to be shed in multimeric form in the patient circulation should be avoided. Of note, our most advanced IgE class therapeutic antibody candidate, MOv18 IgE, is designed against the cell surface tumor antigen FRα which is shed in low levels and in a monomeric form in human sera. To address concerns of potential type 1 hypersensitivity responses upon administration of antibody in patients, we have evaluated the activation of human immune cells involved in systemic allergic responses, such as basophils and mast cells. We conducted these experiments using two ex vivo and in vitro functional readouts of effector cell activation following the addition of therapeutic IgE antibodies in blood and sera from patients with cancer and healthy volunteers. In both of these readouts, we have found a lack of human immune cell activation, even in the presence of soluble forms of tumor antigens. These findings suggest that this approach bears low risk of systemic type 1 hypersensitivity (143). This is likely due to the absence of IgE cross-linking in blood, even in the presence of soluble tumor antigens and circulating tumor cells at the highest reported physiological amounts in patients. These studies provided support for the potential safety of a tumor antigen-specific IgE antibody administered in the patient's circulation (138, 144).

In conclusion, we propose that therapeutic IgE antibodies may harness allergic responses in individuals with cancer, resulting in significant antitumor effects, and that this antibody class has the potential to emerge as an important therapeutic modality to direct IgE immune responses against cancer. We await the testing of the first therapeutic IgE in humans and continue in the design and development of IgE antibodies for the treatment of many malignancies, including breast cancer, ovarian cancer, and melanoma.

CONCLUDING REMARKS AND FUTURE ROLES OF ANTIBODIES IN THERAPY

Key roles of IgE class antibodies in allergic diseases, in the associated allergic inflammation, and in parasitic and infectious diseases have emerged over 4 decades of research. Increased levels of IgE antibodies specific to allergens are central to the pathogenesis, exacerbation, and diagnosis of many allergic conditions. Increased levels of IgE are also associated with sensitivity to infections in patients with HIES, while certain viral infections also trigger class switching and production of IgE that can lead to symptom exacerbations in allergic individuals. On the other hand, IgE antibodies are also thought to confer protective roles in parasitic infections. Potential functions for the IgG class are also reported in some anaphylactic responses, while IgG4 subclass and IgA antibodies are associated with development of natural and specific allergen immunotherapy-induced tolerance to allergen exposure. These provide support for the important contributions of antibodies in allergic and infectious diseases.

Importantly, the approval of omalizumab for the treatment of a number of IgE-mediated allergies constituted a proof-of-principle agent and a significant milestone in the clinical management of patients. Omalizumab has also contributed new understanding of the interactions between IgE, its receptors, and allergens and novel insights into the mechanisms by which these interactions impact on the development of allergic inflammation. These developments have also placed these interactions at the forefront of translational efforts to design novel treatments. Furthermore, they have prompted increased focus on the intelli-

gent design of new more effective therapeutics with improved functional properties or on the design of agents with multimodal actions, all aiming at achieving better efficacy than that shown with application of omalizumab in the clinic. Such strategies would include monoclonal antibodies but also small molecules with the capacity to interfere with IgE-FcεR interactions (145).

The significance of antibodies in the treatment of allergic diseases has also been suggested in a different context, through the pivotal findings that allergen immunotherapy triggers increased levels of protective humoral responses in patients. These responses manifest in the form of IgG4 subclass antibodies. All these developments highlight the central role of antibodies in passive but also active immunotherapy of allergic diseases. Furthermore, the mechanisms by which IgG4 antibodies operate are currently an area of intense research activity and may themselves lead to the rational design of active immunotherapies designed to trigger more effective humoral responses capable of regulating IgE-mediated inflammation. Another potential future strategy may be the design of engineered IgG4 subclass antibody therapeutics capable of passively blocking IgE-mediated responses in patients with allergies.

Finally, IgE antibodies and their potent effector functions, known to confer protection in parasitic infections and to contribute to allergic diseases, may be utilized as therapeutics for cancer. A number of groups have examined the concept of raising IgE antibodies through a number of active immunization approaches and also by harnessing powerful immune effector cell functions against cancer cells through passive immunotherapy with monoclonal antibodies (138, 139, 140, 142, 146, 147, 148, 149, 150, 151, 152, 153). A growing number of studies, including those from our group, demonstrate the promise of activating allergic responses against cancer and have defined the emerging field of AllergoOncology (138, 154, 155). Passive immunotherapy with engineered antibodies has, in our hands, demonstrated considerable efficacy with a number of antibody therapeutic candidates, in different oncological disease settings, and in a number of disease-relevant models (138). Ultimately, the utility of an antibody class such as IgE, commonly associated with the pathogenesis of allergies, may find a new purpose in cancer therapy. Our planned first-in-class clinical study of our anti-FRα IgE antibody will undoubtedly provide new insights into the hypothesis that the potent effector activatory functions of IgE antibodies could be directed against malignancy.

ACKNOWLEDGMENTS

We acknowledge support from Cancer Research UK (C30122/A11527); CR UK/EPSRC/MRC/NIHR KCL/UCL Comprehensive Cancer Imaging Centre (C1519/A10331); KCL Experimental Cancer Medicine Centre, jointly funded by Cancer Research UK, the National Institute for Health Research (NIHR), Welsh Assembly Government, HSC R&D Office for Northern Ireland, and Chief Scientist Office, Scotland. The research was supported by the NIHR Biomedical Research Centre based at Guy's and St. Thomas' National Health Service (NHS) Foundation Trust and King's College London.

Conflicts of interest: We disclose no conflicts.

The views expressed are those of the authors and not necessarily those of the NHS, the NIHR, or the Department of Health.

CITATION

Karagiannis SN, Karagiannis P, Josephs DH, Saul L, Gilbert AE, Upton N, Gould HJ. 2013. IgE and allergy: antibodies in immune inflammation and treatment. Microbiol Spectrum 1(1):AID-0006-2012.

REFERENCES

1. **Galli SJ, Tsai M, Piliponsky AM.** 2008. The development of allergic inflammation. *Nature* **454:**445–454.

2. **Oppenheimer J, Nelson HS.** 2006. Skin testing. *Ann Allergy Asthma Immunol* **96:**S6–S12.

3. **Bernstein IL, Li JT, Bernstein DI, Hamilton R, Spector SL, Tan R, Sicherer S, Golden DB, Khan DA, Nicklas RA, Portnoy JM, Blessing-Moore J, Cox L, Lang DM, Oppenheimer J, Randolph CC, Schuller DE, Tilles SA, Wallace DV, Levetin E, Weber R.** 2008. Allergy diagnostic testing: an updated practice parameter. *Ann Allergy Asthma Immunol* **100:**S1–S148.

4. **Akhabir L, Sandford AJ.** 2011. Genome-wide association studies for discovery of genes involved in asthma. *Respirology* **16:**396–406.

5. **Valenta R, Ball T, Focke M, Linhart B, Mothes N, Niederberger V, Spitzauer S, Swoboda I, Vrtala S, Westritschnig K, Kraft D.** 2004. Immunotherapy of allergic disease. *Adv Immunol* **82:**105–153.

6. **Barnes PJ.** 2011. Pathophysiology of allergic inflammation. *Immunol Rev* **242:**31–50.

7. **Johansson SG, Bennich H.** 1967. Immunological studies of an atypical (myeloma) immunoglobulin. *Immunology* **13:**381–394.

8. **Ishizaka K, Ishizaka T, Hornbrook MM.** 1966. Physico-chemical properties of human reaginic antibody. IV. Presence of a unique immunoglobulin as a carrier of reaginic activity. *J Immunol* **97:**75–85.

9. **Geha RS, Jabara HH, Brodeur SR.** 2003. The regulation of immunoglobulin E class-switch recombination. *Nat Rev Immunol* **3:**721–732.

10. **Gould HJ, Sutton BJ.** 2008. IgE in allergy and asthma today. *Nat Rev Immunol* **8:**205–217.

11. **Galli SJ, Tsai M.** 2012. IgE and mast cells in allergic disease. *Nat Med* **18:**693–704.

12. **Dhaliwal B, Yuan D, Pang MO, Henry AJ, Cain K, Oxbrow A, Fabiane SM, Beavil AJ, McDonnell JM, Gould HJ, Sutton BJ.** 2012. Crystal structure of IgE bound to its B-cell receptor CD23 reveals a mechanism of reciprocal allosteric inhibition with high affinity receptor FcepsilonRI. *Proc Natl Acad Sci USA* **109:**12686–12691.

13. **Kraft S, Kinet JP.** 2007. New developments in FcepsilonRI regulation, function and inhibition. *Nat Rev Immunol* **7:**365–378.

14. **Dullaers M, De Bruyne R, Ramadani F, Gould HJ, Gevaert P, Lambrecht BN.** 2012. The who, where, and when of IgE in allergic airway disease. *J Allergy Clin Immunol* **129:**635–645.

15. **Acharya M, Borland G, Edkins AL, Maclellan LM, Matheson J, Ozanne BW, Cushley W.** 2010. CD23/FcepsilonRII: molecular multi-tasking. *Clin Exp Immunol* **162:**12–23.

16. **Dierks SE, Bartlett WC, Edmeades RL, Gould HJ, Rao M, Conrad DH.** 1993. The oligomeric nature of the murine Fc epsilon RII/CD23.

Implications for function. *J Immunol* **150**: 2372–2382.

17. **Vouldoukis I, Mazier D, Moynet D, Thiolat D, Malvy D, Mossalayi MD.** 2011. IgE mediates killing of intracellular Toxoplasma gondii by human macrophages through CD23-dependent, interleukin-10 sensitive pathway. *PLoS One* **6**: e18289.

18. **Vouldoukis I, Riveros-Moreno V, Dugas B, Ouaaz F, Becherel P, Debre P, Moncada S, Mossalayi MD.** 1995. The killing of Leishmania major by human macrophages is mediated by nitric oxide induced after ligation of the Fc epsilon RII/CD23 surface antigen. *Proc Natl Acad Sci USA* **92**:7804–7808.

19. **Chen HY, Liu FT, Yang RY.** 2005. Roles of galectin-3 in immune responses. *Arch Immunol Ther Exp (Warsaw)* **53**:497–504.

20. **Bax HJ, Keeble AH, Gould HJ.** 2012. Cytokinergic IgE action in mast cell activation. *Front Immunol* **3**:229.

21. **Ziegler SF, Artis D.** 2010. Sensing the outside world: TSLP regulates barrier immunity. *Nat Immunol* **11**:289–293.

22. **Fort MM, Cheung J, Yen D, Li J, Zurawski SM, Lo S, Menon S, Clifford T, Hunte B, Lesley R, Muchamuel T, Hurst SD, Zurawski G, Leach MW, Gorman DM, Rennick DM.** 2001. IL-25 induces IL-4, IL-5, and IL-13 and Th2-associated pathologies in vivo. *Immunity* **15**:985–995.

23. **Schmitz J, Owyang A, Oldham E, Song Y, Murphy E, McClanahan TK, Zurawski G, Moshrefi M, Qin J, Li X, Gorman DM, Bazan JF, Kastelein RA.** 2005. IL-33, an interleukin-1-like cytokine that signals via the IL-1 receptor-related protein ST2 and induces T helper type 2-associated cytokines. *Immunity* **23**:479–490.

24. **Lambrecht BN, Hammad H.** 2010. The role of dendritic and epithelial cells as master regulators of allergic airway inflammation. *Lancet* **376**:835–843.

25. **Sokol CL, Chu NQ, Yu S, Nish SA, Laufer TM, Medzhitov R.** 2009. Basophils function as antigen-presenting cells for an allergen-induced T helper type 2 response. *Nat Immunol* **10**:713–720.

26. **Yoshimoto T, Yasuda K, Tanaka H, Nakahira M, Imai Y, Fujimori Y, Nakanishi K.** 2009. Basophils contribute to T(H)2-IgE responses in vivo via IL-4 production and presentation of peptide-MHC class II complexes to CD4+ T cells. *Nat Immunol* **10**:706–712.

27. **Perrigoue JG, Saenz SA, Siracusa MC, Allenspach EJ, Taylor BC, Giacomin PR, Nair MG, Du Y, Zaph C, van Rooijen N,** Comeau MR, Pearce EJ, Laufer TM, Artis D. 2009. MHC class II-dependent basophil-CD4+ T cell interactions promote T(H)2 cytokine-dependent immunity. *Nat Immunol* **10**:697–705.

28. **Saenz SA, Siracusa MC, Perrigoue JG, Spencer SP, Urban JF Jr, Tocker JE, Budelsky AL, Kleinschek MA, Kastelein RA, Kambayashi T, Bhandoola A, Artis D.** 2010. IL25 elicits a multipotent progenitor cell population that promotes T(H)2 cytokine responses. *Nature* **464**:1362–1366.

29. **Karagiannis SN, Warrack JK, Jennings KH, Murdock PR, Christie G, Moulder K, Sutton BJ, Gould HJ.** 2001. Endocytosis and recycling of the complex between CD23 and HLA-DR in human B cells. *Immunology* **103**:319–331.

30. **Mudde GC, Bheekha R, Bruijnzeel-Koomen CA.** 1995. Consequences of IgE/CD23-mediated antigen presentation in allergy. *Immunol Today* **16**:380–383.

31. **Ying S, Humbert M, Meng Q, Pfister R, Menz G, Gould HJ, Kay AB, Durham SR.** 2001. Local expression of epsilon germline gene transcripts and RNA for the epsilon heavy chain of IgE in the bronchial mucosa in atopic and nonatopic asthma. *J Allergy Clin Immunol* **107**:686–692.

32. **Cameron L, Hamid Q, Wright E, Nakamura Y, Christodoulopoulos P, Muro S, Frenkiel S, Lavigne F, Durham S, Gould H.** 2000. Local synthesis of epsilon germline gene transcripts, IL-4, and IL-13 in allergic nasal mucosa after ex vivo allergen exposure. *J Allergy Clin Immunol* **106**:46–52.

33. **Fawaz LM, Sharif-Askari E, Hajoui O, Soussi-Gounni A, Hamid Q, Mazer BD.** 2007. Expression of IL-9 receptor alpha chain on human germinal center B cells modulates IgE secretion. *J Allergy Clin Immunol* **120**:1208–1215.

34. **Karagiannis SN, Bracher MG, Beavil RL, Beavil AJ, Hunt J, McCloskey N, Thompson RG, East N, Burke F, Sutton BJ, Dombrowicz D, Balkwill FR, Gould HJ.** 2008. Role of IgE receptors in IgE antibody-dependent cytotoxicity and phagocytosis of ovarian tumor cells by human monocytic cells. *Cancer Immunol Immunother* **57**:247–263.

35. **Karagiannis SN, Bracher MG, Hunt J, McCloskey N, Beavil RL, Beavil AJ, Fear DJ, Thompson RG, East N, Burke F, Moore RJ, Dombrowicz DD, Balkwill FR, Gould HJ.** 2007. IgE-antibody-dependent immunotherapy of solid tumors: cytotoxic and phagocytic mechanisms of eradication of ovarian cancer cells. *J Immunol* **179**:2832–2843.

36. **Ishizaka T, Conrad DH, Schulman ES, Sterk AR, Ishizaka K.** 1983. Biochemical analysis of

initial triggering events of IgE-mediated histamine release from human lung mast cells. *J Immunol* **130**:2357–2362.

37. **Dombrowicz D, Flamand V, Brigman KK, Koller BH, Kinet JP.** 1993. Abolition of anaphylaxis by targeted disruption of the high affinity immunoglobulin E receptor alpha chain gene. *Cell* **75**:969–976.

38. **Davey AM, Krise KM, Sheets ED, Heikal AA.** 2008. Molecular perspective of antigen-mediated mast cell signaling. *J Biol Chem* **283**:7117–7127.

39. **MacNeil AJ, Yang YJ, Lin T-J.** 2011. MAPK kinase 3 specifically regulates Fc cpsilonRI-mediated IL-4 production by mast cells. *J Immunol* **187**:3374–3382.

40. **Medina-Tamayo J, Sanchez-Miranda E, Balleza-Tapia H, Ambriz X, Cid ME, Gonzalez-Espinosa D, Gutierrez AA, Gonzalez-Espinosa C.** 2007. Super-oxidized solution inhibits IgE-antigen-induced degranulation and cytokine release in mast cells. *Int Immunopharmacol* **7**:1013–1024.

41. **Nishida K, Yamasaki S, Ito Y, Kabu K, Hattori K, Tezuka T, Nishizumi H, Kitamura D, Goitsuka R, Geha RS, Yamamoto T, Yagi T, Hirano T.** 2005. Fc{epsilon}RI-mediated mast cell degranulation requires calcium-independent microtubule-dependent translocation of granules to the plasma membrane. *J Cell Biol* **170**:115–126. (Erratum, **171**:177.)

42. **Oka T, Sato K, Hori M, Ozaki H, Karaki H.** 2002. FcepsilonRI cross-linking-induced actin assembly mediates calcium signalling in RBL-2H3 mast cells. *Br J Pharmacol* **136**:837–846.

43. **Oettgen HC, Martin TR, Wynshaw-Boris A, Deng C, Drazen JM, Leder P.** 1994. Active anaphylaxis in IgE-deficient mice. *Nature* **370**:367–370.

44. **Miyajima I, Dombrowicz D, Martin TR, Ravetch JV, Kinet JP, Galli SJ.** 1997. Systemic anaphylaxis in the mouse can be mediated largely through IgG1 and Fc gammaRIII. Assessment of the cardiopulmonary changes, mast cell degranulation, and death associated with active or IgE- or IgG1-dependent passive anaphylaxis. *J Clin Investig* **99**:901–914.

45. **Jonsson F, Mancardi DA, Kita Y, Karasuyama H, Iannascoli B, Van Rooijen N, Shimizu T, Daeron M, Bruhns P.** 2011. Mouse and human neutrophils induce anaphylaxis. *J Clin Investig* **121**:1484–1496.

46. **Daeron M.** 1997. Fc receptor biology. *Annu Rev Immunol* **15**:203–234.

47. **Jonsson F, Mancardi DA, Zhao W, Kita Y, Iannascoli B, Khun H, van Rooijen N, Shimizu T, Schwartz LB, Daeron M, Bruhns P.** 2012. Human FcgammaRIIA induces anaphylactic and allergic reactions. *Blood* **119**:2533–2544.

48. **Tsujimura Y, Obata K, Mukai K, Shindou H, Yoshida M, Nishikado H, Kawano Y, Minegishi Y, Shimizu T, Karasuyama H.** 2008. Basophils play a pivotal role in immunoglobulin-G-mediated but not immunoglobulin-E-mediated systemic anaphylaxis. *Immunity* **28**:581–589.

49. **Finkelman FD, Urban JF Jr.** 2001. The other side of the coin: the protective role of the TH2 cytokines. *J Allergy Clin Immunol* **107**:772–780.

50. **Verwaerde C, Joseph M, Capron M, Pierce RJ, Damonneville M, Velge F, Auriault C, Capron A.** 1987. Functional properties of a rat monoclonal IgE antibody specific for Schistosoma mansoni. *J Immunol* **138**:4441–4446.

51. **Capron M, Capron A.** 1994. Immunoglobulin E and effector cells in schistosomiasis. *Science* **264**:1876–1877.

52. **Gounni AS, Lamkhioued B, Ochiai K, Tanaka Y, Delaporte E, Capron A, Kinet JP, Capron M.** 1994. High-affinity IgE receptor on eosinophils is involved in defence against parasites. *Nature* **367**:183–186.

53. **Hagan P, Blumenthal UJ, Dunn D, Simpson AJ, Wilkins HA.** 1991. Human IgE, IgG4 and resistance to reinfection with Schistosoma haematobium. *Nature* **349**:243–245.

54. **Dunne DW, Butterworth AE, Fulford AJ, Ouma JH, Sturrock RF.** 1992. Human IgE responses to Schistosoma mansoni and resistance to reinfection. *Mem Inst Oswaldo Cruz* **87**(Suppl 4):99–103.

55. **Gurish MF, Bryce PJ, Tao H, Kisselgof AB, Thornton EM, Miller HR, Friend DS, Oettgen HC.** 2004. IgE enhances parasite clearance and regulates mast cell responses in mice infected with *Trichinella spiralis*. *J Immunol* **172**:1139–1145.

56. **Watanabe N, Bruschi F, Korenaga M.** 2005. IgE: a question of protective immunity in Trichinella spiralis infection. *Trends Parasitol* **21**:175–178.

57. **Davis SD, Schaller J, Wedgwood RJ.** 1966. Job's Syndrome. Recurrent, "cold," staphylococcal abscesses. *Lancet* **i**:1013–1015.

58. **Freeman AF, Holland SM.** 2009. Clinical manifestations, etiology, and pathogenesis of the hyper-IgE syndromes. *Pediatr Res* **65**:32R–37R.

59. **Woellner C, Gertz EM, Schaffer AA, Lagos M, Perro M, Glocker EO, Pietrogrande MC, Cossu F, Franco JL, Matamoros N, Pietrucha B, Heropolitanska-Pliszka E, Yeganeh M, Moin M, Espanol T, Ehl S, Gennery AR, Abinun M, Breborowicz A, Niehues T, Kilic SS, Junker A, Turvey SE, Plebani A, Sanchez B, Garty BZ, Pignata C, Cancrini C, Litzman J, Sanal O, Baumann U, Bacchetta R, Hsu AP, Davis JN, Hammarstrom L, Davies EG, Eren E, Arkwright PD, Moilanen JS, Viemann D, Khan S, Marodi L,**

Cant AJ, Freeman AF, Puck JM, Holland SM, Grimbacher B. 2010. Mutations in STAT3 and diagnostic guidelines for hyper-IgE syndrome. *J Allergy Clin Immunol* 125:424–432.

60. Su HC, Jing H, Zhang Q. 2011. DOCK8 deficiency. *Ann NY Acad Sci* 1246:26–33.

61. Engelhardt KR, McGhee S, Winkler S, Sassi A, Woellner C, Lopez-Herrera G, Chen A, Kim HS, Lloret MG, Schulze I, Ehl S, Thiel J, Pfeifer D, Veelken H, Niehues T, Siepermann K, Weinspach S, Reisli I, Keles S, Genel F, Kutukculer N, Camcioglu Y, Somer A, Karakoc-Aydiner E, Barlan I, Gennery A, Metin A, Degerliyurt A, Pietrogrande MC, Yeganeh M, Baz Z, Al-Tamemi S, Klein C, Puck JM, Holland SM, McCabe ER, Grimbacher B, Chatila TA. 2009. Large deletions and point mutations involving the dedicator of cytokinesis 8 (DOCK8) in the autosomal-recessive form of hyper-IgE syndrome. *J Allergy Clin Immunol* 124:1289–1302.

62. Freeman AF, Holland SM. 2010. Clinical manifestations of hyper IgE syndromes. *Dis Markers* 29:123–130.

63. Xiong H, Curotto de Lafaille MA, Lafaille JJ. 2012. What is unique about the IgE response? *Adv Immunol* 116:113–141.

64. Minegishi Y, Saito M, Tsuchiya S, Tsuge I, Takada H, Hara T, Kawamura N, Ariga T, Pasic S, Stojkovic O, Metin A, Karasuyama H. 2007. Dominant-negative mutations in the DNA-binding domain of STAT3 cause hyper-IgE syndrome. *Nature* 448:1058–1062.

65. He J, Shi J, Xu X, Zhang W, Wang Y, Chen X, Du Y, Zhu N, Zhang J, Wang Q, Yang J. 2012. STAT3 mutations correlated with hyper-IgE syndrome lead to blockage of IL-6/STAT3 signalling pathway. *J Biosci* 37:243–257.

66. Milner JD, Brenchley JM, Laurence A, Freeman AF, Hill BJ, Elias KM, Kanno Y, Spalding C, Elloumi HZ, Paulson ML, Davis J, Hsu A, Asher AI, O'shea J, Holland SM, Paul WE, Douek DC. 2008. Impaired T(H)17 cell differentiation in subjects with autosomal dominant hyper-IgE syndrome. *Nature* 452:773–776.

67. Dong C. 2008. TH17 cells in development: an updated view of their molecular identity and genetic programming. *Nat Rev Immunol* 8:337–348.

68. Renner ED, Rylaarsdam S, Anover-Sombke S, Rack AL, Reichenbach J, Carey JC, Zhu Q, Jansson AF, Barboza J, Schimke LF, Leppert MF, Getz MM, Seger RA, Hill HR, Belohradsky BH, Torgerson TR, Ochs HD. 2008. Novel signal transducer and activator of transcription 3 (STAT3) mutations, reduced T(H)17 cell numbers, and variably defective STAT3 phosphorylation in hyper-IgE syndrome. *J Allergy Clin Immunol* 122:181–187.

69. Erazo A, Kutchukhidze N, Leung M, Christ AP, Urban JF Jr, Curotto de Lafaille MA, Lafaille JJ. 2007. Unique maturation program of the IgE response in vivo. *Immunity* 26:191–203.

70. Gevaert P, Nouri-Aria KT, Wu H, Harper CE, Takhar P, Fear DJ, Acke F, De Ruyck N, Banfield G, Kariyawasam HH, Bachert C, Durham SR, Gould HJ. 2013. Local receptor revision and class switching to IgE in chronic rhinosinusitis with nasal polyps. *Allergy* 68:55–63.

71. Chularojanamontri L, Wimoolchart S, Tuchinda P, Kulthanan K, Kiewjoy N. 2009. Role of omalizumab in a patient with hyper-IgE syndrome and review of dermatologic manifestations. *Asian Pac J Allergy Immunol* 27:233–236.

72. Imani F, Proud D, Griffin DE. 1999. Measles virus infection synergizes with IL-4 in IgE class switching. *J Immunol* 162:1597–1602.

73. Rager KJ, Langland JO, Jacobs BL, Proud D, Marsh DG, Imani F. 1998. Activation of anti-viral protein kinase leads to immunoglobulin E class switching in human B cells. *J Virol* 72:1171–1176.

74. Johnston SL, Pattemore PK, Sanderson G, Smith S, Lampe F, Josephs L, Symington P, O'Toole S, Myint SH, Tyrrell DA, et al. 1995. Community study of role of viral infections in exacerbations of asthma in 9–11 year old children. *BMJ* 310:1225–1229.

75. Nicholson KG, Kent J, Ireland DC. 1993. Respiratory viruses and exacerbations of asthma in adults. *BMJ* 307:982–986.

76. Murray CS, Poletti G, Kebadze T, Morris J, Woodcock A, Johnston SL, Custovic A. 2006. Study of modifiable risk factors for asthma exacerbations: virus infection and allergen exposure increase the risk of asthma hospital admissions in children. *Thorax* 61:376–382.

77. Green RM, Custovic A, Sanderson G, Hunter J, Johnston SL, Woodcock A. 2002. Synergism between allergens and viruses and risk of hospital admission with asthma: case-control study. *BMJ* 324:763.

78. Zambrano JC, Carper HT, Rakes GP, Patrie J, Murphy DD, Platts-Mills TA, Hayden FG, Gwaltney JM Jr, Hatley TK, Owens AM, Heymann PW. 2003. Experimental rhinovirus challenges in adults with mild asthma: response to infection in relation to IgE. *J Allergy Clin Immunol* 111:1008–1016.

79. Soto-Quiros M, Avila L, Platts-Mills TA, Hunt JF, Erdman DD, Carper H, Murphy

DD, Odio S, James HR, Patrie JT, Hunt W, O'Rourke AK, Davis MD, Steinke JW, Lu X, Kennedy J, Heymann PW. 2012. High titers of IgE antibody to dust mite allergen and risk for wheezing among asthmatic children infected with rhinovirus. *J Allergy Clin Immunol* **129:** 1499–1505.

80. **Corne JM, Marshall C, Smith S, Schreiber J, Sanderson G, Holgate ST, Johnston SL.** 2002. Frequency, severity, and duration of rhinovirus infections in asthmatic and non-asthmatic individuals: a longitudinal cohort study. *Lancet* **359:**831–834.

81. **Message SD, Laza-Stanca V, Mallia P, Parker HL, Zhu J, Kebadze T, Contoli M, Sanderson G, Kon OM, Papi A, Jeffery PK, Stanciu LA, Johnston SL.** 2008. Rhinovirus-induced lower respiratory illness is increased in asthma and related to virus load and Th1/2 cytokine and IL-10 production. *Proc Natl Acad Sci USA* **105:** 13562–13567.

82. **Paul WE, Zhu J.** 2010. How are T(H)2-type immune responses initiated and amplified? *Nat Rev Immunol* **10:**225–235.

83. **Papadopoulos NG, Stanciu LA, Papi A, Holgate ST, Johnston SL.** 2002. Rhinovirus-induced alterations on peripheral blood mononuclear cell phenotype and costimulatory molecule expression in normal and atopic asthmatic subjects. *Clin Exp Allergy* **32:**537–542.

84. **Perez-Yarza EG, Moreno A, Lazaro P, Mejias A, Ramilo O.** 2007. The association between respiratory syncytial virus infection and the development of childhood asthma: a systematic review of the literature. *Pediatr Infect Dis J* **26:**733–739.

85. **Sigurs N, Bjarnason R, Sigurbergsson F, Kjellman B, Bjorksten B.** 1995. Asthma and immunoglobulin E antibodies after respiratory syncytial virus bronchiolitis: a prospective cohort study with matched controls. *Pediatrics* **95:**500–505.

86. **Dakhama A, Lee YM, Ohnishi H, Jing X, Balhorn A, Takeda K, Gelfand EW.** 2009. Virus-specific IgE enhances airway responsiveness on reinfection with respiratory syncytial virus in newborn mice. *J Allergy Clin Immunol* **123:**138–145.

87. **Chang TW.** 2000. The pharmacological basis of anti-IgE therapy. *Nat Biotechnol* **18:**157–162.

88. **Adis International Ltd.** 2002. Omalizumab: anti-IgE monoclonal antibody E25, E25, humanised anti-IgE MAb, IGE 025, monoclonal antibody E25, Olizumab, Xolair, rhuMAb-E25. *BioDrugs* **16:**380–386.

89. **Garman SC, Wurzburg BA, Tarchevskaya SS, Kinet J-P, Jardetzky TS.** 2000. Structure of the Fc fragment of human IgE bound to its high-affinity receptor Fc[epsi]RI[alpha]. *Nature* **406:**259–266.

90. **Beck LA, Marcotte GV, MacGlashan D, Togias A, Saini S.** 2004. Omalizumab-induced reductions in mast cell FcεRI expression and function. *J Allergy Clin Immunol* **114:**527–530.

91. **Prussin C, Griffith DT, Boesel KM, Lin H, Foster B, Casale TB.** 2003. Omalizumab treatment downregulates dendritic cell FcepsilonRI expression. *J Allergy Clin Immunol* **112:**1147–1154.

92. **MacGlashan DW, Bochner BS, Adelman DC, Jardieu PM, Togias A, McKenzie-White J, Sterbinsky SA, Hamilton RG, Lichtenstein LM.** 1997. Down-regulation of Fc(epsilon)RI expression on human basophils during in vivo treatment of atopic patients with anti-IgE antibody. *J Immunol* **158:**1438–1445.

93. **Hunt J, Keeble AH, Dale RE, Corbett MK, Beavil RL, Levitt J, Swann MJ, Suhling K, Ameer-Beg S, Sutton BJ, Beavil AJ.** 2012. A fluorescent biosensor reveals conformational changes in human immunoglobulin E Fc: implications for mechanisms of receptor binding, inhibition, and allergen recognition. *J Biol Chem* **287:**17459–17470.

94. **D'Amato G.** 2006. Role of anti-IgE monoclonal antibody (omalizumab) in the treatment of bronchial asthma and allergic respiratory diseases. *Eur J Pharmacol* **533:**302–307.

95. **Leung DY, Sampson HA, Yunginger JW, Burks AW Jr, Schneider LC, Wortel CH, Davis FM, Hyun JD, Shanahan WR Jr.** 2003. Effect of anti-IgE therapy in patients with peanut allergy. *N Engl J Med* **348:**986–993.

96. **van Neerven RJ, van Roomen CP, Thomas WR, de Boer M, Knol EF, Davis FM.** 2001. Humanized anti-IgE mAb Hu-901 prevents the activation of allergen-specific T cells. *Int Arch Allergy Immunol* **124:**400–402.

97. **Poole JA, Meng J, Reff M, Spellman MC, Rosenwasser LJ.** 2005. Anti-CD23 monoclonal antibody, lumiliximab, inhibited allergen-induced responses in antigen-presenting cells and T cells from atopic subjects. *J Allergy Clin Immunol* **116:**780–788.

98. **Shiung YY, Chiang CY, Chen JB, Wu PC, Hung AF, Lu DC, Pan RL, Chang TW.** 2012. An anti-IgE monoclonal antibody that binds to IgE on CD23 but not on high-affinity IgE. Fc receptors. *Immunobiology* **217:**676–683.

99. **Chu SY, Horton HM, Pong E, Leung IW, Chen H, Nguyen DH, Bautista C, Muchhal US, Bernett MJ, Moore GL, Szymkowski DE, Desjarlais JR.** 2012. Reduction of total IgE by targeted coengagement of IgE B-cell receptor and FcgammaRIIb with Fc-engineered antibody. *J Allergy Clin Immunol* **129:**1102–1115.

100. **Abdulla NE, Ninan MJ, Markowitz AB.** 2012. Rituximab: current status as therapy for malignant and benign hematologic disorders. *BioDrugs* **26**:71–82.

101. **Simon D, Hosli S, Kostylina G, Yawalkar N, Simon HU.** 2008. Anti-CD20 (rituximab) treatment improves atopic eczema. *J Allergy Clin Immunol* **121**:122–128.

102. **Arkwright PD.** 2009. Anti-CD20 or anti-IgE therapy for severe chronic autoimmune urticaria. *J Allergy Clin Immunol* **123**:510–511. (Author's reply, **123**:511.)

103. **Tanaka H, Nagai H, Maeda Y.** 1998. Effect of anti-IL-4 and anti-IL-5 antibodies on allergic airway hyperresponsiveness in mice. *Life Sci* **62**:PL169–PL174.

104. **Steinke JW.** 2004. Anti-interleukin-4 therapy. *Immunol Allergy Clin N Am* **24**:599–614.

105. **Piper E, Brightling C, Niven R, Oh C, Faggioni R, Poon K, She D, Kell C, May RD, Geba GP, Molfino NA.** 2013. A phase 2 placebo-controlled study of tralokinumab in moderate-to-severe asthma. *Eur Respir J* **41**:330–338.

106. **Corren J, Lemanske RF, Hanania NA, Korenblat PE, Parsey MV, Arron JR, Harris JM, Scheerens H, Wu LC, Su Z, Mosesova S, Eisner MD, Bohen SP, Matthews JG.** 2011. Lebrikizumab treatment in adults with asthma. *N Engl J Med* **365**:1088–1098.

107. **Lee JJ, McGarry MP, Farmer SC, Denzler KL, Larson KA, Carrigan PE, Brenneise IE, Horton MA, Haczku A, Gelfand EW, Leikauf GD, Lee NA.** 1997. Interleukin-5 expression in the lung epithelium of transgenic mice leads to pulmonary changes pathognomonic of asthma. *J Exp Med* **185**:2143–2156.

108. **Stein ML, Villanueva JM, Buckmeier BK, Yamada Y, Filipovich AH, Assa'ad AH, Rothenberg ME.** 2008. Anti-IL-5 (mepolizumab) therapy reduces eosinophil activation ex vivo and increases IL-5 and IL-5 receptor levels. *J Allergy Clin Immunol* **121**:1473–1483.

109. **Adis International Ltd.** 2008. Mepolizumab: 240563, anti-IL-5 monoclonal antibody - GlaxoSmithKline, anti-interleukin-5 monoclonal antibody - GlaxoSmithKline, SB 240563. *Drugs R D* **9**:125–130.

110. **Robinson DS.** 2013. Mepolizumab treatment for asthma. *Expert Opin Biol Ther* **13**:295–302.

111. **Walsh GM.** 2009. Reslizumab, a humanized anti-IL-5 mAb for the treatment of eosinophil-mediated inflammatory conditions. *Curr Opin Mol Ther* **11**:329–336.

112. **Busse WW, Katial R, Gossage D, Sari S, Wang B, Kolbeck R, Coyle AJ, Koike M, Spitalny GL, Kiener PA, Geba GP, Molfino NA.** 2010. Safety profile, pharmacokinetics, and biologic activity of MEDI-563, an anti-IL-5 receptor alpha antibody, in a phase I study of subjects with mild asthma. *J Allergy Clin Immunol* **125**:1237–1244.

113. **Kolbeck R, Kozhich A, Koike M, Peng L, Andersson CK, Damschroder MM, Reed JL, Woods R, Dall'acqua WW, Stephens GL, Erjefalt JS, Bjermer L, Humbles AA, Gossage D, Wu H, Kiener PA, Spitalny GL, Mackay CR, Molfino NA, Coyle AJ.** 2010. MEDI-563, a humanized anti-IL-5 receptor alpha mAb with enhanced antibody-dependent cell-mediated cytotoxicity function. *J Allergy Clin Immunol* **125**:1344–1353.

114. **Kearley J, Erjefalt JS, Andersson C, Benjamin E, Jones CP, Robichaud A, Pegorier S, Brewah Y, Burwell TJ, Bjermer L, Kiener PA, Kolbeck R, Lloyd CM, Coyle AJ, Humbles AA.** 2011. IL-9 governs allergen-induced mast cell numbers in the lung and chronic remodeling of the airways. *Am J Respir Crit Care Med* **183**:865–875.

115. **Parker JM, Oh CK, LaForce C, Miller SD, Pearlman DS, Le C, Robbie GJ, White WI, White B, Molfino NA.** 2011. Safety profile and clinical activity of multiple subcutaneous doses of MEDI-528, a humanized anti-interleukin-9 monoclonal antibody, in two randomized phase 2a studies in subjects with asthma. *BMC Pulm Med* **11**:14.

116. **Brightling C, Berry M, Amrani Y.** 2008. Targeting TNF-alpha: a novel therapeutic approach for asthma. *J Allergy Clin Immunol* **121**:5–10.

117. **Wenzel SE, Barnes PJ, Bleecker ER, Bousquet J, Busse W, Dahlen SE, Holgate ST, Meyers DA, Rabe KF, Antczak A, Baker J, Horvath I, Mark Z, Bernstein D, Kerwin E, Schlenker-Herceg R, Lo KH, Watt R, Barnathan ES, Chanez P.** 2009. A randomized, double-blind, placebo-controlled study of tumor necrosis factor-alpha blockade in severe persistent asthma. *Am J Respir Crit Care Med* **179**:549–558.

118. **Ivanciuc O, Schein CH, Braun W.** 2002. Data mining of sequences and 3D structures of allergenic proteins. *Bioinformatics* **18**:1358–1364.

119. **Reisinger J, Horak F, Pauli G, van Hage M, Cromwell O, Konig F, Valenta R, Niederberger V.** 2005. Allergen-specific nasal IgG antibodies induced by vaccination with genetically modified allergens are associated with reduced nasal allergen sensitivity. *J Allergy Clin Immunol* **116**:347–354.

120. **Niederberger V, Horak F, Vrtala S, Spitzauer S, Krauth MT, Valent P, Reisinger J, Pelzmann M, Hayek B, Kronqvist M, Gafvelin G, Gronlund H,**

Purohit A, Suck R, Fiebig H, Cromwell O, Pauli G, van Hage-Hamsten M, Valenta R. 2004. Vaccination with genetically engineered allergens prevents progression of allergic disease. *Proc Natl Acad Sci USA* **101**(Suppl 2):14677–14682.

121. Bordas-Le Floch V, Bussieres L, Airouche S, Lautrette A, Bouley J, Berjont N, Horiot S, Huet A, Jain K, Lemoine P, Chabre H, Batard T, Mascarell L, Baron-Bodo V, Tourdot S, Nony E, Moingeon P. 2012. Expression and characterization of natural-like recombinant Der p 2 for sublingual immunotherapy. *Int Arch Allergy Immunol* **158**:157–167.

122. Chruszcz M, Pomes A, Glesner J, Vailes LD, Osinski T, Porebski PJ, Majorek KA, Heymann PW, Platts-Mills TAE, Minor W, Chapman MD. 2012. Molecular determinants for antibody binding on group 1 house dust mite allergens. *J Biol Chem* **287**:7388–7398.

123. Marsh DG, Lichtenstein LM, Campbell DH. 1970. Studies on "allergoids" prepared from naturally occurring allergens. I. Assay of allergenicity and antigenicity of formalinized rye group I component. *Immunology* **18**:705–722.

124. Ferrari E, Breda D, Longhi R, Vangelista L, Nakaie CR, Elviri L, Casali E, Pertinhez TA, Spisni A, Burastero SE. 2012. In search of a vaccine for mouse allergy: significant reduction of Mus m 1 allergenicity by structure-guided single-point mutations. *Int Arch Allergy Immunol* **157**:226–237.

125. Valenta R, Linhart B, Swoboda I, Niederberger V. 2011. Recombinant allergens for allergen-specific immunotherapy: 10 years anniversary of immunotherapy with recombinant allergens. *Allergy* **66**:775–783.

126. Canonica GW, Bousquet J, Casale T, Lockey RF, Baena-Cagnani CE, Pawankar R, Potter PC, Bousquet PJ, Cox LS, Durham SR, Nelson HS, Passalacqua G, Ryan DP, Brozek JL, Compalati E, Dahl R, Delgado L, van Wijk RG, Gower RG, Ledford DK, Filho NR, Valovirta EJ, Yusuf OM, Zuberbier T, Akhanda W, Almarales RC, Ansotegui I, Bonifazi F, Ceuppens J, Chivato T, Dimova D, Dumitrascu D, Fontana L, Katelaris CH, Kaulsay R, Kuna P, Larenas-Linnemann D, Manoussakis M, Nekam K, Nunes C, O'Hehir R, Olaguibel JM, Onder NB, Park JW, Priftanji A, Puy R, Sarmiento L, Scadding G, Schmid-Grendelmeier P, Seberova E, Sepiashvili R, Sole D, Togias A, Tomino C, Toskala E, Van Beever H, Vieths S. 2009. Sublingual immunotherapy: World Allergy Organization Position Paper 2009. *Allergy* **64**(Suppl 91):1–59.

127. Shamji MH, Ljorring C, Francis JN, Calderon MA, Larche M, Kimber I, Frew AJ, Ipsen H, Lund K, Wurtzen PA, Durham SR. 2012. Functional rather than immunoreactive levels of IgG4 correlate closely with clinical response to grass pollen immunotherapy. *Allergy* **67**:217–226.

128. James LK, Bowen H, Calvert RA, Dodev TS, Shamji MH, Beavil AJ, McDonnell JM, Durham SR, Gould HJ. 2012. Allergen specificity of IgG(4)-expressing B cells in patients with grass pollen allergy undergoing immunotherapy. *J Allergy Clin Immunol* **130**:663–670.

129. Pilette C, Nouri-Aria KT, Jacobson MR, Wilcock LK, Detry B, Walker SM, Francis JN, Durham SR. 2007. Grass pollen immunotherapy induces an allergen-specific IgA2 antibody response associated with mucosal TGF-beta expression. *J Immunol* **178**:4658–4666.

130. Satoguina JS, Weyand E, Larbi J, Hoerauf A. 2005. T regulatory-1 cells induce IgG4 production by B cells: role of IL-10. *J Immunol* **174**:4718–4726.

131. Wood N, Bourque K, Donaldson DD, Collins M, Vercelli D, Goldman SJ, Kasaian MT. 2004. IL-21 effects on human IgE production in response to IL-4 or IL-13. *Cell Immunol* **231**:133–145.

132. van der Neut Kolfschoten M, Schuurman J, Losen M, Bleeker WK, Martinez-Martinez P, Vermeulen E, den Bleker TH, Wiegman L, Vink T, Aarden LA, De Baets MH, van de Winkel JG, Aalberse RC, Parren PW. 2007. Anti-inflammatory activity of human IgG4 antibodies by dynamic Fab arm exchange. *Science* **317**:1554–1557.

133. Passalacqua G, Albano M, Riccio A, Fregonese L, Puccinelli P, Parmiani S, Canonica GW. 1999. Clinical and immunologic effects of a rush sublingual immunotherapy to Parietaria species: a double-blind, placebo-controlled trial. *J Allergy Clin Immunol* **104**:964–968.

134. Savilahti EM, Rantanen V, Lin JS, Karinen S, Saarinen KM, Goldis M, Makela MJ, Hautaniemi S, Savilahti E, Sampson HA. 2010. Early recovery from cow's milk allergy is associated with decreasing IgE and increasing IgG4 binding to cow's milk epitopes. *J Allergy Clin Immunol* **125**:1315–1321.

135. Savilahti EM, Saarinen KM, Savilahti E. 2010. Duration of clinical reactivity in cow's milk allergy is associated with levels of specific immunoglobulin G4 and immunoglobulin A antibodies to beta-lactoglobulin. *Clin Exp Allergy* **40**:251–256.

136. Harada K, Shimoda S, Kimura Y, Sato Y, Ikeda H, Igarashi S, Ren XS, Sato H, Nakanuma Y. 2012. Significance of immunoglobulin G4 (IgG4)-positive cells in extrahepatic cholangiocarcinoma: molecular mechanism of IgG4 reaction in cancer tissue. *Hepatology* **56**:157–164.

137. Karagiannis P, Gilbert AE, Josephs DH, Ali N, Dodev T, Saul L, Correa I, Roberts L, Beddowes E, Koers A, Hobbs C, Ferreira S, Geh JL, Healy C,

Harries M, Acland KM, Blower PJ, Mitchell T, Fear DJ, Spicer JF, Lacy KE, Nestle FO, Karagiannis SN. 2013. IgG4 subclass antibodies impair antitumor immunity in melanoma. *J Clin Investig* **123**:1457–1474.

138. Karagiannis SN, Josephs DH, Karagiannis P, Gilbert AE, Saul L, Rudman SM, Dodev T, Koers A, Blower PJ, Corrigan C, Beavil AJ, Spicer JF, Nestle FO, Gould HJ. 2012. Recombinant IgE antibodies for passive immunotherapy of solid tumours: from concept towards clinical application. *Cancer Immunol Immunother* **61**: 1547–1564.

139. Karagiannis SN, Wang Q, East N, Burke F, Riffard S, Bracher MG, Thompson RG, Durham SR, Schwartz LB, Balkwill FR, Gould HJ. 2003. Activity of human monocytes in IgE antibody-dependent surveillance and killing of ovarian tumor cells. *Eur J Immunol* **33**:1030–1040.

140. Gould HJ, Mackay GA, Karagiannis SN, O'Toole CM, Marsh PJ, Daniel BE, Coney LR, Zurawski VR Jr, Joseph M, Capron M, Gilbert M, Murphy GF, Korngold R. 1999. Comparison of IgE and IgG antibody-dependent cytotoxicity in vitro and in a SCID mouse xenograft model of ovarian carcinoma. *Eur J Immunol* **29**: 3527–3537.

141. Karagiannis SN, Nestle FO, Gould HJ. 2010. IgE interacts with potent effector cells against tumors: ADCC and ADCP, p 185–213. *In* Penichet ML, Jensen-Jarolim E (ed), *Cancer and IgE*. Humana Press, Springer, New York, NY.

142. Karagiannis P, Singer J, Hunt J, Gan SK, Rudman SM, Mechtcheriakova D, Knittelfelder R, Daniels TR, Hobson PS, Beavil AJ, Spicer J, Nestle FO, Penichet ML, Gould HJ, Jensen-Jarolim E, Karagiannis SN. 2009. Characterisation of an engineered trastuzumab IgE antibody and effector cell mechanisms targeting HER2/neu-positive tumour cells. *Cancer Immunol Immunother* **58**:915–930.

143. Rudman SM, Josephs DH, Cambrook H, Karagiannis P, Gilbert AE, Dodev T, Hunt J, Koers A, Montes A, Taams L, Canevari S, Figini M, Blower PJ, Beavil AJ, Nicodemus CF, Corrigan C, Kaye SB, Nestle FO, Gould HJ, Spicer JF, Karagiannis SN. 2011. Harnessing engineered antibodies of the IgE class to combat malignancy: initial assessment of FcεRI-mediated basophil activation by a tumour-specific IgE antibody to evaluate the risk of type I hypersensitivity. *Clin Exp Allergy* **41**:1400–1413.

144. Jensen-Jarolim E, Singer J. 2011. Why could passive immunoglobulin E antibody therapy be safe in clinical oncology? *Clin Exp Allergy* **41**: 1337–1340.

145. CharacterisationSutton BJ, Beavil RL, Beavil AJ. 2000. Inhibition of IgE-receptor interactions. *Br Med Bull* **56**:1004–1018.

146. Nigro EA, Brini AT, Soprana E, Ambrosi A, Dombrowicz D, Siccardi AG, Vangelista L. 2009. Antitumor IgE adjuvanticity: key role of Fc epsilon RI. *J Immunol* **183**:4530–4536.

147. Teng MW, Kershaw MH, Jackson JT, Smyth MJ, Darcy PK. 2006. Adoptive transfer of chimeric FcepsilonRI gene-modified human T cells for cancer immunotherapy. *Hum Gene Ther* **17**:1134–1143.

148. Kershaw MH, Darcy PK, Trapani JA, MacGregor D, Smyth MJ. 1998. Tumor-specific IgE-mediated inhibition of human colorectal carcinoma xenograft growth. *Oncol Res* **10**:133–142.

149. Teo PZ, Utz PJ, Mollick JA. 2012. Using the allergic immune system to target cancer: activity of IgE antibodies specific for human CD20 and MUC1. *Cancer Immunol Immunother* **61**:2295–2309.

150. Spillner E, Plum M, Blank S, Miehe M, Singer J, Braren I. 2012. Recombinant IgE antibody engineering to target EGFR. *Cancer Immunol Immunother* **61**:1565–1573.

151. Daniels TR, Leuchter RK, Quintero R, Helguera G, Rodriguez JA, Martinez-Maza O, Schultes BC, Nicodemus CF, Penichet ML. 2012. Targeting HER2/neu with a fully human IgE to harness the allergic reaction against cancer cells. *Cancer Immunol Immunother* **61**:991–1003.

152. Riemer AB, Untersmayr E, Knittelfelder R, Duschl A, Pehamberger H, Zielinski CC, Scheiner O, Jensen-Jarolim E. 2007. Active induction of tumor-specific IgE antibodies by oral mimotope vaccination. *Cancer Res* **67**:3406–3411.

153. Knittelfelder R, Riemer AB, Jensen-Jarolim E. 2009. Mimotope vaccination--from allergy to cancer. *Expert Opin Biol Ther* **9**:493–506.

154. Jensen-Jarolim E, Achatz G, Turner MC, Karagiannis S, Legrand F, Capron M, Penichet ML, Rodriguez JA, Siccardi AG, Vangelista L, Riemer AB, Gould H. 2008. AllergoOncology: the role of IgE-mediated allergy in cancer. *Allergy* **63**:1255–1266.

155. Jensen-Jarolim E, Pawelec G. 2012. The nascent field of AllergoOncology. *Cancer Immunol Immunother* **61**:1355–1357.

ANTIBODY DISCOVERY APPROACHES

6

Phage and Yeast Display

JARED SHEEHAN[1] and WAYNE A. MARASCO[1]

DISCOVERY OF THERAPEUTIC ANTIBODIES USING PHAGE DISPLAY TECHNOLOGY

Bacteriophage Biology and Antibody Display Method

Bacteriophage (phage) are viruses that infect and replicate within bacterial cells. Filamentous phage particles inject single-stranded DNA into target bacterial cells for subsequent replication and assembly of new virions within the host cytoplasm. The filamentous phage species capable of infecting *Escherichia coli* manifest as long, thin filaments that are secreted from host bacteria without cell lysis. Due to their ease of manipulation and stability in a range of temperatures and pH, F pilus-specific filamentous phage species, including f1, fd, and M13, serve as reliable vehicles for combinatorial technologies, such as phage display (1–4).

A collection of the first human antibody libraries displayed on the phage surface was published in the early 1990s (5–8). This antibody phage display technology is based upon a large collection of human antibody genes subcloned into an *E. coli* expression vector, which is packaged into filamentous phage. Upon production from host bacterial cells, these phage particles display the antibody

[1]Department of Cancer Immunology and AIDS, Dana-Farber Cancer Institute, Harvard Medical School, Boston, MA 02215.

Antibodies for Infectious Diseases
Edited by James E. Crowe, Jr., Diana Boraschi, and Rino Rappuoli
© 2015 American Society for Microbiology, Washington, DC
doi:10.1128/microbiolspec.AID-0028-2014

fragment on its surface as a fusion product with one of the viral coat proteins. This established library must be screened to isolate the phage antibodies of interest. To ensure representation of all immunoglobulin variants within the library, a larger number of phage particles—above the total number of unique antibody sequences—is typically screened. This fold-excess in selection experiments is easily achieved since filamentous phage can produce titers up to 10^{13} particles per ml of culture (1).

The purpose of antibody display library selections is to isolate an antibody variant with the desired functional properties. A purified, heterogeneous population of phage library members is screened to identify and enrich for the antibody sequences of interest. This phage library selection typically involves the capture of the target antigen, either by immobilization on a plastic surface (solid phase) or coupled to magnetic beads (solution phase). When incubated with this captured antigen, the phage surfaces—purified virions in solution—allow binding of specific antibody variants. Multiple washes remove nonbinding phage particles, while attached phage are typically eluted under either low- or high-pH conditions to disrupt the antibody-antigen association. Following this elution step, these phage antibodies are used to infect an *E. coli* culture for amplification of the antigen-reactive library subpopulation. The purified, amplified phage antibodies from this initial selection event are used for subsequent rounds of panning. Due to the possibility of nonspecific binding, at least two to three rounds of this type of iterative library selection are performed to enrich for positive binders and reduce "background" binding events. An overview of this phage library selection procedure is outlined in Fig. 1.

Sources of Antibody Genes for Display Libraries

The quality and diversity of a phage library's total antibody repertoire is dependent upon the source of immunoglobulin genes. To establish the library repertoire, the heterogeneous pool of antibody genes is typically derived from B cell mRNA from healthy donors (naïve library) or immunized donors or animals (immune library) (6–7). The variable fragments from the donated B cell cDNA are amplified using germline gene family-based primers (8). These heavy (V_H) and light (V_L) chain gene copies are randomly associated through cloning methods involving specific expression vectors depending upon the antibody fragment format to be displayed on the phage surface (discussed in "Antibody Phage Display Formats," below). In addition, synthetic libraries may be established through prearranged V, D, and J gene associations and V_H/V_L pairings, based upon desired immunogenetic profiles or biochemical properties.

Naïve Phage Antibody Libraries

While nonimmunized human B cell donor sources are typically peripheral blood mononuclear cells, other sources of a library's antibody gene repertoire include spleen, tonsils, bone marrow, and murine peripheral blood mononuclear cells (7, 9–12). The advantage of the naïve library lies in the diversity of the antigen-unbiased variants, which can be used for selections against a large panel of targets, including self and toxic antigens (7, 10, 13). The quality of monoclonal antibodies (mAbs) isolated from this type of naïve library is dependent upon the total population number, with large, diverse libraries of ~10^{10} unique variants permitting the discovery of human antibodies with subnanomolar binding affinities (10). The availability of large, pre-established collections of nonimmune immunoglobulin gene pools has made the creation of naïve phage antibody libraries more convenient than immune libraries (12).

Immune Phage Antibody Libraries

In addition to these naïve sources, a phage library's antibody gene pool may be created from human donors or animals immunized with an antigen of interest. This type of immune library is enriched for antigen-reactive

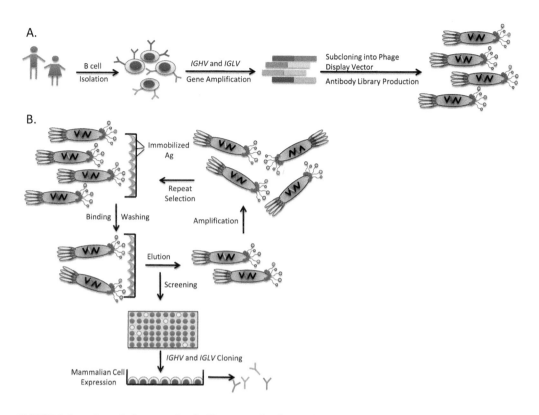

FIGURE 1 Overview of phage antibody library production and selections. (A) The phage antibody library repertoire is derived from the B cells of naïve or immune donors. The amplified *IGHV* and *IGLV/IGKV* genes are subcloned into a phage display vector for *E. coli* expression and library production. (B) The phage antibody library is selected against an immobilized target antigen. After washing to remove nonbinders, the Ag-reactive phage antibodies are eluted, amplified, and reselected through subsequent rounds. ELISA screens identify monoclonal, Ag-binding phage antibodies, whose heavy and light chain antibody genes are subcloned into mammalian expression vectors. doi:10.1128/microbiolspec.AID-0028-2014.f1

variants with populations of affinity matured V_H and V_L gene fragments, due to the host immune system machinery (6, 12, 14). Unlike naïve gene pools, immune phage libraries are comprised of antibody genes that are biased toward the initial antigen. While this antigenic bias limits the scope of targets for this type of library, immune gene pools are composed of a higher frequency of antigen-reactive library members at the onset of selections. Further, immune phage antibody libraries permit the monitoring of natural immunoglobulin responses, functioning as diagnostics in patients with autoimmune disorders and viral infections (15, 16). Compared with hybridoma campaigns, significantly more mAbs can be isolated from a single immunized donor through an immune phage antibody library (12).

Synthetic Phage Antibody Libraries

An antibody gene repertoire is artificially designed, prior to cloning into a phage expression vector, to create a synthetic phage display library. Usually, the *in vitro* assembly of novel immunoglobulin genes involves a designed randomization of complementary determining regions (CDRs) into V, D, and J segments (17). The heavy chain CDR3 is considered the most hypervariable of all antigen-contacting loops, causing this region to be targeted for extensive manipulation (18).

Although several optimized phage libraries are established, two examples of modern, synthetic, and semi-synthetic phage display libraries are frequently described in the literature as discovery tools. One corporation created a phage display library that combines both DNA sequences from synthetic design and naïve human donors. For this semi-synthetic antibody library, donor-sourced fragments comprise the V_H CDR3 and complete V_L, while *in vitro* synthesis of V segment DNA introduces designed diversity in V_H CDR1 and CDR2 (19). Another group developed synthetic phage display libraries by modifying the sequence and length of all six CDRs based upon their context in natural human antibody gene families (20–22).

Antibody Phage Display Formats

Previous reports describe phage display libraries as fusion products with all five of the pIII, pVI, pVII, pVIII, and viral coat proteins (5, 13, 23–26). Fusion products of the minor coat pIII —either a truncated or full-length protein— represent the majority of human antibody display libraries. The surface protein pIII is an integral membrane protein that is necessary for phage particle assembly and release from host cells (2). Since only the pIII C-terminus is necessary for new virion construction, a human antibody or antibody fragment can be expressed as a fusion product with this truncated viral protein (3, 5, 13). Schematics of these phage protein-scFv fusions are detailed in Fig. 2.

Two of the primary pIII antibody display library types involve human single-chain variable fragment (scFv) or fragment antigen-binding (Fab) formats. The human scFv format consists of a heavy chain variable (VH) domain and light chain variable (VL) domain expressed as a single polypeptide connected by a flexible linker region, with no associated constant domains. With Fab libraries, the heavy and light chains are expressed as separate gene products from the same vector with constant heavy 1 and constant light

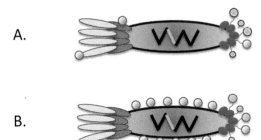

FIGURE 2 **Types of phage antibody display. (A) Monovalent display with the scFv or Fab fusion (green circle) to truncated pIII along with wild-type copies of pIII (purple circles). This monovalent mAb display format can also be used with pVII (olive) or pIX (light blue) separately. (B) Multivalent display with the scFv or Fab fusion to all copies of truncated pIII. Multivalent mAb display is also possible with the major coat protein pVIII (black border) separate from pIII. The pVI (red circles) coat proteins are also present in these diagrams. doi:10.1128/microbiolspec. AID-0028-2014.f2**

domains, respectively (5). The establishment of modern, optimized, human antibody phage display libraries supports the contemporary role of this combinatorial technology in ongoing antibody discovery (19–22).

scFv-pIII Display

Within this scFv-pIII display technology, the single-chain antibodies can be expressed as monovalent or multivalent fusion products on the phage surface. The majority of pIII fusion libraries are based on monovalent (phagemid) vectors compared to multivalent (phage) vectors (27). To "rescue" the viral particles from host bacterial cells, the phagemid vector system requires the addition of other wild-type phage genes and proteins via helper phage infection (28). This helper phage infection introduces a wild-type copy of pIII, which outcompetes the scFv-pIII fusion during particle incorporation. This preference for wild-type pIII results in a recovered phage particle population whose majority displays no scFv-pIII fusion on the viral surface, with the second most-frequent population bearing a single copy of the fusion product (27). Despite this wild-type dominance, the monovalent scFv-pIII display technique allows for the selection of higher-affinity antibodies due to single-copy competition among library variants during iterative rounds of selection. This monovalent competition requires at least two to three successive rounds of panning to enrich for scFv-pIII variants over wild-type pIII phage particles.

A multivalent scFv-pIII library can be created through a helper phage population with a *gene III* deletion, delivery of a helper plasmid, or the subcloning of *scFv* genes into a true phage vector (13, 27, 29–31). The multivalent display of scFv-pIII fusion proteins permits for the selection of library isolates based upon avidity, rather than affinity. In addition, these phage library-derived variants demonstrate a stronger functional affinity when the target antigen is multivalent, such as the environment during solid phase selections (27). An advantage of this multivalent display strategy is the reduced number of iterative rounds of selection required to isolate antigen-reactive clones. Selection campaigns using a multivalent scFv-pIII library yield antigen-binding populations after only a single round of panning, with antigen-reactive frequencies of >30% observed by the second round (27). Similar selections with monovalent phagemid libraries require at least three rounds of selection before reaching this frequency of positive binding events. Despite this accelerated selection process, multivalent phage library vectors suffer poorer transformation efficiencies, resulting in smaller, less diverse antibody gene pools (27).

Fab-pIII Display

Early pioneering work in establishing phage display included libraries expressing Fab fragments for selections (5, 9, 32, 33). Modern phage libraries displaying Fab fragments are well established and engineered for improved biochemical and expression properties for therapeutic discovery (19–22). For displaying Fabs on the phage surface, either the heavy or light chain constant domain—preferably the constant heavy 1 to avoid anchored V_L dimers—is C-terminally fused to pIII. The non-anchored partner chain is secreted into the periplasmic region, where V_H/V_L chain pairing occurs to form a complete Fab on the phage surface (12). While the reduced size of the scFv fragment provides for increased genetic stability over Fab libraries, many scFvs are observed to oligomerize, negatively impacting selection strategies (12, 13).

Structural properties of the Fab fragment have desirable features for certain antibody discovery processes. Specifically, the presence of the constant heavy 1 and constant light domains may influence conformational characteristics of the V_H and V_L fragments. Compared with the scFv format, certain reports have described the increased capacity of selected Fabs to retain antigen specificity when converted to a full-length IgG antibody (34). In addition to favorable biochemical properties, *in vivo* studies demonstrated the biological potential of Fab antibody fragments. Efficacy studies in a rheumatoid arthritis mouse model reported no significant therapeutic difference between Fab or IgG1 treatments (35). In terms of antibody development, one study described the Fab format as a reliable platform during affinity maturation efforts. The improvements in binding characteristics observed in particular Fab conformations were retained following the conversion to full-length IgG. (36). These findings suggest that the Fab format is a successful antibody fragment surrogate for the selection, prediction, and optimization of IgG candidates.

Antibodies for Infectious Diseases Discovered by Phage Display

The continuing emergence of novel strains and drug-resistant microbial pathogens has created persistent threats to public health. The ongoing discovery of mAbs directed against targets of infectious agents presents clinical opportunities for patients. These antimicrobial mAbs are typically well tolerated in patients and demonstrate high specificity for the targeted pathogen, reducing the opportunity for cross-reactivity with host or nontarget agents.

The *in vitro* discovery technology of phage display is one of the most promising vehicles for identifying antimicrobial, therapeutic antibodies. This selection method allows for the opportunity to isolate mAbs against toxic species or antigens, a threatening characteristic not suitable for murine hybridoma campaigns. Previous phage display approaches describe the discovery of antiviral and antibacterial mAbs.

Antiviral mAbs Discovered by Phage Display

The efforts of antiviral research are aimed at a fluid pathogenic landscape whose future characteristics are difficult to predict. Among all human pathogens, viruses are the best-suited pathogens to evade host immune pressure. Viral mutational robustness allows for antigenic drift, where escape mutations within targeted epitopes result in progeny with increased resistance to neutralizing mAbs or small molecules (37). Furthermore, coinfections with two or more viral strains allow for antigenic shift through gene transfer, establishing novel pathogens and complicating vaccine and treatment strategies (38–40). These continuous modes of viral evolution necessitate the development of new treatment options, which include the discovery of antiviral mAbs.

The targets of early antiviral mAb discovery using phage display included human immunodeficiency virus type 1 (HIV-1), respiratory syncytial virus, and herpes simplex virus (14, 16). Surface viral glycoproteins are preferred targets for phage selection campaigns, given their extracellular exposure, typically soluble character, and critical roles in the viral life cycle (41). Viral neutralization is a significant trait under consideration during the characterization of mAbs isolated from selections against viral antigens. This capacity of antiviral mAbs to bind and inactivate viral particles is

initially evaluated through designed *in vitro* experiments. Following these primary bioassays, the *in vivo* protection of lead candidate mAbs is determined through viral challenge studies in animals. Potential mechanisms of viral neutralization include the inhibition of virus attachment to host cell receptors, the blockage of membrane fusion events releasing viral genetic material, and prevention of new virion release from infected cells (42, 43).

Outside of direct inactivation, nonneutralizing antiviral mAbs may bind viral antigens on the cell surface during progeny release, recruiting cytotoxic cells or complement proteins to offer *in vivo* protection. These findings fueled the ongoing debate surrounding the correlation between *in vitro* neutralization and *in vivo* protection for antibodies (41, 44). Since the principal fraction of nonneutralizing mAbs fail to clear viral infections *in vivo*, however, the emphasis during antiviral mAb discovery should be placed on neutralizing immunoglobulins (41). A brief summary of antiviral mAbs discovered using phage antibody libraries is listed in Table 1.

Anti-Influenza mAbs Discovered by Phage Display

One of the most popular targets for recent antiviral mAb discovery is the influenza virus. Due to the absence of a universal vaccine and the ongoing emergence of new strains as human pathogens, the discovery of protective mAbs against influenza remains relevant. Influenza A viruses—the group of influenza viruses most closely associated with human infections—are classified within the classical subtypes of H1-H16 and N1-N9 based upon structural and antigenic characteristics of the hemagglutinin (HA) and neuraminidase viral glycoproteins (45). The HA molecule is the major surface envelope protein and is responsible for mediating attachment to sialic acid on the target cell surface (46). The globular head of HA, which contains the sialic acid binding domain, is amenable to mutations to avoid immune pressure without significant costs to viral fitness (41, 47). The HA stem domain is

TABLE 1 Summary of antiviral antibodies discovered using phage display[a]

Viral family	Virus	Viral target	Ab fragment displayed	Ab source	Reference
Coronaviridae	MERS-CoV	Spike glycoprotein	scFv	Naïve	72
	MERS-CoV	Spike receptor binding domain (RBD)	Fab	Naïve	73
	SARS-CoV	Spike, S1 domain	scFv	Naïve	65
	SARS-CoV	Spike RBD	Fab	Naïve	66
Filoviridae	Ebola virus	Inactivated virus	Fab	Immune	78
Flaviviridae	Dengue virus	mAb-captured dengue virus	scFv	Naïve	76
	Dengue virus	Nonstructural protein 5 (NS5)	Fab	Naïve	77
	West Nile virus	E glycoprotein	scFv	Naïve	74
	West Nile virus	Inactivated virus, VLP, or E glycoprotein	scFv	Immune	75
Herpesviridae	Herpes simplex virus	mAb-captured gB and gD glycoproteins	Fab	Immune	81
Orthomyxoviridae	Influenza A virus	Hemagglutinin (HA)	scFv	Naïve	49–51
	Influenza A virus	HA	scFv	Semi-synthetic	52
	Influenza A virus	HA	scFv	Immune	53
	Influenza A and B viruses	HA	scFv	Immune	51
Paramyxoviridae	Respiratory syncytial virus	F glycoprotein	Fab	Immune	79–80
Retroviridae	HIV-1	gp120	Fab	Immune	59, 60, 63
	HIV-1	gp41	Fab	Immune	61–63

[a]Note: This list is a summary of selected publications and is not to be considered complete.

involved in the pH-dependent endosomal membrane fusion event and is a more conserved region of the viral glycoprotein and is less tolerant of amino acid substitutions (48).

Seminal phage display studies using purified, recombinant HA protein as the selection antigen reported whole panels of broadly neutralizing human mAbs (49–51). The broadly neutralizing mAbs isolated from these phage library selections are overwhelmingly biased toward the conserved stem domain, preventing endosomal membrane fusion but permitting viral attachment. Given the stem region conservation and epitope proximity, the potent neutralization among these phage display-derived mAbs is observed across multiple subtypes of influenza viruses. Following up on these initial studies, selections using a semi-synthetic phage library identified specific immunoglobulin signatures associated with

heterosubtypic neutralization for stem-directed anti-HA mAbs (52).

Phage display experiments using influenza HA as the selection antigen have also identified neutralizing antibodies directed against the globular head of the glycoprotein. While these antibodies are capable of binding HA proteins across multiple viral subtypes, globular head-directed mAbs tend to be less heteroreactive, given the lack of strict conservation among these epitopes. Studies involving phage library selections yielded head-directed mAbs capable of neutralizing single or multiple subtypes, including H1N1, H2N2, and H3N2 viruses (53–54). Despite this limited scope of reactivity, mAbs that are neutralizing to the globular head are typically more potent, a trend likely due to epitope availability on the viral surface (41). Neutralization escape variants are more easily generated by immune pressure on the globular head, however, as the loops and glycosylation sites allow this region to tolerate mutations (55).

Anti-HIV-1 mAbs Discovered by Phage Display

Another well-documented target for phage display library selections is HIV-1. The primary target of anti-HIV-1 humoral responses is the trimeric Env protein of the viral surface. The gp120 protein of this Env complex binds the CD4 molecule and the CCR5 or CXCR5 coreceptors on $CD4^+$ T cells and macrophages. This engagement causes a conformational change in the Env complex to induce the membrane fusion activity of the gp41 component (56). One of the primary challenges in developing an HIV-1 vaccine strategy or broadly neutralizing mAbs is the extensive genetic diversity, with up to 10% *Env* gene variability within a single patient (57). Similar to influenza HA, the HIV-1 Env trimer utilizes several mechanisms to avoid neutralizing mAbs, including masking of critical epitopes, amino acid mutations, and glycan shielding without loss of protein activity (58).

Among the collection of first-generation anti-HIV-1 mAbs, several neutralizing library variants, including mAb b12, were isolated using phage display technology (59, 60). Although these discoveries provided initial data related to the CD4 binding site epitope, these mAbs are limited in their scope of neutralization, with mAb b12 neutralizing only one third of total HIV-1 isolates (41). More recent phage library selections against the viral gp120 and gp41 antigen yielded mAbs neutralizing a diverse collection of primary isolates and subtypes (61–63). In addition, the immunization schedule using HIV-1 antigens influences the selection quality of anti-HIV-1 mAbs from immune phage libraries, consistent with earlier findings regarding immune libraries' capacity for tracking natural humoral responses in humans (64). While these phage display-related studies offered primary mapping data and early vaccine strategies, current anti-HIV-1 mAb discovery efforts rely more

heavily on single B cell sorting or reverse transcriptase PCR techniques and the screening of *in vitro*-activated B cells (41).

Anticoronavirus mAbs Discovered by Phage Display

The severe acute respiratory syndrome coronavirus (SARS-CoV) predated its Middle East respiratory syndrome coronavirus (MERS-CoV) relative as an emerging human pathogen during the early 2000s. A potent neutralizing antibody was identified from panning experiments with purified, truncated S1 domain-only antigen (65). Other selection studies produced a similarly neutralizing mAb (66). These phage display studies using SARS-CoV antigen fragments influenced the future strategies surrounding the current MERS-CoV emerging infectious disease.

A human pathogen recently targeted by phage display studies is the emerging MERS-CoV. Similar to its SARS-CoV *Coronaviridae* family member, the MERS-CoV strains are capable of residing in other mammalian species, including bats and camels (67, 68). The MERS-CoV uses the major envelope spike (S) glycoprotein trimer for attachment and entry into target cells, with the S1 domain containing the dipeptidyl peptidase 4 (DPP4) receptor binding site and the S2 region mediating membrane fusion (69, 70). Previous reports involving infected patients describe the production of S protein-directed neutralizing antibodies (71).

Recently published studies describe phage library selections to identify panels of neutralizing mAbs. Selections against full-length MERS-CoV S protein using scFv-pIII display libraries yielded neutralizing antibodies localizing to the receptor binding domain. Despite the presence of the full-length protein during selections, this campaign resulted in S1 domain-specific mAbs, which neutralized MERS-CoV pseudotyped virus-like particles by blocking the DPP4 binding site on the viral glycoprotein (72). Similarly, Fab-pIII library selections against truncated DPP4 receptor binding domain-only antigen yielded mAbs capable of neutralizing both pseudotyped and live MERS-CoV (73). These studies provide examples of the ongoing relevance of phage display technology in current, emerging infectious diseases.

Other Antiviral mAbs Discovered by Phage Display

In addition to the viruses discussed above, mAbs directed against other viral pathogens are detailed in the literature. Initial studies involving phage library selections against purified West Nile Virus (WNV) envelope E glycoprotein produced neutralizing antibody sequences (74). Additional neutralizing mAbs were isolated from phage library selections using inactivated WNV or virus-like particles as well as immobilized E glycoprotein (75). A total of nine unique antibody sequences were identified from phage library selections against Ab-captured dengue virus particles; all members of this mAb panel demonstrated some degree of cross-reactivity among the four dengue virus serotypes (76). Recent phage library panning experiments using purified dengue nonstructural protein 5 generated a collection of cross-reactive mAbs intended for future mechanistic studies of the viral replication machinery (77).

Outside of flaviviruses and coronaviruses, other viral pathogens previously served as targets of early phage display campaigns. Experiments involving inactivated Ebola virus isolates generated one antiglycoprotein mAb capable of neutralizing the virus *in vitro* (78). Neutralizing mAbs showing *in vivo* protection against respiratory syncytial virus were isolated from preliminary Fab library selections against the viral F glycoprotein (79–80). Similarly, neutralizing mAbs preventing the cell-to-cell transmission of herpes simplex virus were discovered from pannings against glycoprotein D (81).

Antibacterial mAbs Discovered by Phage Display

The ongoing development of bacterial resistance to antimicrobial agents continues to pose global threats to both healthy individuals and infected patients. Specifically, the misuse of antimicrobial drugs drives bacterial evolution such that antibiotics are becoming increasingly ineffective among Gram-negative and Gram-positive strains (82–85). Previous clinical observations support the role of passive immunotherapy as prophylactic and therapeutic strategies against bacterial pathogens and their toxins (86).

Phage display technologies allow for antibody library selections against bacterial antigens, infectious agents which are impractical for *in vivo* approaches such as hybridoma campaigns. Unlike approaches with viral pathogens, successful phage display efforts surrounding antibacterial mAb discovery involve secreted toxins as selection antigens, rather than surface or structural proteins. These species-specific exotoxins cause patient symptoms including diarrhea, renal failure, paralysis, and death (87).

In terms of these secreted toxins, mAb-based antibacterial therapies offer several advantages over antibiotic compounds. These antibiotic drugs do not demonstrate the ability to eliminate pro-inflammatory bacterial factors or cell fragments, which can be neutralized or cleared through mAb binding. This outcome may permit disease progression despite the removal of the bacterial pathogen. Further, toxin neutralization mechanisms create more feasible preclinical models for evaluating novel mAbs, accelerating their discovery (87). A brief summary of antibacterial mAbs discovered using phage antibody libraries is listed in Table 2.

Antibotulinum mAbs Discovered by Phage Display

The *Clostridium* genus encompasses a group of Gram-positive bacteria species capable of secreting toxins. *Clostridium botulinum* produces botulinum neurotoxins (BoNTs) of serotypes A-G, with the A, B, and E serotypes most frequently causing human botulism (88). These BoNTs act at cholinergic nerve endings to prevent acetylcholine release, providing the

TABLE 2 Summary of antibacterial antibodies discovered using phage display[a]

Bacterial family	Bacterial species	Bacterial target	Ab fragment displayed	Ab source	Reference
Bacillaceae	Bacillus anthracis	Protective antigen	scFv	Naïve	94
	Bacillus anthracis	Lethal factor	scFv	Immune	95
	Bacillus anthracis	Edema factor	Fab	Immune	96
Clostridiaceae	Clostridium botulinum	Botulinum neurotoxin (BoNT) subtypes A–E	scFv	Immune and naïve	88
	Clostridium botulinum	BoNT/A heavy chain	scFv	Immune	90
	Clostridium difficile	Toxin B	scFv	Immune	97
	Clostridium tetani	Tetanus toxoid	Fab	Naïve	98
Staphylococcaceae	Staphylococcus aureus	GrfA peptide fragments	scFv	Immune	99

[a]Note: This list is a summary of selected publications and is not to be considered complete.

paralytic effects of these exotoxins (89). Phage library selections against BoNT serotypes A-E produced neutralizing mAbs, with the successful clones preferentially isolated from immune sources (88, 90). The most potent of these neutralizing mAbs were directed against the BoNT heavy chain C-terminus. The administration of any mAb pair recognizing nonoverlapping heavy chain epitopes provided complete protection during murine *in vivo* toxin neutralization experiments, while single antibody delivery resulted in significant viability loss (91). The ongoing mAb discovery surrounding BoNTs remains important, given their classification as high-risk agents as bioweapons (91).

Antianthrax mAbs Discovered by Phage Display

Similar to the *C. botulinum* BoNTs, the Gram-positive *Bacillus anthracis*, the causative agent of anthrax, is considered a public safety threat because of its use as a biological weapon (92). Upon establishing an infection within lymph nodes, dividing bacilli release three exotoxins: protective antigen (PA), lethal factor (LF), and edema factor (EF). The PA toxin binds cellular receptors for delivery of LF or EF into the host cytosol. The PA toxin may combine with LF to form lethal toxin or EF to create the edema toxin, both of which induce the toxic symptoms associated with anthrax disease (93).

Phage library selections against recombinant PA resulted in the discovery of raxibacumab (ABthrax), a human IgG1 mAb that binds PA to inhibit cellular delivery of LF and EF to prevent and treat inhalational anthrax (94). Prior to FDA approval, this anti-PA mAb demonstrated *in vivo* protection in both rabbits and monkeys. An anti-LF scFv produced from phage library panning demonstrated *in vitro* toxin neutralization and *in vivo* protection (95). Phage library selections against recombinant EF yielded an anti-EF mAb that protected mice from edema and death during lethal dose administration (96). These phage display studies continue to be valuable in defining protective, biodefense strategies.

Other Antibacterial mAbs Discovered by Phage Display

Bacterial pathogens other than *C. botulinum* and *B. anthracis* are described as targets of phage display experiments. A relative of *C. botulinum*, the *Clostridium difficile* pathogen is the leading cause of antibiotic-associated diarrhea, with increasing severity due to the ongoing emergence of hypervirulent strains (87). Disease onset occurs by production of toxins A and B following intestinal colonization. Phage library panning experiments against *C. difficile* toxin B generated a mAb, with improved affinity over the parent antibody, intended for use as a novel immunodiagnostic agent (97). *Clostridium tetani*, another member of this *Clostridium* genus, establishes infection through open wounds and secretes tetanus toxoid to induce painful muscle rigidity and spasms. A mAb isolated from library selections against tetanus toxoid demonstrated *in vitro* neutralization of this exotoxin (98).

While the majority of successful phage library panning campaigns involve exotoxins, less successful experiments involving bacterial surface proteins are described in the literature. *Staphylococcus aureus* continues to present major challenges in clinical settings due to the tendency of this species to develop antibiotic resistance, such as methicillin-resistant *S. aureus* (MRSA). Phage library selections against peptide fragments of the GrfA surface macromolecule transporter from MRSA resulted in a lead candidate scFv (Aurograb), which eventually failed in clinical trials (87, 99). Given the spread of MRSA strains among hospitals, its elevated resistance rate to antibiotics, and the current failure of available human antibodies, the continued development of new mAb selection strategies will create improved therapeutic alternatives during patient infections.

DISCOVERY OF THERAPEUTIC ANTIBODIES USING YEAST DISPLAY TECHNOLOGY

Yeast Biology and Antibody Display System

Yeast are eukaryotic, unicellular organisms comprising a variety of strains belonging to the kingdom *Fungi*. The budding yeast *Saccharomyces cerevisiae* possesses a rigid cell wall approximately 200 nm thick, primarily composed of mannoproteins and β-linked glucans (100). The budding yeast cell wall surface agglutinins function as adhesion proteins, promoting aggregation of opposite mating types during mating events (101). The Aga2p subunit, which binds the agglutinin proteins of the opposite mating type, is tethered to the

yeast cell wall through two disulfide bonds to Aga1p (100). The cell wall of each yeast cell can display 10^4 to 10^5 agglutinins (100, 102). Since the development of the yeast display technology, *S. cerevisiae* has served as the most commonly used species in this combinatorial strategy.

To establish a yeast antibody display library, the heterogeneous immunoglobulin gene pool is cloned into the yeast display plasmid and expressed as fusion products with the Aga2p protein. The human antibody fragments are typically fused to the C-terminus of the Aga2p subunit (100). While the scFvs are the most frequently used format in yeast display, other antibody fragments may be displayed on the yeast surface, including Fabs, whole IgG1s, and camelid domain antibodies (102). The Aga1p cell wall protein is stably expressed from a chromosomal locus. The expression of both Aga1p and the mAb-Aga2p product are under the control of the galactose-inducible GAL1 promoter (102, 103). A diagram detailing the yeast surface display system is shown in Fig. 3.

In the presence of galactose, the yeast cell displays the antibody fragment fused to the C-terminus of the Aga2p subunit. Variations in the surface density of this combinatorial complex can be monitored and normalized using immunofluorescent labeling of either the HA or c-Myc tags bordering the scFv or Fab. Since protein expression is induced following cell growth, the GAL1 promoter protects potentially toxic antibody fragments from negative selection. Following the subcloning of the antibody gene repertoire into the yeast display vector, the typical established library consists of 10^7 to 10^9 unique variants (100, 103).

Although the early studies with yeast display predominantly involved affinity maturation of existing antibody sequences, recent discovery campaigns show the successful isolation of novel, *de novo* immunoglobulins. Both magnetic assisted cell sorting (MACS) and fluorescence activated cell sorting (FACS) procedures are employed during isolation of antibody clones from yeast libraries (103). Due

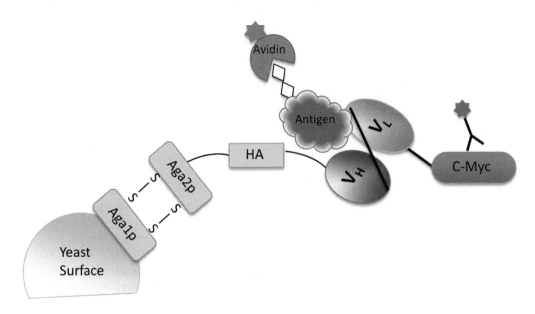

FIGURE 3 **Overview of yeast antibody display. The scFv (or Fab) is displayed as a fusion product with the** *Saccharomyces* **Aga2p protein (light blue). This fusion product can be detected and normalized by fluorescent signaling through the HA tags (orange) and c-Myc tags (dark blue). During FACS selections, the Ag-reactive library variants are detected through the fluorescent avidin tag (pink) on the biotinylated target antigen (red). doi:10.1128/microbiolspec.AID-0028-2014.f3**

to the flow cytometry rate limitations of 10^7 to 10^8 cells per hour, the MACS steps are used to remove nonbinding mAb fragments to reduce the cell input number for subsequent FACS selection. These MACS separations mimic the panning process from phage display to remove nonbinding yeast cells. Even less successful MACS selections can reduce the nonreactive background by approximately 100 times, permitting reasonable yeast cell numbers for FACS screening (102).

Following this MACS-based depletion, the antigen-reactive population is screened by FACS to enrich for candidate clones. The antigen concentration during yeast library screening is kept at 10-fold excess above the desired dissociation constant (K_D) of individual clones to allow the majority of the displayed mAb fragments to be engaged at equilibrium. Further, this antigen excess prevents the titration of target by antibody binding (102). These MACS-selected yeast cells are labeled for the simultaneous detec-

tion of scFv or Fab expression (using the c-Myc tag) and antigen binding (using the biotin label on this target). During this first round of FACS selection, the top 5% of this double-positive population is typically collected to protect diversity, with the selection gate narrowed to the top 0.1 to 1% in subsequent rounds of flow cytometry screening (103). Following three to five rounds of these FACS selections, the plasmid DNA is isolated from this heterogeneous, sorted population and used to transform competent *E. coli* cells. Plasmid DNA is isolated from a selection of these *E. coli* transformants for antibody sequence analysis.

Yeast Display versus Phage Display Technologies

Both advantages and drawbacks exist when comparing yeast and phage antibody library technologies, although their gene repertoires may arise from the same sources (see "Sources of Antibody Genes for Display Libraries," above). The most immediate advantage of yeast display is the accurate control over selection parameters during FACS screening. The collected population percentage, signal normalization, and desired binding affinities can be fixed by the flow cytometry boundaries. This ability to define binding criteria during the selection process represents an advantage over phage display platforms, where variant discrimination is dependent on washing steps rather than real-time kinetic observations (102). In other words, this systematic bias toward desired binding properties available during yeast library selections is not available during phage library campaigns.

Other advantages surrounding yeast display technologies are rooted in the quality of antibody fragment displayed. Yeast libraries make use of the eukaryotic, posttranslational modifications to display scFvs or Fabs in a similar fashion as mammalian cells. Yeast cells employ similar glycosylation patterns as mammalian systems, improving antibody solubility as well as removing a future unknown attribute during full-length IgG expression in mammalian systems. In addition, proper folding events within the yeast endoplasmic reticulum, in the presence of chaperone proteins, protect library diversity by permitting expression of clones too complex for prokaryotic processing used by *E. coli* cells during phage display (102).

While this eukaryotic translation machinery offers expression advantages over phage display libraries, certain drawbacks exist in yeast display approaches. The total number of unique antibody clones in yeast libraries is always several orders of magnitude lower than phage libraries, due to the lower transformation efficiency observed in yeast cells. Yeast antibody libraries possess a theoretical limit of 1×10^7 to 1×10^9 total clones, with phage display libraries capable of representing 1×10^6 to 1×10^{11} variants (103). However, recent advances in transformation optimization allow for the routine generation of yeast antibody display libraries with 1×10^{10} total unique clones (104).

Another disadvantage of the yeast display system involves the number of antibody copies displayed per cell. Since each yeast cell displays 1×10^4 to 1×10^5 scFv or Fab copies, the selection events are based upon antibody avidity, rather than affinity. This property is emphasized during selections against oligomeric antigens, where the multicopy yeast display profile allows for multivalent binding (102). This antibody density on the yeast cell surface may result in the isolation of variants with lower affinity than those discovered from monovalent phage display methods.

A modern selection strategy makes use of both phage and yeast selections. In this study, two rounds of phage selections against *Mycobacterium tuberculosis* Ag85 were performed. Following this naïve phage library selection, this antigen-enriched population was subcloned into a yeast display system for minilibrary construction, which yielded over 100 unique mAbs (105). This combined selection approach takes advantage of the strengths of both technologies: the large library size and affinity-based selections of phage display and the controlled, defined collection of variants from yeast display. This powerful, two-system strategy should be considered in future discovery efforts, given the larger panel of valuable mAbs isolated through the strengths of both technologies.

Antibodies for Infectious Diseases Discovered by Yeast Display

Although the previously discussed aspects of yeast display highlight the capacity of this combinatorial technology as an effective selection system, the use of yeast libraries for novel antibody discovery is relatively new compared with the history of phage display libraries. Since the initial application of yeast display technologies focused on epitope mapping and affinity maturation, the current employment of yeast surface display in the field of antibody discovery for infectious disease remains biased toward these structural and functional characterization studies (102).

Compared to phage display approaches, the published list of antiviral and antibacterial mAbs isolated from yeast libraries is limited.

Antiviral mAb Discovery Involving Yeast Display

Ongoing research surrounding the discovery of novel antiviral mAbs is supported by the yeast display technology. Unlike phage display, epitope mapping serves as the most popular application of yeast libraries in the development of antiviral mAbs. Typically, mAbs isolated from phage libraries or murine hybridoma campaigns are mapped to specific epitopes on the target antigen by yeast display techniques. However, certain reports describe the use of yeast library selections for the discovery of novel antiviral mAbs. Despite this efficacy, fewer antiviral mAb discovery efforts using yeast display have been published. The

most common viral targets for yeast display studies include HIV-1 and flaviviruses. As this yeast display platform continues to develop, additional viral pathogens should be targeted using yeast antibody libraries. A brief summary of antiviral mAb discovery efforts using yeast antibody libraries is listed in Table 3.

Anti-HIV-1 mAbs Discovered by Yeast Display

Separate selection campaigns against recombinant HIV-1 gp120 using yeast and phage display systems provided a comparative study examining the collection of selected antibodies. These libraries were created from the same immune donor pool and screened using the same antigen, limiting the investigation to display system differences (106). These yeast library selections produced at least twice as many unique antibody variants as the phage

TABLE 3 Summary of antiviral antibodies discovered using yeast display[a]

Viral family	Virus	Viral target	Ab fragment or Ag displayed	Ab source	Library application	Reference
Flaviviridae	Dengue virus (DENV)	DENV-1 E glycoprotein	DENV-1 E DIII mutants	N/A	Epitope mapping	108
	Dengue virus	DENV-2 E glycoprotein	DENV-2 E DI-DIII mutants	N/A	Epitope mapping	109
	Dengue virus	DENV-3 E glycoprotein	DENV-3 E wild-type and mutant DIII fragments	N/A	Epitope mapping	110
	Dengue virus	DENV-4 E glycoprotein	DENV-4 E ectodomain and DI-DIII fragments	N/A	Epitope mapping	111
	Dengue virus	DENV DIII fragments	Fab	Naïve	mAb selections	112
	West Nile virus	E glycoprotein	WNV E ectodomain and mutant DIII fragments	N/A	Epitope mapping	72, 107
Orthomyxoviridae	Influenza A virus	HA	Wild-type HA0, HA1, and HA2 subunits; HA1 subunit mutants	N/A	Epitope mapping	113
	Influenza A virus	HA	Wild-type HA fragments and HA1 subunit fragments	N/A	Epitope mapping	114
Retroviridae	HIV-1	gp120	scFv	Immune	mAb selections	106

[a]Note: This list is a summary of selected publications and is not to be considered complete.

selections, including all the mAbs identified from the phage library. The authors attributed this difference in antibody recovery to the eukaryotic expression of the scFv fragment as the primary factor between yeast and phage display. This increased sensitivity in selecting against gp120 supports the demand for future yeast library technology in antiviral antibody isolation.

Anti-Flavivirus mAb Discovery Involving Yeast Display

Among the flaviviruses, WNV is targeted for protective antibody discovery. Antibody-mediated neutralization of WNV involves recognition of the E glycoprotein. This WNV surface E protein is characterized by three separate structural domains. Yeast display experiments using hybridoma-derived mAbs provided the molecular basis for their neutralization activity (107). The majority of the mAbs characterized in this study localized to domain III (DIII) of the viral E antigen. In addition, yeast surface display mapped a panel of E-selected neutralizing mAbs from a phage library to specific domains of the viral glycoprotein (72). These phage library-derived scFvs selectively bound DI/DII, with no interaction with DIII. These yeast-library mapped variations in E glycoprotein epitope localization may be rooted in the different antibody selection methods. These yeast display-detailed protective epitopes are projected to influence ongoing vaccine strategies against WNV.

Similar to WNV, the four serotypes of dengue virus (DENV1-4) possess a surface E glycoprotein composed of three distinct domains. Yeast display strategies using a series of mutant DIII fragments from the DENV-1 E protein revealed the single or combinations of residues for the binding of seven mAbs isolated from murine hybridomas (108). Likewise, panels of neutralizing mAbs against DENV-2, DENV-3, and DENV-4 were finely mapped across all three domains of the E antigen using yeast libraries (109–111).

Recent selections isolated human antibodies against dengue E protein from yeast display libraries (112). These novel, competitive yeast library selections were based upon cross-reactive, neutralizing epitope determinants provided from yeast mapping studies (109). Competitive FACS sorting in the presence of a mutant DIII fragment expressed as an Fc fusion protein produced several wild-type DIII-Fc-reactive populations. The observation of these wild-type antigen-binding subpopulations suggests the mutant protein competition influenced yeast library selections. This unique strategy of competing antigens during selections offers a novel method for isolating epitope-defined variants from yeast antibody display libraries.

Anti-Influenza mAb Discovery Involving Yeast Display

Previous fine epitope mapping studies for anti-influenza mAbs describe the use of yeast display libraries. Broad domain mapping for independent panels of anti-influenza mAbs are described from yeast libraries displaying full-length, precursor influenza HA (HA0) or the HA1 and HA2 subunits separately (113, 114). After confirming binding and domain localization, sublibraries of mutant HA fragments were generated by error-prone PCR for fine epitope mapping. Loss of binding to particular mutant HA subunits indicated particular residues on the viral envelope protein required for mAb binding. These investigations provided structural neutralization determinants for separate mAb panels against surface HA from high-pathogenic influenza strains.

Antibacterial mAb Discovery Involving Yeast display

The advantages surrounding yeast surface display for antibacterial mAb discovery offer the same strengths as phage libraries, namely the elimination of *in vivo* obstacles imposed by hybridoma campaigns and the rapid, high throughput selection of whole antibody libraries. Similar to the discovery work with phage libraries, the primary success with yeast library selections involves soluble, secreted exotoxins, rather than bacterial cell wall– or membrane-associated antigens. In keeping with the trends discussed concerning antiviral mAb discovery, the majority of published yeast library studies describe epitope mapping or affinity maturation. While recent studies describe success with novel antibacterial mAb isolation from yeast libraries, the shorter history of these technologies results in a shorter catalog of published discovery data. A brief summary of bacterial mAb discovery efforts using yeast antibody libraries is listed in Table 4.

Antibotulinum mAb Discovery Involving Yeast Display

Recent selection efforts using yeast display libraries report the successful discovery of novel mAbs binding to *C. botulinum* neurotoxin subtype A (BoNT/A). This campaign yielded three lead candidate scFv clones demonstrating high-affinity binding to full-length BoNT/A (115). To identify novel epitopes, yeast clones were screened against BoNT/A after labeling with previously characterized mAbs recognizing the neurotoxin heavy chain to mask this domain during library selection.

In addition to novel mAb discovery, yeast surface display approaches are used for affinity maturation of known anti-BoNT antibodies. Yeast display V_L shuffled libraries of two previously identified scFvs were sorted on decreasing concentrations of BoNT/B, E, or F and produced improved mAbs with broadened high affinity binding to additional subtypes beyond the parent clone (116). Similarly, V_L shuffling through haploid yeast mating methods generated affinity-matured Fabs from the parent scFvs isolated from an immune yeast library (117).

Antianthrax mAb Discovery Involving Yeast Display

Fine epitope mapping studies using yeast surface display provided the structural requirements for mAbs neutralizing *B. anthracis* toxin components. The screening of a yeast display library composed of mutant edema factor DIII fragments identified critical residues for neutralization of an anthrax toxin (118). These yeast display efforts revealed that the heavy chain CDR3 of an EF-neutralizing mAb competes for an epitope shared with calmodulin, which serves as an enzymatic activator of *B. anthracis* edema factor. In the same fashion, a yeast library displaying mutants of the N-terminal region of the protective antigen (PA_{20}) defined the contact residues of a known, neutralizing mAb (119). These mapping data indicated that the published mAb prevents the furin-mediated activation of PA,

TABLE 4 Summary of antibacterial antibodies discovered using yeast display[a]

Bacterial family	Bacterial species	Bacterial target	Ab fragment or Ag displayed	Ab source	Library application	Reference
Bacillaceae	*Bacillus anthracis*	Edema factor	Mutant EF DIII fragments	N/A	Epitope mapping	118
	Bacillus anthracis	Protective antigen (PA)	Mutant N-terminal PA fragments (PA_{20})	N/A	Epitope mapping	119
Clostridiaceae	*Clostridium botulinum*	Botulinum neurotoxin (BoNT) subtype A	scFv	Naïve	mAb selections	115
	Clostridium botulinum	BoNT subtypes B, E, and F	Fab	Immune	Affinity maturation	116
	Clostridium botulinum	BoNT subtypes A and B	scFv and Fab	Immune	mAb selections and affinity maturation	117

[a]Note: This list is a summary of selected publications and is not to be considered complete.

despite the contact residues being distant from the furin recognition sequence.

CONCLUSIONS

This article details the development and use of the phage and yeast display technologies for the discovery of novel mAbs for infectious diseases. Through the application of these combinatorial methods, the successful isolation of unique antibodies as treatment options and vaccine development tools continues to be reported. The discovery of pathogen-specific mAbs alleviates the clinical challenges posed by the enduring development of microbial resistance, which is provided through escape mutations and evolution of resistant strains. These isolated mAbs offer nontoxic, target-specific treatment options and vaccine strategy determinants for viral and bacterial pathogens.

The selection of high-affinity (within and below the nanomolar range) antibodies across formats (scFv and Fab) and degrees of valency (mono- and multivalent) describes the flexibility of the phage and yeast display approaches. The continued improvement of phage library quality has maintained the relevance of this discovery platform for today's emerging infectious diseases. In addition, the ongoing success of antibody selections using yeast display libraries drives the expansion of this approach beyond its early epitope mapping and affinity maturation applications. These microbial surface display technologies offer powerful platforms for antibody drug discovery and vaccine development within and beyond infectious diseases.

ACKNOWLEDGMENT

Conflicts of interest: We declare no conflicts.

CITATION

Sheehan J, Marasco WA. 2015. Phage and yeast display. Microbiol Spectrum 3(1):AID-0028-2014.

REFERENCES

1. **Rakonjac J, Bennett NJ, Spagnuolo J, Gagic D, Russel M.** 2011. Filamentous bacteriophage: biology, phage display and nanotechnology applications. *Curr Issues Mol Biol* **13:**51–76.
2. **Boeke JD, Model P.** 1982. A prokaryotic membrane anchor sequence: carboxyl terminus of bacteriophage f1 gene III protein retains it in the membrane. *Proc Natl Acad Sci USA* **79:** 5200–5204.
3. **Rakonjac J, Feng J, Model P.** 1999. Filamentous phage are released from the bacterial membrane by a two-step mechanism involving a short C-terminal fragment of pIII. *J Mol Biol* **289:**1253–1265.
4. **Loeb T.** 1960. Isolation of a bacteriophage for the F plus and Hfr mating types of *Escherichia coli* K-12. *Science* **131:**932–933.
5. **Barbas CF III, Kang AS, Lerner RA, Benkovic SJ.** 1991. Assembly of combinatorial antibody libraries on phage surfaces: the gene III site. *Proc Natl Acad Sci USA* **88:**7978–7982.
6. **Clackson T, Hoogenboom HR, Griffiths AD, Winter G.** 1991. Making antibody fragments using phage display libraries. *Nature* **352:**624–628.
7. **Marks JD, Hoogenboom HR, Bonnert TP, McCafferty J, Griffiths AD, Winter G.** 1991. By-passing immunization. Human antibodies from V-gene libraries displayed on phage. *J Mol Biol* **222:**581–597.
8. **Marks JD, Tristem M, Karpas A, Winter G.** 1991. Oligonucleotide primer for polymerase chain reaction amplification of human immunoglobulin variable genes and design of family-specific oligonucleotide probes. *Eur J Immunol* **21:**985–991.
9. **de Haard HJ, van Neer N, Reurs A, Hufton SE, Roovers RC, Henderikx P, de Bruïne AP, Arends JW, Hoogenboom HR.** 1999. A large non-immunized human Fab phage library that permits rapid isolation and kinetic analysis of high affinity antibodies. *J Biol Chem* **274:**18218–18230.
10. **Vaughan TJ, Williams AJ, Pritchard K, Osbourn JK, Pope AR, Earnshaw JC, McCafferty J, Hodits RA, Wilton J, Johnson KS.** 1996. Human antibodies with sub-nanomolar affinities isolated from a large non-immunized phage display library. *Nat Biotechnol* **14:**309–314.
11. **Gram H, Marconi LA, Barbas CF 3rd, Collet TA, Lerner RA, Kang AS.** 1992. *In vitro* selection and affinity maturation of antibodies from a naïve combinatorial immunoglobulin library. *Proc Natl Acad Sci USA* **89:**3576–3580.
12. **Hoogenboom HR.** 2002. Overview of antibody phage-display technology and its applications,

p 1–38. *In* O'Brien PM, Aitken R (ed), *Antibody Phage Display, Methods and Protocols. Methods in Molecular Biology*, **Vol. 178**. Humana Press, Totowa, NJ.

13. **Griffiths AD, Malmqvist M, Marks JD, Bye JM, Embleton MJ, McCafferty J, Baier M, Holliger KP, Gorick BD, Hughes-Jones NC.** 1993. Human anti-self antibodies with high specificity from phage display libraries. *EMBO J* **12**:725–734.

14. **Burton DR, Barbas CF 3rd, Persson MA, Koenig S, Chanock RM, Lerner RA.** 1991. A large array of human monoclonal antibodies to type 1 human immunodeficiency virus from combinatorial libraries of asymptomatic seropositive individuals. *Proc Natl Acad Sci USA* **88**:10134–10137.

15. **de Wildt RM, Finnern R, Ouwehand WH, Griffiths AD, van Venrooij WJ, Hoet RM.** 1996. Characterization of human variable domain antibody fragments against the U1 RNA-associated A protein, selected from a synthetic and a patient-derived combinatorial V gene library. *Eur J Immunol* **26**:629–639.

16. **Barbas CF 3rd, Burton DR.** 1996. Selection and evolution of high-affinity human anti-viral antibodies. *Trends Biotechnol* **14**:230–234.

17. **Hoogenboom HR, Winter G.** 1992. By-passing immunization. Human antibodies from synthetic repertoires of germline VH segments rearranged in vitro. *J Mol Biol* **227**:381–388.

18. **Zhu K, Day T.** 2013. *Ab initio* structure prediction of the antibody hypervariable H3 loop. *Proteins* **81**:1081–1089.

19. **Hoet RM, Cohen EH, Kent RB, Rookey K, Schoonbroodt S, Hogan S, Rem L, Frans N, Daukandt M, Pieters H, van Hegelsom R, Neer NC, Nastri HG, Rondon IJ, Leeds JA, Hufton SE, Huang L, Kashin I, Devlin M, Kuang G, Steukers M, Viswanathan M, Nixon AE, Sexton DJ, Hoogenboom HR, Ladner RC.** 2005. Generation of high-affinity human antibodies by combining donor-derived and synthetic complementarity-determining-region diversity. *Nat Biotechnol* **23**:344–348.

20. **Rothe C, Urlinger S, Löhning C, Prassler J, Stark Y, Jäger U, Hubner B, Bardroff M, Pradel I, Boss M, Bittlingmaier R, Bataa T, Frisch C, Brocks B, Honegger A, Urban M.** 2008. The human combinatorial antibody library HuCAL GOLD combines diversification of all six CDRs according to the natural immune system with a novel display method for efficient selection of high-affinity antibodies. *J Mol Biol* **376**:1182–1200.

21. **Knappik A, Ge L, Honegger A, Pack P, Fischer M, Wellnhofer G, Hoess A, Wölle J, Plückthun A, Virnekäs B.** 2000. Fully synthetic human combinatorial antibody libraries (HuCAL) based on modular consensus frameworks and CDRs randomized with trinucleotides. *J Mol Biol* **11**:57–86.

22. **Tiller T, Schuster I, Deppe D, Siegers K, Strohner R, Herrmann T, Berenguer M, Poujol D, Stehle J, Stark Y, Heßling M, Daubert D, Felderer K, Kaden S, Kölln J, Enzelberger M, Urlinger S.** 2013. A fully synthetic human Fab antibody library fixed on VH/VL framework pairings with favorable biophysical properties. *MAbs* **5**:445–470.

23. **Gao C, Mao S, Lo CH, Wirsching P, Lerner RA, Janda KD.** 1999. Making artificial antibodies: a format for phage display of combinatorial heterodimeric arrays. *Proc Natl Acad Sci USA* **96**:6025–6030.

24. **Jespers LS, De Keyser A, Stanssens PE.** 1996. LambdaZLG6: a phage lambda vector for high-efficiency cloning and surface expression of cDNA libraries on filamentous phage. *Gene* **173**:179–181.

25. **Iannolo G, Minenkova O, Petruzzelli R, Cesareni G.** 1995. Modifying filamentous phage capsid: limits in the size of the major capsid protein. *J Mol Biol* **248**:835–844.

26. **Zwick MB, Shen J, Scott JK.** 2000. Homodimeric peptides displayed by the major coat protein of filamentous phage. *J Mol Biol* **300**:307–320.

27. **O'Connell D, Becerril B, Roy-Burman A, Daws M, Marks JD.** 2002. Phage versus phagemid libraries for generation of human monoclonal antibodies. *J Mol Biol* **312**:49–56.

28. **Marks JD, Hoogenboom HR, Griffiths AD, Winter G.** 1992. Molecular evolution of proteins on filamentous phage. Mimicking the strategy of the immune system. *J Biol Chem* **267**:16007–16010.

29. **de Wildt RM, Tomlinson IM, Ong JL, Holliger P.** 2002. Isolation of receptor-ligand pairs by capture of long-lived multivalent interaction complexes. *Proc Natl Acad Sci USA* **99**:8530–8535.

30. **Rakonjac J, Jovanovic G, Model P.** 1997. Filamentous phage infection-mediated gene expression: construction and propagation of the gIII deletion mutant helper phage R408d3. *Gene* **198**:99–103.

31. **Chasteen L, Ayriss J, Pavlik P, Bradbury AR.** 2006. Eliminating helper phage from phage display. *Nucleic Acid Res* **34**:e145.

32. **Hoogenboom HR, Griffiths AD, Johnson KS, Chiswell DJ, Hudson P, Winter G.** 1991. Multi-subunit proteins on the surface of filamentous phage: methodologies for displaying antibody (Fab) heavy and light chains. *Nucleic Acids Res* **19**:4133–4137.

33. **Garrard LJ, Yang M, O'Connell MP, Kelley RF, Henner DJ.** 1991. Fab assembly and enrichment in a monovalent phage system. *Biotechnology* **9**:1373–1377.

34. **Chan CE, Chan AH, Lim AP, Hanson BJ.** 2011. Comparison of the efficiency of antibody selection from semi-synthetic scFv and non-immune Fab phage display libraries against protein targets for rapid development of diagnostic immunoassays. *J Immunol Methods* **373**:79–88.

35. **Qi J, Ye X, Ren G, Kan F, Zhang Y, Guo M, Zhang Z, Li D.** 2014. Pharmacological efficacy of anti-IL-1β scFv, Fab, and full-length antibodies in treatment of rheumatoid arthritis. *Mol Immunol* **57**:59–65.

36. **Steinwand M, Droste P, Frenzel A, Hust M, Dübel S, Schirrmann T.** 2014. The influence of antibody fragment format on phage display based affinity maturation of IgG. *MAbs* **6**:204–218.

37. **Lauring AS, Frydman J, Andino R.** 2013. The role of mutational robustness in RNA virus evolution. *Nat Rev Microbiol* **11**:327–336.

38. **Balmer O, Tanner M.** 2011. Prevalence and implications of multiple-strain infections. *Lancet Infect Dis* **11**:868–878.

39. **Leye N, Vidal N, Ndiaye O, Diop-Ndiaye H, Wade AS, Mboup S, Delaporte E, Toure-Kane C, Peeters M.** 2013. High frequency of HIV-1 infections with multiple HIV-1 strains in men having sex with men (MSM) in Senegal. *Infect Genet Evol* **20**:206–214.

40. **Yewdell JW, Spiro DJ, Golding H, Quill H, Mittelman A, Nabel GJ.** 2013. Getting to the heart of influenza. *Sci Transl Med* **5**:e191ed8.

41. **Corti D, Lanzavecchia A.** 2013. Broadly neutralizing antiviral antibodies. *Annu Rev Immunol* **31**:705–742.

42. **Marasco WA, Sui J.** 2007. The growth and potential of human antiviral monoclonal antibody therapeutics. *Nat Biotechnol* **25**:1421–1434.

43. **Thie H, Meyer T, Schirrmann T, Hust M, Dübel S.** 2008. Phage display derived therapeutic antibodies. *Curr Pharm Biotechnol* **9**:439–446.

44. **Jegaskanda S, Job ER, Kramski M, Laurie K, Isitman G, de Rose R, Winnall WR, Stratov I, Brooks AG, Reading PC, Kent SJ.** 2013. Cross-reactive influenza-specific antibody-dependent cellular cytotoxicity antibodies in the absence of neutralizing antibodies. *J Immunol* **190**:1837–1848.

45. **Gamblin SJ, Skehel JJ.** 2010. Influenza hemagglutinin and neuraminidase membrane glycoproteins. *J Biol Chem* **285**:38403–38409.

46. **Skehal JJ, Wiley DC.** 2000. Receptor binding and membrane fusion in virus entry: the influenza hemagglutinin. *Annu Rev Biochem* **69**:531–569.

47. **Wiley DC, Wilson IA, Skehel JJ.** 1981. Structural identification of the antibody-binding sites of Hong Kong influenza haemagglutinin and their involvement in antigenic variation. *Nature* **289**:373–378.

48. **Both GW, Sleigh MJ, Cox NJ, Kendal AP.** 1983. Antigenic drift in influenza virus H3 hemagglutinin from 1968 to 1980: multiple evolutionary pathways and sequential amino acid changes at key antigenic sites. *J Virol* **48**:52–60.

49. **Sui J, Hwang WC, Perez S, Wei G, Aird D, Chen LM, Santelli E, Stec B, Cadwell G, Ali M, Wan H, Murakami A, Yammanuru A, Han T, Cox NJ, Bankston LA, Donis RO, Liddington RC, Marasco WA.** 2009. Structural and functional bases for broad-spectrum neutralization of avian and human influenza A viruses. *Nat Struct Mol Biol* **16**:265–273.

50. **Throsby M, van den Brink E, Jongeneelen M, Poon LL, Alard P, Cornelissen L, Bakker A, Cox F, van Deventer E, Guan Y, Cinatl J, ter Meulen J, Lasters I, Carsetti R, Peiris M, de Kruif J, Goudsmit J.** 2008. Heterosubtypic neutralizing monoclonal antibodies cross-protective against H5N1 and H1N1 recovered from human IgM+ memory B cells. *PLoS One* **3**:e3942. doi:10.1371/journal.pone.0003942.

51. **Dreyfus C, Laursen NS, Kwaks T, Zuijdgeest D, Khayat R, Ekiert DC, Lee JH, Metlagel Z, Bujny MV, Jongeneelen M, van der Vlugt R, Lamrani M, Korse HJ, Geelen E, Sahin Ö, Sieuwerts M, Brakenhoff JP, Vogels R, Li OT, Poon LL, Peiris M, Koudstaal W, Ward AB, Wilson IA, Goudsmit J, Friesen RH.** 2012. Highly conserved protective epitopes on influenza B viruses. *Science* **337**:1343–1348.

52. **Avnir Y, Tallarico AS, Zhu Q, Bennett AS, Connelly G, Sheehan J, Sui J, Fahmy A, Huang CY, Cadwell G, Bankston LA, McGuire AT, Stamatatos L, Wagner G, Liddington RC, Marasco WA.** 2014. Molecular signatures of hemagglutinin stem-directed heterosubtypic human neutralizing antibodies against influenza A viruses. *PLoS Pathog* **10**:e1004103. doi:10.1371/journal.ppat.1004103.

53. **Ekiert DC, Kashyap AK, Steel J, Rubrum A, Bhabha G, Khayat R, Lee JH, Dillon MA, O'Neil RE, Faynboym AM, Horowitz M, Horowitz L, Ward AB, Palese P, Webby R, Lerner RA, Bhatt RR, Wilson IA.** 2012. Cross-neutralization of influenza A viruses mediated by a single antibody loop. *Nature* **489**:526–532.

54. **Iba Y, Fujii Y, Ohshima N, Sumida T, Kubota-Koketsu R, Ikeda M, Wakiyama M, Shirouzu M, Okada J, Okuno Y, Kurosawa Y, Yokoyama S.** Conserved neutralizing epitope at globular head of hemagglutinin in H3N2 influenza viruses. *J Virol* **88:**7130–7144.

55. **Caton AJ, Brownlee GG, Yewdell JW, Gerhard W.** 1982. The antigenic structure of the influenza virus A/PR/8/34 hemagglutinin (H1 subtype). *Cell* **31:**417–427.

56. **Bartesaghi A, Merk A, Borgnia MJ, Milne JL, Subramaniam S.** 2013. Prefusion structure of trimeric HIV-1 envelope glycoprotein determined by cryo-electron microscopy. *Nat Struct Mol Biol* **20:**1352–1357.

57. **Taylor BS, Sobieszczyk ME, McCutchan FE, Hammer SM.** The challenge of HIV-1 subtype diversity. *N Engl J Med* **358:**1590–1602.

58. **Quakkelaar ED, Bunnik EM, van Alphen FP, Boeser-Nunnink BD, van Nuenen AC, Schuitemaker H.** 2007. Escape of human immunodeficiency virus type 1 from broadly neutralizing antibodies is not associated with a reduction of viral replicative capacity *in vitro*. *Virology* **363:**447–453.

59. **Burton DR, Barbas CF 3rd, Persson MA, Koenig S, Chanock RM, Lerner RA.** 1991. A large array of human monoclonal antibodies to type 1 human immunodeficiency virus from combinatorial libraries of asymptomatic seropositive individuals. *Proc Natl Acad Sci USA* **88:**10134–10137.

60. **Burton DR, Pyati J, Kodrui R, Sharp SJ, Thornton GB, Parren PW, Sawyer LA, Hendry RM, Dunlop N, Nara PL, Lamacchia M, Garratty E, Stiehm ER, Bryson YJ, Cao Y, Moore JP, Ho DD, Barbas CF 3rd.** 1994. Efficient neutralization of primary isolates of HIV-1 by a recombinant human monoclonal antibody. *Science* **266:**1024–1027.

61. **Zwick MB, Labrijn AF, Wang M, Spenlehauer C, Saphire EO, Binley JM, Moore JP, Stiegler G, Katinger H, Burton DR, Parren PW.** 2001. Broadly neutralizing antibodies targeted to the membrane-proximal external region of human immunodeficiency virus type 1 glycoprotein gp41. *J Virol* **75:**10892–10905.

62. **Zhu Z, Qin HR, Chen W, Zhao Q, Shen X, Schutte R, Wang Y, Ofek G, Streaker E, Prabakaran P, Fouda GG, Liao HX, Owens J, Louder M, Yang Y, Klaric KA, Moody MA, Mascola JR, Scott JK, Kwong PD, Montefiori D, Haynes BF, Tomaras GD, Dimitrov DS.** 2011. Cross-reactive HIV-1-neutralizing human monoclonal antibodies identified from a patient with 2F5-like antibodies. *J Virol* **85:**11401–11408.

63. **Choudhry V, Zhang MY, Sidorov IA, Louis JM, Harris I, Dimitrov AS, Bouma P, Cham F, Choudhary A, Rybak SM, Fouts T, Montefiori DC, Broder CC, Quinnan GV Jr, Dimitrov DS.** 2007. Cross-reactive HIV-1 neutralizing monoclonal antibodies selected by screening of an immune human phage library against an envelope glycoprotein (gp140) isolated from a patient (R2) with broadly HIV-1 neutralizing antibodies. *Virology* **363:**79–90.

64. **Yoshikawa M, Mukai Y, Tsunoda S, Tsutsumi Y, Yoshioka Y, Okada N, Nakagawa S.** 2011. Modifying the antigen-immunization schedule improves the variety of monoclonal antibodies obtained from immune-phage antibody libraries against HIV-1 Nef and Vif. *J Biosci Bioeng* **111:**597–599.

65. **Sui J, Li W, Murakami A, Tamin A, Matthews LJ, Wong SK, Moore MJ, Tallarico AS, Olurinde M, Choe H, Anderson LJ, Bellini WJ, Farzan M, Marasco WA.** 2004. Potent neutralization of severe acute respiratory syndrome (SARS) coronavirus by a human mAb to S1 protein that blocks receptor association. *Proc Natl Acad Sci USA* **101:**2536–2541.

66. **Prabakaran P, Gan J, Feng Y, Zhu Z, Choudhry V, Xiao X, Ji X, Dimitrov DS.** 2006. Structure of severe acute respiratory syndrome coronavirus receptor-binding domain complexed with neutralizing antibody. *J Biol Chem* **281:**15829–15836.

67. **Ferguson NM, Van Kerkhove MD.** 2014. Identification of MERS-CoV in dromedary camels. *Lancet Infect Dis* **14:**93–94.

68. **Memish ZA, Mishra N, Olival KJ, Fagbo SF, Kapoor V, Epstein JH, Alhakeem R, Durosinloun A, Al Asmari M, Islam A, Kapoor A, Briese T, Daszak P, Al Rabeeah AA, Lipkin WI.** 2013. Middle East respiratory syndrome coronavirus in bats, Saudi Arabia. *Emerg Infect Dis* **19:**1819–1823.

69. **Raj VS, Mou H, Smits SL, Dekkers DH, Müller MA, Dijkman R, Muth D, Demmers JA, Zaki A, Fouchier RA, Thiel V, Drosten C, Rottier PJ, Osterhaus AD, Bosch BJ, Haagmans BL.** Dipeptidyl pepetidase 4 is a functional receptor for the emerging human coronavirus-EMC. *Nature* **495:**251–254.

70. **Graham RL, Donaldson EF, Baric RS.** A decade after SARS: strategies for controlling emerging coronaviruses. *Nat Rev Microbiol* **11:**836–848.

71. **Gierer S, Bertram S, Kaup F, Wrensch F, Heurich A, Krämer-Kühl A, Welsch K, Winkler M, Meyer B, Drosten C, Dittmer U, von Hahn T, Simmons G, Hofmann H, Pöhlmann S.** 2013. The spike protein of the emerging coronavirus EMC uses a novel coronavirus receptor for entry, can be activated by TMPRSS2, and is targeted by neutralizing antibodies. *J Virol* **87:**5502–5511.

72. Tang XC, Agnihothram SS, Jiao Y, Stanhope J, Graham RL, Peterson EC, Avnir Y, Tallarico AS, Sheehan J, Zhu Q, Baric RS, Marasco WA. 2014. Identification of human neutralizing antibodies against MERS-CoV and their role in virus adaptive evolution. *Proc Natl Acad Sci USA* **111**:E2018–E2026.

73. Ying T, Du L, Ju TW, Prabakaran P, Lau CC, Lu L, Liu Q, Wang L, Feng Y, Wang Y, Zheng BJ, Yuen KY, Jiang S, Dimitrov DS. 2014. Exceptionally potent neutralization of Middle East respiratory syndrome coronavirus by human monoclonal antibodies. *J Virol* **88**:7796–7805.

74. Gould LH, Sui J, Foellmer H, Oliphant T, Wang T, Ledizet M, Murakami A, Noonan K, Lambeth C, Kar K, Anderson JF, de Silva AM, Diamond MS, Koski RA, Marasco WA, Fikrig E. 2005. Protective and therapeutic capacity of human single-chain Fv-Fc fusion proteins against West Nile Virus. *J Virol* **79**:14606–14613.

75. Throsby M, Geuijen C, Goudsmit J, Bakker AQ, Korimbocus J, Kramer RA, Clijsters-van der Horst M, de Jong M, Jongeneelen M, Thijsse S, Smit R, Visser TJ, Bijl N, Marissen WE, Loeb M, Kelvin DJ, Preiser W, ter Meulen J, de Kruif J. 2006. Isolation and charactertization of human monoclonal antibodies from individuals infected with West Nile Virus. *J Virol* **80**:6982–6992.

76. Cabezas S, Rojas G, Pavon A, Alvarez M, Pupo M, Guillen G, Guzman MG. 2008. Selection of phage-displayed human antibody fragments on dengue virus particles captured by a monoclonal antibody: application to the four serotypes. *J Virol Methods* **147**:235–243.

77. Zhao Y, Moreland NJ, Tay MY, Lee CC, Swaminathan K, Vasudevan SG. 2014. Identification and molecular characterization of human antibody fragments specific for dengue NS5 protein. *Virus Res* **179**:225–230.

78. Maruyama T, Rodriguez LL, Jahrling PB, Sanchez A, Khan AS, Nichol ST, Peters CJ, Parren PW, Burton DR. 1999. Ebola virus can be effectively neutralized by antibody produced in natural human infection. *J Virol* **73**:6024–6030.

79. Barbas CF 3rd, Crowe JE Jr, Cababa D, Jones TM, Zebedee SL, Murphy BR, Chanock RM, Burton DR. 1992. Human monoclonal Fab fragments derived from a combinatorial library bind to respiratory syncytial virus F glycoprotein and neutralize infectivity. *Proc Natl Acad Sci USA* **89**:10164–10168.

80. Crowe JE Jr, Murphy BR, Chanock RM, Williamson RA, Barbas CF 3rd, Burton DR. 1994. Recombinant human respiratory syncytial virus (RSV) monoclonal antibody Fab is effective therapeutically when introduced directly into the lungs of RSV-infected mice. *Proc Natl Acad Sci USA* **91**:1386–1390.

81. Burioni R, Williamson RA, Sanna PP, Bloom FE, Burton DR. 1994. Recombinant human Fab to glycoprotein D neutralizes infectivity and prevents cell-to-cell transmission of herpes simplex viruses 1 and 2 *in vitro*. *Proc Natl Acad Sci USA* **91**:355–359.

82. Christensen DJ, Gottlin EB, Benson RE, Hamilton PT. 2001. Phage display for target-based antibacterial drug discovery. *Drug Discov Today* **6**:721–727.

83. Lee HS, Loh YX, Lee JJ, Liu CS, Chu C. 2014. Antimicrobial consumption and resistance in five Gram-negative bacterial species in a hospital from 2003 to 2011. *J Microbiol Immunol Infect* **S1684**:1182(14)00074-7. doi:10.1016/j.jmii.2014.04.009.

84. Velayati AA, Masjedi MR, Farnia P, Tabarsi P, Ghanavi J, Ziazarifi AH, Hoffner SE. 2009. Emergence of new forms of totally drug-resistant tuberculosis bacilli: super extensively drug-resistant tuberculosis or totally drug-resistant strains in Iran. *Chest* **136**:420–425.

85. Ford C, Yusim K, Ioerger T, Feng S, Chase M, Greene M, Korber B, Fortune S. 2012. *Mycobacterium tuberculosis*—heterogeneity revealed through whole genome sequencing. *Tuberculosis (Edinb)* **92**:194–201.

86. Gronski P, Seiler FR, Schwick HG. 1991. Discovery of antitoxins and development of antibody preparations for clinical uses from 1890 to 1990. *Mol Immunol* **28**:1321–1332.

87. Oleksiewicz MB, Nagy G, Nagy E. 2012. Antibacterial monoclonal antibodies: back to the future? *Arch Biochem Biophys* **526**:124–131.

88. Amersdorfer P, Wong C, Smith T, Chen S, Deshpande S, Sheridan R, Marks JD. 2002. Genetic and immunological comparison of anti-botulinum type A antibodies from immune and non-immune human phage libraries. *Vaccine* **20**:1640–1648.

89. Rossetto O, Pirazzini M, Bolognese P, Rigoni M, Montecucco C. 2011. An update of the mechanism of action of tetanus and botulinum neurotoxins. *Acta Chim Slov* **58**:702–707.

90. Amersdorfer P, Wong C, Chen S, Smith T, Deshpande S, Sheridan R, Finnern R, Marks JD. 1997. Molecular charactertization of murine humoral immune response to botulinum neurotoxin type A binding domain as assessed by using phage antibody libraries. *Infect Immun* **65**:3743–3752.

91. Marks JD. 2004. Deciphering antibody properties that lead to potent botulinum neurotoxin neutralization. *Mov Disord* **19**(Suppl 8):S101–S108.

92. **Jernigan DB, Raghunathan PL, Bell BP, Brechner R, Bresnitz EA, Butler JC, Cetron M, Cohen M, Doyle T, Fischer M, Greene C, Griffith KS, Guarner J, Hadler JL, Hayslett JA, Meyer R, Petersen LR, Phillips M, Pinner R, Popovic T, Quinn CP, Reefhuis J, Reissman D, Rosenstein N, Schuchat A, Shieh WJ, Siegal L, Swerdlow DL, Tenover FC, Traeger M, Ward JW, Weisfuse I, Wiersma S, Yeskey K, Zaki S, Ashford DA, Perkins BA, Ostroff S, Hughes J, Fleming D, Koplan JP, Gerberding JL.** 2002. Investigation of bioterrorism-related anthrax, United States, 2001: epidemiologic findings. *Emerg Infect Dis* **8:**1019–1028.

93. **Chen Z, Moayeri M, Purcell R.** 2011. Monoclonal antibody therapies against anthrax. *Toxins (Basel)* **3:**1004–1019.

94. **Migone TS, Subramanian GM, Zhong J, Healey LM, Corey A, Devalaraja M, Lo L, Ullrich S, Zimmerman J, Chen A, Lewis M, Meister G, Gillum K, Sanford D, Mott J, Bolmer SD.** 2009. Raxibacumab for the treatment of inhalational anthrax. *N Engl J Med* **361:** 135–144.

95. **Pelat T, Hust M, Laffly E, Condemine F, Bottex C, Vidal D, Lefranc MP, Dübel S, Thullier P.** 2007. High-affinity, human antibody-like antibody fragment (single-chain variable fragment) neutralizing the lethal factor (LF) of *Bacillus anthracis* by inhibiting protective antigen-LF complex formation. *Antimicrob Agents Chemother* **51:**2758–2764.

96. **Chen Z, Moayeri M, Zhao H, Crown D, Leppla SH, Purcell RH.** 2009. Potent neutralization of anthrax edema toxin by a humanized monoclonal antibody that competes with calmodulin for edema factor binding. *Proc Natl Acad Sci USA* **106:**13487–13492.

97. **Deng XK, Nesbit LA, Morrow KJ Jr.** 2003. Recombinant single-chain variable fragment antibodies directed against *Clostridium difficile* toxin B produced by use of an optimized phage display system. *Clin Diagn Lab Immunol* **10:**587–595.

98. **Neelakantam B, Sridevi NV, Shukra AM, Sugumar P, Samuel S, Rajendra L.** 2014. Recombinant human antibody fragment against tetanus toxoid produced by phage display. *Eur J Microbiol Immunol (Bp)* **4:**45–55.

99. **Burnie JP, Matthews RC, Carter T, Beaulieu E, Donohoe M, Chapman C, Williamson P, Hodgetts SJ.** 2000. Identification of an immunodominant ABC transporter in methicillin-resistant *Staphylococcus aureus* infections. *Infect Immun* **68:**3200–3209.

100. **Gera N, Hussain M, Rao BM.** 2013. Protein selection using yeast surface display. *Methods* **60:**15–26.

101. **Lipke PN, Kurjan J.** 2000. Sexual agglutination in budding yeasts: structure, function, and regulation of adhesion glycoproteins. *Microbiol Rev* **56:**180–194.

102. **Boder ET, Raeeszadeh-Sarmazdeh M, Price JV.** 2012. Engineering antibodies by yeast display. *Arch Biochem Biophys* **526:**99–106.

103. **Chao G, Lau WL, Hackel BJ, Sazinsky SL, Lippow SM, Wittrup KD.** 2006. Isolating and engineering human antibodies using yeast surface display. *Nat Protoc* **1:**755–768.

104. **Benatuil L, Perez JM, Belk J, Hsieh CM.** 2010. An improved yeast transformation method for the generation of very large human antibody libraries. *Protein Eng Des Sel* **23:**155–159.

105. **Ferrara F, Naranjo LA, Kumar S, Gaiotto T, Mukundan H, Swanson B, Bradbury AR.** 2012. Using phage and yeast display to select hundreds of monoclonal antibodies: application to antigen 85, a tuberculosis marker. *PLoS One* **7:**e49535. doi:10.1371/journal.pone.0049535.

106. **Bowley DR, Labrijn AF, Zwick MB, Burton DR.** 2007. Antigen selection from an HIV-1 immune antibody library displayed on yeast yields many novel antibodies compared to selection from the same library displayed on phage. *Protein Eng Des Sel* **20:**81–90.

107. **Oliphant T, Engle M, Nybakken GE, Doane C, Johnson S, Huang L, Gorlatov S, Mehlhop E, Marri A, Chung KM, Ebel GD, Kramer LD, Fremont DH, Diamond MS.** 2005. Development of a humanized monoclonal antibody with therapeutic potential against West Nile virus. *Nat Med* **11:**522–530.

108. **Shrestha B, Brien JD, Sukupolvi-Petty S, Austin SK, Edeling MA, Kim T, O'Brien KM, Nelson CA, Johnson S, Fremont DH, Diamond MS.** 2010. The development of therapeutic antibodies that neutralize homologous and heterologous genotypes of dengue virus type 1. *PLoS Pathog* **6:** e1000823. doi:10.1371/journal.ppat.1000823.

109. **Sukupolvi-Petty S, Austin SK, Engle M, Brien JD, Dowd KA, Williams KL, Johnson S, Rico-Hesse R, Harris E, Pierson TC, Fremont DH, Diamond MS.** 2010. Structure and function analysis of therapeutic monoclonal antibodies against dengue virus type 2. *J Virol* **84:**9227–9239.

110. **Brien JD, Austin SK, Sukupolvi-Petty S, O'Brien KM, Johnson S, Fremont DH, Diamond MS.** 2010. Genotype-specific neutralization and protection by antibodies against dengue virus type 3. *J Virol* **84:**10630–10643.

111. **Sukupolvi-Petty S, Brien JD, Austin SK, Shrestha B, Swayne S, Kahle K, Doranz BJ, Johnson S, Pierson TC, Fremont DH, Diamond MS.** 2013. Functional analysis of antibodies against dengue virus type 4 reveals strain-

dependent epitope exposure that impacts neutralization and protection. *J Virol* **87**:8826–8842.

112. **Puri V, Streaker E, Prabakaran P, Zhu Z, Dimitrov DS.** 2013. Highly efficient selection of epitope specific antibody through competitive yeast display library sorting. *MAbs* **5**:533–539.

113. **Han T, Sui J, Bennett AS, Liddington RC, Donis RO, Zhu Q, Marasco WA.** 2011. Fine epitope mapping of monoclonal antibodies against hemagglutinin of a highly pathogenic H5N1 influenza virus using yeast surface display. *Biochem Biophys Res Commun* **409**:253–259.

114. **Hu H, Voss J, Zhang G, Buchy P, Zuo T, Wang L, Wang F, Zhou F, Wang G, Tsai C, Calder L, Gamblin SJ, Zhang L, Deubel V, Zhou B, Skehel JJ, Zhou P.** 2012. A human antibody recognizing a conserved epitope of H5 hemagglutinin broadly neutralizes highly pathogenic avian influenza. *J Virol* **86**:2978–2989.

115. **Gray SA, Barr JR, Kalb SR, Marks JD, Baird CL, Cangelosi GA, Miller KD, Feldhaus MJ.** 2011. Synergistic capture of *Clostridium botulinum* type A neurotoxin by scFv antibodies to novel epitopes. *Biotechnol Bioeng* **108**:2456–2467.

116. **Garcia-Rodriguez C, Geren IN, Lou J, Conrad F, Forsyth C, Wen W, Chakraborti S, Zao H, Manzanarez G, Smith TJ, Brown J, Tepp WH, Liu N, Wijesuriya S, Tomic MT, Johnson EA, Smith LA, Marks JD.** 2011. Neutralizing human monoclonal antibodies binding multiple serotypes of botulinum neurotoxin. *Protein Eng Des Sel* **24**:321–331.

117. **Lou J, Geren I, Garcia-Rodriguez C, Forsyth CM, Wen W, Knopp K, Brown J, Smith T, Smith LA, Marks JD.** 2010. Affinity maturation of human botulinum neurotoxin antibodies by light chain shuffling via yeast mating. *Protein Eng Des Sel* **23**:311–319.

118. **Makiya M, Dolan M, Agulto L, Purcell R, Chen Z.** 2012. Structural basis of anthrax edema factor neutralization by a neutralizing antibody. *Biochem Biophys Res Commun* **417**:324–329.

119. **Reason D, Liberato J, Sun J, Camacho J, Zhou J.** 2011. Mechanism of lethal toxin neutralization by a human monoclonal antibody specific for the PA(20) region of *Bacillus anthracis* protective antigen. *Toxins (Basel)* **3**:979–990.

Efficient Methods To Isolate Human Monoclonal Antibodies from Memory B Cells and Plasma Cells

7

DAVIDE CORTI[1,2] and ANTONIO LANZAVECCHIA[2]

MANY WAYS TO MAKE HUMAN MONOCLONAL ANTIBODIES

Today, several methods are available to isolate human monoclonal antibodies. The first efficient method described was the panning of phage display libraries constructed from the Ig variable genes of immunized or infected individuals (1) or from random synthetic libraries (2). While this method has led to the isolation of several neutralizing antibodies against multiple pathogens, the resulting antibodies do not represent necessarily the natural antibody repertoire, since the antibody fragments are generated from the random pairing of immunoglobulin VH and VL variable regions. Thus, in the case of phage libraries, it is unlikely that a given VH/VL pair went through a selection process, including the negative selection for self-reactivity. Another significant drawback is that target antigens must be known a priori, since the selection is based on binding to a purified antigen, rather than for instance neutralization. Consequently, this system is not suitable to identify new neutralizing targets within complex pathogens. In addition, selection for high-affinity binding does not necessarily translate into higher protection if the epitope recognized is not readily available on the viral spikes. An additional problem of this approach that was frequently

[1]Humabs BioMed SA, 6500 Bellinzona, Switzerland; [2]Institute for Research in Biomedicine, 6500 Bellinzona, Switzerland.

Antibodies for Infectious Diseases
Edited by James E. Crowe, Jr., Diana Boraschi, and Rino Rappuoli
© 2015 American Society for Microbiology, Washington, DC
doi:10.1128/microbiolspec.AID-0018-2014

encountered is that the antibodies isolated in *Escherichia coli* or yeasts may be expressed suboptimally in mammalian cells.

Mice that carry human immunoglobulin loci produce fully human antibodies in response to immunization with the significant advantage that, being mice, they can be immunized and make antibodies to human antigens (3). This system has become the method of choice for the isolation of antibodies specific for human antigens such as cytokines or cell surface molecule. However, it is less suitable to make antibodies against human pathogens such as HIV, hepatitis C virus (HCV), hepatitis B virus (HBV), cytomegalovirus (CMV), that do not infect mice. In addition, the immune response of mice is often suboptimal, possibly owing to the mismatch between human Ig and mouse Fc receptors. Thus, the isolation of antibodies from immune donors offers the advantage of fully exploiting the strength of the human antibody response to a human pathogen.

An important advance in this field was represented by the use of single-cell reverse transcription (RT)-PCR to isolate the immunoglobulin heavy and light chain variable gene pairs from single B cells, followed by expression of the full antibody by transfection of H and L chain genes in 293 cells (4). The single-cell RT-PCR and expression approach has been also used to isolate antibodies from plasma cells isolated soon after a booster vaccination (5), and from memory B cells, which can be isolated according to their capacity to bind fluorescently labeled antigens (6). The latter approach has been particularly successful in the isolation of broadly neutralizing antibodies against the CD4 binding site of gp120. However, staining and sorting B cells with labeled antigens is not generally feasible whenever the target antigen is not available or unknown. In conclusion, the single-cell RT-PCR and expression approach has been very useful, especially when antigen binding can be used to enrich for specific cells or when specific cells are highly represented in the population, as is the case for plasma cells

collected after antigenic boost. A significant limitation of this approach is that the cloning and expression of individual antibodies is very labor intensive, and, consequently, the throughput has been generally limited to a few hundred clones. However, recent technological advances using nanofluidic devices have considerably increased the throughput of this approach (7).

A simple and effective alternative to the single-cell RT-PCR and expression method is the direct screening of the antibodies produced by plasma cells or by activated or immortalized memory B cells. This can be achieved by using methods based on cell cultures, such as those described in this article, that allow instead the interrogation of the cell-derived monoclonal antibodies in their natural secreted form (Fig. 1). In 2004, we reported an efficient method of memory B-cell immortalization using EBV and CpG (8), and, in 2011, we demonstrated the feasibility of culturing single plasma cells and identifying those producing antibodies with special properties (9). These methods will be described in detail below. In 2008, Spits and coworkers developed an alternative method to immortalize human memory B cells by using retroviruses encoding the antiapoptotic factors Bcl-6 and Bcl-xL (10). Memory B cells are transduced under polyclonal conditions (typically 100 cells per well) in the presence of IL-21, and CD40L-expressing cells differentiate into long-lived antibody-secreting cells that still expressed their B-cell receptor on the cell surface. These cells also maintained a low-level activation-induced cytidine deaminase-mediated mutation activity that represents a possible source of antibody clone instability, but which can also be used to increase antibody affinity through an *in vitro* iterative selection process. In 2009, Walker et al. described the isolation of an HIV-1 broadly neutralizing antibody able to recognize the Env protein only in the trimeric native form by using another approach that relied on the *in vitro* activation and expansion of

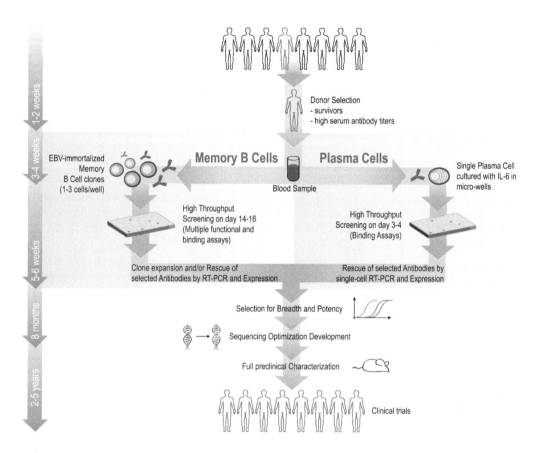

FIGURE 1 Interrogation of human memory B cells and plasma cell repertoires using high-throughput cellular screens. Shown is a timeline of the process that goes from the selection of donors to the isolation, characterization, and development of the antibodies. doi:10.1128/microbiolspec.AID-0018-2014.f1

human memory B cells for approximately 10 days, followed by the screening of culture supernatant and lysis of all expanded cells (11). The details of this method have not been disclosed, but Connors and colleagues have recently described and published in detail a similar approach (12). The antibody-containing supernatants are used in functional sensitive assays to identify the wells from which the antibody genes can be retrieved for cloning and expression in 293 cells. A significant drawback of the latter two methods is related to the low levels of antibodies produced in the culture supernatants. In the Bcl-6/Bcl-xL transduction and the polyclonal stimulation technologies, the average productivities are claimed to be ~0.1 to 1 ×g/ml and 0.01 to 0.1 ×g/

ml, respectively. The low antibody levels might limit the testing and identification of antibodies in several types of functional assays that could require higher levels of antibody.

EFFICIENT IMMORTALIZATION OF MEMORY B CELLS BY USING EBV AND CPG

Memory B cells are readily accessible in peripheral blood and persist for the lifetime of an individual and are therefore an excellent source to isolate monoclonal antibodies. Work in the late 1970s showed that human memory B cells could be immortalized with EBV and that this method could be used to isolate human monoclonal antibodies (13). However, the efficiency of B-cell immortalization was low, typically in the order of 0.1%, and therefore did not allow an efficient interrogation of the human memory repertoire. In 2004, we reported that the efficiency of EBV immortalization could be dramatically increased by the addition of a toll-like receptor (TLR) agonist, in particular, CpG or R848 that trigger TLR9 and TLR7, which are expressed at high levels on human B cells (8, 14).

The basis for the powerful synergy between EBV and TLR stimulation was clarified in a subsequent study where we examined the requirements for the activation of human B cells (15). In this study, we reported that maximal stimulation of B cells requires three distinct signals: signal 1 delivered by B-cell receptor (BCR) stimulation, signal 2 delivered by T-helper cells primarily via CD40L/CD40 interaction, and signal 3 delivered by a TLR agonist (Fig. 2A). In particular, while BCR cross-linking and cognate interaction with activated T cells provided a suboptimal stimulus, addition of CpG or R848 potently boosted B-cell proliferation and differentiation to antibody-producing cells. Interestingly, EBV is known to activate B cells by expressing two proteins, LMP2A and LMP1, that mimic activated BCR and CD40, respectively, but there is no evidence that EBV may activate TLR as well (16). Thus, the three-signal model of B-cell activation is consistent with the potent synergy that TLR agonists have on B-cell immortalization (Fig. 2B).

The method has been adapted to high-throughput cultures performed in 384 plates. In a typical experiment, memory B cells are isolated by positive or negative selection according to the isotype expressed (IgG or IgA), incubated with EBV and CpG, and seeded in multiple 384 plates in the presence of irradiated allogeneic peripheral blood mononuclear cells (PBMCs) as feeder cells. The efficiency of immortalization, as demonstrated by the production of high levels of IgG is close to 30% (Fig. 2C). Given an efficiency immortalization of 20 to 30%, we typically seed 3 cells/well in order to have clonal growth. This procedure allows the avoidance or minimization of the need to subclone positive cultures and the easy rescue of the few clones that may show poor growth *in vitro*. Using this method and taking advantage of an automated liquid-handling system and fully integrated immunoassays, we can typically screen repertoires of >10^4 IgG memory B cells. An even higher number of cells can be screened by plating higher numbers of cells per culture (up to 30 to 100). In the latter case, subcloning of positive cultures will be required in order to isolate a clone making the desired antibody. Importantly, in all cases, the antibody is present at high concentrations in the culture supernatant so that multiple assays can be performed in parallel, including functional assays such as virus neutralization or bacterial opsonophagocytosis killing assays. An example of a screening by neutralization is provided in Fig. 2D. Of almost 50,000 culture supernatants of immortalized B cells from three donors, several were found to protect cells from the cytopathic effect of metapneumovirus (MPV), and one clone, named MPE8, was found in a parallel assay to neutralize respiratory syncytial virus (RSV) as well. Another example (Fig. 2E) shows how it is possible to rapidly identify in B cells obtained from an individual immunized with the pandemic H1N1 strain so-called heterosubtypic antibodies that bind to H1 and cross-react with the heterologous H5 hemagglutinin.

A significant advantage of the EBV-based method is that the immortalized B cells secrete high amounts of antibodies but also maintain expression of BCR, although at a low and variable level. Consequently, antigen-specific cells can be selected from a polyclonal population by panning or staining with isotype- or light chain-specific antibodies or with the specific antigen. In addition, we never found evidence of ongoing somatic mutations in EBV-immortalized clones. EBV-immortalized B-cell clones maintain constant productivity with antibodies typically

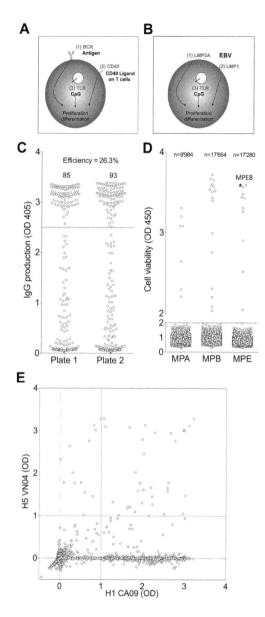

recovered in the culture supernatants at concentrations ranging from 5 to 50 μg/ml in static cultures. Thus, antibodies can be easily prepared from the culture supernatant in milligram amounts. In the past 10 years, the EBV+CpG immortalization method has been used in our laboratory to interrogate memory B and isolate monoclonal antibodies specific for a variety of human pathogens, toxins, and self-antigens (Table 1).

LONG-TERM CULTURE OF SINGLE PLASMA CELLS AND THEIR INTERROGATION USING MULTIPLE ASSAYS

We originally reported that antigen-specific plasma cells appear in high numbers in peripheral blood 1 week after booster immunization (17) when they may account for up to 40 to 90% of total Ig-secreting cells (17). While other laboratories have used this source of specific plasma cells to clone VH/VL pairs by RT-PCR and produce the antibodies

1 cell/well in 384 culture plates containing irradiated allogeneic PBMC. Shown is the concentration of IgG in culture supernatants on day 10. Positive values above 2.5 OD correspond to IgG concentrations >1 μg/ml. The efficiency was calculated according to the Poisson distribution. (D) Example of a primary screening for MPV-neutralizing antibodies. In preliminary experiments, culture conditions were defined to achieve cytopathic effect by using primary MPV isolates. Culture supernatants were incubated with MPV followed by addition of LLC-MK2 cells. Living cells were measured by using a colorimetric assay on day 8. Several antibodies were isolated, including one (MPE8) that neutralizes four different paramyxoviruses. Shown is the total numbers of cultures screened. (E) Blood was collected from an immune donor 2 weeks after vaccination with a seasonal vaccine, and IgG memory cells were immortalized and plated at 3 cells/well in 384-well plates. The supernatants were screened for the presence of antibodies that bind to either H1 HA (CA09) present in the vaccine or to H5 HA (VN04) that represents a heterologous group 1 HA. doi:10.1128/microbiolspec.AID-0018-2014.f2

FIGURE 2 Efficient immortalization of human memory B cells by combination of EBV and CpG and isolation of rare neutralizing antibodies. (A) BCR stimulation mediated by antigen, T-cell help mediated by CD40L/CD40 interaction, and TLR stimulation provide three synergistic stimuli for activation of human B cells (15). (B) EBV encodes LMP2a and LMP1 that mimic constitutively activated BCR and CD40, thus providing signal 1 and signal 2. Addition of TLR agonists potently synergizes with the viral genes leading to efficient activation and immortalization (8). (C) Immortalization efficiency of IgG+ memory B cells plated at

TABLE 1 Examples of human monoclonal antibodies isolated by using high-throughput cellular screens

Target	Findings	Reference
SARS-CoV[a]	Potent and broadly neutralizing antibodies	8, 22
Diphtheria toxin	Substoichiometric neutralization of the toxin	Unpublished
Anthrax protective antigen	Substoichiometric neutralization of the toxin	Unpublished
HIV-1	Neutralizing antibodies targeting different sites including heptad repeat 1	23, 24
Influenza A virus	Broadly neutralizing and pan-influenza-A-neutralizing antibodies	9, 25
HCMV	Extremely potent neutralizing antibodies targeting the gHgLpUL pentameric complex	19
RSV/MPV/PVM/BRSV[b]	An antibody that neutralizes 4 paramyxoviruses	20
Plasmodium falciparum	Antibodies to VAR2 CSA, MSP2, and p27. Fc-dependent killing of parasites	26, 27
Norovirus	Analysis of the GII.4 norovirus evolution	28
Dengue virus	Fc-engineered antibodies neutralizing all 4 serotypes and effective in an ADE mouse model	29, 30
Rabies virus	Potent and broadly neutralizing antibodies covering all 7 lyssavirus genotypes	Unpublished
Staphylcoccus aureus	Anti-MSCRAMMs and other target molecule antibodies with therapeutic potential	Unpublished
Avian flu (H5N1)	Potent and broadly neutralizing antibodies	31
Ebola virus	Potent antibody neutralizing all Ebola species	Unpublished
Pemphigus	Fine specificity, mechanism of action, and role of somatic mutations	32
GM-CSF[c]	Fine specificity, mechanism of action, and role of somatic mutations	Unpublished
Citrullinated proteins	Specificity and role of somatic mutations	Unpublished
HBV	Potent neutralizing antibodies against HBsAg covering all genotypes and drug selected mutants	Unpublished
HCV	Potent and broadly neutralizing antibodies	Unpublished
MERS-CoV[d]	Potent and broadly neutralizing antibody	Unpublished

[a]SARS, severe acute respiratory syndrome.
[b]PVM, pneumonia virus of mice; BRSV, bovine-RSV.
[c]GM-CSF, granulocyte-macrophage colony-stimulating factor.
[d]MERS, Middle East respiratory syndrome.

recombinantly (5), we were interested to develop a method that would allow us to rapidly focus on rare antibodies, for instance, capable of binding two different viruses. We reasoned that if single plasma cells could be maintained in culture for enough time in a small volume, the antibody released in the supernatant could reach concentrations sufficient to perform several parallel assays. We found that single plasma cells isolated from blood or bone marrow could be maintained in culture for several weeks when cultured on a monolayer of immortalized stromal cells. In these conditions, single plasma cells secreted Ig at a constant rate of approximately 100 pg/cell/day (Fig. 3A). We also found that, in the absence of stromal cells, recombinant IL-6 was sufficient to maintain plasma cell viability at least for 3 to 4 days (9).

The plating efficiency in IL-6-dependent cultures is high, ranging from 50 to 100% (Fig. 3B). In a typical experiment, we isolate $CD138^+ CD27^{hi}$ cells by cell sorting and seed them in 384 well plates at 1 cell/well in 50 μl of complete medium supplemented with IL-6. After 3 to 4 days, the supernatants are removed and tested in multiple parallel assays by using an automated liquid-handling system. The throughput and efficiency of the method is illustrated by the finding that the FI6 pan-influenza-neutralizing antibody was isolated every year for 5 consecutive years from the same donor from plasma cells collected after infection or vaccination (D. Corti, unpublished data). An example of the high throughput of this method is shown in Fig. 3C and D, where 13,000 plasma cell cultures were screened to determine the fraction of hemagglutinin (HA)-

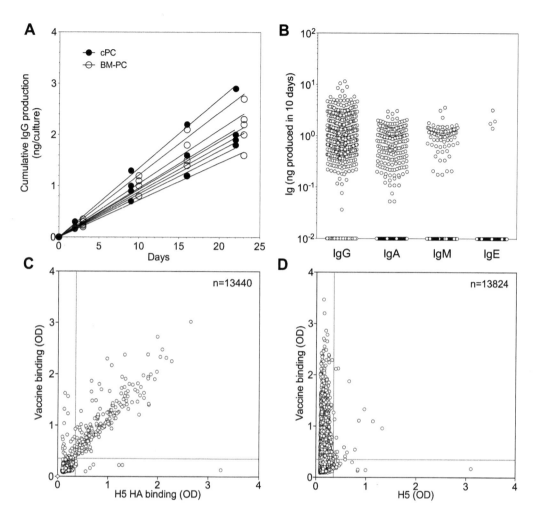

FIGURE 3 Cultures of single plasma cells are instrumental for the rapid identification of rare antibodies. **(A)** Survival of single CD138$^+$ plasma cells isolated from peripheral blood (open circles) or bone marrow (filled circles) in the presence of IL-6 and stromal cell monolayers. Shown is the cumulative production of IgG in cultures containing single plasma cells. **(B)** Plasma cells were isolated from peripheral blood as CD38$^+$ CD138$^+$ and plated at 0.5 cell/well in the presence of IL-6. IgG, IgA, IgM, and IgE levels were measured in each culture supernatant. The efficiency of cloning as estimated from the frequency of Ig-containing cultures was estimated to be approximately 70%. **(C), (D)** HA-specific antibodies produced by plasma cells isolated in 2009 following infection with H1N1 CA09 cross-react extensively with H5-HA (VN04). **(C)** In contrast, plasma cells isolated from the same donor in 2010 following vaccination with the seasonal trivalent vaccine are largely vaccine specific **(D)**. doi:10.1128/microbiolspec.AID-0018-2014.f3

specific antibodies that cross-react with the heterologous H5 HA. This same method was used to clone rare IgE antibodies from an allergic individual.

Once identified, the positive cultures are subjected to single-cell RT-PCR and the specific VH/VL pairs are isolated, and the recombinant antibodies are expressed by using appropriate vectors. This high frequency of somatic mutations might represent a potential problem to antibody sequencing, because the mutated sequences may no longer be complementary to the oligos used for VH/VL gene amplification. To overcome this potential problem, we use, in a stepwise fashion, multiple sets of primers spanning different regions of the variable region leader sequence that allow us to obtain, with almost 100% efficiency, VH and VL sequences from all isolated plasma cell clones.

A TARGET-AGNOSTIC APPROACH FOR ANTIGEN DISCOVERY FOR VACCINE DESIGN

The high throughput of the cell-based screens and the possibility of directly assessing the function of the antibody (rather than just binding) are essential elements to implement a target-agnostic approach that aims at the identification of the most effective antibodies

and, through the analysis of their specificity, of the most promising targets for vaccine design. This approach was originally proposed by Dennis Burton as a way to identify conserved epitopes in the highly variable viral glycoproteins, such as the Env of HIV-1 (18), but in a broader sense can be also used to identify in complex pathogens the molecules that induce the most potent neutralizing response, without prior knowledge of their nature.

A relevant example is provided by human cytomegalovirus (HCMV), a herpes virus that uses several glycoproteins to infect human cells. Previous studies focused on gB or gHgL, which are abundant proteins that were known to be targeted by neutralizing antibodies. Using a target-agnostic approach, we isolated from immune donors

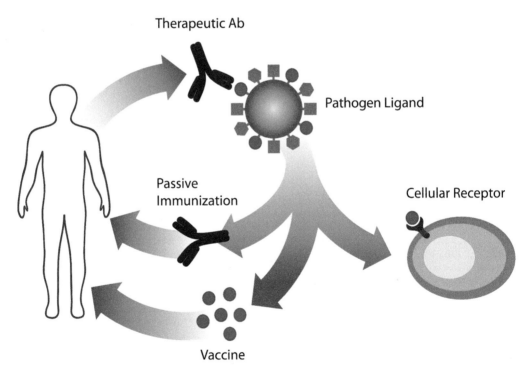

FIGURE 4 A target-agnostic approach to antibody discovery and vaccine design. In analytic vaccinology, donors that have developed a protective response are identified and memory B cells/plasma cells are interrogated to identify the most effective neutralizing antibodies in terms of potency and breadth. The antibodies are then used to identify the target antigen and to probe its correct conformation when the latter is produced as a recombinant vaccine. The vaccine is expected to elicit antibodies of the same quality as those originally isolated. In addition, the recombinant molecules can be used to identify cellular receptors. doi:10.1128/microbiolspec.AID-0018-2014.f4

a large panel of antibodies based on their capacity to neutralize infection of fibroblasts or epithelial cells by a primary HCMV isolate and identified a group of unusually potent antibodies that selectively neutralized infection of epithelial, endothelial, and myeloid cells at concentrations 1,000-fold lower than antibodies specific for gB or ghgL (19). We found that these antibodies recognize multiple antigenic sites on a pentameric complex of gH/gL/pUL128/pUL130/pUL131A, which was previously described to be required for infection of endothelial epithelial and myeloid cells but was not known to be the target of neutralizing antibodies. We then produced a soluble pentameric complex that correctly displays all the neutralizing epitopes and elicits in mice very high titers of neutralizing antibodies. In addition, the soluble recombinant pentamer produced is used to identify the cellular receptors and dissect the mechanisms of virus entry in different cell types. We refer to this process as analytic vaccinology, since it is essentially based on the analysis of the antibody response to the pathogen (Fig. 4).

Another example of analytic vaccinology is provided by the analysis of the neutralizing antibody response to the F protein of RSV (20). Previous studies suggested that the postfusion F protein could be developed as a vaccine, since it was recognized by palivizumab, a neutralizing monoclonal antibody that is used to prevent RSV infection in newborns (21). In contrast, we found that, of 30 neutralizing antibodies tested, only 4 bound to the postfusion protein while the remaining, including the MPE8 antibody that cross-neutralizes four paramyxoviruses, were specific for the prefusion F conformation. These findings suggest that the prefusion protein should be considered as the most effective vaccine capable of inducing a broad spectrum of antibodies that neutralize but fail to react with the abundant postfusion F protein. Efforts to produce a stabilized prefusion form will be facilitated by the use of the antibodies that can be used as probes to test the conformation and stability of different constructs.

ACKNOWLEDGMENT

Conflicts of interest: We disclose no conflicts.

CITATION

Corti D, Lanzavecchia A. 2014. Efficient methods to isolate human monoclonal antibodies from memory B cells and plasma cells. Microbiol Spectrum 2(5):AID-0018-2014.

REFERENCES

1. **Burton DR, Barbas CF.** 1994. Human antibodies from combinatorial libraries. *Adv Immunol* **57:**191–280.
2. **Hoogenboom HR.** 2002. Overview of antibody phage-display technology and its applications. *Methods Mol Biol* **178:**1–37.
3. **Green LL.** 1999. Antibody engineering via genetic engineering of the mouse: XenoMouse strains are a vehicle for the facile generation of therapeutic human monoclonal antibodies. *J Immunol Methods* **231:**11–23.
4. **Wardemann H, Yurasov S, Schaefer A, Young J, Meffre E, Nussenzweig M.** 2003. Predominant autoantibody production by early human B cell precursors. *Science* **301:**1374–1377.
5. **Wrammert J, Smith K, Miller J, Langley WA, Kokko K, Larsen C, Zheng N-Y, Mays I, Garman L, Helms C, James J, Air GM, Capra JD, Ahmed R, Wilson PC.** 2008. Rapid cloning of high-affinity human monoclonal antibodies against influenza virus. *Nature* **453:**667–671.
6. **Scheid JF, Mouquet H, Feldhahn N, Seaman MS, Velinzon K, Pietzsch J, Ott RG, Anthony RM, Zebroski H, Hurley A, Phogat A, Chakrabarti B, Li Y, Connors M, Pereyra F, Walker BD, Wardemann H, Ho D, Wyatt RT, Mascola JR, Ravetch JV, Nussenzweig MC.** 2009. Broad diversity of neutralizing antibodies isolated from memory B cells in HIV-infected individuals. *Nature* **458:**636–640.
7. **Dekosky BJ, Ippolito GC, Deschner RP, Lavinder JJ, Wine Y, Rawlings BM, Varadarajan N, Giesecke C, Dörner T, Andrews SF, Wilson PC, Hunicke-Smith SP, Willson CG, Ellington AD, Georgiou G.** 2013. High-throughput sequencing of the paired human immunoglobulin heavy and light chain repertoire. *Nat Biotechnol* **31:**166–169.
8. **Traggiai E, Becker S, Subbarao K, Kolesnikova L, Uematsu Y, Gismondo MR, Murphy BR, Rappuoli R, Lanzavecchia A.** 2004. An efficient method to make human monoclonal antibodies

from memory B cells: potent neutralization of SARS coronavirus. *Nat Med* **10**:871–875.

9. **Corti D, Voss J, Gamblin SJ, Codoni G, Macagno A, Jarrossay D, Vachieri SG, Pinna D, Minola A, Vanzetta F, Silacci C, Fernandez-Rodriguez BM, Agatic G, Bianchi S, Giacchetto-Sasselli I, Calder L, Sallusto F, Collins P, Haire LF, Temperton N, Langedijk JPM, Skehel JJ, Lanzavecchia A.** 2011. A neutralizing antibody selected from plasma cells that binds to group 1 and group 2 influenza A hemagglutinins. *Science* **333**:850–856.

10. **Kwakkenbos MJ, Diehl SA, Yasuda E, Bakker AQ, van Geelen CMM, Lukens MV, van Bleek GM, Widjojoatmodjo MN, Bogers WMJM, Mei H, Radbruch A, Scheeren FA, Spits H, Beaumont T.** 2010. Generation of stable monoclonal antibody-producing B cell receptor-positive human memory B cells by genetic programming. *Nat Med* **16**:123–128.

11. **Walker LM, Phogat SK, Chan-Hui P-Y, Wagner D, Phung P, Goss JL, Wrin T, Simek MD, Fling S, Mitcham JL, Lehrman JK, Priddy FH, Olsen OA, Frey SM, Hammond PW, Kaminsky S, Zamb T, Moyle M, Koff WC, Poignard P, Burton DR.** 2009. Broad and potent neutralizing antibodies from an African donor reveal a new HIV-1 vaccine target. *Science* **326**:285–289.

12. **Huang J, Doria-Rose NA, Longo NS, Laub L, Lin C-L, Turk E, Kang BH, Migueles SA, Bailer RT, Mascola JR, Connors M.** 2013. Isolation of human monoclonal antibodies from peripheral blood B cells. *Nat Protoc* **8**:1907–1915.

13. **Steinitz M, Klein G, Koskimies S, Makel O.** 1977. EB virus-induced B lymphocyte cell lines producing specific antibody. *Nature* **269**:420–422.

14. **Bernasconi N, Onai N.** 2003. A role for Toll-like receptors in acquired immunity: up-regulation of TLR9 by BCR triggering in naive B cells and constitutive expression in memory B cells. *Blood* **101**:4500–4504.

15. **Ruprecht CR, Lanzavecchia A.** 2006. Toll-like receptor stimulation as a third signal required for activation of human naive B cells. *Eur J Immunol* **36**:810–816.

16. **Thorley-Lawson DA.** 2001. Epstein-Barr virus: exploiting the immune system. *Nat Rev Immunol* **1**:75–82.

17. **Bernasconi NL, Traggiai E, Lanzavecchia A.** 2002. Maintenance of serological memory by polyclonal activation of human memory B cells. *Science* **298**:2199–2202.

18. **Burton D.** 2002. Antibodies, viruses and vaccines. *Nat Rev Immunol* **2**:706–713.

19. **Macagno A, Bernasconi NL, Vanzetta F, Dander E, Sarasini A, Revello MG, Gerna G, Sallusto F, Lanzavecchia A.** 2010. Isolation of human monoclonal antibodies that potently neutralize human cytomegalovirus infection by targeting different epitopes on the gH/gL/UL128-131A complex. *J Virol* **84**:1005–1013.

20. **Corti D, Bianchi S, Vanzetta F, Minola A, Perez L, Agatic G, Guarino B, Silacci C, Marcandalli J, Marsland BJ, Piralla A, Percivalle E, Sallusto F, Baldanti F, Lanzavecchia A.** 2013. Cross-neutralization of four paramyxoviruses by a human monoclonal antibody. *Nature* **501**:439–443.

21. **The-IMPACT-RSV-Study-Group.** 1998. Palivizumab, a humanized respiratory syncytial virus monoclonal antibody, reduces hospitalization from respiratory syncytial virus infection in high-risk infants. *Pediatrics* **102**:531–537.

22. **Rockx B, Corti D, Donaldson E, Sheahan T, Stadler K, Lanzavecchia A, Baric R.** 2008. Structural basis for potent cross-neutralizing human monoclonal antibody protection against lethal human and zoonotic severe acute respiratory syndrome coronavirus challenge. *J Virol* **82**:3220–3235.

23. **Corti D, Langedijk JPM, Hinz A, Seaman MS, Vanzetta F, Fernandez-Rodriguez BM, Silacci C, Pinna D, Jarrossay D, Balla-Jhagjhoorsingh S, Willems B, Zekveld MJ, Dreja H, O'Sullivan E, Pade C, Orkin C, Jeffs SA, Montefiori DC, Davis D, Weissenhorn W, McKnight A, Heeney JL, Sallusto F, Sattentau QJ, Weiss RA, Lanzavecchia A.** 2010. Analysis of memory B cell responses and isolation of novel monoclonal antibodies with neutralizing breadth from HIV-1-infected individuals. *PLoS One* **5**:e8805. doi:10.1371/journal.pone.0008805.

24. **Sabin C, Corti D, Buzon V, Seaman MS, Lutje Hulsik D, Hinz A, Vanzetta F, Agatic G, Silacci C, Mainetti L, Scarlatti G, Sallusto F, Weiss R, Lanzavecchia A, Weissenhorn W.** 2010. Crystal structure and size-dependent neutralization properties of HK20, a human monoclonal antibody binding to the highly conserved heptad repeat 1 of gp41. *PLoS Pathog* **6**:e1001195. doi:10.1371/journal.ppat.1001195.

25. **Corti D, Suguitan AL, Pinna D, Silacci C, Fernandez-Rodriguez BM, Vanzetta F, Santos C, Luke CJ, Torres-Velez FJ, Temperton NJ, Weiss RA, Sallusto F, Subbarao K, Lanzavecchia A.** 2010. Heterosubtypic neutralizing antibodies are produced by individuals immunized with a seasonal influenza vaccine. *J Clin Invest* **120**:1663–1673.

26. **Barfod L, Bernasconi NL, Dahlbäck M, Jarrossay D, Andersen PH, Salanti A, Ofori MF, Turner L, Resende M, Nielsen MA, Theander TG, Sallusto F, Lanzavecchia A, Hviid L.** 2007. Human pregnancy-associated malaria-specific B

cells target polymorphic, conformational epitopes in VAR2CSA. *Mol Microbiol* **63:**335–347.

27. **Stubbs J, Olugbile S, Saidou B, Simpore J, Corradin G, Lanzavecchia A.** 2011. Strain-transcending Fc-dependent killing of Plasmodium falciparum by merozoite surface protein 2 allele-specific human antibodies. *Infect Immun* **79:**1143–1152.

28. **Lindesmith LC, Beltramello M, Donaldson EF, Corti D, Swanstrom J, Debbink K, Lanzavecchia A, Baric RS.** 2012. Immunogenetic mechanisms driving norovirus GII.4 antigenic variation. *PLoS Pathog* **8:**e1002705. doi:10.1371/journal.ppat.1002705.

29. **Beltramello M, Williams KL, Simmons CP, Macagno A, Simonelli L, Quyen NTH, Sukupolvi-Petty S, Navarro-Sanchez E, Young PR, de Silva AM, Rey FA, Varani L, Whitehead SS, Diamond MS, Harris E, Lanzavecchia A, Sallusto F.** 2010. The human immune response to Dengue virus is dominated by highly cross-reactive antibodies endowed with neutralizing and enhancing activity. *Cell Host Microbe* **8:**271–283.

30. **Williams KL, Sukupolvi-Petty S, Beltramello M, Johnson S, Sallusto F, Lanzavecchia A, Diamond MS, Harris E.** 2013. Therapeutic efficacy of antibodies lacking FcγR against lethal dengue virus infection is due to neutralizing potency and blocking of enhancing antibodies. *PLoS Pathog* **9:**e1003157. doi:10.1371/journal.ppat.1003157.

31. **Simmons CP, Bernasconi NL, Suguitan AL, Mills K, Ward JM, Chau NVV, Hien TT, Sallusto F, Ha DQ, Farrar J, de Jong MD, Lanzavecchia A, Subbarao K.** 2007. Prophylactic and therapeutic efficacy of human monoclonal antibodies against H5N1 influenza. *PLoS Med* **4:**e178. doi:10.1371/journal.pmed.0040178.

32. **Di Zenzo G, Di Lullo G, Corti D, Calabresi V, Sinistro A, Vanzetta F, Didona B, Cianchini G, Hertl M, Eming R, Amagai M, Ohyama B, Hashimoto T, Sloostra J, Sallusto F, Zambruno G, Lanzavecchia A.** 2012. Pemphigus autoantibodies generated through somatic mutations target the desmoglein-3 cis-interface. *J Clin Invest* **122:**3781–3790.

Use of Human Hybridoma Technology To Isolate Human Monoclonal Antibodies

8

SCOTT A. SMITH[1] and JAMES E. CROWE, JR.[2]

HISTORY OF HYBRIDOMAS

Monoclonal antibodies (mAbs) have revolutionized the conduct of science since their first description in 1975 (1). The use of these specific reagents also has made possible improved clinical diagnostics in the medical arena, and many antibodies have found their way to clinical use as prophylactic or therapeutic agents. Nevertheless, the potential of mAbs derived specifically from technology based on human hybridomas remains largely unfulfilled. The principal reason for the lack of a large number of hybridoma-derived mAb therapeutics has simply been the technical difficulty in generating stable hybridomas that secrete human mAbs of high affinity and functional activity. This chapter reviews recent efforts to develop and employ novel methods for the efficient generation of human hybridomas secreting human mAbs for clinical use.

The principal advantage of the use of human hybridoma technology for mAb generation is that this approach preserves the authentic sequence and pairing of antibody DNA from a natural B cell for the expression of a naturally occurring full-length human mAb. There are significant theoretical advantages for expressing cDNAs encoding authentic heavy and light

[1]Vanderbilt Vaccine Center and Department of Medicine, Vanderbilt University Medical Center, Nashville, TN 37232; [2]Vanderbilt Vaccine Center and Departments of Pediatrics and Pathology, Microbiology, and Immunology, Vanderbilt University Medical Center, Nashville, TN 37232.

Antibodies for Infectious Diseases
Edited by James E. Crowe, Jr., Diana Boraschi, and Rino Rappuoli
© 2015 American Society for Microbiology, Washington, DC
doi:10.1128/microbiolspec.AID-0027-2014

chains with chains that are paired using the coding sequence as it was generated naturally through B cell selection, class switch, and affinity maturation. No genetic modification of these sequences is required. Since antibody expression is typically very stable in hybridomas, sequence amplification of antibody variable genes is achieved easily if recombinant production or manipulation is desired. The resulting recombinant mAb retains most features of naturally occurring human antibodies, as the clone retains the native amino acid sequence and heavy/light chain pairing. Since the native constant region of the antibody in the original human B cell is retained in the mAb expressed by the resulting hybridoma, the functional properties of the particular Fc region can be studied for Fc-mediated activities, such as antibody-dependent cellular cytotoxicity.

Despite the advantages inherent to making natural human mAbs, the low efficiency of the hybridoma isolation process historically was a technical drawback that was too great to overcome, and many other methods of producing human mAbs have been used instead in recent years to meet the demand for generation of therapeutic antibodies. The principal disadvantage of the hybridoma method is low fusion efficiency. Over the last several decades, however, this problem has been overcome slowly through improvements in several technical features of the process. These improvements will be discussed in more detail throughout this article. Currently, human hybridomas can be generated with great efficiency and throughput. Panels of antigen-specific human hybridomas secreting full-length naturally occurring mAbs to a large number of targets have been developed recently using human peripheral blood mononuclear cells as the starting material.

FIRST HUMAN HYBRIDOMAS

The prospect of using human mAbs for the prevention or treatment of human diseases was evident early on and was the driving force behind intense effort put into the development of human hybridoma methods. Initial studies were done in the early 1970s using mouse myeloma cells, fusing them with primary human B cells (2). A human tetraploid hybridoma also was made through the fusion of two human lymphocyte lines (3). It was not until 1980, however, that the first successful human mAb was produced (4). This feat was achieved by fusing lymphoid cells harvested from spleens obtained during staging laparotomy from patients with Hodgkin's lymphoma with the human myeloma cell line U266. This accomplishment was a large step toward the use of human hybridomas to make mAbs, as it proved the feasibility of the method. The large numbers of lymphoid cells used in that fusion process were sufficient to overcome the low fusion efficiency at the time. The challenge of identifying antigen-specific cells and expanding them to numbers that enabled researchers to overcome the barrier of low fusion efficiency would, however, require several more decades of investigation.

One significant obstacle to the generation of human hybridomas over the years was the inability to consistently expand desired populations of antigen-specific B cells. Antigen-specific memory B cells generally circulate at low frequencies in the peripheral blood, typically in a range that centers around 1 in 10,000 B cells or lower. For example, precursor frequencies of anti-tetanus toxoid-specific B cells were initially reported following immunization as being approximately 1 per 10,000 peripheral blood mononuclear cells (PBMCs) (5). Fusion efficiencies typically have not been sufficient to immortalize enough cells from the number of B cells that can be obtained from humans by routine phlebotomy. When combined with a fusion efficiency of 1 in 100,000 B cells in the suspension, as is typical of polyethylene glycol (PEG)-mediated cell fusion, one would need approximately 1 liter of blood to obtain a single tetanus toxoid-specific human hybridoma under these circumstances. Consequently, the generation of human hybridoma cells secreting desirable human mAbs without expanding the frequency or number of antigen-specific B cell populations was difficult.

Human B cells can be immortalized by methods using Epstein-Barr virus (EBV) transformation (6, 7). EBV transformation is often carried out on samples containing large numbers of B cells, either from PBMCs or cells obtained from lymphatic tissues such as tonsil cells. These EBV-transformed B cell lines, which contain many clones of differing specificities, must be grown for a considerable period of time to allow for the emergence of immortalized lines. Since immortalization does not occur with every clone of transformed B cells, production of antigen-specific clones was historically very difficult. Moreover, EBV-transformed B cells generally grow poorly, often secrete low amounts of antibodies, and can exhibit chromosomal instability (6, 8–10). Recently, the addition of CpG oligonucleotide a toll-like receptor (TLR) 9 agonist during B cell transformation was shown to greatly facilitate the transformation process (11–13). This stimulation significantly improved the efficiency of transformation and has been used to expand antigen-specific B cells for the clonal amplification of their antibody variable sequences by reverse transcriptase PCR (13).

The prospect of using EBV-transformed B cells for the generation of human hybridomas was first realized in the early 1980s. This method was achieved initially by fusing a human EBV-transformed B cell line producing antigen-specific mAb with a murine myeloma to produce a stable heterohybridoma secreting mAb (14, 15). This procedure resulted in a more stable, higher-producing clone. Hypoxanthine phosphoribosyl transferase-deficient variant EBV-transformed B cell lines also were developed for use as human fusion partners (16). The use of an immortalized EBV-transformed B cell clone to create a stable fully human hybridoma was described in 1984 (17). A fully human hybridoma was generated successfully by fusing a cytomegalovirus-specific EBV-immortalized B cell line with a hypoxanthine phosphoribosyl transferase-deficient human lymphoblastoid partner created previously. Many groups have now used variations of these techniques to employ EBV transformation to expand populations of antigen-specific B cells. These methods have improved mAb yield and hybridoma generation throughput considerably. In fact, EBV transformation continues to be used to this day to expand B cells prior to human hybridoma generation.

B CELL SOURCE

One of the critical factors underlying the difficulty in generating human hybridomas is the low frequency of antigen-specific B cells in peripheral blood under normal circumstances. Typically, antigen-specific B cells are present in peripheral blood at a frequency of ≤0.1%. Therefore, large numbers of PBMCs are required from individuals to obtain a significant number of antigen-specific B cells. For example, if a desired antigen-specific B cell occurs at a frequency of 1 in 1,000, and PBMCs contain 10% B cells, then 1 million PBMCs contain only 100 antigen-specific B cells. Several strategies have been devised to enrich and/or expand antigen-specific B cell populations prior to fusion.

The most readily available source of antigen-specific B cells is peripheral blood. For the most part, directly fusing PBMCs with a myeloma partner is not productive in generating a desired antigen-specific human hybridoma, due to the limited number of antigen-specific cells in circulation. Enrichment of antigen-specific B cells from large samples of PBMCs using either fluorescence activated cell sorting or other cell isolation techniques (such as magnetic bead separation) often results in only modest improvement in the yield of functional cells.

The use of various cytokines, or cell lines made to express B cell cytokines, to amplify single B cells in culture has been described in the B cell field, principally using CD40-ligand (CD40L or CD154) expressing cells and recombinant human cytokines (interleukin 2 [IL-2], IL-4, and IL-10) (18). Synergy was also noted with the combination of CD40L and IL-21 (19). Feeder cell lines have also been used, based on their ability to support primary human B cell growth, frequently following gamma irradiation to prevent them from dividing. Several feeder cell lines have been described for this purpose: a fibroblast cell line transfected with the human CD40L molecule (20), an immortalized cell line FDC-H1 with features of human follicular dendritic cells (21), the U-937 human macrophage-like cell line (ATCC-CRL-1593.2) (22), and the EL4-B5 mutant thymoma cell line (23).

In addition to human CD40L, B lymphocyte stimulating factor (BLyS), also known as BAFF (for B cell activating factor belonging to the tumor necrosis factor family) (24), has been used to support primary B cells in culture providing costimulatory signals. BAFF is a relatively new member of the tumor necrosis factor family that was simultaneously identified by four different laboratories and named BAFF, BLyS, TALL-1, THANK, and zTNF4. The cytokine is expressed abundantly in monocytes and macrophages and is upregulated by interferon gamma. Endogenous BAFF is processed intracellulary by a protease of the furin family of proprotein convertases. Secreted BAFF acts as a potent B cell growth factor. BAFF plays an important role as costimulator of B cell proliferation and function. Using soluble cytokines or feeder cells able to provide costimulator function and/or cytokines, single B cells can be expanded to clones of a few hundred cells in several weeks. Antigen-specific B cell clones can be confirmed by testing cell supernatant specificity using enzyme-linked immunosorbent assay. The expanded antigen-specific cells then can be immortalized by fusion with a myeloma to form a hybridoma.

The simplest and most common strategy for the amplification of B cell populations using PBMCs is to use EBV transformation (25). Freshly isolated or cryopreserved PBMCs, obtained from an individual or individuals who have been identified as possessing B cells of the desired antigen specificity, can be expanded in an oligoclonal manner using EBV transformation. Using culture supernatant of the marmoset cell line B95.8, which contains high titers of EBV, B cells can be infected via complement receptor 2 (CD21), and transformants emerge over the course of 1 to 2 weeks, forming large colonies of cells known as lymphoblastoid cells (often abbreviated LCLs) (26). Cultures can be supplemented with cyclosporin A to inhibit EBV-specific T cells, which are present in many individuals, from killing B cell transformants (27). The overall efficiency of EBV transformation was improved dramatically through the use of CpG oligonucleotide, increasing transformation of B cell populations from <10% to >30% (13) (see Fig. 1).

Recently it was shown that by adding an inhibitor of EBV-associated apoptosis, a pharmacologic inhibitor of the serine/threonine-protein kinase 2, which is required for checkpoint-mediated cell cycle arrest, results in further improvement in lymphoblastoid cell survival and expansion (28, 29). In the end, increased numbers of lymphoblastoid cells result in a greater probability of successfully producing hybridomas secreting antibodies of interest. Next, EBV-transformed

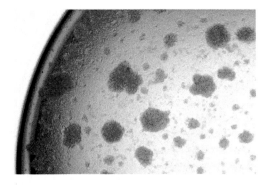

FIGURE 1 **Lymphoblastoid cell formation from PBMCs. doi:10.1128/microbiolspec.AID-0027-2014.f1**

B cell cultures are screened for antigen-specific antibody production using enzyme-linked immunosorbent assay or other multiwall plate assays. Cultures producing the desired antibody then are fused with a myeloma cell line in an oligoclonal manner. The resulting oligoclonal hybridoma lines are then biologically cloned by a physical method to isolate single cells, using one of the methods discussed later in this article, to produce a human hybridoma secreting an antigen-specific mAb.

FUSION METHODS

The most difficult and critical step in the production of human hybridomas is the ability to efficiently fuse desired populations of lymphocytes with a myeloma partner. There are three basic techniques used to generate hybridomas for the purpose of mAb production: (i) the use of chemical agents such as PEG, (ii) fusogenic viruses, and (iii) electrical cytofusion. The first method used to study cell fusion took advantage of viruses, principally Sendai virus, capable of fusing together the membranes of two cells. The most common technique, however, employed in the 1975 seminal paper by Kohler and Milstein (1), with variations of the theme still commonly used today, involves chemical fusion using PEG. Finally, protocols based on the use of electrical currents to align and fuse the membrane of cells for the efficient generation of hybridomas were developed and optimized.

Viruses were first used as a means to fuse cells in the 1960s and early 1970s (30). There are several viruses, or their fusion proteins, which have been used successfully for the purpose of hybridoma generation. The two most commonly used are Sendai virus and vesicular stomatitis virus. Sendai virus, also referred to as murine parainfluenza virus type 1 or hemagglutinating virus of Japan, is a paramyxovirus which was the first animal virus whose mode of infection was elucidated (31). The viral fusion protein, or F protein, makes up part of the exposed spikes on the envelope of the virus and inserts into the cell

membrane, allowing for introduction of the viral nucleocapsid into the cytoplasm of the host cell. The use of Sendai virus for cell fusion was described thoroughly by Okada in 1993 (32). One advantage of using Sendai virus is its broad tropism, which is mediated by the hemagglutinin-neuraminidase protein that recognizes sialic acid as a receptor on the host cell membrane. Kits containing inactivated Sendai virus are commercially available for the generation of murine hybridomas. The second virus that has been used for the fusion of cells to generate hybridomas for mAb secretion is vesicular stomatitis virus (33). In a study performed by Nagata et al., the efficiencies of hybridoma generation were compared using Sendai virus, vesicular stomatitis virus, and PEG-mediated cell fusion (34). Interestingly, their results suggested that the isotypes of antibodies obtained were influenced by the fusion method, as vesicular stomatitis virus-mediated fusion resulted in greater production of IgG mAbs (34). A related method that has been used is to transduce cells with viral fusogenic proteins. Unfortunately, the resulting cells often continue to fuse for as long as the proteins are expressed, which makes this method less optimal.

The most common method used to produce hybridomas takes advantage of the fusogenic properties of PEG, discovered by Kao and Michayluk in 1974 (35). The exact mechanism by which PEG-mediated cell fusion occurs is not known. Most experts believe that the mechanism primarily involves volume exclusion, driving adjacent cell membranes together (36). Unfortunately PEG is quite toxic to cells, as it can fuse multiple cells, resulting in giant polykaryons, and can even result in the fusion of intracellular membrane structures (37). The fusion process, however, is relatively simple and cheap. B cells are mixed with a myeloma fusion partner and suspended in a solution containing PEG in a drop-wise fashion. After a short incubation, fusion solution is removed and the cells are washed and resuspended in selection medium. Different PEG preparations have been shown to result in different efficiencies of cell fusion (38). The main problem with using PEG for the generation of human hybridomas is its low efficiency of fusion. Estimates of average fusion efficiencies are in the order of 1 hybridoma generated per 100,000 starting B cells. When fusing murine splenocytes from hyper-immunized animals (which can possess about 10^8 B cells), an extremely low inefficiency can be tolerated if one simply aims to find one or several mAbs that bind to an antigen. However, when using human samples such as blood (yielding about 1×10^6 PBMCs or about 50,000 B cells per ml of blood), or more precious samples such as tumor infiltrating lymphocytes, such inefficiencies make success unlikely.

The most efficient method of cell fusion and hybridoma generation is electrical cytofusion. This method of cell fusion is an essential step in the most innovative techniques in modern human hybridoma protocols and has been optimized for the purpose of human hybridoma generation (39). At the center of this membrane fusion technique is the concept of electroporation. The application of high-intensity electric field pulses to cells causes transient membrane permeabilization. The extent of permeabilization is thought to depend on several physical parameters associated with the technique such as pulse intensity, number, duration, shape, and interval. Electric field intensity is the most critical parameter in the induction of permeabilization. The intensity must exceed a critical threshold for membrane permeabilization to be induced. The electric field intensity delivered depends on the cell size. The extent of permeabilization (which correlates experimentally with the flow rate across the membrane) is controlled by both pulse number and duration (40). Increasing the electric field intensity above the critical threshold needed for permeabilization results in an increase in the area of the membrane that is involved. Permeabilization is transient and disappears with time after delivery of the electric field pulses. The half-life of permeabilization may be under the control of the electric field parameters. The rate of resealing of the pore in the membrane may be influenced by both pulse duration and number but is independent of the electric field intensity that creates the permeabilization (40). Therefore, optimal evaluation of critical parameters for membrane permeabilization requires flexible control over each aspect of the electrical field. One of the more recent innovations in the electroporation hardware used for this purpose is that many of these parameters can be controlled and varied independently. Previously designed electroporators did not have such precise control of all variables, thereby likely introducing uncontrolled variation in experiments.

Membrane effects of applied electrical fields in electrofusion are similar to those in electroporation except that membranes in close contact can fuse together during the process of pore formation. Therefore, electric field intensities used in electrofusion are similar to those used in electroporation. Electrofusion is performed in a sequence of steps. First, cells are brought into contact with other cells. Cell-cell contact can be achieved by several methods, although none has been sufficiently optimized in our estimation. Chemical methods such as avidin-biotin bridging have been used to bring together two cell types specifically (41–44). Chemical methods require more manipulation than other methods but can be useful in certain circumstances. Physical methods such as centrifugation can bring cells into contact prior to (or after) the fusion pulse (45). Electroacoustic fusion of cells in sugar solutions and of cells brought into contact in an ultrasonic standing wave field has been described (46). In fact, simple centrifugation followed by electroporation can be used to create cell fusion. The most commonly described effective method for bringing cells into contact prior to electrofusion, however, is termed dielectrophoresis. Dielectrophoresis is achieved within a suspension of cells using an alternating current electrical field.

In any fusion method, sufficient force must be applied to each cell to overcome the negative surface charge. If electricity is used, merely applying a uniform electric field will not move a cell because the net charge of the cell is zero. Thus, from the definition of electric field there is no force applied. However, a nonuniform field moves the positive ions inside each cell to one side and the negative ions to the opposite side, producing a dipole. Once the dipole is induced, a net force is exerted on the cell because the intensity of the field is greater on one side than the other. The movement of cells in one direction causes the cells to concentrate in an area. Since the cells are now dipoles, the negative side of one cell will attract the positive side of another cell, overcoming the negative surface charge. A photomicrograph illustrating pearl chain formation is shown in Fig. 2.

The second step in electrofusion is to apply one or more high-voltage pulses to the cells, inducing membrane fusion. The voltage required must be above a threshold to induce membrane breakdown and below a maximum voltage that causes cell death. The threshold voltage is approximately one volt across the cell membrane or two volts across two membranes (47). The voltage across a cell is equal to 1.5 times the cell radius times the electric field strength times the cosine of the angle of the membrane in relation of the direction of the field. This is the same formula used for electroporation. Multiple fusion pulses may be more efficient than a single pulse.

The last step in the electrofusion process (when using dielectrophoresis as an alignment tool) is postfusion alignment using alternating current fields. Electrofusion is a process that continues to occur over some time after the fusion pulse is applied. Reapplying dielectrophoresis after the fusion pulse allows maturation of the fusion process by holding cells in optimal alignment and contact.

Optimizing of dielectrophoresis and electrofusion parameters has been achieved partly via observable events through the use of a microscope slide or coaxial electrode. "Pearl chain length" (length of aligned cells) can be increased by increasing the voltage or increasing the time of prefusion sine wave application. Increased pearl chain length may not always be advantageous, however. It is unclear at this point whether long pearl chains are advantageous or not. According to Zimmermann (47), the fusion of adjacent cell membranes of cells in a pearl chain is a stochastic process. Thus, the electroporation conditions generate a probability of fusion of adjacent cell membranes. This means that it is possible to select electrofusion conditions that generate predominantly two cell fusions, even if pearl chain length is long in contrast to two-cell-only pearl chains.

The goal of electrofusion, at least as applied to hybridoma formation, is to generate

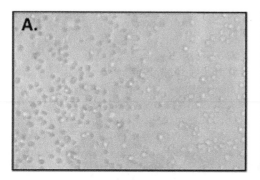 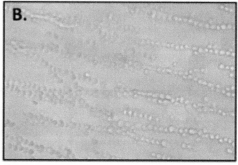

FIGURE 2 (A) Pre- and (B) post-pearl chain formation. doi:10.1128/microbiolspec.AID-0027-2014.f2

the most B cell-myeloma hybridomas. Through the use of selective medium preparations, fusions of like cells (either B cells or myeloma cells) are not productive. Likewise, unfused B cells and myeloma cells are also unable to survive. This selection is achieved through the use of medium containing HAT (hypoxanthine-aminopterin-thymidine) and ouabain. Unfused myeloma cells or fused myeloma cells that do not contain a B cell nucleus are killed by aminopterin. Without being fused to a B cell, the myeloma fusion partner is not able to perform *de novo* synthesis of DNA and is forced to undergo apoptosis. The B cell possesses the ability to overcome this blockade by performing the salvage pathway, for which hypoxanthine and thymidine are used as raw material for building DNA. Unfused B cells or fused B cells that do not contain a myeloma cell nucleus are killed by ouabain. Without being fused to the ouabain-resistant myeloma cell, the B cell (particularly transformed B cells) is highly susceptible to the plasma membrane sodium pump inhibiting effects of ouabain, and apoptosis is induced. The only products of fusion to survive in the selective medium are the B cell-myeloma hybridomas.

FUSION PARTNERS

Murine myeloma cells, originally developed for the production of mouse mAbs, were not suitable as fusion partners for human B cells, as they produced unstable heterospecific hybrids, often resulting in rejection of the relevant human chromosomes. The development and refinement of suitable fusion partners has been an ongoing and instrumental part of the human hybridoma technology. Investigators have been developing myeloma cell lines suitable for fusion with human B cells since the early 1980s. In general, these lines can be divided into two major types: fully human and heterohybridomas constructed by fusing murine myeloma cells with human cells. Several of the myeloma cell lines suitable

for fusion with human B cells are available at the American Type Culture Collection.

A number of fully human myeloma cell lines have been used successfully in fusion for the generation of human hybridomas. The most studied of these is the human myeloma U266 and its derived lines. U266 was originally isolated from a patient with multiple myeloma and found to secrete IgE (48). This myeloma was made HAT-sensitive and used as the first human fusion partner to generate fully human hybridomas (4, 49). The U266-derived SKO-007 line, made to be 8-azaguanine sensitive, was also used to generate some of the first fully human hybridomas (50–52). The human line LICR-LON-HMy2, also derived from malignant patient cells, was compared to SKO-007 and found to be superior (51, 53). LICR-LON-HMy2 was used to generate a hybridoma secreting mAb through the fusion of lymph node lymphocytes from a patient with breast cancer (54). The human myeloma line RPMI 8226, which expressed free light chain, was also used in the initial attempts to make fully human hybridomas (55, 56). The human myeloma-like cell line KR12 was generated by fusion of the human plasmacytoma line RPMI8226 with the human lymphoblastoid cell line KR-4 (14, 57). A more recently isolated human myeloma fusion partner, designated Karpas 707H, was developed for the purpose of making human hybridomas (58). Like U266, Karpas 707H was established from a patient with multiple myeloma. It was made to be both HAT-sensitive and ouabain-resistant, so it could be used with EBV-transformed B cells. Unfortunately, many laboratories attempting to make human hybridomas using these myeloma lines met with only limited success.

A larger group of fusion partners, themselves being heterohybridomas, have been developed by fusing murine myeloma cell lines with human cells. These fusion partners are nonsecreting mouse-human hybrids that are often made resistant to ouabain so they can produce stable hybridomas upon fusion with human EBV-transformed B cells. Since the heterohybridoma partner does not secrete an antibody, antibody secreted from the resulting hybridoma is encoded by the nucleus of the fused B cell. Ostberg and Pursch described the production of heterohybridomas made resistant to 8-azaguanine and used to generate human hybridomas secreting anti-influenza mAbs (59). One of these heteromyeloma fusion lines, SPAZ-4, was used later to generate human mAbs with specificities to various malignancies by fusion with lymph node lymphocytes from patients with carcinoma (60, 61). Two heterohybridoma cell lines, SHM-D33 and HMMA 2.5, continue to be used for production of human mAbs. SHM-D33 was generated by fusing the mouse myeloma cell line P3X63Ag8 with human myeloma cell line FU-266 (62). This fusion partner has been used very successfully to generate large panels of naturally occurring human anti-HIV mAbs (63–65). Another heterohybridoma fusion partner that has been very productive is HMMA 2.5 (66), which was generated using a multistep process. The parental line, HMMA2.11TG/O, was made by first fusing bone marrow mononuclear cells from a patient with IgA myeloma with the mouse myeloma cell line P3X63Ag8.653. HMMA 2.5 is a subclone that then was selected for optimal fusion efficiency after passaging in 6-thioguanosine. Cell line HMMA 2.5 was found to achieve the highest fusion efficiency when it was compared to six other myeloma cell lines using electrofusion (39). This heterohybridoma has been used to generate large panels of naturally occurring fully human mAbs to many viruses, including influenza and dengue viruses (29, 67–69).

Another heterohybridoma line used to successfully generate human hybridomas is K6H6/B5 (70–72). This line was developed by fusing malignant lymphoid cells isolated from a patient with nodular lymphoma with the mouse myeloma cell line NS-1-Ag4. K6H6/B5 was used to successfully create human hybridomas that secrete mAbs to hepatitis C virus (73). A very unique hetero-

hybridoma fusion partner denoted SPYMEG was developed by fusion of Sp2 murine myeloma cells and MEG-01 human megakaryoblastic leukemia cells (74). Recently, SPYMEG was employed for the production of anti-influenza mAbs, generated by fusing PBMCs from influenza-vaccinated and naturally infected volunteers (75, 76). It was also used successfully to make human hybridomas secreting anti-HIV neutralizing mAbs by fusion with PBMCs obtained from HIV-1-infected individuals (77). A more recently created line, MFP-2, is a trioma that was generated by fusing a murine myeloma cell line with a human myeloma cell line, yielding the intermediate heteromyeloma B6B11. This heterohybridoma was then fused with a human lymphocyte to generate the MFP-2 trioma line (78). The authors used this partner to develop mAbs with specificity to breast cancer tissue and cell lines (78, 79). The MFP-2 fusion partner was also used to produce several anti-West Nile virus mAbs (80).

Recently, a heterohybridoma fusion partner cell line was derived from the murine myeloma cell line Sp2 and modified to coexpress genes encoding murine interleukin-6 and human telomerase catalytic subunit (TERT) (81). The expression of murine IL-6 directly stimulates proliferation as well as immunoglobulin production from the resulting hybridoma. Human TERT can lengthen telomeres, thereby providing cells with unlimited replication capability and promoting karyotypic stability. The Sp2/mIL-6/hTERT heterohybridoma line then was demonstrated to produce stable hybridomas able to secrete fully human mAbs by fusing splenic B cells from a patient immunized with a *Streptococcus pneumoniae* vaccine. The authors succeeded in creating hybridomas that secrete human mAbs specific for *S. pneumoniae* antigens (81).

BIOLOGICAL CLONING METHODS

The final step in the generation of a human hybridoma is to isolate successful fusion products as clones derived from single cells, a process often referred to as biological cloning. There are several advantages to isolating individual hybridomas early and growing them in a clonal manner. Frequently, mixed populations of mAb-producing hybridomas are created following fusion. Depending on the experiment, there may be hundreds or even thousands of different clones produced. Cell cloning is an essential step in ensuring that a monoclonal antibody is ultimately generated. Also, hybridoma clones that produce the greatest quantity of mAbs are relatively rare following fusion and consume a greater amount of energy and nutrients. Because of this, high-producing clones often grow slower and can be overgrown easily by low- or nonproducing hybridoma clones (82). There are now several methods that can be used to perform biological cloning of human hybridomas. Traditionally, this was accomplished by limiting dilution plating. More recently, advances in flow cytometric automated single-cell sorting, with indexing capabilities, have allowed for fast, accurate, and versatile single-cell plating. Finally, semisolid medium preparations can be used to grow single hybridoma cells as isolated, suspended colonies. With special clone-picking devices, this process can be highly automated and can also be performed in an antigen-specific and semi-quantitative fashion for selection and biological cloning of high-producing human hybridomas (83) (Fig. 3).

The most common method to generate biological clones of hybridomas is limiting dilution cloning. This technique, and variations thereof, is based on the Poisson distribution (84). The Poisson distribution is a discrete frequency distribution that describes the probability of a number of independent events occurring in a fixed interval of time. If a known number of viable cells are added to a plate with a given number of wells, this model can be used to provide the probability that any given well would contain a given number of cells, for example, if one were to plate 0.8 cells/well

by counting the total number of cells to be added to a given number of wells, such as adding approximately 77 cells to a 96-well culture plate. By using the Poisson distribution, this dilution provides that approximately 36% of wells will contain 1 cell/well. By the same probability distribution, approximately 45% will contain 0 cells, 14% will contain 2 cells, 4% will contain 3 cells, and approximately 1% of wells will contain 4 cells. Thus, by using this method, one would expect that 19% of wells would contain >1 cell. Since hybridomas vary greatly in their ability to survive and make antibody, this calculation is often an overestimation of final growth and mAb expression. Limiting dilution plating is often performed using multiple plates and repeated for several rounds to improve the likelihood of isolating a true clone that is both stable and produces a high level of mAb. If greater cloning stringency is desired, hybridomas are plated at 0.3 cells/well, resulting in the percent of wells with >1 cell being only 3.3%, and this process can be repeated in a serial fashion two or three times. This method has the advantage of being simple and relatively inexpensive in terms of equipment. However, it is very time consuming and labor intensive, it has low throughput, and obtaining clonality is never guaranteed (85, 86). One cannot be certain that the starting population of hybridomas is in a homogenous single-cell suspension, as some clones may stick together. Additionally, since only a few hundred to a few thousand clones can be interrogated, the prospect of identifying a high-producing clone is low.

An alternative related approach used by many laboratories is to perform serial dilutions such that the cell concentration is diluted down and across the cell culture plate. By adding a known number of cells to the A1 position well, diluting down the A column, then diluting the A column across the plate with a multichannel pipette, one can achieve adequate separation of cells. This method has the advantage of near

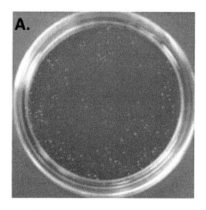 

FIGURE 3 **Cloning in (A) semi-solid medium and (B) final human hybridoma. doi:10.1128/microbiolspec. AID-0027-2014.f3**

infinite variability, which may be important in isolating poor-growing or low-viability clones. The clear disadvantage is that only a handful of wells that are likely to contain isolated clones can be assessed in each dilution plate. Multiple rounds of dilution plating are often used as an attempt to ensure clonality.

Increasingly, laboratories have turned to sterile single-cell sorting of hybridomas using a flow cytometer outfitted with an automated single-cell deposition unit to accomplish the task of biological cloning. Methods that use flow cytometry and cell sorting greatly increase the number of cells that can be screened and can almost ensure that clonality is achieved. This technique of biological cloning is in many ways superior to limiting dilution methods but requires access to an expensive instrument, which may not be available. For those with access to cell sorting, the added expense of using the instrument is often offset by saving time and resources needed to perform multiple rounds of limiting dilution cloning. By staining for viability and using forward and side scatter to eliminate doublets and clumps, a single cell can be accurately and consistently placed into culture medium, even within a 384-well plate platform. This approach results in a considerable increase in throughput, and thus the quantity of hybridomas that can

be effectively interrogated is dramatically amplified. Ideally, single-cell cloning could be coupled to selection of hybridomas based on antigen specificity and antibody quantity.

Methods for using flow cytometry to single-cell sort hybridomas on the basis of their antigen specificity have been developed and in some cases are commercially available. The use of flow cytometric sorting to select high-producing Chinese hamster ovary (CHO) cell clones was described initially (87) and then applied shortly thereafter to hybridomas (88). Cell sorting to identify and isolate clones also has been used for bispecific hybridomas and isotype-switch variants, and even for identifying variants with higher antibody avidity (89–91). One important limitation in the ability to use flow cytometric sorting for isolating antigen-specific hybridomas is the differential expression levels of native surface antibodies. The B cell receptor is not expressed at high levels on the surface of all hybridomas, making it difficult to selectively sort antigen-specific hybridomas after fusion. For this reason, several strategies have been developed to sort cells for antigen specificity or level of production by employing the secreted antibody.

One method uses an artificial affinity matrix to capture antibody, which has been secreted from the cell and is directly retained on the surface of the cell (92). The secreted molecules are bound to the secreting cell and can be subsequently labeled for flow cytometric analysis. This method is accomplished by first directly biotinylating the secreting cells, adding an avidin conjugated capture antibody, and then isolating cells within a protein-impermeable matrix to prevent cross-contamination of the secreted protein. The captured antibody then can be labeled fluorescently. This method has been used successfully in the isolation of hybridoma cells by flow cytometric sorting (93).

A related method, which is commercially available for use, is the gel microdroplet encapsulation technique. This strategy uses an agarose droplet to encapsulate the secreting cells. The agarose matrix itself is biotinylated so that an avidin bridge forms with biotinylated anti-immunoglobulin antibody, which can capture the antibody secreted from the cell (94, 95). This technique has been employed successfully to use flow cytometric sorting and sort hybridomas based on their secreted mAb (95–97). The agarose matrix is able to prevent secreted antibody from cross-contaminating neighboring encapsulated cells. Unlike the direct biotinylation method described previously, the droplet encapsulation method requires removal of the agarose matrix after the cell(s) is/are selected. Unfortunately, both methods are challenging and require considerable optimization.

Another method used for biological cloning and growth of hybridomas involves embedding in semisolid medium. When cells are plated, often following fusion, in semisolid medium containing methylcellulose and the HAT selection components, hybridomas grow in suspended isolated colonies (83, 98). Hybridoma colonies can be picked into growth medium with a high probability of being clonal. Building on this method, manufacturers have developed instruments (for example, ClonePix [Molecular Devices LLC]) that isolate, detect, and measure relative secretion of monoclonal antibody from hybridomas. With methylcellulose semisolid HAT medium and the ability to pick fluorescent colonies in a fully automated manner, high-producing clones can be obtained in many cases by means of a single culture step following fusion. A complete hybridoma generation procedure that incorporates methylcellulose embedding, fluorescent antigen labeling, and clone picking was described recently (99).

ACKNOWLEDGMENT

Conflicts of interest: We disclose no conflicts.

CITATION

Smith SA, Crowe JE, Jr. 2015. Use of human hybridoma technology to isolate human monoclonal antibodies. Microbiol Spectrum 3(1):AID-0027-2014.

REFERENCES

1. **Kohler G, Milstein C.** 1975. Continuous cultures of fused cells secreting antibody of predefined specificity. *Nature* **256:**495–497.
2. **Schwaber J, Cohen EP.** 1973. Human x mouse somatic cell hybrid clone secreting immunoglobulins of both parental types. *Nature* **244:**444–447.
3. **Bloom AD, Nakamura FT.** 1974. Establishment of a tetraploid, immunoglobulin producing cell line from the hybridization of two human lymphocyte lines. *Proc Natl Acad Sci USA* **71:**2689–2692.
4. **Olsson L, Kaplan HS.** 1980. Human–human hybridomas producing monoclonal antibodies of predefined antigenic specificity. *Proc Natl Acad Sci USA* **77:**5429–5431.
5. **Stevens RH, Macy E, Morrow C, Saxon A.** 1979. Characterization of a circulating subpopulation of spontaneous anti-tetanus toxoid antibody producing B cells following *in vivo* booster immunization. *J Immunol* **122:**2498–2504.
6. **Casali P, Inghirami G, Nakamura M, Davies TF, Notkins AL.** 1986. Human monoclonals from antigen-specific selection of B lymphocytes and transformation by EBV. *Science* **234:**476–479.
7. **Kozbor D, Roder JC.** 1981. Requirements for the establishment of high titered human monoclonal antibodies against tetanus toxoid using the Epstein-Barr virus technique. *J Immunol* **127:**1275–1280.

8. **Crawford DH, Ando I.** 1986. EB virus induction is associated with B-cell maturation. *Immunology* **59:**405–409.

9. **Roder JC, Cole SP, Kozbor D.** 1986. The EBV-hybridoma technique. *Methods Enzymol* **121:** 140–167.

10. **Steinitz M, Koskimies S, Klein G, Makela O.** 1978. Establishment of specific antibody producing human lines by antigen preselection and EBV transformation. *Curr Top Microbiol Immunol* **81:**156–163.

11. **Bernasconi NL, Traggiai E, Lanzavecchia A.** 2002. Maintenance of serological memory by polyclonal activation of human memory B cells. *Science* **298:**2199–2202.

12. **Hartmann G, Krieg AM.** 2000. Mechanism and function of a newly identified CpG DNA motif in human primary B cells. *J Immunol* **164:**944–953.

13. **Traggiai E, Becker S, Subbarao K, Kolesnikova L, Uematsu Y, Gismondo MR, Murphy BR, Rappuoli R, Lanzavecchia A.** 2004. An efficient method to make human monoclonal antibodies from memory B cells: potent neutralization of SARS coronavirus. *Nat Med* **10:**871–875.

14. **Kozbor D, Roder JC, Chang TH, Steplewski Z, Koprowski H.** 1982. Human anti-tetanus toxoid monoclonal antibody secreted by EBV-transformed human B cells fused with murine myeloma. *Hybridoma* **1:**323–328.

15. **Foung SK, Perkins S, Raubitschek A, Larrick J, Lizak G, Fishwild D, Engleman EG, Grumet FC.** 1984. Rescue of human monoclonal antibody production from an EBV-transformed B cell line by fusion to a human-mouse hybridoma. *J Immunol Methods* **70:**83–90.

16. **Chiorazzi N, Wasserman RL, Kunkel HG.** 1982. Use of Epstein-Barr virus-transformed B cell lines for the generation of immunoglobulin-producing human B cell hybridomas. *J Exp Med* **156:**930–935.

17. **Emanuel D, Gold J, Colacino J, Lopez C, Hammerling U.** 1984. A human monoclonal antibody to cytomegalovirus (CMV). *J Immunol* **133:**2202–2205.

18. **Lagerkvist AC, Furebring C, Borrebaeck CA.** 1995. Single, antigen-specific B cells used to generate Fab fragments using CD40-mediated amplification or direct PCR cloning. *Biotechniques* **18:**862–869.

19. **Ding BB, Bi E, Chen H, Yu JJ, Ye BH.** 2013. IL-21 and CD40L synergistically promote plasma cell differentiation through upregulation of Blimp-1 in human B cells. *J Immunol* **190:**1827–1836.

20. **Cocks BG, de Waal Malefyt R, Galizzi JP, de Vries JE, Aversa G.** 1993. IL-13 induces proliferation and differentiation of human B cells activated by the CD40 ligand. *Int Immunol* **5:**657–663.

21. **Orscheschek K, Merz H, Schlegelberger B, Feller AC.** 1994. An immortalized cell line with features of human follicular dendritic cells. Antigen and cytokine expression analysis. *Eur J Immunol* **24:**2682–2690.

22. **Nilsson K, Sundström C.** 1974. Establishment and characteristics of two unique cell lines from patients with lymphosarcoma. *Int J Cancer* **13:**808–823.

23. **Zubler RH, Erard F, Lees RK, Van Laer M, Mingari C, Moretta L, MacDonald HR.** 1985. Mutant EL-4 thymoma cells polyclonally activate murine and human B cells via direct cell interaction. *J Immunol* **134:**3662–3668.

24. **Moore PA, Belvedere O, Orr A, Pieri K, LaFleur DW, Feng P, Soppet D, Charters M, Gentz R, Parmelee D, Li Y, Galperina O, Giri J, Roschke V, Nardelli B, Carrell J, Sosnovtseva S, Greenfield W, Ruben SM, Olsen HS, Fikes J, Hilbert DM.** 1999. BLyS: member of the tumor necrosis factor family and B lymphocyte stimulator. *Science* **285:**260–263.

25. **Gorny MK.** 1994. Production of human monoclonal antibodies via fusion of Epstein-Barr virus-transformed lymphocytes with heteromyeloma, p 276–281. *In* Celis JE (ed), *Cell Biology: A Laboratory Handbook*, 2nd ed. Academic Press, San Diego, CA.

26. **Miller G, Lipman M.** 1973. Release of infectious Epstein-Barr virus by transformed marmoset leukocytes. *Proc Natl Acad Sci USA* **70:**190–194.

27. **Wallace LE, Young LS, Rowe M, Rowe D, Rickinson AB.** 1987. Epstein-Barr virus-specific T-cell recognition of B-cell transformants expressing different EBNA 2 antigens. *Int J Cancer* **39:**373–379.

28. **Nikitin PA, Yan CM, Forte E, Bocedi A, Tourigny JP, White RE, Allday MJ, Patel A, Dave SS, Kim W, Hu K, Guo J, Tainter D, Rusyn E, Luftig MA.** 2010. An ATM/Chk2-mediated DNA damage-responsive signaling pathway suppresses Epstein-Barr virus transformation of primary human B cells. *Cell Host Microbe* **8:**510–522.

29. **Smith SA, Zhou Y, Olivarez NP, Broadwater AH, de Silva AM, Crowe JE Jr.** 2012. Persistence of circulating memory B cell clones with potential for dengue virus disease enhancement for decades following infection. *J Virol* **86:**2665–2675.

30. **Okada Y.** 1962. Analysis of giant polynuclear cell formation caused by HVJ virus from Ehrlich's ascites tumor cells. I. Microscopic

observation of giant polynuclear cell formation. *Exp Cell Res* **26**:98–128.

31. **Morgan C, Howe C.** 1968. Structure and development of viruses as observed in the electron microscope. IX. Entry of parainfluenza I (Sendai) virus. *J Virol* **2**:1122–1132.

32. **Okada Y.** 1993. Sendai virus-induced cell fusion. *Methods Enzymol* **221**:18–41.

33. **Nagata S, Yamamoto K, Ueno Y, Kurata T, Chiba J.** 1991. Production of monoclonal antibodies by the use of pH-dependent vesicular stomatitis virus-mediated cell fusion. *Hybridoma* **10**:317–322.

34. **Nagata S, Yamamoto K, Ueno Y, Kurata T, Chiba J.** 1991. Preferential generation of monoclonal IgG-producing hybridomas by use of vesicular stomatitis virus-mediated cell fusion. *Hybridoma* **10**:369–378.

35. **Kao KN, Michayluk MR.** 1974. A method for high-frequency intergeneric fusion of plant protoplasts. *Planta* **115**:355–367.

36. **Lentz BR.** 2007. PEG as a tool to gain insight into membrane fusion. *Eur Biophys J* **36**:315–326.

37. **Kerkis AY, Zhdanova NS.** 1992. Formation and ultrastructure of somatic cell hybrids. *Electron Microsc Rev* **5**:1–24.

38. **Lane RD, Crissman RS, Lachman MF.** 1984. Comparison of polyethylene glycols as fusogens for producing lymphocyte-myeloma hybrids. *J Immunol Methods* **72**:71–76.

39. **Yu X, McGraw PA, House FS, Crowe JE Jr.** 2008. An optimized electrofusion-based protocol for generating virus-specific human monoclonal antibodies. *J Immunol Methods* **336**:142–151.

40. **Rols MP, Teissie J.** 1990. Electropermeabilization of mammalian cells. Quantitative analysis of the phenomenon. *Biophys J* **58**:1089–1098.

41. **Lo MM, Tsong TY, Conrad MK, Strittmatter SM, Hester LD, Snyder SH.** 1984. Monoclonal antibody production by receptor-mediated electrically induced cell fusion. *Nature* **310**:792–794.

42. **Wojchowski DM, Sytkowski AJ.** 1986. Hybridoma production by simplified avidin-mediated electrofusion. *J Immunol Methods* **90**:173–177.

43. **Hewish DR, Werkmeister JA.** 1989. The use of an electroporation apparatus for the production of murine hybridomas. *J Immunol Methods* **120**:285–289.

44. **Bakker Schut TC, Kraan YM, Barlag W, de Leij L, de Grooth BG, Greve J.** 1993. Selective electrofusion of conjugated cells in flow. *Biophys J* **65**:568–572.

45. **Teissie J, Rols MP.** 1986. Fusion of mammalian cells in culture is obtained by creating the contact between cells after their electropermeabilization. *Biochem Biophys Res Commun* **140**:258–266.

46. **Bardsley DW, Liddell JE, Coakley WT, Clarke DJ.** 1990. Electroacoustic production of murine hybridomas. *J Immunol Methods* **129**:41–47.

47. **Neil GA, Zimmermann U.** 1993. Electrofusion. *Methods Enzymol* **220**:174–196.

48. **Nilsson K, Bennich H, Johansson SG, Pontén J.** 1970. Established immunoglobulin producing myeloma (IgE) and lymphoblastoid (IgG) cell lines from an IgE myeloma patient. *Clin Exp Immunol* **7**:477–489.

49. **Olsson L, Kaplan HS.** 1983. Human–human monoclonal antibody-producing hybridomas: technical aspects. *Methods Enzymol* **92**:3–16.

50. **Brodin T, Olsson L, Sjögren HO.** 1983. Cloning of human hybridoma, myeloma and lymphoma cell lines using enriched human monocytes as feeder layer. *J Immunol Methods* **60**:1–7.

51. **Cote RJ, Morrissey DM, Houghton AN, Beattie EJ Jr, Oettgen HF, Old LJ.** 1983. Generation of human monoclonal antibodies reactive with cellular antigens. *Proc Natl Acad Sci USA* **80**:2026–2030.

52. **Olsson L.** 1983. Monoclonal antibodies in clinical immunobiology. Derivation, potential, and limitations. *Allergy* **38**:145–154.

53. **Sikora K, Alderson T, Ellis J, Phillips J, Watson J.** 1983. Human hybridomas from patients with malignant disease. *Br J Cancer* **47**:135–145.

54. **Hibi N, Arii S, Iizumi T, Nemoto T, Chu TM.** 1986. Human monoclonal antibody recognizing liver-type aldolase B. *Biochem J* **240**:847–856.

55. **Matsuoka Y, Moore GE, Yagi Y, Pressman D.** 1967. Production of free light chains of immunoglobulin by a hematopoietic cell line derived from a patient with multiple myeloma. *Proc Soc Exp Biol Med* **125**:1246–1250.

56. **Pickering JW, Gelder FB.** 1982. A human myeloma cell line that does not express immunoglobulin but yields a high frequency of antibody-secreting hybridomas. *J Immunol* **129**:406–412.

57. **Kozbor D, Tripputi P, Roder JC, Croce CM.** 1984. A human hybrid myeloma for production of human monoclonal antibodies. *J Immunol* **133**:3001–3005.

58. **Karpas A, Dremucheva A, Czepulkowski BH.** 2001. A human myeloma cell line suitable for the generation of human monoclonal antibodies. *Proc Natl Acad Sci USA* **98**:1799–1804.

59. **Ostberg L, Pursch E.** 1983. Human X (mouse X human) hybridomas stably producing human antibodies. *Hybridoma* **2**:361–367.

60. **Goldstein NI, Nagle R, Villar H, Hersh E, Fisher PB.** 1990. Isolation and characterization of a human monoclonal antibody which reacts with breast and colorectal carcinoma. *Anticancer Res* **10:**1491–1500.

61. **Freedman RS, Ioannides CG, Tomasovic B, Patenia R, Zhang HZ, Liang JC, Edwards CL.** 1991. Development of a cell surface reacting human monoclonal antibody recognizing ovarian and certain other malignancies. *Hybridoma* **10:**21–33.

62. **Teng NN, Lam KS, Calvo Riera F, Kaplan HS.** 1983. Construction and testing of mouse–human heteromyelomas for human monoclonal antibody production. *Proc Natl Acad Sci USA* **80:**7308–7312.

63. **Gorny MK, Xu JY, Karwowska S, Buchbinder A, Zolla-Pazner S.** 1993. Repertoire of neutralizing human monoclonal antibodies specific for the V3 domain of HIV-1 gp 120. *J Immunol* **150:**635–643.

64. **Gorny MK, Wang XH, Williams C, Volsky B, Revesz K, Witover B, Burda S, Urbanski M, Nyambi P, Krachmarov C, Pinter A, Zolla-Pazner S, Nadas A.** 2009. Preferential use of the VH5-51 gene segment by the human immune response to code for antibodies against the V3 domain of HIV-1. *Mol Immunol* **46:**917–926.

65. **Gorny MK.** 2012. Human hybridoma technology. *Antibody Technol J* **2:**1–5.

66. **Posner MR, Elboim H, Santos D.** 1987. The construction and use of a human–mouse myeloma analogue suitable for the routine production of hybridomas secreting human monoclonal antibodies. *Hybridoma* **6:**611–625.

67. **Yu X, Tsibane T, McGraw PA, House FS, Keefer CJ, Hicar MD, Tumpey TM, Pappas C, Perrone LA, Martinez O, Stevens J, Wilson IA, Aguilar PV, Altschuler EL, Basler CF, Crowe JE Jr.** 2008. Neutralizing antibodies derived from the B cells of 1918 influenza pandemic survivors. *Nature* **455:**532–536.

68. **Smith SA, de Alwis R, Kose N, Durbin AP, Whitehead SS, de Silva AM, Crowe JE Jr.** 2013. Human monoclonal antibodies derived from memory B cells following live attenuated dengue virus vaccination or natural infection exhibit similar characteristics. *J Infect Dis* **207:**1898–1908.

69. **Smith SA, de Alwis AR, Kose N, Harris E, Ibarra KD, Kahle KM, Pfaff JM, Xiang X, Doranz BJ, de Silva AM, Austin SK, Sukupolvi-Petty S, Diamond MS, Crowe JE Jr.** 2013. The potent and broadly neutralizing human dengue virus-specific monoclonal antibody 1C19 reveals a unique cross-reactive epitope on the bc loop of domain II of the envelope protein. *MBio* **4:**e00873–913. doi:10.1128/mBio.00873-13.

70. **Carroll WL, Thielemans K, Dilley J, Levy R.** 1986. Mouse x human heterohybridomas as fusion partners with human B cell tumors. *J Immunol Methods* **89:**61–72.

71. **Carroll WL, Lowder JN, Streifer R, Warnke R, Levy S, Levy R.** 1986. Idiotype variant cell populations in patients with B cell lymphoma. *J Exp Med* **164:**1566–1580.

72. **Brown S, Dilley J, Levy R.** 1980. Immunoglobulin secretion by mouse X human hybridomas: an approach for the production of anti-idiotype reagents useful in monitoring patients with B cell lymphoma. *J Immunol* **125:**1037–1043.

73. **da Silva Cardoso M, Siemoneit K, Sturm D, Krone C, Moradpour D, Kubanek B.** 1998. Isolation and characterization of human monoclonal antibodies against hepatitis C virus envelope glycoproteins. *J Med Virol* **55:**28–34.

74. **Ogura M, Morishima Y, Ohno R, Kato Y, Hirabayashi N, Nagura H, Saito H.** 1985. Establishment of a novel human megakaryoblastic leukemia cell line, MEG-01, with positive Philadelphia chromosome. *Blood* **66:**1384–1392.

75. **Kubota-Koketsu R, Mizuta H, Oshita M, Ideno S, Yunoki M, Kuhara M, Yamamoto N, Okuno Y, Ikuta K.** 2009. Broad neutralizing human monoclonal antibodies against influenza virus from vaccinated healthy donors. *Biochem Biophys Res Commun* **387:**180–185.

76. **Pan Y, Sasaki T, Kubota-Koketsu R, Inoue Y, Yasugi M, Yamashita A, Ramadhany R, Arai Y, Du A, Boonsathorn N, Ibrahim MS, Daidoji T, Nakaya T, Ono K, Okuno Y, Ikuta K, Watanabe Y.** 2014. Human monoclonal antibodies derived from a patient infected with 2009 pandemic influenza A virus broadly cross-neutralize group 1 influenza viruses. *Biochem Biophys Res Commun* **450:**42–48.

77. **Akapirat S, Avihingsanon A, Ananworanich J, Schuetz A, Ramasoota P, Luplertlop N, Ono K, Ikuta K, Utachee P, Kameoka M, Leaungwutiwong P.** 2013. Variables influencing anti-human immunodeficiency virus type 1 neutralizing human monoclonal antibody (NhMAb) production among infected Thais. *Southeast Asian J Trop Med Public Health* **44:**825–841.

78. **Kalantarov GF, Rudchenko SA, Lobel L, Trakht I.** 2002. Development of a fusion partner cell line for efficient production of human monoclonal antibodies from peripheral blood lymphocytes. *Hum Antibodies* **11:**85–96.

79. **Kirman I, Kalantarov GF, Lobel LI, Hibshoosh H, Estabrook A, Canfield R, Trakht I.** 2002. Isolation of native human

monoclonal autoantibodies to breast cancer. *Hybrid Hybridomics* 21:405–414.

80. **Calvert AE, Kalantarov GF, Chang GJ, Trakht I, Blair CD, Roehrig JT.** 2011. Human monoclonal antibodies to West Nile virus identify epitopes on the prM protein. *Virology* **410**:30–37.

81. **Dessain SK, Adekar SP, Stevens JB, Carpenter KA, Skorski ML, Barnoski BL, Goldsby RA, Weinberg RA.** 2004. High efficiency creation of human monoclonal antibody-producing hybridomas. *J Immunol Methods* **291**:109–122.

82. **Kromenaker SJ, Srienc F.** 1994. Stability of producer hybridoma cell lines after cell sorting: a case study. *Biotechnol Prog* 10:299–307.

83. **Mann CJ.** 2007. Rapid isolation of antigen-specific clones from hybridoma fusions. *Nat Methods* 4:1–2.

84. **Haight FA.** 1967. *Handbook of the Poisson Distribution.* John Wiley & Sons, New York, NY.

85. **Coller HA, Coller BS.** 1986. Poisson statistical analysis of repetitive sub-cloning by the limiting dilution technique as a way of assessing hybridoma monoclonality. *Methods Enzymol* **121**:412–417.

86. **Underwood PA, Bean PA.** 1987. Hazards of the limiting dilution methods of cloning hybridomas. *J Immunol Methods* **107**:119–128.

87. **Brezinsky SCG, Chiang GG, Szilvasi A, Mohan S, Shapiro RI, MacLean A, Sisk W, Thill G.** 2003. A simple method for enriching populations of transfected CHO cells for cells of higher specific productivity. *J Immunol Methods* 277:141–155.

88. **Parks DR, Bryan VM, Oi VT, Herzenberg LA.** 1979. Antigen-specific identification and cloning of hybridomas with a fluorescence-activated cell sorter. *Proc Natl Acad Sci USA* **76**:1962–1966.

89. **Jantscheff P, Winkler L, Karawajew L, Kaiser G, Böttger V, Micheel B.** 1993. Hybrid hybridomas producing bispecific antibodies to CEA and peroxidase isolated by a combination of HAT medium selection and fluorescence activated cell sorting. *J Immunol Methods* **163**:91–97.

90. **Dangl JL, Parks DR, Oi VT, Herzenberg LA.** 1982. Rapid isolation of cloned isotype switch variants using fluorescence activated cell sorting. *Cytometry* 2:395–401.

91. **Martel F, Bazin R, Verrette S, Lemieux R.** 1988. Characterization of higher avidity monoclonal antibodies produced by murine B-cell hybridoma variants selected for increased antigen binding of membrane Ig. *J Immunol* **141**:1624–1629.

92. **Manz R, Assenmacher M, Pflüger E, Miltenyi S, Radbruch A.** 1995. Analysis and sorting of live cells according to secreted molecules, relocated to a cell-surface affinity matrix. *Proc Natl Acad Sci USA* **92**:1921–1925.

93. **Holmes P, Al-Rubeai M.** 1999. Improved cell line development by a high throughput affinity capture surface display technique to select for high secretors. *J Immunol Methods* **230**:141–147.

94. **Weaver J, Williams G, Klibanov A, Demain A.** 1988. Gel microdroplets: rapid detection and enumeration of individual microorganisms by their metabolic activity. *Nat Biotechnol* **6**:1084–1089.

95. **Powell KT, Weaver JC.** 1990. Gel microdroplets and flow cytometry: rapid determination of antibody secretion by individual cells within a cell population. *Nat Biotechnol* 8:333–337.

96. **Kenney JS, Gray F, Ancel MH, Dunne JF.** 1995. Production of monoclonal antibodies using a secretion capture report web. *Nat Biotechnol* **13**:787–790.

97. **Gray F, Kenney JS, Dunne JF.** 1995. Secretion capture and report web: use of affinity derivatised agarose microdroplets for the selection of hybridoma cells. *J Immunol Methods* **182**:155–163.

98. **Davis JM, Pennington JE, Kubler AM, Conscience JF.** 1982. A simple, single-step technique for selecting and cloning hybridomas for the production of monoclonal antibodies. *Immunol Methods* **50**:161–171.

99. **Yokoyama WM, Christensen M, Dos Santos G, Miller D, Ho J, Wu T, Dziegelewski M, Neethling FA.** 2013. Production of monoclonal antibodies. *Curr Protoc Immunol* **102**:1–29.

Humanized Mice for Studying Human Immune Responses and Generating Human Monoclonal Antibodies

9

RAMESH AKKINA[1]

INTRODUCTION

The potential uses of human pathogen-specific antibodies are enormous in terms of both diagnostics and therapeutics. Early applications used polyclonal sera for prophylaxis and therapies, but problems such as allergic reactions, cost, and difficulty in their generation have led to the use of mouse-derived monoclonal antibodies that were humanized by various methods (1). These methods involved substituting part or all of the murine antibody backbone with its human equivalent to derive chimeric or fully humanized antibodies. Less labor-intensive methods used transgenic mice harboring human immunoglobulin genes for immunization to derive human antibodies (2). While this has hastened human antibody generation, some limitations exist, such as differences in the maturation processes between the mouse B cells expressing human antibodies and human B cells secreting human antibodies. Therefore, an ideal way to produce authentic affinity-matured human antibodies is to identify and harness the specific antibody-producing human B-cell clones themselves. Conventional methods involved immortalizing antigen-specific B cells from individuals who either recovered from a disease or were vaccinated with a desired antigen to derive stable antibody-producing cells. Alternatively, more recent high-throughput

[1]Department of Microbiology, Immunology and Pathology, Colorado State University, Fort Collins, CO 80523.
Antibodies for Infectious Diseases
Edited by James E. Crowe, Jr., Diana Boraschi, and Rino Rappuoli
© 2015 American Society for Microbiology, Washington, DC
doi:10.1128/microbiolspec.AID-0003-2012

methods involved rescuing the specific antibody genes from either specific plasma cells or memory B cells (3). While these methods have now become routine, they both require collecting B cells from suitable human subjects. In addition to the paucity of specific pathogen-exposed human subjects when needed and the existence of low numbers of antigen-specific cells, there are other practical and ethical considerations. One such consideration is the derivation of antibodies against dangerous pathogens such as Ebola virus. These limitations pointed out the need for a more practical experimental system that permits isolation of large quantities of antigen-specific B cells against any pathogen or antigen of interest. In this regard, newer-generation humanized mice harboring a transplanted human immune system with a capacity to yield antigen-specific B and plasma cells are expected to fill this need (4, 5, 6) and are discussed here.

IMMUNODEFICIENT MOUSE STRAINS FOR HUMAN CELL RECONSTITUTION

A common denominator for all humanized immune system mouse models is the transplantation of mature or progenitor human hematopoietic cells by various routes into immunodeficient mice receptive to xenografts without graft rejection. In this regard, there has been a gradual evolution and improvements in the generation of immunodeficient mouse strains (7). Early strains such as nude mice, while lacking T cells and thus having defects in T-cell responses, still harbored mouse B cells and NK cells and therefore were not permissive for human cell reconstitution. The availability of severe combined immunodeficiency (SCID) mice that lacked both T and B cells allowed human cell reconstitution and led to the creation of hu-peripheral blood lymphocyte (PBL)-SCID and SCID-hu mouse models (see below). Later improvements gave rise to nonobese diabetic (NOD)-SCID mice that have a lower level of

NK cells and other innate immune defects that permit higher levels of human cell and tissue engraftments but were still less than ideal. A major advancement was the targeted disruption of the interleukin-2 (IL-2) receptor common gamma chain (IL2-Rcγ) coding for the common and essential signaling component for the action of cytokines IL-2, IL-4, IL-7, IL-9, IL-15, and IL-21 (7, 8). Impairment of IL-7 and IL-15 signaling blocks native mouse NK-cell development, thus permitting enhanced human cell engraftment. This mutation, when introduced together with the SCID, NOD, RAG1, or RAG2 gene mutations in different combinations by selective breeding, yielded a number of new-generation severely immunocompromised recipient mice for far superior human cell engraftment (6). These include Rag2$^{-/-}$ c$\gamma^{-/-}$, Rag1$^{-/-}$ c$\gamma^{-/-}$ (RG), NOD/shi-scid/c$\gamma^{-/-}$ null (NOG), and NOD/SCID/c$\gamma^{-/-}$ (NSG) mice. Ongoing efforts are being directed toward introducing HLA class I and II human immune system and cytokine genes to generate new transgenic mice to permit more robust human antibody and cellular immune responses (see below).

HUMANIZED MOUSE MODELS WITH HUMAN IMMUNE SYSTEM

A variety of Hu mice are made by using different strains of immunodeficient mice as well as by using different human cells and tissues. These are summarized in Table 1 and a broad description is provided below.

Hu-PBL Mice

Hu-PBL mice are generated by the transplantation of human mature peripheral blood mononuclear cells (PBMCs) via the intraperitoneal (i.p.) route into SCID mice (9). More recent versions use either NSG or RG mice. The transplanted human immune cells persist for several weeks and show effector functions. These mice can be productively infected by viruses such as HIV-1 that target

TABLE 1 **Summary of current Hu mouse models**

Model	Generation/mice used	Advantages	Disadvantages
Hu-PBL	i.p. injection of human PBMC. SCID, NOD-SCID, NSG, NOG.	Easy to prepare. Immediate use. Good T-cell engraftment.	No multilineage hematopoiesis. No primary immune response. Graft versus host disease.
Hu-HSC	Intrahepatic injection of CD34+ HSC into neonates. Intravenous injection of CD34$^+$ HSC into adults. Rag2$^{-/-}$ c$\gamma^{-/-}$, NSG, NOG.	Easy to prepare. Multilineage hematopoiesis. Primary immune response.	No human HLA restriction.
SCID-hu	Coimplantation of human fetal liver and thymic fragments under kidney capsule. SCID or NOD-SCID.	Abundant T-cell lymphopoiesis.	Surgery needed. Requires human fetal tissue. No multilineage hematopoiesis. No primary immune response. Poor peripheral T-cell engraftment.
BLT	Coimplantation of human fetal liver and thymic fragments under kidney capsule with additional injection of autologous CD34$^+$ HSC. Rag2$^{-/-}$ c$\gamma^{-/-}$, NOD-SCID, NSG.	Multilineage hematopoiesis. T-cell education in autologous thymus. HLA restriction.	Surgery needed. Requires human fetal tissue.

cells of the human hematopoietic system. Human memory B cells continue to produce antibodies from previous antigen exposure; however, there is no multilineage human hematopoietic cell generation and consequently no primary immune response. While graft versus host disease (GVHD) by the injected T cells is a drawback, this model is ideal for studying xeno-GVHD.

SCID-Hu MICE

Coimplantation of human fetal thymus and liver (containing hematopoietic stem cells) fragments under the SCID mouse renal capsule generate mice that harbor a functional human thymus (called the thy/liv organoid) (10). These mice primarily produce human thymocytes and naive T cells. These T cells predominantly reside in the thy/liv organoid, and there is poor peripheral T-cell circulation. Because of the insufficient generation of a full spectrum of immune cells, they lack the capacity to generate a human immune response. Nevertheless, these models have been instrumental in the study of some key aspects of viral pathogenesis with viruses such as HIV and HTLV and laid the foundation for the generation of new humanized mouse models (11).

Hu-HSC Mice

This model involves transplantation of hematopoietic stem cells (HSCs) into a variety of immunodeficient mice and has evolved substantially over the years (7, 12, 13). Early versions involved the injection of hematopoietic progenitor cells (CD34$^+$ cells) (also termed SCID repopulating cells) into conditioned adult SCID mice by intravenous (i.v.) or intrafemoral routes. While there was de novo lymphopoiesis, T-cell development was poor. Use of new-generation IL-2 c$\gamma^{-/-}$ that encompasses RG, NOG, or NSG mice led to better engraftment. There are two versions of these with important differences. One is the injection of HSCs into adult irradiated NSG/NOG mice. While multiple hematopoietic lineages are generated, there is a poor yield of T cells. The second is intrahepatic injection of HSC into conditioned newborn RG, NSG, or NOG mice that results in superior human cell engraftment and the generation of T cells, B cells, macrophages, NK cells, and dendritic cells (6, 13). Infection of both versions of these mice with different pathogens or immunization with different antigens gives rise to human immune responses (see below). There is also mucosal human cell engraftment permitting HIV-1 infection by mucosal routes (14).

BLT Mice

This model is a slight modification and consequent improvement of the earlier SCID-hu mouse model. The name derives from transplantation of bone marrow, liver, and thymus (BLT); the main difference from SCID-hu mouse model is the additional transplantation of autologous HSCs purified from fetal liver (13, 15, 16). The original BLT version used NOD-SCID mice, whereas the new improved versions use NSG, NOG, or RG mice (17, 18). Superior human cell engraftment with the generation of T cells, B cells, macrophages, NK cells, and dendritic cells is seen. The presence of autologous human thymus permits appropriate T-cell education and human T-cell restriction.

Hu-Liver-HSC Mice

The models described above are restricted to human immune system transplantation with the generation of human immune cell subsets. As noted, human pathogens that infect the human hematopoietic system can be studied in addition to generating human immune responses against a variety of antigens. To further broaden their application in infectious disease research, a recent development is the derivation of Hu-HSC mice that permits infection with other human-specific pathogens with a predilection to infect other human organ systems such as the liver. Transgenic mice that simultaneously permit human hepatocyte and HSC engraftment were recently developed (19). This permitted creation of Hu-liver-HSC mice susceptible to the hepatitis C virus and with a capacity for human immune response.

OVERVIEW OF Hu MOUSE PREPARATION, INFECTION, AND IMMUNIZATION

A general outline of Hu mouse preparations is depicted in Fig. 1. Preparation of Hu-HSC mice is not technically intensive since no surgery is involved (13). Immunodeficient mouse strains, namely RG, NOG, and NSG, are commonly used (6, 20, 21, 22, 23). Injection of HSC into neonatal mice versus adult mice gives far superior engraftment with the generation of human immune-competent mice that harbor all four needed immune cell subsets, namely T cells, B cells, macrophages, and dendritic cells. Newborn mice, preferably within 3 days of birth, are injected with $CD34^+$ HSCs from different sources that include cord blood, fetal liver, or human bone marrow. Of these, the efficiency and duration of engraftment appear to be better with the fetal liver-derived $CD34^+$ cells because of their more primitive lineage status in development. The following protocol is routinely used in our laboratory and yields well-engrafted mice. Single-cell suspension is prepared from fragments of human fetal liver (16 to 20 weeks gestation) by enzymatic digestion with collagenase, DNase, and hyaluronidase. The cells are incubated with CD34 antibody and later subjected to immunomagnetic bead-based positive section. The purity of $CD34^+$ cells generally ranges between 90% and 99% after two successive cycles of selection. The purified cells are cultured overnight in a human cytokine media mix containing IL-3, IL-6, and stem cell factor (25 ng of each per ml). Preferably, fresh cells are injected into neonates, although previously frozen cells can also be used. The neonatal mice are irradiated at 350 rads 2 to 4 hours before cell injections. We routinely use 5×10^5 human fetal liver-derived $CD34^+$ cells per mouse pup to ensure consistent engraftment, although lower numbers of cells can be used. Cells are injected via insulin syringe in a 25-μl volume intrahepatically by visualizing the dark area occupied by the liver under the relatively transparent skin (Fig. 2). Postinjection, pups are returned to their mothers and weaned 3 weeks later. Mice are housed in BSL-2 conditions. The engrafted mice are screened to determine the levels of human $CD45^+$ cells in peripheral blood at approximately 12 weeks of age. In general, we obtain mice with 40%

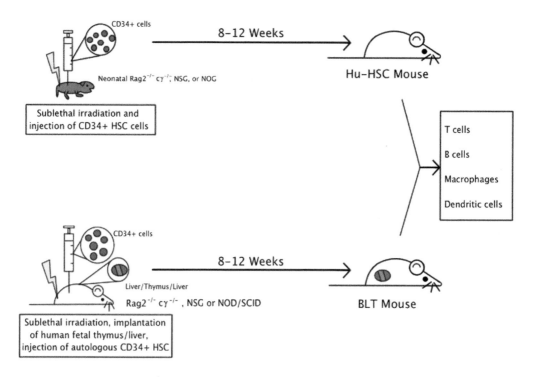

FIGURE 1 Schematic for generation of Hu-HSC RG (Rag-hu) and BLT mice. doi:10.1128/microbiolspec.AID-0003-2012.f1.

to 90% human cell engraftment. Human cell engraftment is seen in primary and secondary lymphoid organs. In addition, mucosal engraftment with human cells is also seen in the female reproductive tract as well as in the gut, permitting HIV-1 mucosal transmission. In general, 20 to 30 Hu-HSC mice can be made with a typical batch of fetal liver derived CD34+ cells.

Original preparations of BLT mice used NOD-SCID mice, and these have been effectively used in many experimental settings including HIV-1 mucosal viral transmission (15, 16, 24). Owing to far superior engraftment, more recent protocols use NSG mice (17, 25, 26). Male mice are preferred for surgical tissue implantation because of their larger kidney size. Adult mice are conditioned by sublethal whole body irradiation at 325 rads before transplantation. Human fetal thymic and liver tissues are dissected into 1-mm fragments and introduced together under the left kidney capsule of anesthetized mice by the

use of a trocar. Later, each of the mice is injected (i.v., tail route) with autologous 2.5×10^5 CD34+ HSC purified from the remaining fetal liver. The reconstituted mice are evaluated for human cell engraftment at 12 to16 weeks posttransplantation before the use for various experiments. In general, 15 to 20 mice can be made with a typical set of fetal tissues.

While different human pathogens and different immunogens are studied in Hu mice based on the need of the investigator and the types of human tissues transplanted, the following general scheme provides a broad overview of these protocols. Viral pathogens such as HIV-1, dengue, and Epstein-Barr virus (EBV) have been studied more frequently to date in these new models. With HIV-1, the most common route of experimental infection is via the i.p. route for pathogenesis and therapeutic studies. A typical infection involves either the CCR5-tropic viral strain BaL or the CXCR4-tropic strain NL4-3. Injection with 1×10^5 IU gives rise to viremia within a week

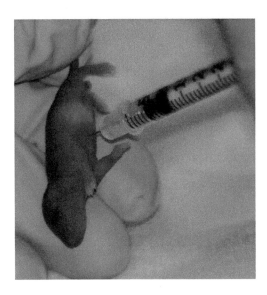

FIGURE 2 **Intrahepatic injection of CD34⁺ hematopoietic stem cells (HSCs) into newborn immunodeficient RG mouse. doi:10.1128/microbiolspec. AID-0003-2012.f2.**

and persistent life-long infection, based on the maintenance of human cell engraftment that in turn depends on the quality of the HSC injected (22, 27). For dengue viral infection, the viral inoculum is delivered by i.p., subcutaneous, or intradermal routes (28, 29). Infected mice develop acute viremia generally lasting for 3 weeks. With EBV 1×10^5 to 1×10^6 RIU are injected i.p., and immune responses are assayed at 4 to 10 weeks. With HIV-1, antibody responses are monitored at approximately 4 to 6 weeks. IgM responses can be seen with dengue viral infection within 2 weeks at the earliest, whereas IgG responses take much longer, usually about 8 weeks. For experimental immunizations, a variety of antigens have been used. These include tetanus toxoid (TT), hepatitis B virus (HBV), HIV-1, and West Nile virus envelope (WNV-E) antigens among others (7, 17, 21). With regard to human vaccine preparations, three doses each of HBV or TT vaccine (each corresponding to 1/10 the human dose) are given intramuscularly (i.m.) 2 weeks apart to Hu-HSC RG mice (21), and antibody responses are evaluated starting 2 weeks later. In a recent

protocol using BLT mice, recombinant HIV-1 envelope or WNV-E protein were mixed with a synthetic adjuvant IC31 and injected i.m. in both quadriceps muscles (17). Three doses were given on days 0, 21, and 45, and mice were monitored for immune responses for 90 days.

HUMAN CELL RECONSTITUTION AND ANTIBODY RESPONSES IN Hu MICE

A number of reports documented the generation of antigen-specific human antibody responses in Hu-HSC mice (29, 30, 31, 32, 33, 34, 35, 36). Both IgM and IgG responses were reported by different investigators, although, in general, IgG responses were found to be weak. Human antibody repertoire in Hu-HSC RG mice by analysis of the length of the CDR3 hypervariable regions revealed that the IgM B-cell repertoire was similar to that seen in normal healthy individuals, thus indicating no obvious limitations to generate a wide spectrum of human antibodies of various specificities (21). However, immunizations of Hu-HSC RG mice with TT and HBV vaccines gave a predominantly IgM response with limited antigen-specific IgG production, indicating a general failure to class switch. The paucity of antigen-specific IgG is puzzling given that these mice do accumulate total serum IgG efficiently. One study used PBMC transfected with a human T-cell receptor specific for influenza *hemagglutinin* (HA) peptide and bearing an HLA matched with that of the transplanted HSC used to prepare the Hu mice. When these T cells were transferred into the respective mice, anti-HA human IgG response was observed, suggesting that isotype switch deficiency is not due to an intrinsic defect in the B cells but rather to impairment in T-cell cooperation (37). This impairment may be due to human T-cell restriction by murine major histocompatibility complex (MHC) in addition to a potential T-cell dysfunction. When IgD⁺CD19⁺ naive B cells from Hu-HSC mice were treated in vitro with anti-CD40 antibodies, IL-2, and IL-21 in the presence of antigen, they became activated and secreted IgG, again confirming the functionality of the B cells in these mice. In evaluating T-cell help, another study using HLA-DR4 (MHC class II) transgenic mice and reconstitution with matching HSC reported improved immune responses that included IgG class switching and higher levels of IgG production (38). A more recent phenotypic analysis of B cells from Hu-HSC mice prepared by using adult NSG mice indicated a normal B-cell developmental pathway (39). However, molecular analysis of single B cells indicated that, while the overall distribution of Vh genes reflected a normal human antibody repertoire, mature B-cell subsets showed autoimmune characteristics (39). Overall, the wide variations seen in Hu-HSC mice with regard to antibody production and class switch could be attributed to a number of factors. These include lack of proper human T-cell restriction and help as well as differences in protocols, including utilizing neonatal mice versus adult mice for HSC transplantation and HSC sources, namely cord blood and fetal liver. In any case, additional improvements are necessary as discussed below. SCID-hu mice have been further improved to generate BLT mice that provide a more appropriate thymic microenvironment for human T-cell development and improved T-B cell cooperation (15, 16). This resulted in a more robust T-cell development and multilineage hematopoiesis including the generation of B cells, macrophages, and dendritic cells. The lineage-specific differentiation, positive and negative selection of T cells is expected to occur in the autologous human thymus. T cells in these mice were shown to generate MHC class I and II restricted human immune responses and offer T-cell help to the antigen-stimulated B cells (16, 40). A number of early studies have shown both IgM and IgG antigen-specific responses, albeit with varied robustness. However, later studies failed to show antibody class switching despite repeated booster immunizations (41).

A recent study evaluated BLT mice more thoroughly to determine the antigen-specific antibody responses by immunization with adjuvanted HIV-1 and WNV envelope antigens (17). Profound differences were noted both in terms of B-cell composition and antibody responses in comparison with healthy human immune responses. Even repeated booster immunizations did not result in secondary responses characterized by generation of IgG. Unlike in the human, there was an abundance of a "B-1 like" B-cell population (CD19$^+$ CD5$^+$). The predominant antibody response characterized by the IgM phenotype and lack of IgG is attributed to the CD5$^+$ B-cell subset that is believed to produce "natural antibody" by using a T-cell-independent pathway.

T-CELL RESPONSES AND HLA RESTRICTION IN HU MICE

Initial reports showed induction of antigen-specific T-cell responses in Hu-HSC mice against various human pathogens (14, 42, 43). Immune control of HIV-1 and EBV infection was abolished by the depletion of CD8 T cells in Hu-HSC mice, thus providing additional indirect evidence for their role in protection (44, 45). However, other studies reported deficiencies in T-cell responses (37, 46, 47). While polyclonal stimulation of Hu-HSC mouse splenocytes by phytohemagglutinin, anti-CD3/anti-CD28 antibodies, and phorbol myristate acetate/ionomycin lead to cell proliferation and cytokine secretion, they were 10-fold less than what is seen with human PBMC, suggesting a functional defect. Moreover, human T cells responded poorly to *in vivo* immunizations as shown by the lack of interferon-γ or IL-4 secretion after specific antigen restimulation *ex vivo*. Specific CD4 and CD8 responses were measured by cytokine secretion assays, cell proliferation assays, or cytotoxic assays *in vitro* by restimulation of cells from mice infected with either HIV-1 or EBV. Even in reports showing immune activity, the responses are low and are attributed to several factors. The overall low level of T cells is believed to result from a potential lymphopenia-induced T-cell activation among other causes. Another reason for low levels of T cells in Hu-HSC mice is thought to be a lack of HLA restriction, since T-cell selection is happening in xenogenic mouse thymus in a H-2-restricted fashion, which might not be efficient for human cells. Furthermore, the low numbers of T cells generated also display poor survival in the periphery owing to their suboptimal interactions with mouse APCs and weak signaling (30). Supporting these possibilities, it was recently reported that when RG mice transgenic for HLA-DR4 were reconstituted with matching HLA DR4 CD34 cord blood cells, the number of thymic and peripheral T cells was drastically increased. Shultz et al generated class I HLA-A2 transgenic mice and reconstituted them with matched HSC (6). These mice showed HLA restricted cellular immune responses to EBV. Based on these data, it has now become evident that enforced expression of HLA-A2 and HLA-DR4 enables HLA-restricted T-cell functions which also correlate with improved cytokine secretion and IgG production. Another desirable alteration in these mouse models is to knock out the murine MHC expression such that unwanted H-2-restricted responses can be avoided by the transplanted human immune cells. T-cell responses in BLT mice appear to be more normal because of reconstitution with autologous human thymus and HSC, thus permitting HLA restriction of T-cell responses and more efficient T- and B-cell interactions and cooperation. HIV-1 infection in BLT mice demonstrated epitope-specific T-cell responses to HIV antigens in a class I restricted manner in a recent study (48). Anti-HIV-1 CD8 responses were found to mimic those in humans in terms of their specificity, kinetics, and immunodominance. Furthermore, it was found that mice expressing the particular HLA class allele HLA-B 57 showed enhanced control of HIV infection as seen in humans that bear the same allele.

GENERATION OF HUMAN MONOCLONAL ANTIBODIES IN Hu MICE

Since humanized mice are shown to harbor a normal human antibody repertoire, they can be exploited to generate a broad spectrum of antibodies, both neutralizing and nonneutralizing. The scope of their use is further broadened by the creation of new models, such as those harboring human liver, so that agents like hepatitis viruses can also be used to generate specific antibodies. A general schematic summarizing different methods of deriving human monoclonal antibodies in Hu mice is presented in Fig. 3. The broad scheme would involve either infection or vaccination with a desired antigen with or without an adjuvant. At the peak time of immune response, the splenocytes containing the B cells are harvested for later selection, expansion, and immortalization. Alternatively, antigen-specific individual B cells can be sorted postimmunization, and their antibody genes can be cloned and later incorporated into an expression system to yield large quantities of antibodies. Furthermore, the specific antibody gene sequences can also be class switched based on what type of antibody is desired for therapeutic purposes by the use of molecular techniques. Following some of these lines, one recent report described the entire process of generating human monoclonal antibodies by using Hu-HSC RG mice (21). This is summarized in brief here as a basis for broader applications. Mice were immunized with commercially available TT and HBc vaccines as described above. Postvaccination, memory B cells expressing surface immunoglobulins were fluorescence-activated cell sorter sorted from splenic and mesenteric lymph node single-cell suspensions. The sorted B cells were immortalized by transduction with a retroviral vector encoding BCL6 and BCL-XL genes and cultured in the presence of CD40L and IL-2. Another novel method that can be used is STAT5 overexpression to immortalize B cells (49). Supernatants from the immortalized B-cell pools cultured in microtiter

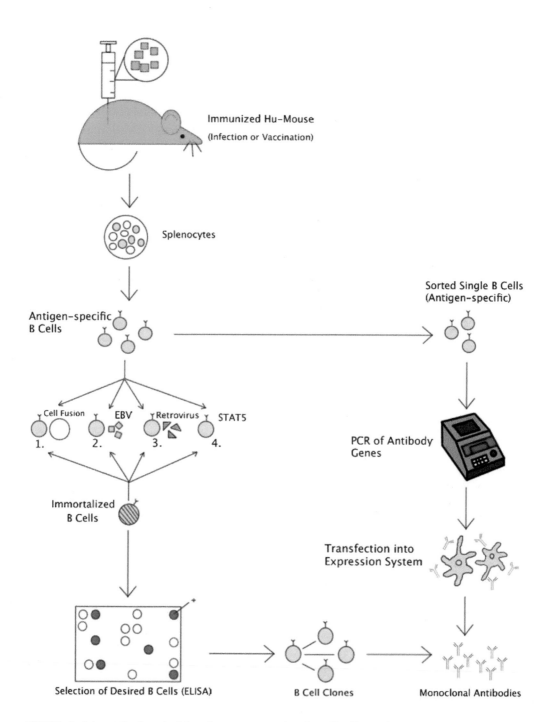

FIGURE 3 Schematic for deriving human monoclonal antibodies using Hu mice. doi:10.1128/microbiolspec.AID-0003-2012.f3.

plates were tested by enzyme-linked immuno-sorbent assay to identify specific antibody-producing wells. Cells from the desired anti-body-positive wells were subjected to limiting dilution culturing to obtain monoclonal B-cell lines. In this study, only IgM antibody-secreting B-cell clones could be obtained, although IgG responses were seen in the immunized mice, albeit at lower levels. Thus, further improvements in the protocol are necessary to capture and immortalize these rare IgG-producing B cells. Other options available for efficient B-cell immortalization involve transformation of antibody-producing B cells activated by TLR9 agonists like CpG followed by high-efficiency electrofusion with myeloma cells (50). Alternatively, using a molecular cloning approach, antigen-specific antibody genes can be rescued from the respective B cells for high-efficiency expression in a surrogate system, as has been accomplished with a number of antigens (51).

HUMAN PATHOGENS AND OTHER ANTIGENS STUDIED IN Hu MICE

A variety of human pathogens, particularly viruses, have been studied in new-generation Hu mice. HIV-1 is by far the most widely studied pathogen (22, 36, 47). Hu mice have also been used to study HTLV-1 proviral integration and the induction of T-cell lymphomas (52, 53). Studies of other virus families have also been gaining momentum. A number of studies focusing on dengue viral infection showed viremia with concomitant humoral and cellular responses (28, 29). Hu mice with human hepatocyte reconstitution allowed infection with hepatotropic viruses such as hepatitis C virus and HBV inducing pathologies and immune responses (19, 54). A variety of human herpes viruses have also been studied. These reports documented HLA-restricted adaptive T-cell immune responses to EBV, cytomegalovirus reactivation from latency, protective innate and adaptive immune responses against intravaginal HSV-2, and gen-eration of an anti-Kaposi's sarcoma-associated herpesvirus-antibody immune response (16, 43, 55, 56, 57). More recent studies have expanded the use of Hu mice to other nonviral pathogens. These encompass work with drug-resistant *Salmonella enterica* serovar Typhimurium (58, 59), persistent infection with the malaria parasite *Plasmodium falciparum* (60), and detection of Hu mouse adaptive and innate immune responses against *Leishmania* (61). In addition to live pathogens, a number of antigens and human vaccine preparations have also been tested to evaluate Hu mouse human immune responses. Immunization with DNP (23)-KLH antigen generated human T-cell proliferation and human IgG responses (40). Toxic shock syndrome toxin 1 caused an expansion of human T cells and activation of human dendritic cells (16). Administration of a variety of vaccines demonstrated adaptive immune responses including influenza-specific human CD8$^+$ T cells, human IgM antibody responses to tetanus toxoid and HBV (21, 62). This list is only a partial representation of that reported in the current literature which is expected to grow because the use of these mouse models is expected to become more widespread.

ADVANTAGES AND DISADVANTAGES OF DIFFERENT Hu MOUSE MODELS

From the standpoint of generating human monoclonal antibodies, there are advantages and disadvantages with each of the two new Hu-HSC and BLT mouse models. With regard to the ease of preparation, the Hu-HSC model is relatively easy to create since only a quick intrahepatic injection of HSC is needed and does not involve surgery. Additionally, human HSC from easily procurable sources such as cord blood can be used, and larger cohorts of mice from a single donor can be made. However, a disadvantage with this model is the lack of proper human T-cell restriction and ideal T- and B-cell cooperation because of the absence of an autologous human thymus.

Coexpression of HLA class I and II genes by transgenesis will overcome this deficiency. A particular advantage with the BLT mouse model is the presence of transplanted human thymus, thus permitting proper T-cell education and T-cell restriction thus offering a better T- and B-cell cooperation. Both IgM and IgG responses are seen, although the IgG responses are found to be weaker, akin to that seen with the hu-HSC model. Major disadvantages are the complicated surgery required to implant human fetal tissues under the kidney capsule, and the number of mice that can be generated from a single fetal donor tissue is limited. Large-scale exploitation of this model also poses challenges owing to the requirement for fetal tissues that are limited in supply and often difficult to procure.

LIMITATIONS TO BE OVERCOME, CURRENT ADVANCES, AND FUTURE PROSPECTS

While the current human immunocompetent mouse models have come a long way since the description of the original human-mouse chimeras, there are several limitations that need to be overcome (9). These encompass (i) residual innate immunity in the immunodeficient mouse strains, thus requiring irradiation and prior conditioning; (ii) less than ideal T-cell numbers and lack of full maturation of B cells; (iii) lack of human HLA class I and class II restriction in hu-HSC mouse models and lack of appropriate levels of HLA APCs in the BLT mouse model; (iv) deficiencies in T- and B-cell cooperation resulting in low levels of antibody responses and inefficient immunoglobulin class switch; and, finally, (v) poorly cross-reactive native murine cytokines and required growth factors.

Some of these deficiencies are currently being tackled and rectified as detailed below. In addition to T cells, B cells, and NK cells, macrophages are also found to contribute to xenograft rejection in Hu mice. Mouse macrophages expressing native SIRPα recep-

tor remove xenografted human cells that do not express the cognate ligand CD47 ("don't eat me" marker of self) (63, 64). In this context, it has been recently shown that human SIRPα transgenic mice exhibit improved human cell reconstitution (65). Conversely, human HSC stably transduced with murine CD47 ligand encoding lentiviral vectors also showed increased engraftment (66). Thus, improvement of constitutive CD47-SIRPα interactions in Hu mice will enhance the survival of human cells in the mouse environment and will provide more robust and lasting human cell engraftment. As mentioned above, the expression of human HLA-DR4 in transgenic mice also leads to increased T-cell numbers in reconstituted mice. Coexpression of HLA class I and class II in doubly transgenic mice is likely to further improve human T-cell reconstitution and T-B cell cooperation, as well as help and mediate HLA-restricted immune responses (30). The knock-in of the human HLA class I and class II genes in mouse MHC loci will preclude the unwanted mouse H-2-restricted human cell immune responses. Since many murine cytokines and growth factors are poorly cross-reactive with their corresponding human cell receptors, thus contributing to suboptimal human cell development and maintenance, supplying these *in trans* either by injection or by transgenesis overcomes these deficiencies. These cytokines include granulocyte-macrophage colony-stimulating factor (GM-CSF), IL-4, macrophage colony-stimulating factor (M-CSF) for monocyte/macrophage, IL-7 for T cells, IL-15 for NK cells, and erythropoietin for erythrocytes (67). Knock-in replacement of mouse cytokine genes with their human equivalents in respective loci has an additional advantage of their constitutive expression governed by the mouse regulatory elements. Indeed, with the use of this approach, respective transgenic mouse strains have been developed. Expression of human thrombopoietin resulted in higher human cell engraftment and better HSC maintenance (68). Transgenic mice with human IL-3, GM-CSF (67), and M-CSF

(69) knock-in genes exhibited improved mycloid differentiation and function, thus demonstrating the benefits of these enabling strategies. Thus, as can be seen from above, the current ongoing intensive work in different areas of generating Hu mice has identified several areas for improving the existing human immunocompetent models. However, these different strategies need to converge to yield a better mouse model. This will involve breeding a composite recipient mouse strain incorporating all desirable attributes. Such a mouse should permit ideal engraftment of human HSC and give rise to a Hu mouse capable of a robust human antibody response encompassing immunoglobulin class switching and high-affinity maturation. Given the recent rapid progress, such an ideal system will soon be available.

ACKNOWLEDGMENTS

I thank members of my laboratory for their contributions to Hu mouse research and Jonathan LeCureux for assistance with the manuscript. Work in my laboratory is supported by NIH grants AI073255, AI095101, AI100845, HL074704, HL94257, U54AI065357, and PO1AI099783.

Conflicts of interest: I declare no conflicts.

CITATION

Akkina R. 2014. Humanized mice (Hu mice) for studying human immune responses and generating human monoclonal antibodies. Microbiol Spectrum 2(2):AID-0003-2012.

REFERENCES

1. **Presta LG.** 2008. Molecular engineering and design of therapeutic antibodies. *Curr Opin Immunol* **20:**460–470.
2. **Lonberg N.** 2005. Human antibodies from transgenic animals. *Nat Biotechnol* **23:**1117–1125.
3. **Jakobovits A, Amado RG, Yang X, Roskos L, Schwab G.** 2007. From XenoMouse technology to panitumumab, the first fully human antibody product from transgenic mice. *Nat Biotechnol* **25:**1134–1143.
4. **Berges BK, Rowan MR.** 2011. The utility of the new generation of humanized mice to study HIV-1 infection: transmission, prevention, pathogenesis, and treatment. *Retrovirology* **8:**65. doi:10.1186/1742-4690-8-65.
5. **Nischang M, Gers-Huber G, Audige A, Akkina R, Speck RF.** 2012. Modeling HIV infection and therapies in humanized mice. *Swiss Med Wkly* **142:**w13618. doi:10.4414/smw.2012.13618.
6. **Shultz LD, Brehm MA, Bavari S, Greiner DL.** 2011. Humanized mice as a preclinical tool for infectious disease and biomedical research. *Ann N Y Acad Sci* **1245:**50–54.
7. **Akkina R.** 2013. Human immune responses and potential for vaccine assessment in humanized mice. *Curr Opin Immunol* **25:**403–409.
8. **Ito M, Kobayashi K, Nakahata T.** 2008. NOD/Shi-scid IL2rgamma(null) (NOG) mice more appropriate for humanized mouse models. *Curr Top Microbiol Immunol* **324:**53–76.
9. **Mosier DE.** 2000. Human xenograft models for virus infection. *Virology* **271:**215–219.
10. **McCune JM.** 1996. Development and applications of the SCID-hu mouse model. *Semin Immunol* **8:**187–196.
11. **Jamieson BD, Zack JA.** 1999. Murine models for HIV disease. *AIDS* **13**(Suppl A)**:**S5–S11.
12. **Legrand N, Ploss A, Balling R, Becker PD, Borsotti C, Brezillon N, Debarry J, de Jong Y, Deng H, Di Santo JP, Eisenbarth S, Eynon E, Flavell RA, Guzman CA, Huntington ND, Kremsdorf D, Manns MP, Manz MG, Mention JJ, Ott M, Rathinam C, Rice CM, Rongvaux A, Stevens S, Spits H, Strick-Marchand H, Takizawa H, van Lent AU, Wang C, Weijer K, Willinger T, Ziegler P.** 2009. Humanized mice for modeling human infectious disease: challenges, progress, and outlook. *Cell Host Microbe* **6:**5–9.
13. **Akkina R.** 2013. New generation humanized mice for virus research: comparative aspects and future prospects. *Virology* **435:**14–28.
14. **Berges BK, Akkina SR, Folkvord JM, Connick E, Akkina R.** 2008. Mucosal transmission of R5 and X4 tropic HIV-1 via vaginal and rectal routes in humanized Rag2–/– gammac –/– (RAG-hu) mice. *Virology* **373:**342–351.
15. **Lan P, Tonomura N, Shimizu A, Wang S, Yang YG.** 2006. Reconstitution of a functional human immune system in immunodeficient mice through combined human fetal thymus/liver and CD34$^+$ cell transplantation. *Blood* **108:** 487–492.
16. **Melkus MW, Estes JD, Padgett-Thomas A, Gatlin J, Denton PW, Othieno FA, Wege AK, Haase AT, Garcia JV.** 2006. Humanized mice mount specific adaptive and innate immune responses to EBV and TSST-1. *Nat Med* **12:**1316–1322.

17. Biswas S, Chang H, Sarkis PT, Fikrig E, Zhu Q, Marasco WA. 2011. Humoral immune responses in humanized BLT mice immunized with West Nile virus and HIV-1 envelope proteins are largely mediated via human CD5[+] B cells. *Immunology* **134**:419–433.

18. Stoddart CA, Maidji E, Galkina SA, Kosikova G, Rivera JM, Moreno ME, Sloan B, Joshi P, Long BR. 2011. Superior human leukocyte reconstitution and susceptibility to vaginal HIV transmission in humanized NOD-scid IL-2R $\gamma^{-/-}$ (NSG) BLT mice. *Virology* **417**:154–160.

19. Washburn ML, Bility MT, Zhang L, Kovalev GI, Buntzman A, Frelinger JA, Barry W, Ploss A, Rice CM, Su L. 2011. A humanized mouse model to study hepatitis C virus infection, immune response, and liver disease. *Gastroenterology* **140**:1334–1344.

20. Akkina R, Berges BK, Palmer BE, Remling L, Neff CP, Kuruvilla J, Connick E, Folkvord J, Gagliardi K, Kassu A, Akkina SR. 2011. Humanized Rag1$^{-/-}$ γc$^{-/-}$ mice support multilineage hematopoiesis and are susceptible to HIV-1 infection via systemic and vaginal routes. *PloS One* **6**:e20169. doi:10.1371/journal.pone. 0020169.

21. Becker PD, Legrand N, van Geelen CM, Noerder M, Huntington ND, Lim A, Yasuda E, Diehl SA, Scheeren FA, Ott M, Weijer K, Wedemeyer H, Di Santo JP, Beaumont T, Guzman CA, Spits H. 2010. Generation of human antigen-specific monoclonal IgM antibodies using vaccinated "human immune system" mice. *PloS One* **5**:e13137. doi:10.1371/journal.pone.0013137.

22. Berges BK, Wheat WH, Palmer BE, Connick E, Akkina R. 2006. HIV-1 infection and CD4 T cell depletion in the humanized Rag2$^{-/-}$ γc$^{-/-}$ (RAG-hu) mouse model. *Retrovirology* **3**:76. doi:10.1186/1742-4690-3-76.

23. McDermott SP, Eppert K, Lechman ER, Doedens M, Dick JE. 2010. Comparison of human cord blood engraftment between immunocompromised mouse strains. *Blood* **116**:193–200.

24. Denton PW, Garcia JV. 2011. Humanized mouse models of HIV infection. *AIDS Rev* **13**:135–148.

25. Denton PW, Olesen R, Choudhary SK, Archin NM, Wahl A, Swanson MD, Chateau M, Nochi T, Krisko JF, Spagnuolo RA, Margolis DM, Garcia JV. 2012. Generation of HIV latency in humanized BLT mice. *J Virol* **86**:630–634.

26. Marsden MD, Kovochich M, Suree N, Shimizu S, Mehta R, Cortado R, Bristol G, An DS, Zack JA. 2012. HIV latency in the humanized BLT mouse. *J Virol* **86**:339–347.

27. Berges BK, Akkina SR, Remling L, Akkina R. 2010. Humanized Rag2$^{-/-}$ γc$^{-/-}$ (RAG-hu) mice can sustain long-term chronic HIV-1 infection lasting more than a year. *Virology* **397**: 100–103.

28. Jaiswal S, Pazoles P, Woda M, Shultz LD, Greiner DL, Brehm MA, Mathew A. 2012. Enhanced humoral and HLA-A2-restricted dengue virus-specific T-cell responses in humanized BLT NSG mice. *Immunology* **136**:334–343.

29. Kuruvilla JG, Troyer RM, Devi S, Akkina R. 2007. Dengue virus infection and immune response in humanized RAG2$^{-/-}$ γc$^{-/-}$ (RAG-hu) mice. *Virology* **369**:143–152.

30. Garcia S, Freitas AA. 2012. Humanized mice: current states and perspectives. *Immunol Lett* **146**:1–7.

31. Gorantla S, Sneller H, Walters L, Sharp JG, Pirruccello SJ, West JT, Wood C, Dewhurst S, Gendelman HE, Poluektova L. 2007. Human immunodeficiency virus type 1 pathobiology studied in humanized BALB/c-Rag2$^{-/-}$$\gamma$c$^{-/-}$ mice. *J Virol* **81**:2700–2712.

32. Ishikawa F, Yasukawa M, Lyons B, Yoshida S, Miyamoto T, Yoshimoto G, Watanabe T, Akashi K, Shultz LD, Harada M. 2005. Development of functional human blood and immune systems in NOD/SCID/IL2 receptor {gamma} chain(null) mice. *Blood* **106**:1565–1573.

33. Matsumura T, Kametani Y, Ando K, Hirano Y, Katano I, Ito R, Shiina M, Tsukamoto H, Saito Y, Tokuda Y, Kato S, Ito M, Motoyoshi K, Habu S. 2003. Functional CD5[+] B cells develop predominantly in the spleen of NOD/SCID/γc^{null} (NOG) mice transplanted either with human umbilical cord blood, bone marrow, or mobilized peripheral blood CD34[+] cells. *Exp Hematol* **31**:789–797.

34. Shultz LD, Saito Y, Najima Y, Tanaka S, Ochi T, Tomizawa M, Doi T, Sone A, Suzuki N, Fujiwara H, Yasukawa M, Ishikawa F. 2010. Generation of functional human T-cell subsets with HLA-restricted immune responses in HLA class I expressing NOD/SCID/IL2r gamma(null) humanized mice. *Proc Natl Acad Sci USA* **107**:13022–13027.

35. Traggiai E, Chicha L, Mazzucchelli L, Bronz L, Piffaretti JC, Lanzavecchia A, Manz MG. 2004. Development of a human adaptive immune system in cord blood cell-transplanted mice. *Science* **304**:104–107.

36. Watanabe S, Terashima K, Ohta S, Horibata S, Yajima M, Shiozawa Y, Dewan MZ, Yu Z, Ito M, Morio T, Shimizu N, Honda M, Yamamoto N. 2007. Hematopoietic stem cell-engrafted NOD/SCID/IL2Rγ^{null} mice develop human lymphoid systems and induce long-lasting HIV-1 infection with specific humoral immune responses. *Blood* **109**:212–218.

37. Watanabe Y, Takahashi T, Okajima A, Shiokawa M, Ishii N, Katano I, Ito R, Ito M, Minegishi M, Minegishi N, Tsuchiya S,

Sugamura K. 2009. The analysis of the functions of human B and T cells in humanized NOD/shi-scid/γc^{null} (NOG) mice (hu-HSC NOG mice). *Int Immunol* **21**:843–858.

38. Danner R, Chaudhari SN, Rosenberger J, Surls J, Richie TL, Brumeanu TD, Casares S. 2011. Expression of HLA class II molecules in humanized NOD.Rag1KO.IL2RgcKO mice is critical for development and function of human T and B cells. *PloS One* **6**:e19826. doi:10.1371/journal.pone.0019826.

39. Chang H, Biswas S, Tallarico AS, Sarkis PT, Geng S, Panditrao MM, Zhu Q, Marasco WA. 2012. Human B-cell ontogeny in humanized NOD/SCID γc^{null} mice generates a diverse yet auto/poly- and HIV-1-reactive antibody repertoire. *Genes Immun* **13**:399–410.

40. Tonomura N, Habiro K, Shimizu A, Sykes M, Yang YG. 2008. Antigen-specific human T-cell responses and T cell-dependent production of human antibodies in a humanized mouse model. *Blood* **111**:4293–4296.

41. Rajesh D, Zhou Y, Jankowska-Gan E, Roenneburg DA, Dart ML, Torrealba J, Burlingham WJ. 2010. Th1 and Th17 immunocompetence in humanized NOD/SCID/IL2rgammanull mice. *Hum Immunol* **71**:551–559.

42. Hiramatsu H, Nishikomori R, Heike T, Ito M, Kobayashi K, Katamura K, Nakahata T. 2003. Complete reconstitution of human lymphocytes from cord blood CD34+ cells using the NOD/SCID/gammacnull mice model. *Blood* **102**:873–880.

43. Strowig T, Gurer C, Ploss A, Liu YF, Arrey F, Sashihara J, Koo G, Rice CM, Young JW, Chadburn A, Cohen JI, Munz C. 2009. Priming of protective T cell responses against virus-induced tumors in mice with human immune system components. *J Exp Med* **206**:1423–1434.

44. Gorantla S, Makarov E, Finke-Dwyer J, Gebhart CL, Domm W, Dewhurst S, Gendelman HE, Poluektova LY. 2010. CD8+ cell depletion accelerates HIV-1 immunopathology in humanized mice. *J Immunol* **184**:7082–7091.

45. Yajima M, Imadome K, Nakagawa A, Watanabe S, Terashima K, Nakamura H, Ito M, Shimizu N, Yamamoto N, Fujiwara S. 2009. T cell-mediated control of Epstein-Barr virus infection in humanized mice. *J Infect Dis* **200**:1611–1615.

46. An DS, Poon B, Ho Tsong Fang R, Weijer K, Blom B, Spits H, Chen IS, Uittenbogaart CH. 2007. Use of a novel chimeric mouse model with a functionally active human immune system to study human immunodeficiency virus type 1 infection. *Clin Vaccine Immunol* **14**:391–396.

47. Baenziger S, Tussiwand R, Schlaepfer E, Mazzucchelli L, Heikenwalder M, Kurrer MO, Behnke S, Frey J, Oxenius A, Joller H, Aguzzi A, Manz MG, Speck RF. 2006. Disseminated and sustained HIV infection in CD34+ cord blood cell-transplanted Rag2$^{-/-}$$\gamma_c^{-/-}$ mice. *Proc Natl Acad Sci USA* **103**:15951–15956.

48. Dudek TE, No DC, Seung E, Vrbanac VD, Fadda L, Bhoumik P, Boutwell CL, Power KA, Gladden AD, Battis L, Mellors EF, Tivey TR, Gao X, Altfeld M, Luster AD, Tager AM, Allen TM. 2012. Rapid evolution of HIV-1 to functional CD8(+) T cell responses in humanized BLT mice. *Sci Transl Med* **4**:143ra98. doi:10.1126/scitranslmed.3003984.

49. Scheeren FA, van Geelen CM, Yasuda E, Spits H, Beaumont T. 2011. Antigen-specific monoclonal antibodies isolated from B cells expressing constitutively active STAT5. *PloS One* **6**:e17189. doi:10.1371/journal.pone.0017189.

50. Crowe JE Jr. 2009. Recent advances in the study of human antibody responses to influenza virus using optimized human hybridoma approaches. *Vaccine* **27**(Suppl 6):G47–G51.

51. Smith K, Garman L, Wrammert J, Zheng NY, Capra JD, Ahmed R, Wilson PC. 2009. Rapid generation of fully human monoclonal antibodies specific to a vaccinating antigen. *Nat Protoc* **4**:372–384.

52. Banerjee P, Tripp A, Lairmore MD, Crawford L, Sieburg M, Ramos JC, Harrington W Jr, Beilke MA, Feuer G. 2010. Adult T-cell leukemia/lymphoma development in HTLV-1-infected humanized SCID mice. *Blood* **115**:2640–2648.

53. Yamamoto I, Takajo I, Umeki K, Morishita K, Hatakeyama K, Kataoka H, Nomura H, Okayama A. 2010. Multiple integrations of human T-lymphotropic virus type 1 proviruses in the engrafted cells from the asymptomatic carriers in NOD/SCID/gammacnull mice. *Intervirology* **53**:229–239.

54. He Z, Zhang H, Zhang X, Xie D, Chen Y, Wangensteen KJ, Ekker SC, Firpo M, Liu C, Xiang D, Zi X, Hui L, Yang G, Ding X, Hu Y, Wang X. 2010. Liver xeno-repopulation with human hepatocytes in Fah-/-Rag2-/- mice after pharmacological immunosuppression. *Am J Pathol* **177**:1311–1319.

55. Kwant-Mitchell A, Ashkar AA, Rosenthal KL. 2009. Mucosal innate and adaptive immune responses against herpes simplex virus type 2 in a humanized mouse model. *J Virol* **83**:10664–10676.

56. Parsons CH, Adang LA, Overdevest J, O'Connor CM, Taylor JR Jr, Camerini D, Kedes DH. 2006. KSHV targets multiple leukocyte lineages during long-term productive infection in NOD/SCID mice. *J Clin Invest* **116**:1963–1973.

57. **Smith MS, Goldman DC, Bailey AS, Pfaffle DL, Kreklywich CN, Spencer DB, Othieno FA, Streblow DN, Garcia JV, Fleming WH, Nelson JA.** 2010. Granulocyte-colony stimulating factor reactivates human cytomegalovirus in a latently infected humanized mouse model. *Cell Host Microbe* 8:284–291.

58. **Firoz Mian M, Pek EA, Chenoweth MJ, Ashkar AA.** 2011. Humanized mice are susceptible to Salmonella typhi infection. *Cell Mol Immunol* 8:83–87.

59. **Libby SJ, Brehm MA, Greiner DL, Shultz LD, McClelland M, Smith KD, Cookson BT, Karlinsey JE, Kinkel TL, Porwollik S, Canals R, Cummings LA, Fang FC.** 2010. Humanized nonobese diabetic-*scidIL2r*γ^{null} mice are susceptible to lethal *Salmonella* Typhi infection. *Proc Natl Acad Sci USA* 107:15589–15594.

60. **Arnold L, Tyagi RK, Meija P, Swetman C, Gleeson J, Perignon JL, Druilhe P.** 2011. Further improvements of the *P. falciparum* humanized mouse model. *PLoS One* 6:e18045. doi:10.1371/journal.pone.0018045.

61. **Wege AK, Florian C, Ernst W, Zimara N, Schleicher U, Hanses F, Schmid M, Ritter U.** 2012. Leishmania major infection in humanized mice induces systemic infection and provokes a nonprotective human immune response. *PLoS Negl Trop Dis* 6:e1741. doi:10.1371/journal.pntd.0001741.

62. **Yu CI, Gallegos M, Marches F, Zurawski G, Ramilo O, Garcia-Sastre A, Banchereau J, Palucka AK.** 2008. Broad influenza-specific CD8[+] T-cell responses in humanized mice vaccinated with influenza virus vaccines. *Blood* 112:3671–3678.

63. **Ide K, Wang H, Tahara H, Liu J, Wang X, Asahara T, Sykes M, Yang YG, Ohdan H.** 2007. Role for CD47-SIRPalpha signaling in xenograft rejection by macrophages. *Proc Natl Acad Sci USA* 104:5062–5066.

64. **van den Berg TK, van der Schoot CE.** 2008. Innate immune 'self' recognition: a role for CD47-SIRPalpha interactions in hematopoietic stem cell transplantation. *Trends Immunol* 29:203–206.

65. **Strowig T, Rongvaux A, Rathinam C, Takizawa H, Borsotti C, Philbrick W, Eynon EE, Manz MG, Flavell RA.** 2011. Transgenic expression of human signal regulatory protein alpha in Rag2–/–gamma(c)–/– mice improves engraftment of human hematopoietic cells in humanized mice. *Proc Natl Acad Sci USA* 108:13218–13223.

66. **Legrand N, Huntington ND, Nagasawa M, Bakker AQ, Schotte R, Strick-Marchand H, de Geus SJ, Pouw SM, Bohne M, Voordouw A, Weijer K, Di Santo JP, Spits H.** 2011. Functional CD47/signal regulatory protein alpha (SIRPα) interaction is required for optimal human T- and natural killer- (NK) cell homeostasis in vivo. *Proc Natl Acad Sci USA* 108:13224–13229.

67. **Willinger T, Rongvaux A, Strowig T, Manz MG, Flavell RA.** 2011. Improving human hemato-lymphoid-system mice by cytokine knock-in gene replacement. *Trends Immunol* 32:321–327.

68. **Rongvaux A, Willinger T, Takizawa H, Rathinam C, Auerbach W, Murphy AJ, Valenzuela DM, Yancopoulos GD, Eynon EE, Stevens S, Manz MG, Flavell RA.** 2011. Human thrombopoietin knockin mice efficiently support human hematopoiesis in vivo. *Proc Natl Acad Sci USA* 108:2378–2383.

69. **Rathinam C, Poueymirou WT, Rojas J, Murphy AJ, Valenzuela DM, Yancopoulos GD, Rongvaux A, Eynon EE, Manz MG, Flavell RA.** 2011. Efficient differentiation and function of human macrophages in humanized CSF-1 mice. *Blood* 118:3119–3128.

Antibodies: Computer-Aided Prediction of Structure and Design of Function

10

ALEXANDER M. SEVY[1] and JENS MEILER[1]

INTRODUCTION

The central role antibodies play in our immune system makes them important targets for computation-based structural modeling. Antibodies consist of a "constant" and a "variable" region (Fig. 1). The constant region is virtually identical in all antibodies of the same isotype, while the variable region differs from one B-cell-derived antibody to the next. The variable region of an antibody is the "business end," the region that recognizes its antigen via so-called complementarity-determining regions (CDRs). Their large size (~150 kDa) and inherent variability, in particular in the CDRs, make antibodies a formidable challenge for molecular modeling. Before we begin to model antibodies, it is useful to briefly review their overall structure.

Relation of Antibody Sequence, Structure, and Function

The fundamental unit within an antibody is an immunoglobulin (IG) domain of around 70 to 110 amino acids that adopts the characteristic IG β-sandwich fold. Antibodies are homodimers of heterodimers, where each

[1]Department of Chemistry and Center for Structural Biology, Vanderbilt University, Nashville, TN 37212.
Antibodies for Infectious Diseases
Edited by James E. Crowe, Jr., Diana Boraschi, and Rino Rappuoli
© 2015 American Society for Microbiology, Washington, DC
doi:10.1128/microbiolspec.AID-0024-2014

heterodimer consists of one heavy and one light chain (Fig. 1) (1), each chain having multiple IG domains. A mammalian antibody light chain consists of two IG domains, the C-terminal one called "constant" and the N-terminal one, "variable." The mammalian antibody heavy chain consists of four or five IG domains, the most N-terminal one being variable, and all others constant. The two N-terminal IG domains of the heavy chain interact with the two IG domains of a light chain to form heterodimers. These heterodimers homo-dimerize via the C-terminal IG domains of the heavy chain to form

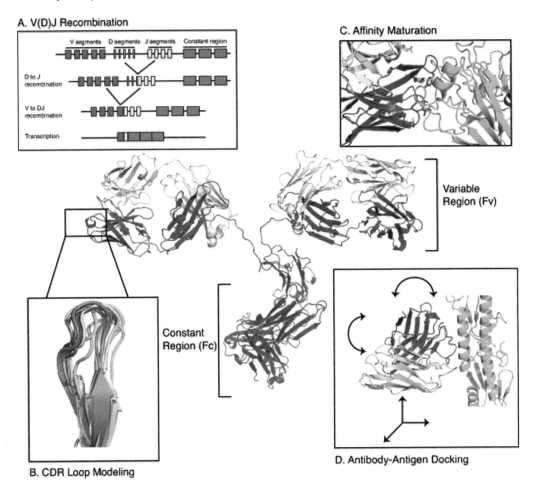

FIGURE 1 **Challenges in antibody modeling. Though all antibodies share a common core structure (center panel, PDB ID 1IGT [1]; heavy chains in magenta, light chains in yellow), slight differences in variable regions and especially CDR loops can have a great effect on function. The vast sequence space generated by genetic recombination in V, D, and J genes (A) results in many different CDR loop conformations. Modeling of CDR loops from sequence information alone is a necessary computational task for accurate structure prediction (B). The ability to simulate the affinity maturation process *in silico* is another important task that can be used to generate an antibody with either increased higher affinity for its native target, or for a completely novel target (C) (matured residues shown in cyan). Accurate antibody modeling requires not only the ability to model an antibody alone, but also the ability to model its interaction with a given antigen. Computational docking techniques achieve this by sampling different positions of an antibody on its target to find the most favorable position (D). doi:10.1128/microbiolspec. AID-0024-2014.f1**

the final antibody. This domain arrangement ensures that the variable domains of heavy and light chains colocalize in space to form the so-called paratope.

Each of these variable domains contains three CDRs that are the second (CDR1), fourth (CDR2), and sixth (CDR3) loop regions of the β-sandwich, locating the CDRs on the same end of the IG fold. The amino acid sequence within the CDRs is determined by a process called somatic recombination, where an IG domain is assembled by combining randomly chosen gene segments—V and J for the light chain and V, D, and J for the heavy chain (Fig. 1A). This process generates a large number of antibody sequences, as there are multiple copies of each gene type-somatic recombination combined with "junctional diversity" at the joints of the gene segments creates a theoretical limit of around 10^{11} unique V(D)J sequences. In particular, CDR3 of the heavy chain (HCDR3), encoded by the D-gene, is highly variable in length, structure, and dynamics (Fig. 1C). These "germline" antibodies are further modified in a process called affinity maturation (Fig. 1D). During B cell proliferation the genes encoding the variable domains experience an increased rate of point mutation. This "somatic hypermutation" causes amino acid changes in the paratopes of daughter B cells, a process that allows tighter interaction with the "epitope" region of the antigen, i.e., affinity maturation.

Motivations for Antibody Modeling

The large number of theoretically possible antibodies and the large number of antibodies actually present in humans prohibit a comprehensive experimental characterization of antibody structure and dynamics. While great progress has been made in antibody structure determination via crystallization (currently around 2,000 depositions in the Protein Data Bank [PDB] contain the phrase "antibody"), the number of experimental structures available in the PDB will always be small compared to the total immune repertoire, leaving room for structure prediction of important antibodies with unknown structure. As antibody structures in the PDB have increased exponentially in recent years (Fig. 2), computational biologists have gained a greater understanding of the molecular determinants of proper loop folding and antigen binding, ultimately allowing high-throughput, accurate structural modeling on a scale infeasible for experimental methods alone. Understanding the structural determinants of antibody-antigen interaction (i.e., how the paratope engages the epitope) is critical for understanding antibody function and processes such as affinity maturation. As the number of cocrystal structures of antibody and antigen will always be small, computational docking algorithms can provide models for antibody-antigen complexes that are not experimentally determined (Fig. 1D). Note that computational structure prediction usually does not replace the experiment but complements experimental data. For examples, starting from an experimental structure of antibody and antigen, their interaction could be modeled; starting from one antibody-antigen complex, models for affinity-matured antibody-antigen complexes can be constructed; or modeling can add atomic detail not present in lower-resolution electron density maps obtained, for example, through electron microscopy (EM). Computational design of antibody-antigen complexes can be used, for example, to study the process of affinity maturation *in silico* or identify antibodies with novel sequences not present or not yet observed in nature (Fig. 1B). Computational antibody engineering is also applied to humanize or stabilize therapeutic antibodies.

Challenges for Antibody Modeling

Challenges when predicting the structures of antibodies via comparative modeling include how changes in IG sequence change the relative orientation of the two variable IG domains in the complex and therefore influence the paratope structure. Obviously,

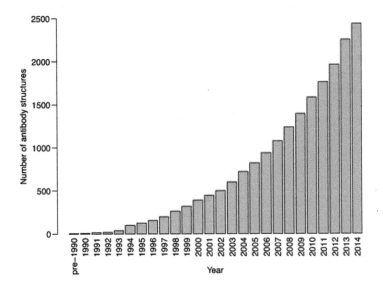

FIGURE 2 Exponential growth of structurally determined antibodies. Total antibody structures in the Protein Data Bank (PDB) are shown by year. The increase in structures enables more accurate computational approaches to antibody modeling and engineering. doi:10.1128/microbiolspec.AID-0024-2014.f2

modeling the conformation of CDR loops is a substantial challenge, in particular for CDR3, which has an average length of around 15 amino acids in humans and can be as long as 30 residues or more—well beyond the loop lengths tested in a typical loop construction benchmark (4, 8, and 12 amino acids). The plasticity of the paratope with the often flexible CDRs presents a formidable challenge to antibody/antigen docking simulations, as they require flexibility of both paratope and epitope, creating a huge conformational search space. When engineering antibodies, these challenges are multiplied by the enormous number of possible antibody sequences and the resulting gigantic size of the sequence space that needs to be sampled, in addition to the conformational space. These challenges result in another formidable motivation for modeling antibodies: the benchmarking of new computational techniques. The challenges related to modeling antibodies combined with the availability of many experimental structures make antibody structure prediction and functional design an important playground to test new algorithms.

COMPARATIVE MODELING OF ANTIBODIES

Given the large number of theoretically possible and actually existing antibodies, experimental structure determination will remain reserved to a small fraction of particularly important antibodies. Therefore, computational construction of a structural model is of central importance. A particular focus of comparative modeling techniques is accurate modeling of the CDRs.

Canonical Structure of CDRs

The concept of canonical structures of light CDR (LCDR) and heavy CDR (HCDR) loops can be traced back to seminal work by Chothia, Thornton, Lesk, and others in the 1980s and 1990s describing the conformational space sampled by all CDR loops with known structure and linking these to conserved residues among these sequences (2–4). Formally, the canonical structure hypothesis states that the CDR loops of antibodies typically adopt one of a discrete set of conformations and that these conformations can be inferred from the amino acid sequence. This concept has been pursued to discretize the conformational space of CDRs and predict a loop conformation based on its primary sequence. The set of canonical conformations has been relatively well defined for all LCDR loops and for the heavy HCDR1 and 2 loops. However, the HCDR3 loop is by far the most variable in sequence and length, drastically increasing the conformational space it can sample. As the number of experimentally determined antibody structures has exploded since the initial reports of canonical structures, attempts to group CDR loops and create a definitive set of loop conformations have continued to add new clusters to the known set. While it is likely that this trend will continue for some time, the fact that the number of clusters is still orders of magnitude lower than the known antibody repertoire validates the original canonical structure hypothesis by Chothia et al. for CDRs other than HCDR3 (2).

Studies of canonical non-HCDR3 loop conformations have focused on clustering known structures and deriving common characteristics in primary sequence to enable *a priori* prediction of a loop conformation based on sequence alone. The number of canonical loop conformations has increased along with experimental structures available for analysis; initial studies using only 17 structures identified 18 non-HCDR3 clusters (2), whereas more recent studies using ~1,200 structures have increased the number of non-HCDR3 clusters to 72 (5). Clusters are identified by their loop type and length, with the majority of non-HCDR3 loops falling between 8 and 13 residues in length. Though the number of non-HCDR3 loop clusters has increased with each subsequent analysis, the overall clustering pattern still maintains a high degree of uniformity and predictability. Figure 3 shows median loop structures of loops deriving from the largest cluster for each of the CDR L1, L2, L3, H1, and H2 loops (5). Studies have consistently reported 85 to 90%

accuracy in predicting the structure of non-HCDR3 loops based on their gene source and primary sequence, lending credibility to the use of cluster analysis in non-HCDR3 loop modeling.

Predicting the Conformation of HCDR3

Prediction of HCDR3 loop conformations presents a considerably larger challenge, as they are much more structurally diverse and tend to be longer, ranging usually from 5 to 26 residues, with an average of 16 residues (6). In rare cases they can be substantially longer. HCDR3 loops are generally divided into "torso" and "head" regions for clustering purposes (7), and loops are characterized by either a bulged or extended beta-sheet conformation in the torso region. Since HCDR3 loops cannot typically be placed into a conformational cluster based on sequence alone, recent work has focused on developing a set of rules to predict certain aspects of the conformation based on key residue positions (8). The more stable bulged conformation tends to be preferred by HCDR3 loops, stabilized by a hydrogen bond between a conserved tryptophan and a backbone carbonyl. One rule dictates that an aspartate residue two positions upstream of the conserved tryptophan is sufficient to displace this hydrogen bond and results in a shift to the extended conformation. Another states that the position of a basic residue opposite this aspartate dictates the formation of a bulged or extended conformation. Taken together, these rules are able to correctly predict torso conformation with ~85% accuracy, comparable to that of non-HCDR3 loops.

Though the torso conformation of HCDR3 loops can be predicted by sequence analysis, the antigen-binding head region of the loop remains intractable to clustering, leading to considerable efforts to use *de novo* modeling to predict HCDR3 conformation. Currently, software packages such as Rosetta (9) and Prime (10) have been adapted to predict low-energy loop conformations, either based on peptide

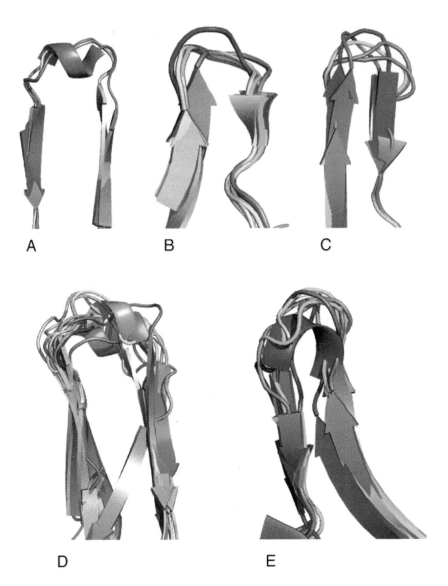

FIGURE 3 Canonical CDR loop conformations. Pictured above are median loop structures representing the largest cluster of (A) CDR L1, (B) L2, (C) L3, (D) H1, and (E) H2. Light and heavy chain loop variability varies widely between the CDR loops, with heavy chain loops tending to be more variable. doi:10.1128/ microbiolspec.AID-0024-2014.f3

fragments gleaned from the PDB or generated *de novo*. These protocols have achieved varying degrees of success: HCDR3 loops shorter than 12 to 14 residues can be consistently predicted within a reasonable margin of error (~2 Å), while longer loops are less predictable and tend to have higher deviation. As the average HCDR3 loop is ~16 residues in length,

current algorithms for *de novo* modeling remain insufficient to address a large proportion of important antibodies. However, the recent advances in predicting the conformation of the HCDR3 base via clustering and improvements in *de novo* loop construction promise to enable more reliable HCDR3 prediction in the near future.

Programs, Platforms, and Servers Dedicated to Antibody Modeling

Because of the large number of antibody-based therapeutics, there is substantial interest in determining the structure of antibodies in a high-throughput, accurate manner. Experimental methods such as X-ray crystallography and nuclear magnetic resonance (NMR) spectroscopy, while highly informative, are labor-, time-, and resource-intensive. In addition, complete antibodies tend to be too large for NMR spectroscopy. X-ray crystallography, in the absence of the antigen, often struggles to determine the conformation of a long HCDR3 loop in the biologically relevant conformation needed to engage the antigen. Sometimes the HCDR3 loop can be locked into a different conformation by crystal packing or its coordinates cannot be determined because of flexibility. Therefore, many groups have worked on automated protocols to computationally model antibody variable region structures to predict the conformational space including the conformation needed for binding. This has resulted in a number of publicly accessible antibody-modeling servers, which use a combination of comparative modeling, *de novo* structure prediction, and energy minimization to generate an ensemble of potential conformations. Recently, organized efforts such as the Antibody Modeling Assessment (AMA) have focused on comparing these modeling servers and determining the accuracy of antibody-modeling techniques relative to one another (11, 12).

Antibody-modeling servers typically rely on comparative modeling to model framework regions and CDR loops, with the notable exception of HCDR3. Framework regions are well conserved between antibodies, and a suitable template can usually be found among antibodies with experimentally determined structures in the PDB. One concern with comparative modeling is the issue of generating chimeras, combining heavy and light chain frameworks and CDR loops from different templates to use the template with the highest sequence homology. The relative orientation of the heavy and light chain V domains has a significant impact on the antigen-binding properties of an antibody (13). Although the framework regions are well conserved, combining heavy and light chain frameworks from different templates results in just one and possibly incorrect relative orientation of the heavy and light chain V domains, introducing error into the predicted antibody structure. In addition, although LCDR loops and HCDR1 and 2 have canonical conformations, grafting these loops onto a disparate framework can result in errors in the relative placement of these loops and their interactions. To address these problems, modeling servers have introduced several different solutions. Some servers such as PIGS allow the user a great deal of input regarding the manner in which chimeras are built, allowing the user to tune these parameters for each model (14). The MOE and WAM modeling servers build an ensemble of chimeras built from different templates and use force field energy minimization algorithms to relieve clashes and determine the most likely conformation (15, 16). RosettaAntibody takes a similar approach but uses a knowledge-based potential rather than molecular mechanics force field to relieve clashes in framework and loop placements (17).

Another major challenge is modeling the noncanonical HCDR3 loop. The sequence and structural variability of this loop make it difficult to model it simply by homology in most cases. The PIGS server attempts to model HCDR3 in the same manner as it models the other loops, by sequence homology to known HCDR3 structures (14). This approach can be effective in cases where a similar HCDR3 exists in the PDB, and as more structures are added, this likelihood increases. The MOE server also grafts HCDR3 loops from a template, followed by a more complicated protocol of HCDR3 clustering, force field energy minimization to build an ensemble of structures (16). However, the variability of the HCDR3 loop is such that a

more sophisticated modeling technique is necessary in many cases. Other notable approaches
for HCDR3 loop modeling involve either
fragment-based or *de novo* modeling. Rosetta
Antibody uses a fragment-based approach,
pulling short peptide fragments from the
PDB and using robotics-based algorithms in
conjunction with knowledge-based potentials
to close the HCDR3 loop in an energetically
favorable conformation (17). WAM uses a
similar approach, modeling based on PDB-
derived peptides based on different parameters
of the HCDR3, such as length and predicted
kinked conformation. However, the server
follows fragment assembly with a force field-
based minimization to achieve a local energy
minimum (15).

Since the introduction of these antibody-
modeling servers, a standing question has
been which method is most effective—in
user friendliness, structural accuracy, and
transparency of results. To this end, the
Antibody Modeling Assessment has held a
biannual blinded study to give groups the
chance to model the structures of unpublished antigen-binding fragment (Fab) X-
ray structures to assess the state of the field.
The assessments in 2011 and 2014 involved
blind prediction of 9 and 11 Fab fragments,
respectively, and analyzed the results by a
number of parameters, including total root
mean square deviation (RMSD), loop and
framework-specific RMSD, and overall
structural integrity. Overall RMSD values
for all servers are generally within 1.0 to
1.5 Å, with results varying between framework and CDR loops. Framework regions
were generally predicted most accurately,
with RMSD values consistently within 1.0 Å.
The highest deviation was seen for HCDR3
loops, with RMSD values ranging from 0.5
to 8.0 Å and predictive ability depending
heavily on the details of individual Fab fragments. Overall, the servers are comparable
in their modeling accuracy, with variation
dependent on particulars of the Fab fragment and metric used to analyze accuracy
(11, 12, 18).

ANTIBODY DOCKING AND EPITOPE MAPPING

Another significant challenge in modeling
antibody-antigen complexes is docking the
antibody onto its epitope on the surface of
the antigen. Though general protein-protein
docking has been successful in many cases,
antibody-antigen docking represents a special
challenge among protein-protein docking cases.
Although useful in other protein-protein docking problems, shape complementarity is not a
good determinant of correct antibody placement, as epitopes and paratopes are typically
flat. Binding affinity is instead determined
by hydrophobic "hot spot" and electrostatic
interactions (19, 20). Short, aggregation-prone
regions are common in many antibodies, consisting of mainly aromatic residues and concentrated in HCDR2 loops, and can contribute
significantly to buried surface area in antibody-antigen interactions (21). In addition,
the model for the antibody used as a starting
point for docking might have to be altered
when the epitope is engaged: if a single conformation is used, conformation of CDR loops
or the relative orientation of the V domains
might have to be changed when engaging the
epitope. If an ensemble of states is used, the
best conformation needs to be selected and
possibly refined further for optimal binding
(22, 23). Additionally, if the location of the
epitope is unknown, a global search needs to
be performed. This adds another degree of
complexity by requiring the docking algorithm
to sample epitopes across the entire surface
of the antigen. Several approaches have been
implemented to address these challenges, such
as algorithms to remodel antibody loop conformations in the presence of the antigen and
application of experimental data to inform
the energy evaluation of docked models.

Antibody Docking Algorithms

One docking algorithm that has had success
in the realm of antibody-antigen docking
is the RosettaDock algorithm, originally

described by Gray et al. (24). The algorithm uses alternating rounds of low-resolution rigid body perturbations and high-resolution side-chain and backbone minimization to generate a model of the docked complex. The RosettaDock protocol relies on random perturbation of the complex and creates large numbers ($\sim 10^5$) of models to capture a global energy minimum. The original protocol was able to recover native conformations with an RMSD on the order of 5 to 10 Å for local searches, with a higher error for global searches. Encouragingly, the antibody-antigen docked complexes showed a strong energy funnel, with low energy structures corresponding to a low RMSD to the native structure. This funnel validates the creation of a large number of complexes, with confidence that those with the lowest scores are most likely to recover the native conformation.

Since its original publication, the Rosetta-Dock protocol has been benchmarked thoroughly with large numbers of both native and homology-modeled structures. Advances in comparative antibody-modeling capabilities beg the question of how well these comparative models can be docking into their native antigens to produce a native-like structure. In general, antibody-modeling servers provide similar results in terms of success in docking comparative models. However, since scores fail to correlate perfectly with RMSD values, with the lowest RMSD model frequently not being the best scoring and vice versa, the best results have been obtained with ensemble docking models, using multiple models from the lower end of the energy landscape as inputs for docking. Using such an ensemble approach has been shown to flatten the energy funnel and increase the proportion of models deemed high and medium quality (9).

Additional docking protocols have been published based on the core algorithm in Rosetta-Dock but tailored specifically to antibody-antigen complexes. In particular, the SnugDock algorithm has been shown to increase docking accuracy for antibody-antigen complexes (25). This algorithm uses the same approach of alternating low- and high-resolution perturbation and minimization steps. However, it adds additional perturbation moves that are specific to antibody-binding motifs, such as CDR loop remodeling and reorientation of the angle between the V domains. This addresses the issue of antibody CDR loops adopting alternate conformations in the bound and free states, and the algorithm is designed to accommodate slight errors in comparative modeling that may disrupt adoption of the native conformation during docking. Although Snug-Dock benchmarking shows similar results to RosettaDock when using the lowest energy models for docking, ensemble docking using SnugDock shows a marked improvement of the energy funnel and increase of high- and medium-quality structures. This result is consistent with a conformational selection paradigm for the initial antibody-antigen interaction with a subsequent induced fit.

Incorporation of Experimental Data To Guide Antibody Docking and Epitope Mapping

The ability to identify a precise binding epitope of an antibody with its corresponding antigen is of obvious use for any antibody being studied. The knowledge of a binding epitope at the individual residue level allows more detailed analysis of the nature of an antibody's interaction with its antigen, including prediction of the mechanism of neutralization of an antibody, escape mutations that may evade binding, specificity of an antibody in binding-related antigens, etc. However, epitope mapping is an area that has relied on low- and medium-throughput experimental techniques, which can make it difficult to map the epitopes of large numbers of antibodies.

Experimental methods such as EM, NMR spectroscopy chemical shift mapping, competitive enzyme-linked immunosorbent assays, site-directed mutagenesis, force spectroscopy, and hydrogen-deuterium exchange have made it possible to obtain structural information on the antibody-antigen complex, including epitope and paratope, without the need for a crystal structure (26–31). Each technique faces its own challenges that make high-throughput epitope mapping difficult (32), but these data have been used successfully to create reliable computational models. A comprehensive example of integrating experimental data into computational modeling is shown in Fig. 4: data from EM, hydrogen-deuterium exchange, and site-directed mutagenesis were used to create a high-resolution model of an antibody-antigen complex for an influenza hemagglutinin directed antibody (33).

Computational methods have also made great strides in recent years to enable the large-scale, rapid mapping of binding epitope. As with experimental methods, computational approaches come with their own disadvantages and cannot be used reliably in isolation. However, various hybrid methods that use different types of experimental data to reduce the complexity of computational searches have shown great promise in providing a feasible approach to the epitope mapping problem. A promising approach to increase the accuracy of docking predictions is the incorporation of experimental data to supplement *in silico* epitope prediction. RosettaDock, in particular, has been benchmarked on both local and global searches and predictably shows better results when perturbations are kept to a minimum and the antibody is placed in the vicinity of the epitope to begin with. Such approaches reduce the conformational space that needs to be sampled.

In addition to reducing sampling space, limited experimental data can also be used to improve scoring. One major issue with docking using current methods is that a near-native conformation is frequently present in the large set of models, but the distinguishing power of the energy function is not sufficient to identify the near-native conformation without any *a priori* knowledge of the structure. Low-resolution epitope mapping using experimental methods can provide an extra distinguishing feature to eliminate incorrect models and identify those that are most likely to adopt the native conformation. Simonelli et al. have validated this hypothesis by using NMR chemical shift mapping to identify an epitope before the start of computational docking (26). Models that do not agree with the experimental results can be discarded, and lower scoring models are more likely to represent the native conformation.

Docking algorithms have been adapted to incorporate experimental data, which increases the accuracy of the final docked complex and the residues involved in the antibody-antigen interface. There are many different steps during the docking protocol in which experimental data can be incorporated.

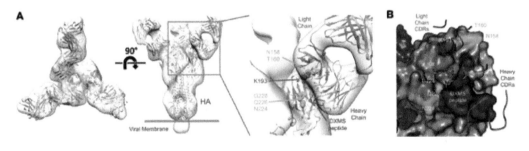

FIGURE 4 Integrating experimental data to aid computational modeling. (A) Low-resolution cryo-EM maps, **(A and B)** combined with hydrogen-deuterium exchange (DXMS) data and site-directed mutagenesis, were used to generate a docked model of a potent anti-influenza antibody. Reprinted from *Journal of Clinical Investigation* (33) with permission from the publisher. doi:10.1128/microbiolspec. AID-0024-2014.f4

Mutagenesis data and cryo-EM density maps have been used to constrain the initial placement of the antibody on the surface of the antigen prior to docking, allowing for a more limited search and resulting in more native-like contacts (33–35). In addition, complex scores can be weighted such that residues experimentally shown to interact are encouraged to do so during the docking protocol (34, 35). This approach drives the formation of models that contain the correct residue pairwise interactions across the interface, while allowing for the creation of new interacting pairs within this framework. Final models can then be clustered and analyzed visually for adherence to experimental data, eliminating those that do not contain key residues at the interface or have topologies inconsistent with EM data.

Another source of experimental data that has been used to improve computational epitope prediction is hydrogen-deuterium exchange (36). This technique involves the dissociation of amide hydrogens on a protein backbone and replacement with deuterium from a solvent. The extent of exchange can then be quantified using NMR or mass spectrometry. Antibody binding to its antigen causes a decrease in solvent accessibility of peptides at the epitope and a concomitant decrease in deuterium incorporation. Epitopes of many different antibodies have been mapped using this technique, with higher throughput than other methods such as X-ray crystallography or mutagenesis (27, 28, 37). Several studies have taken advantage of this phenomenon to improve docking predictions by constraining the initial placement of the antibody and rewarding residue interactions that agree with hydrogen-deuterium exchange data (33, 38).

Other approaches to epitope mapping have moved away from docking and instead use bioinformatics strategies to identify interacting regions. One such approach uses binding of randomly created peptide libraries to determine motifs that are important for antibody recognition (39). The algorithm then identifies pairs of residues within peptide fragments that covary with the binding by the target antibody, allowing for identification of key residues both proximal and distal to the epitope. This method has been validated using antibodies targeting viral protein gp120 from HIV and is beneficial as a complement to docking. Another similar approach uses neutralization data of an antibody with different viral strains varying by sequence. This algorithm identifies mutations that tend to correlate with a decrease in neutralization and proposes these as the binding epitope. In addition, the algorithm can incorporate structural data to eliminate purported epitope residues on the basis of solvent-accessible surface area (40, 41). This method can be beneficial in cases where a large body of neutralization data already exists in the literature for an antibody, as extra experimental data do not have to be collected solely for use by the algorithm.

ANTIBODY DESIGN

The computational design of antibodies is not only the most stringent test of our understanding of the rules that govern antibody structure and interaction, but it also has exciting applications in designing an antibody optimized for a given epitope (affinity maturation) or an antibody that recognizes multiple similar target epitopes (broad neutralization). Through this approach the relation between the sequence, structure, and activity of antibodies can be better understood, as the sequence and structural space can be explored in a more comprehensive manner than possible by analysis of naturally occurring antibodies only. Recently, an important proof-of-principle experiment for computer-aided epitope-focused vaccine design was reported (42). For this paradigm to reach its full potential, knowledge of the optimal antibodies to engage an epitope and the relation between sequence, structure, and activity inferred from computational design must be integrated. Besides the obvious application for the development of better therapeutic antibodies, computational antibody engineering also has the potential for formulation and humanization of therapeutic antibodies (43–46).

Broad Neutralization versus Affinity Maturation

Affinity maturation is a process by which the variable region of an antibody undergoes somatic hypermutation to introduce point mutations in the framework and CDR loops to select for a variant with increased binding affinity for its target. Along with V(D)J recombination and junctional diversity, it is a fundamental reason why a finite set of antibody sequences is able to recognize a virtually infinite array of antigens (47). Experimental methods can be used to re-create maturation in an *ex vivo* context to create an antibody with higher affinity for a given target. For example, phage display combined with random mutagenesis can screen for mutations in a high-throughput manner to create new, tighter-binding antibodies (48). This form of "directed evolution" has been successfull in the maturation of many types of antibodies (48). Additionally, computational algorithms have been developed that mimic the process of directed evolution to produce similar results. Computational methods have been successful in both studying the nature of affinity maturation in germline and matured antibodies and in further refining matured antibodies to increase affinity even more.

Affinity maturation can be simulated *in silico* to analyze compromises in an antibody sequence that lead to a decrease in polyspecificity with a concomitant increase in specificity for a single partner. For example, a general computational method for the design of antibody CDR loops for targeted epitope binding was introduced by Pantazes and Maranas (49). Computational methods such as multistate design are capable of determining the protein sequence optimal for binding an

arbitrary number of binding partners (50, 51). This technique has been applied to explore the changes in antibody sequence and conformation responsible for the shift from a polyspecific, germline antibody to one with higher affinity for a single target. In complementary work, Babor and Kortemme and Willis et al. used multistate design to show that antibody germline sequences are optimal for conformational flexibility of both CDR loops and framework residues, allowing the binding of multiple targets, whereas affinity-matured antibodies have decreased flexibility (52, 53). These authors have also identified the key residues responsible for either mono- or polyspecificity for several commonly seen germline genes. These studies validate the biological relevance of design algorithms, since sequences can be both computationally matured and reverted to germline by using different sets of antigens as inputs.

In silico Affinity Maturation

The understanding of the nature of affinity maturation, as well as the ability to selectively modify the specificity of antibody sequences, has led to advances in antibody engineering that enable maturing antibodies *in silico* to create new sequences with higher affinity. In one case, Clark et al. were able to use computational design to mature an antibody and generate candidate sequences with higher predicted affinity (54). Using a combination of side chain repacking and electrostatic optimization, a triple mutant was created with 10 times higher affinity. A comparable increase in affinity was achieved by Lippow et al. by redesigning an antilysozyme antibody along with the therapeutic antibody cetuximab (55). The design protocol was also able to predict mutations in bevacizumab that had been previously shown to increase affinity. The designed mutations primarily affected the electrostatic nature of the binding interface, either by removing a poorly satisfied polar residue at the interface or by adding a polar residue at the solvent-facing periphery of the interface (55). A similar approach has been taken to increase the species cross-reactivity of an antibody, rather than increasing affinity for a previously targeted antigen. By analyzing sequence differences between two serine protease orthologs, Farady et al. created novel antibody designs by restricting the search space to positions that contact points of difference between orthologs (56). In this manner they were able to target positions that would be most likely to establish new contacts across the binding interface to enable interaction at a reasonable affinity. This method was able to create antibody mutants with increases in affinity of over two orders of magnitude.

One significant limitation of most computational design protocols is that they require a high-resolution crystal structure of the antibody-antigen complex, or alternatively high-resolution structures of each component separately. However, several antibody designs have been made for complexes that do not have a solved structure available, using a combination of comparative modeling, protein-protein docking, and design. Barderas et al. used experimental epitope mapping data to dock a comparative model of an antigastrin antibody onto the surface of its target (57). They then used the docked models to estimate regions of antibody-antigen interaction and created mutants using both phage display and *in silico* affinity maturation to mutagenize antibody residues in contact with the antigen and produce designs with high predicted affinity. In several cases the *in silico* suggested mutations matched the mutations seen by directed evolution, and overall the designs were able to increase affinity to nanomolar levels. Another case used docking of an antidengue antibody with an NMR-mapped epitope to identify and rationally design mutations in the antibody CDR loops (58). The authors used this information to create several types of antibody mutations, including those that abolish binding, those that increase affinity for a single target, and those that increase the breadth of binding to multiple serotypes.

Eliciting Neutralizing Antibodies through Antigen Design

Although much focus has been directed at engineering antibodies with desired properties, recent work has targeted the opposite side of the problem: engineering an antigen that can elicit a desired antibody in an effective and reproducible manner. This comes with the ultimate goal of the rational design of antigens to be used in vaccination that can elicit antibodies targeting a precise, conserved, and neutralizing epitope. Giles et al. attempted to create a broadly reactive antigen by identifying divergent sequences between different clades of influenza hemagglutinin and clustering the consensus sequences. In this way they created a compromise antigen, incorporating elements of various clades designed to elicit antibodies binding all of them (59). This strategy was validated with the finding that the broadly reactive antigen was capable of eliciting greater antibody breadth than a polyvalent virus-like particle displaying the native antigens (60). Wu et al. pursued a similar goal, instead using HIV surface protein gp120 as the antigen. This group used computational design to engineer a modified gp120 that maintained the structure of the neutralizing portion of the molecule while eliminating other antigenic regions that may elicit non-neutralizing antibodies (61). Since the antigenic region of gp120 they targeted was the CD4 binding site, a highly conserved region among divergent HIV strains, they used this engineered antigen as a vaccine to elicit broadly neutralizing antibodies and successfully identified two novel antibodies with a high level of breadth of reactivity (61).

Epitope Grafting To Elicit Neutralizing Antibodies

A complementary task to antigen design is so-called epitope grafting—removing an epitope from its native antigen and grafting it onto a protein structure that can present it to immune receptors in a way that maximizes the immune response. This design task encompasses several unique challenges, the most difficult of which is the selection of an appropriate peptide onto which the epitope can be placed, known as the scaffold. This scaffold must maintain the native conformation of the desired epitope and have minimal immunogenicity in its off-epitope regions, all while maintaining favorable biophysical properties. Advances in scaffold selection and design have made this problem tractable and have shown promise in immunization.

Early work in this field focused on placing a neutralizing linear epitope on a stable scaffold that could maintain the native conformation while enhancing presentation of this epitope. HIV has been widely used as a test case, since there are well-characterized broadly neutralizing antibodies with high-resolution crystal structures available (62). Two independent groups were able to graft the linear epitopes of two broadly neutralizing anti-HIV antibodies, 4E10 and 2F5, onto scaffolds to enhance their presentation and affinity for the desired antibodies (63, 65). These groups used similar approaches of searching the PDB for scaffolds with a region of backbone conformation with high structural similarity to the epitope and using Rosetta Design to place epitope side chains onto the backbone scaffold and minimize the energy of side chain packing. This protocol resulted in several designed peptides with nanomolar affinity for their respective antibody targets and the ability to elicit broadly neutralizing sera upon immunization (63–65). These earlier studies provided an important proof-of-principle for vaccine-based antigen design.

One major limitation of initial reports on epitope grafting is the nature of the scaffold selection process. Since it relies on placing epitope side chains on a backbone with a high degree of similarity to the epitope backbone, success is highly dependent on the presence of a suitable scaffold among structurally determined proteins. In cases where there is no template with structural similarity, this procedure is ineffective. To address this concern, Azoitei et al. published a backbone grafting method wherein they select a structurally similar template and, rather than transfer individual epitope side chains to a template, remove the epitope-mimetic region en masse and transplant the entire epitope backbone region from the native antigen (66). This protocol was benchmarked and shown to produce peptides with higher affinity than the previously described side-chain grafting method, with the added advantage that backbone grafting can be applied to templates with lower structural similarity.

Another challenge in the pursuit of a generalizable epitope grafting method is that initial reports focused on linear, continuous epitopes, even though many neutralizing epitopes are discontinuous. Azoitei et al. developed a more aggressive scaffold search and design method to identify scaffolds that can accommodate multiple discontinuous epitope peptides while maintaining their conformations and relative orientations and minimizing steric clashes (67). The result of this protocol was an epitope scaffold that accurately recapitulates the conformation of the epitope and interactions necessary for antibody-antigen interactions. McLellan et al. pursued a similar strategy to create a discontinuous epitope-presenting scaffold with a respiratory syncytial virus (RSV) epitope (68). In addition to the selection of an appropriate scaffold, there has also been work in redesigning a scaffold to reduce unwanted, nonepitope immunogenicity. Correia et al. showed that epitope scaffolds can be further optimized by flexible backbone remodeling and resurfacing to enhance thermostability, increase binding affinity, and reduce immune reactivity (64).

To circumvent the problem of scaffold selection, Correia et al. recently described a method to build a *de novo* scaffold for optimal epitope presentation of an RSV epitope (42). They selected a three-helix bundle as a template topology and used extensive rounds of sequence optimization and minimization to create an optimized conformation for presentation. These scaffolds were purified and shown to be thermodynamically stable, with affinities in the picomolar range (42). The purified scaffolds were then used to immunize macaques and were shown to induce neutralizing titers comparable to natural RSV infection, a significant landmark for the epitope-grafting methodology.

CONCLUSION

Computational approaches to predict the structure of antibodies and antibody-antigen complexes are of critical importance, as the large number of naturally occurring antibodies restricts experimental characterization to the most important cases. While computational methods are already sufficiently accurate to be useful, it remains a focus of future research to develop better sampling methods and more accurate energy functions. The existing limitations in modeling antibodies make computational methods most useful when applied in a tight feedback loop with experimental data, a situation that is expected to continue for the foreseeable future. The increasing throughput in methods to collect limited experimental data on antibodies and antibody-antigen complexes will further increase the need for computational methods to add atomic detail not present in these datasets. The rapidly increasing availability of high-resolution crystal structures of antibodies and antibody-antigen complexes is expected to improve computational prediction algorithms, for example, through increasing the accuracy of knowledge-based potentials and through further completing the conformational clusters of CDR loop conformations. Ultimately, the reliable computational design of antibodies that recognize a target epitope is a long-term goal for computational structural biology. Given the even larger number of theoretically possible antibody sequences, computational prioritization of the ones to characterize

experimentally is imperative. Computational design of the tightest or most broadly neutralizing antibodies is not only important for the development of optimal therapeutic antibodies or the development of vaccines. Antibody design is also the most stringent test of our understanding of the rules that govern antibody structure and interaction.

ACKNOWLEDGMENT

Conflicts of interest: We disclose no conflicts.

CITATION

Sevy AM, Meiler J. 2014. Antibodies: computer-aided prediction of structure and design of function. Microbiol Spectrum 2(6):AID-0024-2014.

REFERENCES

1. **Harris LJ, Larson SB, Hasel KW, McPherson A.** 1997. Refined structure of an intact IgG2a monoclonal antibody. *Biochemistry* **36**:1581–1597.
2. **Chothia C, Lesk AM.** 1987. Canonical structures for the hypervariable regions of immunoglobulins. *J Mol Biol* **196**:901–917.
3. **Martin AC, Thornton JM.** 1996. Structural families in loops of homologous proteins: automatic classification, modelling and application to antibodies. *J Mol Biol* **263**:800–815.
4. **Al-Lazikani B, Lesk AM, Chothia C.** 1997. Standard conformations for the canonical structures of immunoglobulins. *J Mol Biol* **273**:927–948.
5. **North B, Lehmann A, Dunbrack RL Jr.** 2011. A new clustering of antibody CDR loop conformations. *J Mol Biol* **406**:228–256.
6. **Briney BS, Willis JR, Crowe JE Jr.** 2012. Location and length distribution of somatic hypermutation-associated DNA insertions and deletions reveals regions of antibody structural plasticity. *Genes Immun* **13**:523–529.
7. **Morea V, Tramontano A, Rustici M, Chothia C, Lesk AM.** 1998. Conformations of the third hypervariable region in the VH domain of immunoglobulins. *J Mol Biol* **275**:269–294.
8. **Kuroda D, Shirai H, Kobori M, Nakamura H.** 2008. Structural classification of CDR-H3 revisited: a lesson in antibody modeling. *Proteins* **73**:608–620.
9. **Sivasubramanian A, Sircar A, Chaudhury S, Gray JJ.** 2009. Toward high-resolution homology

modeling of antibody Fv regions and application to antibody-antigen docking. *Proteins* **74**:497–514.

10. **Zhu K, Day T.** 2013. *Ab initio* structure prediction of the antibody hypervariable H3 loop. *Proteins* **81**:1081–1089.

11. **Teplyakov A, Luo J, Obmolova G, Malia TJ, Sweet R, Stanfield RL, Kodangattil S, Almagro JC, Gilliland GL.** 2014. Second antibody modeling assessment. II. Structures and models. *Proteins* **82**:1563–1582. doi:10.1002/prot.24554.

12. **Almagro JC, Beavers MP, Hernandez-Guzman F, Maier J, Shaulsky J, Butenhof K, Labute P, Thorsteinson N, Kelly K, Teplyakov A, Luo J, Sweet R, Gilliland GL.** 2011. Antibody modeling assessment. *Proteins* **79**:3050–3066.

13. **Narayanan A, Sellers BD, Jacobson MP.** 2009. Energy-based analysis and prediction of the orientation between light- and heavy-chain antibody variable domains. *J Mol Biol* **388**:941–953.

14. **Marcatili P, Rosi A, Tramontano A.** 2008. PIGS: automatic prediction of antibody structures. *Bioinformatics* **24**:1953–1954.

15. **Whitelegg NR, Rees AR.** 2000. WAM: an improved algorithm for modelling antibodies on the WEB. *Protein Eng* **13**:819–824.

16. **Maier JKY, Labute P.** 2014. Assessment of fully automated antibody homology modeling protocols in MOE. *Proteins* **82**:1599–1610.

17. **Sircar A, Kim ET, Gray JJ.** 2009. Rosetta-Antibody: antibody variable region homology modeling server. *Nucleic Acids Res* **37**:W474–W479.

18. **Almagro JC, Teplyakov A, Luo J, Sweet RW, Kodangattil S, Hernandez-Guzman F, Gilliland GL.** 2014. Second antibody modeling assessment (AMA-II). *Proteins* **82**:1553–1562.

19. **Sundberg EJ, Urrutia M, Braden BC, Isern J, Tsuchiya D, Fields BA, Malchiodi EL, Tormo J, Schwarz FP, Mariuzza RA.** 2000. Estimation of the hydrophobic effect in an antigen-antibody protein-protein interface. *Biochemistry* **39**:15375–15387.

20. **Moreira IS, Fernandes PA, Ramos MJ.** 2007. Hot spot computational identification: application to the complex formed between the hen egg white lysozyme (HEL) and the antibody HyHEL-10. *Int J Quantum Chem* **107**:299–310.

21. **Wang X, Singh SK, Kumar S.** 2010. Potential aggregation-prone regions in complementarity-determining regions of antibodies and their contribution towards antigen recognition: a computational analysis. *Pharm Res* **27**:1512–1529.

22. **Vajda S.** 2005. Classification of protein complexes based on docking difficulty. *Proteins* **60**:176–180.

23. **Brenke R, Hall DR, Chuang GY, Comeau SR, Bohnuud T, Beglov D, Schueler-Furman O, Vajda S, Kozakov D.** 2012. Application of asymmetric statistical potentials to antibody-protein docking. *Bioinformatics* **28**:2608–2614.

24. **Gray JJ, Moughon S, Wang C, Schueler-Furman O, Kuhlman B, Rohl CA, Baker D.** 2003. Protein-protein docking with simultaneous optimization of rigid-body displacement and side-chain conformations. *J Mol Biol* **331**:281–299.

25. **Sircar A, Gray JJ.** 2010. SnugDock: paratope structural optimization during antibody-antigen docking compensates for errors in antibody homology models. *PLoS Comput Biol* **6**:e1000644. doi:10.1371/journal.pcbi.1000644.

26. **Simonelli L, Beltramello M, Yudina Z, Macagno A, Calzolai L, Varani L.** 2010. Rapid structural characterization of human antibody-antigen complexes through experimentally validated computational docking. *J Mol Biol* **396**:1491–1507.

27. **Sevy AM, Healey JF, Deng W, Spiegel PC, Meeks SL, Li R.** 2013. Epitope mapping of inhibitory antibodies targeting the C2 domain of coagulation factor VIII by hydrogen-deuterium exchange mass spectrometry. *J Thromb Haemost* **11**:2128–2136.

28. **Coales SJ, Tuske SJ, Tornasso JC, Hamuro Y.** 2009. Epitope mapping by amide hydrogen/deuterium exchange coupled with immobilization of antibody, on-line proteolysis, liquid chromatography and mass spectrometry. *Rapid Commun Mass Spectrom* **23**:639–647.

29. **Meeks SL, Healey JF, Parker ET, Barrow RT, Lollar P.** 2007. Antihuman factor VIIIC2 domain antibodies in hemophilia A mice recognize a functionally complex continuous spectrum of epitopes dominated by inhibitors of factor VIII activation. *Blood* **110**:4234–4242.

30. **Chaves RC, Teulon JM, Odorico M, Parot P, Chen SWW, Pellequer JL.** 2013. Conformational dynamics of individual antibodies using computational docking and AFM. *J Mol Recognit* **26**:596–604.

31. **Gogolinska A, Nowak W.** 2013. Molecular basis of lateral force spectroscopy nano-diagnostics: computational unbinding of autism related chemokine MCP-1 from IgG antibody. *J Mol Model* **19**:4773–4780.

32. **Sharon J, Rynkiewicz MJ, Lu ZH, Yang CY.** 2014. Discovery of protective B-cell epitopes for development of antimicrobial vaccines and antibody therapeutics. *Immunology* **142**:1–23.

33. **Thornburg NJ, Nannemann DP, Blum DL, Belser JA, Tumpey TM, Deshpande S, Fritz GA, Sapparapu G, Krause JC, Lee JH, Ward AB, Lee DE, Li S, Winarski KL, Spiller BW, Meiler J, Crowe JE Jr.** 2013. Human antibodies that neutralize respiratory droplet transmissible H5N1 influenza viruses. *J Clin Invest* **123**:4405–4409.

34. McKinney BA, Kallewaard NL, Crowe JE Jr, Meiler J. 2007. Using the natural evolution of a rotavirus-specific human monoclonal antibody to predict the complex topography of a viral antigenic site. *Immunome Res* **3**:8.

35. Schneider S, Zacharias M. 2012. Atomic resolution model of the antibody Fc interaction with the complement C1q component. *Mol Immunol* **51**:66–72.

36. Percy AJ, Rey M, Burns KM, Schriemer DC. 2012. Probing protein interactions with hydrogen/deuterium exchange and mass spectrometry: a review. *Anal Chim Acta* **721**:7–21.

37. Baerga-Ortiz A, Hughes CA, Mandell JG, Komives EA. 2002. Epitope mapping of a monoclonal antibody against human thrombin by R/D-exchange mass spectrometry reveals selection of a diverse sequence in a highly conserved protein. *Protein Sci* **11**:1300–1308.

38. Aiyegbo MS, Sapparapu G, Spiller BW, Eli IM, Williams DR, Kim R, Lee DE, Liu T, Li S, Woods VL Jr, Nannemann DP, Meiler J, Stewart PL, Crowe JE Jr. 2013. Human rotavirus VP6-specific antibodies mediate intracellular neutralization by binding to a quaternary structure in the transcriptional pore. *PLoS One* **8**:e61101. doi:10.1371/journal.pone.0061101.

39. Bublil EM, Yeger-Azuz S, Gershoni JM. 2006. Computational prediction of the cross-reactive neutralizing epitope corresponding to the monoclonal antibody b12 specific for HIV-1 gp120. *FASEB J* **20**:1762–1774.

40. Chuang GY, Acharya P, Schmidt SD, Yang Y, Louder MK, Zhou T, Kwon YD, Pancera M, Bailer RT, Doria-Rose NA, Nussenzweig MC, Mascola JR, Kwong PD, Georgiev IS. 2013. Residue-level prediction of HIV-1 antibody epitopes based on neutralization of diverse viral strains. *J Virol* **87**:10047–10058.

41. Chuang GY, Liou D, Kwong PD, Georgiev IS. 2014. NEP: web server for epitope prediction based on antibody neutralization of viral strains with diverse sequences. *Nucleic Acids Res* **42**:W64–W71.

42. Correia BE, Bates JT, Loomis RJ, Baneyx G, Carrico C, Jardine JG, Rupert P, Correnti C, Kalyuzhniy O, Vittal V, Connell MJ, Stevens E, Schroeter A, Chen M, Macpherson S, Serra AM, Adachi Y, Holmes MA, Li Y, Klevit RE, Graham BS, Wyatt RT, Baker D, Strong RK, Crowe JE Jr, Johnson PR, Schief WR. 2014. Proof of principle for epitope-focused vaccine design. *Nature* **507**:201–206.

43. Hinton PR, Johlfs MG, Xiong JM, Hanestad K, Ong KC, Bullock C, Keller S, Tang MT, Tso JY, Vasquez M, Tsurushita N. 2004. Engineered human IgG antibodies with longer serum half-lives in primates. *J Biol Chem* **279**:6213–6216.

44. Igawa T, Tsunoda H, Tachibana T, Maeda A, Mimoto F, Moriyama C, Nanami M, Sekimori Y, Nabuchi Y, Aso Y, Hattori K. 2010. Reduced elimination of IgG antibodies by engineering the variable region. *Protein Eng Des Sel* **23**:385–392.

45. Kanduc D, Lucchese A, Mittelman A. 2001. Individuation of monoclonal anti-HPV16 E7 antibody linear peptide epitope by computational biology. *Peptides* **22**:1981–1985.

46. Tsurushita N, Hinton PR, Kumar S. 2005. Design of humanized antibodies: from anti-Tac to Zenapax. *Methods* **36**:69–83.

47. Teng G, Papavasiliou FN. 2007. Immunoglobulin somatic hypermutation. *Annu Rev Genet* **41**:107–120.

48. Filpula D. 2007. Antibody engineering and modification technologies. *Biomol Eng* **24**:201–215.

49. Pantazes RJ, Maranas CD. 2010. OptCDR: a general computational method for the design of antibody complementarity determining regions for targeted epitope binding. *Protein Eng Des Sel* **23**:849–858.

50. Leaver-Fay A, Jacak R, Stranges PB, Kuhlman B. 2011. A generic program for multistate protein design. *PLoS One* **6**:e20937. doi:10.1371/journal.pone.0020937.

51. Havranek JJ, Harbury PB. 2003. Automated design of specificity in molecular recognition. *Nat Struct Biol* **10**:45–52.

52. Willis JR, Briney BS, DeLuca SL, Crowe JE Jr, Meiler J. 2013. Human germline antibody gene segments encode polyspecific antibodies. *PLoS Comput Biol* **9**:e1003045. doi:10.1371/journal.pcbi.1003045.

53. Babor M, Kortemme T. 2009. Multi-constraint computational design suggests that native sequences of germline antibody H3 loops are nearly optimal for conformational flexibility. *Proteins* **75**:846–858.

54. Clark LA, Boriack-Sjodin PA, Eldredge J, Fitch C, Friedman B, Hanf KJ, Jarpe M, Liparoto SF, Li Y, Lugovskoy A, Miller S, Rushe M, Sherman W, Simon K, Van Vlijmen H. 2006. Affinity enhancement of an *in vivo* matured therapeutic antibody using structure-based computational design. *Protein Sci* **15**:949–960.

55. Lippow SM, Wittrup KD, Tidor B. 2007. Computational design of antibody-affinity improvement beyond *in vivo* maturation. *Nat Biotechnol* **25**:1171–1176.

56. Farady CJ, Sellers BD, Jacobson MP, Craik CS. 2009. Improving the species cross-reactivity of an antibody using computational design. *Bioorg Med Chem Lett* **19**:3744–3747.

57. Barderas R, Desmet J, Timmerman P, Meloen R, Casal JI. 2008. Affinity maturation of antibodies assisted by *in silico* modeling. *Proc Natl Acad Sci USA* **105**:9029–9034.

58. **Simonelli L, Pedotti M, Beltramello M, Livoti E, Calzolai L, Sallusto F, Lanzavecchia A, Varani L.** 2013. Rational engineering of a human anti-dengue antibody through experimentally validated computational docking. *PloS One* **8**: e55561. doi:10.1371/journal.pone.0055561.

59. **Giles BM, Ross TM.** 2011. A computationally optimized broadly reactive antigen (COBRA) based H5N1 VLP vaccine elicits broadly reactive antibodies in mice and ferrets. *Vaccine* **29**:3043–3054.

60. **Giles BM, Bissel SJ, DeAlmeida DR, Wiley CA, Ross TM.** 2012. Antibody breadth and protective efficacy are increased by vaccination with computationally optimized hemagglutinin but not with polyvalent hemagglutinin-based H5N1 virus-like particle vaccines. *Clin Vaccine Immunol* **19**:128–139.

61. **Wu X, Yang ZY, Li Y, Hogerkorp CM, Schief WR, Seaman MS, Zhou T, Schmidt SD, Wu L, Xu L, Longo NS, McKee K, O'Dell S, Louder MK, Wycuff DL, Feng Y, Nason M, Doria-Rose N, Connors M, Kwong PD, Roederer M, Wyatt RT, Nabel GJ, Mascola JR.** 2010. Rational design of envelope identifies broadly neutralizing human monoclonal antibodies to HIV-1. *Science* **329**:856–861.

62. **Stamatatos L, Morris L, Burton DR, Mascola JR.** 2009. Neutralizing antibodies generated during natural HIV-1 infection: good news for an HIV-1 vaccine? *Nat Med* **15**:866–870.

63. **Correia BE, Ban YE, Holmes MA, Xu H, Ellingson K, Kraft Z, Carrico C, Boni E, Sather DN, Zenobia C, Burke KY, Bradley-Hewitt T, Bruhn-Johannsen JF, Kalyuzhniy O, Baker D, Strong RK, Stamatatos L, Schief WR.** 2010. Computational design of epitope-scaffolds allows induction of antibodies specific for a poorly immunogenic HIV vaccine epitope. *Structure* **18**:1116–1126.

64. **Correia BE, Ban YE, Friend DJ, Ellingson K, Xu H, Boni E, Bradley-Hewitt T, Bruhn-Johannsen JF, Stamatatos L, Strong RK, Schief WR.** 2010. Computational protein design using flexible backbone remodeling and resurfacing: case studies in structure-based antigen design. *J Mol Biol* [Epub ahead of print.] doi:10.1016/j.jmb.2010.09.061.

65. **Ofek G, Guenaga FJ, Schief WR, Skinner J, Baker D, Wyatt R, Kwong PD.** 2010. Elicitation of structure-specific antibodies by epitope scaffolds. *Proc Natl Acad Sci USA* **107**: 17880–17887.

66. **Azoitei ML, Ban YE, Julien JP, Bryson S, Schroeter A, Kalyuzhniy O, Porter JR, Adachi Y, Baker D, Pai EF, Schief WR.** 2012. Computational design of high-affinity epitope scaffolds by backbone grafting of a linear epitope. *J Mol Biol* **415**:175–192.

67. **Azoitei ML, Correia BE, Ban YE, Carrico C, Kalyuzhniy O, Chen L, Schroeter A, Huang PS, McLellan JS, Kwong PD, Baker D, Strong RK, Schief WR.** 2011. Computation-guided backbone grafting of a discontinuous motif onto a protein scaffold. *Science* **334**:373–376.

68. **McLellan JS, Pancera M, Carrico C, Gorman J, Julien JP, Khayat R, Louder R, Pejchal R, Sastry M, Dai K, O'Dell S, Patel N, Shahzad-ul-Hussan S, Yang Y, Zhang B, Zhou T, Zhu J, Boyington JC, Chuang GY, Diwanji D, Georgiev I, Kwon YD, Lee D, Louder MK, Moquin S, Schmidt SD, Yang ZY, Bonsignori M, Crump JA, Kapiga SH, Sam NE, Haynes BF, Burton DR, Koff WC, Walker LM, Phogat S, Wyatt R, Orwenyo J, Wang LX, Arthos J, Bewley CA, Mascola JR, Nabel GJ, Schief WR, Ward AB, Wilson IA, Kwong PD.** 2011. Structure of HIV-1 gp120 V1/V2 domain with broadly neutralizing antibody PG9. *Nature* **480**:336–343.

PATHOGEN-SPECIFIC ANTIBODIES

Antibodies Targeting the Envelope of HIV-1

11

LUZIA M. MAYR[1] and SUSAN ZOLLA-PAZNER[2,3]

INTRODUCTION

HIV continues to be a major global public health issue, with an estimated 35 million people living with the virus and more than 2 million new infections occurring yearly (1). As part of the natural immune response, antibodies (Abs) exert immune pressure on HIV and play a key role both in controlling the virus and in driving escape mutations in the viral envelope glycoproteins. Therefore, and because the elicitation of Abs is believed to be crucial for an effective vaccine against HIV, Abs targeting HIV have been the focus of intense research in the past years.

ANTIBODY RESPONSE TO HIV

Upon infection with HIV, a strong Ab response occurs in essentially all infected individuals. These Abs are directed against several viral proteins, including the gp120 and gp41 envelope proteins that are found on the surface of the virus particles. While in many viral diseases, such as influenza and polio, the Abs against surface antigens can establish protective

[1]INSERM U1109, Université de Strasbourg, 67000 Strasbourg, France; [2]New York Veterans Affairs Harbor Healthcare System, New York, NY 10010; [3]New York University School of Medicine, New York, NY 10016.
Antibodies for Infectious Diseases
Edited by James E. Crowe, Jr., Diana Boraschi, and Rino Rappuoli
© 2015 American Society for Microbiology, Washington, DC
doi:10.1128/microbiolspec.AID-0025-2014

immunity, many HIV envelope-specific Abs have little neutralizing capacity due to the many complex escape mechanisms employed by the surface viral glycoproteins that occur as sparse trimeric spikes in the virus envelope (2). These virus escape mechanisms include the following.

Glycan Shield

One of the reasons why HIV is a difficult target for Abs that prevent infection is the dense glycosylation of the envelope proteins gp120 and gp41. With approximately 25 N-linked glycosylation sites, gp120 is one of the most heavily glycosylated viral proteins described. These glycans are large, complex carbohydrate structures that shield vulnerable epitopes on the surface of HIV, leading to viral escape from Abs (3). The function of glycans can be demonstrated by the removal of certain glycosylation sites, leading to a significant increase in neutralization sensitivity of the virus (4, 5).

High Mutation Rate

The high mutation rate of HIV-1 is another obstacle for the development of immune protection by neutralizing Abs. With an *in vitro* mutation rate of approximately 2.2×10^{-5} to 5.4×10^{-5} per nucleotide base per replication cycle, the virus continuously and rapidly evolves to escape neutralization (6). In an attempt to recognize the mutated virus, neutralizing Abs (nAbs) evolve in tandem with the virus, resulting in successive waves of nAb maturation followed by viral escape. This leads to the phenomenon of nAbs often being able to neutralize virus from months earlier, but not concurrent circulating variants (7–9).

The high mutation rate and the fact that billions of new viral particles are produced daily within each patient leads to an enormous diversity of HIV-1 variants. Based on their sequence, the variants have been divided into nine distinct subtypes, or clades, designated by the letters A, B, C, D, F, G, H, J, and K. Overall, the amino acid sequence of the different subtypes can vary by as much as 30% from one clade to another, but in certain genomic regions the genetic variability can be as high as 42%. Further complicating the HIV landscape are recombinant forms of the virus in which heterologous virus strains combine segments of their genome during reverse transcription to produce genetically divergent new virus forms. Countless recombinants of virtually every virus strain combination have been identified worldwide, and their prevalence differs by geographic regions (10). A protective vaccine will need to induce Abs that target this tremendous viral diversity.

Conformational Masking

The envelope spike is a heterotrimer consisting of three gp120 molecules noncovalently anchored to the viral membrane via three gp41 molecules. In an attempt to shield neutralization-sensitive domains, the elements of the envelope spike adopt a quaternary conformation where domains of neighboring gp120 subunits can interact. For example, it was suggested that in the apex of the three-dimensional envelope spike, intersubunit contact between the V1, V2, and V3 loops occurs, protecting adjacent regions from recognition by Abs (11).

To enter its target cells, HIV must bind sequentially to cellular receptors, including CD4 and one of two chemokine receptors (CXCR4 or CCR5). The regions of gp120 that are involved with binding to these receptors must, therefore, be conserved to maintain the infectious potential of the virus. The CD4 binding site (CD4bs) and chemokine receptor binding sites on gp120 would thus appear to be good targets for Abs; however, while able to bind to some exceptional Abs (9, 12, 13), the CD4bs is partially obscured by glycans and variable regions and undergoes conformational reorganization, allowing it to evade neutralization by conventional CD4bs-specific Abs.

Thus, the virus places an energetic barrier to Ab binding (14).

It is believed that dynamic conformational changes also play a role in masking conserved epitopes on chemokine receptor binding sites (15); regions of gp120 that are involved in binding to the chemokine receptor—the V3 loop and the $\beta20/\beta21$ strands of the bridging sheet—form an exposed surface only after binding to CD4 and are thus exposed to Abs only transiently (16).

TYPES OF ANTIBODIES

Conventional Abs

Abs that commonly occur during HIV infection and that are present in the majority of infected individuals are here defined as "conventional Abs." These Abs do not exhibit unusual structural or genetic characteristics, and their immunoglobulin genes undergo relatively little somatic hypermutation from germline (17, 18). Conventional Abs have long been known to protect against infection in animal systems. This was established with passive immunization of chimpanzees using IgG preparations from the blood of HIV-infected individuals (19). Thus, the proof of principle was established more than two decades ago that Abs alone from unselected HIV-infected individuals could provide sterilizing immunity.

Conventional Abs are elicited as early as two weeks after seroconversion in acutely infected individuals; however, they display very limited neutralization breadth (20): using a standardized reference pseudovirus panel that represents genetically diverse subsets of viruses, conventional Abs targeting gp120 were shown to neutralize up to 50% of tier 1 pseudoviruses, but ≤ 9% of tier 2 pseudoviruses, suggesting that these Abs target epitopes exposed on a minority of viruses and tend to be specific for the virus infecting the host. Conventional neutralizing Abs (nAbs) also have a limited neutralizing potency *in vitro*, and while most tier 1 pseudoviruses

are neutralized with low levels of nAbs (<<1 to 10 μg/ml), often >10 ×g/ml are required to neutralize tier 2 pseudoviruses (21, 22).

The Thai clinical HIV-1 vaccine trial RV144 provided additional support for the role of conventional Abs in protection: high levels of V1V2 and V3 IgG Ab levels, especially those of the IgG3 subclass, were found to be significantly associated with the reduced infection rate (estimated 31% vaccine efficacy) in vaccine recipients (23–28). Monoclonal Abs isolated from the RV144 vaccinees showed very low mutation rates from germline genes encoding the variable region of the heavy chain (VH)—mutation rate range of 1.5 to 4.5% (29, 30), which is even lower than that noted after influenza immunization (mean VH mutation rate of 8.1% [31]). These data further uphold the concept that conventional Abs can be associated with reduced infection rates.

Thus, even though conventional nAbs are limited in their breadth and potency, they are commonly made by HIV-positive individuals (32), by immunized humans (24), and by immunized animals (33, 34), and the previously mentioned studies suggest that they can reduce infection rates. Therefore, such Abs, induced by vaccines, have substantial potential for influencing the course of the HIV epidemic.

Exceptional, Broadly Neutralizing Abs

Unlike conventional HIV Abs, broadly neutralizing Abs (bNAbs) are found in relatively rare HIV-infected subjects (35), with the most broad and potent serum Abs being identified in only ~1% of "elite neutralizers" (36). Most of the broadly neutralizing monoclonal Abs (bNmAbs) have been developed in the last few years (37–41). In addition to wide breadth (neutralization of 100% of tier 1 viruses and 72 to 100% of tier 2 viruses), bNmAbs are very potent, and *in vitro* assays have shown that very small amounts are sufficient for neutralization of tier 1 and tier 2 viruses (<1 μg/ml and 0.02 to 27.0 μg/ml, respectively) (17).

For bNABs to acquire their impressive breadth and potency, extensive somatic hypermutation is required—particularly in the variable heavy chain (VH) genes and in some framework regions—a process that usually requires more than a year of exposure to the virus after HIV infection (42, 43). Several additional unique characteristics of bNmAbs have been described, such as frequent auto- and/or poly-reactivity for host antigens and long heavy chain complementarity-determining region 3 (HCDR3) sequences composed of 20 to 34 residues, which stand in stark contrast to the length of HCDR3s produced by human B cells, which averages 16 residues (44–47). These features contribute to the rarity of bNAbs and pose a major challenge for the development of an HIV-1 vaccine designed to induce such Abs.

While bNmAbs are exceptionally potent and provide protection in animal models (48–51), all attempts to elicit bNAb responses by vaccination have so far been unsuccessful, and it is believed that a panel of special immunogens which will both stimulate suitable naïve B cells and guide them through lineage maturation will be required to achieve this goal (52); this process of Ab maturation appears to be long and complex.

To design these immunogens, bNmAbs from infected donors are being isolated and sequenced to reconstruct the lineage of the Abs, including the sequence of the probable common unmutated ancestor of a given bNmAb. The envelope glycoproteins recognized by the Abs in the bNmAb lineage are being expressed, and these will serve as immunogens to be used sequentially to engage the naïve B cell receptor and to stimulate and guide the evolution of the nAb response (44).

While the ultimate success of this path toward the design of a prophylactic vaccine is unknowable at this point, there is, nevertheless, great potential for the use of bNmAbs for passive immunization to protect against and treat HIV infection. Thus, treatment of macaques with bNmAbs has been shown to completely protect against infection with simian/HIV when these Abs are present at serum concentrations as low as 30 μg/ml (53–55). Broadly neutralizing mAbs are also being developed for treatment of established HIV infection, a process in which bNmAbs will be infused into HIV-infected individuals to decrease and/or eliminate virus. Success has already been achieved in this area as demonstrated by treatment of humanized mice and macaques infected with HIV and simian/HIV, respectively (56–58).

There is also great interest in whether passively transferred bNmAbs can contribute to the prevention of mother-to-child-transmission of HIV-1, the continuing cause of a significant percentage of new infections in the developing world. During pregnancy, HIV-specific Abs can pass from an HIV-infected mother to the fetus through the placenta. These Abs, however, are not effective against later HIV infection, for example, during the breast feeding phase. Moreover, the transmitted virus variants have fewer potential N-linked glycosylation sites, a fact that could impact positively on the interaction of glycan-dependent bNAb with transmitter/founder viruses recognition (59). Indeed, transmitted HIV variants were shown to be susceptible to various bNmAbs, but a combination of potent bNmAbs targeting diverse epitopes might be needed to successfully protect against HIV infection in the mother-to-child-transmission context (60).

VACCINE DEVELOPMENT AND IMMUNOGEN DESIGN

As a result of the extensive data summarized above, the elicitation of Abs is clearly indicated as a requirement for a successful HIV vaccine. As noted, this is a challenging task. The effort to develop vaccine candidates capable of inducing protective Abs has accelerated dramatically since the Thai vaccine trial RV144 revealed that Abs were associated with a reduced rate of infection (24–26, 28).

Several envelope-based immunogens have been tested for their ability to induce nAbs. Monomeric gp120 is relatively easy to produce and has been widely used in animal studies. Initial human vaccine trials elicited only weak nAbs, and no protection against HIV infection was achieved (61, 62). The RV144 vaccine trial, however, demonstrated a beneficial effect of monomeric gp120 in combination with a canarypox prime (63). It was suggested that the epitopes exposed on monomeric gp120 are poor neutralization targets because they are occluded on the native envelope trimer (64), and therefore immunogens were designed that better mimic the native envelope spike. Since the trimeric envelope is highly unstable and difficult to produce, a variety of different immunogens using gp140, the ectodomain of trimeric gp160, have been made (65–67). To date, immunizations using trimeric envelope immunogens have not been successful in the induction of potent nAbs (68, 69). Recent studies, monitoring the coevolution of virus and bNAbs in patients during natural infection, demonstrated that a tight interplay between Ab maturation and subsequent viral escape drives the development of bNAb responses (9, 70, 71). These studies provide important new insights into the elicitation of bNAbs and will advance the development of better immunogens.

Rather than using whole Env monomers or trimers, another approach to vaccine design is the use of recombinant immunogens that target the Ab response to particular epitopes. Computationally designed vaccines that mimic viral and bacterial epitopes have been shown to induce potent conventional protective nAbs against various viruses and bacterial pathogens (72, 73). This same approach is being applied to the design of recombinant vaccines that target specific HIV epitopes. At the present time, the type of epitopes to be targeted by conventional Abs include the glycan-independent V1V2 and V3 regions of the HIV envelope, whereas the type of epitopes to be targeted by bNAbs include

"sites of vulnerability" (74) defined as the glycan-dependent V2 epitope (see "V2q epitope" in the list below), the glycan-dependent epitope at the base of V3, the CD4 binding site in gp120, and the membrane proximal external region (MPER) in gp41.

Abs Targeting Variable Loops 1 and 2 (V1V2)

Electron tomography, cryo-electron microscopy, and biochemical studies have shown that the V1V2 domain is localized at the apex of the trimeric HIV-1 Env structures, and therefore at least some of the V1V2 epitopes are accessible to Abs (75, 76). V2 loop sequences differ in length, but the majority of amino acids are highly conserved, suggesting conserved structural elements (77). The V1V2 region forms four antiparallel β-strands (A, B, C, and D) which are linked via disulfide bonds (78). Via a conserved tripeptide, the ^{179}LDV/I^{181} binding motif, V2 can bind to $\alpha4\beta7$, an integrin expressed on activated CD4$^+$ T cells that is required for the homing of CD4$^+$ T cells to the gut mucosa (79).

Abs targeting the V1V2 region were associated with a lower risk of infection in the RV144 clinical vaccine trial, thus making this area a promising target for vaccine development and the focus of intense research (24–26). To date, three different epitope types have been defined in the V1V2 region:

V2i epitope. A group of seven human mAbs recognizes a conformation-dependent epitope, designated V2i since these Abs target the disordered region in V2 that connects the C and D strands and includes the $\alpha4\beta7$-integrin binding site (hence the term "V2i") (80, 81). The structure of this region has so far not been solved, suggesting that it is highly flexible and dynamic. Abs targeting V2i are highly cross-reactive in binding to monomeric gp120 but do not neutralize HIV well (18), suggesting that the epitope is mostly occluded from Ab recognition in the trimeric envelope.

V2p epitope. This epitope is defined by two mAbs (CH58 and CH59) that were isolated from an RV144 vaccinee. The epitope is glycan-independent, and these mAbs bind V2 peptides (thus, "V2p") and selected monomeric gp120, recognizing an epitope composed of helical or helical-coil structures in the C strand of V1V2 (30, 82).

V2q epitope. This is a quaternary epitope, which is preferentially expressed on the trimeric structure of the gp120 spike. Crystallographic studies with a V1V2-fusion protein show that broad and potently neutralizing V2q mAbs bind to relatively conserved residues within V2 as well as to N-linked glycans—most importantly the N160 glycan. Earlier studies also showed that the binding of V2q-specific mAbs was influenced by residues in V3 (37, 83, 84). V2q-specific bNmAbs, including PG9, PG16, and CH01, are extremely potent and broad in their reactivity and have long CDRH3 loops that interact with N-linked glycans and reach around them to contact amino acids of V2. These V2q mAbs are highly mutated from germline (44).

Abs Targeting Variable Loop 3 (V3)

The V3 loop is located in close proximity to the V1V2 domain at the apex of the envelope trimer (85) and is involved in CCR5 or CXCR4 coreceptor tropism and binding. It thus plays an important role in virus entry into the host cell, and it is required for infectivity since V3-deleted mutants are noninfectious (86).

While, by definition, there is considerable amino acid sequence variation in V3, about 60% of the amino acids are conserved, and the variation occurs at restricted positions (87, 88). The region is characterized by a conserved length of 34 to 35 amino acids, the presence of N-linked glycosyla-

tion sites at its N- and C-terminal ends, and several conserved structural features. The V3 loop can be divided into three structural regions: (i) a base region that is located in the gp120 core and includes a disulfide bond, (ii) a flexible stem region, and (iii) a distal crown that contains the highly conserved GPGR/Q motif at its tip. The recognition of conserved V3 elements contributes to the broad cross-reactivity of V3-specific Abs (89, 90).

V3 Abs are present in essentially all infected individuals (91), and V3 Abs have been elicited by several types of vaccines (4, 92, 93). Moreover, the first demonstration of the successful use of "reverse vaccinology," i.e., the design of vaccines based on epitopes recognized by biologically active mAbs, was achieved using V3-scaffold immunogens which targeted the immune response to this single epitope of the HIV envelope. For this, the V3 loop was spliced into a conformationally correct site on the highly immunogenic protein, cholera toxin subunit B, a protein which forms a pentameric structure and therefore presents five copies of V3 (94), serving as a particularly strong antigen for induction of Abs (95). High anti-V3 Ab titers were elicited in rabbits with one or a combination of V3-cholera toxin subunit B immunogens, and these immune sera were able to neutralize numerous diverse HIV strains (33, 94).

Just as Abs to V2 target three regions (V2i, V2p, and V2q), three types of V3 Abs have been described.

Glycan-independent "ladle-like" V3 Abs

The V3 crown is an immunodominant region, and Abs targeting the epitopes in the crown are made by essentially all HIV-infected individuals (91). Abs to this region are glycan-independent. The ladle-like anti-V3 mAbs bind to the tip of the V3 crown which sits in the "bowl" of the ladle while the N-terminal V3 beta-strand adheres to the "handle" of the ladle. Representative mAbs of this type include 447-52D, where the long CDRH3 forms the handle of the ladle that interacts with the main chain of the N-terminal beta-chain of the V3 crown.

Glycan-independent "cradle-like" V3 Abs

The second type of V3 Ab uses an antigen-binding mode typified by mAb 2557. In such cradle-like Abs the antigen binding site consists of a groove in the Fab fragment, and the epitope lies in this groove, resembling a baby in a cradle; in this case, the major binding site is the hydrophobic core of the V3 crown, usually composed of hydrophobic, conserved residues 307, 309, and 317 (89, 96, 97).

Both types of glycan-independent Abs specific for the V3 crown can neutralize most laboratory-adapted HIV-1 strains and tier 1 viruses but neutralize relatively few tier 2 viruses using standard neutralization assays (21, 98, 99). This is largely due to masking of the V3 loop by glycans (100) and by the V1V2 domain that is situated atop the trimer. Deletion of V1V2 leads to a better exposure of V3 epitopes and thus better neutralization by V3 mAbs (101, 102). Importantly, it was recently shown that anti-V3 Abs are effective against tier 2 viruses if the Ab and virus are coincubated for several hours rather than for 1 to 2 hours, which is the norm in standard neutralization assays (103). These results suggest that the V3 loop is meta-stable on the virus surface, flickering between a cryptic and exposed conformation, the latter being both required for interaction with the chemokine receptor and available for Ab binding leading to neutralization. Additionally, CD4 binding induces a conformational change in gp120, releasing the V3 crown from the surface of the envelope trimer and thus augmenting V3 epitope exposure and sensitivity to V3 Ab neutralization (90).

Glycan-dependent V3 Abs

The base of V3 is poorly immunogenic, eliciting Abs in a relatively small proportion of infected individuals. Nonetheless, mAbs that target this region, such as the PGT121-like and the PGT128-like Ab families, are extremely potent and broadly reactive. These mAbs are highly somatically mutated and require specific glycan interactions, particularly at position N332 (38, 104). The crystal structure of PGT128 in complex with an engineered outer domain of gp120 recently showed that this Ab also interacts with the N301 oligomannose glycan, a position that is not recognized by PGT121-like Abs (104). Even though the two Ab families are suggested to approach gp120 from different angles, both block HIV-1 infection by interfering with CD4 binding through allosteric mechanisms (105).

Abs Targeting the CD4 Binding Site (CD4bs)

The CD4bs is functionally highly conserved and thus seems to be an ideal target for Abs. However, it is well hidden by surrounding glycans and variable regions (74), and Abs are obstructed from binding due to steric and conformational hindrance (see section on conformational masking, above). Studies have shown that many CD4bs mAbs can bind with high affinity to recombinant gp120 but cannot access the CD4bs on the envelope trimer. The mAb b12 was the first neutralizing mAb discovered to successfully target the CD4bs, but its breadth and potency are restricted due to amino acid variation both within and outside of the CD4bs (44, 106, 107).

More recently, several bNmAbs have been isolated that mimic binding of CD4 to gp120 and as a result neutralize HIV-1 potently and with broad reactivity. These CD4bs-specific bNmAbs, isolated from various HIV-infected individuals, share several genetic and structural characteristics. First, their heavy chains all derive from the VH1-2 or the closely related VH1-46 germline genes. These Abs are also highly somatically mutated, with ~20 to 30% of nucleotide changes in their heavy chains compared to germline. However, attempts to induce these CD4bs bNAbs have been problematic, even using "engineered gp120" and recombinant "designer immunogens" modeled on the structure of the epitopes contacted by the very effective bNmAbs (108–110). Cross-clade nAbs were induced in rabbits via the reverse vaccinology approach. Immunogens were designed based on the epitope recognized by the mAb IgG1b12. Thus, fragments of gp120 containing 70% of the b12 epitope were used for priming of rabbits. The animals received a boost with full-length gp120 after 16 and 51 weeks. Cross-clade neutralizing HIV-specific Abs were elicited in the rabbits, which neutralized tier 1, 2, and 3 viruses (111), providing a maximum geometric mean of IC50 titers against five tier 2 and 3 viruses of 1:134.

Abs Targeting the Membrane-Proximal External Region (MPER)

The MPER consists of the last 24 C-terminal amino acids of the gp41 ectodomain. Its sequence is highly conserved, contains many hydrophobic residues, and is usually rich in tryptophans. It is believed that the MPER undergoes significant conformational changes during viral entry (112–114).

Different epitopes have been described in the MPER: the very potent human mAb 10E8 recognizes an α-helix in this region, while other human mAbs, including 2F5 and 4E10, target an overlapping region that additionally includes residues of the transmembrane spanning domain. As opposed to mAbs 2F5 and 4E10, bNmAb 10E8 can neutralize ~95% of viruses tested and lacks detectable reactivity with self-antigens, a feature of the less potent 2F5 and 4E10 (40, 44).

Like the bNAbs targeting gp120, bNAbs specific for the MPER of gp41 have been extremely difficult to induce with vaccines (115). They are present in only a minority of HIV-infected individuals (35, 116), suggesting that this is a poorly immunogenic region. This is supported by the finding that MPER mAbs such as 2F5 and 4E10 appear to mimic self antigens, and therefore the responses of B cells with MPER specificity are down-modulated (46).

CONCLUSIONS

Three decades of study have established the important role of Abs in protecting against HIV infection. However, it has become quite clear that HIV uses many mechanisms to protect itself from the biologic effects of Abs that would block infectivity. Design of an effective vaccine must take into account the presence of glycans and masking phenomena to induce Abs that can penetrate or circumvent these protective shields employed by the virion. Current immunogen design is affected profoundly by whether the aim is to induce conventional Abs or exceptional broadly neutralizing Abs. Induction of exceptional Abs with a vaccine may require the use of a series of immunogens that "guide" the immune response through the mutations required for the specificities displayed by broad and potent neutralizing Abs. However desirable this goal is, whether it is achievable has yet to be established. Alternatively, conventional Abs, while not as broad or as potent as exceptional Abs have already been elicited by vaccine trials and are correlated with a reduced rate of infection in the RV144 phase III clinical vaccine trial. Induction of conventional protective Abs is therefore possible. The vaccine regimens and reagents to be used in vaccine development are many, ranging from DNA and viral vector priming immunogens to proteins representing the trimeric envelope proteins or portions thereof spliced onto immunogenic scaffolds. Many more clinical trials for safety, immunogenicity, and protection are required to establish which of these many regimens and reagents will result in a prophylactic vaccine.

ACKNOWLEDGMENT

Conflicts of interest: We disclose no conflicts.

CITATION

Mayr LM, Zolla-Pazner S. 2015. Antibodies targeting the envelope of HIV-1. Microbiol Spectrum 3(1):AID-0025-2014.

REFERENCES

1. UNAIDS. 2013. *UNAIDS report on the global AIDS epidemic.* http://www.unaids.org/sites/default/files/en/media/unaids/contentassets/documents/epidemiology/2013/gr2013/UNAIDS_Global_Report_2013_cn.pdf.
2. **Mascola JR, Montefiori DC.** 2003. HIV-1: nature's master of disguise. *Nat Med* **9:**393–394.
3. **Wei X, Decker JM, Wang S, Hui H, Kappes JC, Wu X, Salazar-Gonzalez JF, Salazar MG, Kilby JM, Saag MS, Komarova NL, Nowak MA, Hahn BH, Kwong PD, Shaw GM.** 2003. Antibody neutralization and escape by HIV-1. *Nature* **422:**307–312.
4. **Kumar R, Tuen M, Liu J, Nadas A, Pan R, Kong X, Hioe CE.** 2013. Elicitation of broadly reactive antibodies against glycan-modulated neutralizing V3 epitopes of HIV-1 by immune complex vaccines. *Vaccine* **31:**5413–5421.
5. **Hioe CE, Kumar R, Hu S-L.** 2014. The influence of HIV envelope glycosylation on adaptive immune response, p 59–83. *In* Pantophlet R (ed), *HIV Glycans in Infection and Immunity.* Springer Science + Business Media, New York, NY.
6. **Robertson DL, Sharp PM, McCutchan FE, Hahn BH.** 1995. Recombination in HIV-1. *Nature* **374:**124–126.
7. **Richman DD, Wrin T, Little SJ, Petropoulos CJ.** 2003. Rapid evolution of the neutralizing antibody response to HIV type 1 infection. *Proc Natl Acad Sci USA* **100:**4144–4149.
8. **Moore PL, Ranchobe N, Lambson BE, Gray ES, Cave E, Abrahams MR, Bandawe G, Mlisana K, Abdool Karim SS, Williamson C, Morris L.** 2009. Limited neutralizing antibody specificities drive neutralization escape in early HIV-1 subtype C infection. *PLoS Pathog* **5:**e1000598. doi:10.1371/journal.ppat.1000598.
9. **Liao HX, Lynch R, Zhou T, Gao F, Alam SM, Boyd SD, Fire AZ, Roskin KM, Schramm CA, Zhang Z, Zhu J, Shapiro L, Mullikin JC, Gnanakaran S, Hraber P, Wiehe K, Kelsoe G, Yang G, Xia SM, Montefiori DC, Parks R, Lloyd KE, Scearce RM, Soderberg KA, Cohen M, Kamanga G, Louder MK, Tran LM, Chen Y, Cai F, Chen S, Moquin S, Du X, Joyce MG, Srivatsan S, Zhang B, Zheng A, Shaw GM, Hahn BH, Kepler TB, Korber BT, Kwong PD,**

Mascola JR, Haynes BF. 2013. Co-evolution of a broadly neutralizing HIV-1 antibody and founder virus. *Nature* **496:**469–476.
10. **Hemelaar J.** 2012. Implications of HIV diversity for the HIV-1 pandemic. *J Infect* **66:**391–400.
11. **Rusert P, Krarup A, Magnus C, Brandenberg OF, Weber J, Ehlert AK, Regoes RR, Gunthard HF, Trkola A.** 2011. Interaction of the gp120 V1V2 loop with a neighboring gp120 unit shields the HIV envelope trimer against cross-neutralizing antibodies. *J Exp Med* **208:**1419–1433.
12. **Zhou T, Georgiev I, Wu X, Yang ZY, Dai K, Finzi A, Kwon YD, Scheid JF, Shi W, Xu L, Yang Y, Zhu J, Nussenzweig MC, Sodroski J, Shapiro L, Nabel GJ, Mascola JR, Kwong PD.** 2010. Structural basis for broad and potent neutralization of HIV-1 by antibody VRC01. *Science* **329:**811–817.
13. **Wu X, Zhou T, Zhu J, Zhang B, Georgiev I, Wang C, Chen X, Longo NS, Louder M, McKee K, O'Dell S, Perfetto S, Schmidt SD, Shi W, Wu L, Yang Y, Yang ZY, Yang Z, Zhang Z, Bonsignori M, Crump JA, Kapiga SH, Sam NE, Haynes BF, Simek M, Burton DR, Koff WC, Doria-Rose NA, Connors M, Mullikin JC, Nabel GJ, Roederer M, Shapiro L, Kwong PD, Mascola JR.** 2011. Focused evolution of HIV-1 neutralizing antibodies revealed by structures and deep sequencing. *Science* **333:**1593–1602.
14. **Kwong PD, Doyle ML, Casper DJ, Cicala C, Leavitt SA, Majeed S, Steenbeke TD, Venturi M, Chaiken I, Fung M, Katinger H, Parren PW, Robinson J, Van Ryk D, Wang L, Burton DR, Freire E, Wyatt R, Sodroski J, Hendrickson WA, Arthos J.** 2002. HIV-1 evades antibody-mediated neutralization through conformational masking of receptor-binding sites. *Nature* **420:**678–682.
15. **Korkut A, Hendrickson WA.** 2012. Structural plasticity and conformational transitions of HIV envelope glycoprotein gp120. *PLoS One* **7:**e52170. doi:10.1371/journal.pone.0052170.
16. **Shrivastava IH, Wendel K, LaLonde JM.** 2012. Spontaneous rearrangement of the beta20/beta21 strands in simulations of unliganded HIV-1 glycoprotein, gp120. *Biochemistry* **51:**7783–7793.
17. **Zolla-Pazner S.** 2014. A critical question for HIV vaccine development: which antibodies to induce? *Science* **345:**167–168.
18. **Gorny MK, Pan R, Williams C, Wang XH, Volsky B, O'Neal T, Spurrier B, Sampson JM, Li L, Seaman MS, Kong XP, Zolla-Pazner S.** 2012. Functional and immunochemical cross-reactivity of V2-specific monoclonal antibodies from HIV-1-infected individuals. *Virology* **427:**198–207.

19. Prince AM, Reesink H, Pascual D, Horowitz B, Hewlett I, Murthy KK, Cobb KE, Eichberg JW. 1991. Prevention of HIV infection by passive immunization with HIV immunoglobulin. *AIDS Res Hum Retroviruses* 7:971–973.

20. Bar KJ, Tsao CY, Iyer SS, Decker JM, Yang Y, Bonsignori M, Chen X, Hwang KK, Montefiori DC, Liao HX, Hraber P, Fischer W, Li H, Wang S, Sterrett S, Keele BF, Ganusov VV, Perelson AS, Korber BT, Georgiev I, McLellan JS, Pavlicek JW, Gao F, Haynes BF, Hahn BH, Kwong PD, Shaw GM. 2012. Early low-titer neutralizing antibodies impede HIV-1 replication and select for virus escape. *PLoS Pathog* 8:e1002721. doi:10.1371/journal.ppat.1002721.

21. Hioe CE, Wrin T, Seaman MS, Yu X, Wood B, Self S, Williams C, Gorny MK, Zolla-Pazner S. 2010. Anti-V3 monoclonal antibodies display broad neutralizing activities against multiple HIV-1 subtypes. *PLoS One* 5:e10254. doi:10.1371/journal.pone.0010254.

22. Li L, Wang XH, Banerjee S, Volsky B, Williams C, Virland D, Nadas A, Seaman MS, Chen X, Spearman P, Zolla-Pazner S, Gorny MK. 2012. Different pattern of immunoglobulin gene usage by HIV-1 compared to non-HIV-1 antibodies derived from the same infected subject. *PLoS One* 7:e39534. doi:10.1371/journal.pone.0039534.

23. Karasavvas N, Billings E, Rao M, Williams C, Zolla-Pazner S, Bailer RT, Koup RA, Madnote S, Arworn D, Shen X, Tomaras GD, Currier JR, Jiang M, Magaret C, Andrews C, Gottardo R, Gilbert P, Cardozo TJ, Rerks-Ngarm S, Nitayaphan S, Pitisuttithum P, Kaewkungwal J, Paris R, Greene K, Gao H, Gurunathan S, Tartaglia J, Sinangil F, Korber BT, Montefiori DC, Mascola JR, Robb ML, Haynes BF, Ngauy V, Michael NL, Kim JH, de Souza MS. 2012. The Thai Phase III HIV Type 1 Vaccine trial (RV144) regimen induces antibodies that target conserved regions within the V2 loop of gp120. *AIDS Res Hum Retroviruses* 28:1444–1457.

24. Haynes BF, Gilbert PB, McElrath MJ, Zolla-Pazner S, Tomaras GD, Alam SM, Evans DT, Montefiori DC, Karnasuta C, Sutthent R, Liao HX, DeVico AL, Lewis GK, Williams C, Pinter A, Fong Y, Janes H, DeCamp A, Huang Y, Rao M, Billings E, Karasavvas N, Robb ML, Ngauy V, de Souza MS, Paris R, Ferrari G, Bailer RT, Soderberg KA, Andrews C, Berman PW, Frahm N, De Rosa SC, Alpert MD, Yates NL, Shen X, Koup RA, Pitisuttithum P, Kaewkungwal J, Nitayaphan S, Rerks-Ngarm S, Michael NL, Kim JH. 2012. Immune-correlates analysis of an HIV-1 vaccine efficacy trial. *N Engl J Med* 366:1275–1286.

25. Zolla-Pazner S, deCamp AC, Cardozo T, Karasavvas N, Gottardo R, Williams C, Morris DE, Tomaras G, Rao M, Billings E, Berman P, Shen X, Andrews C, O'Connell RJ, Ngauy V, Nitayaphan S, de Souza M, Korber B, Koup R, Bailer RT, Mascola JR, Pinter A, Montefiori D, Haynes BF, Robb ML, Rerks-Ngarm S, Michael NL, Gilbert PB, Kim JH. 2013. Analysis of V2 antibody responses induced in vaccinees in the ALVAC/AIDSVAX HIV-1 vaccine efficacy trial. *PLoS One* 8:e53629. doi:10.1371/journal.pone.0053629.

26. Zolla-Pazner S, deCamp A, Gilbert PB, Williams C, Yates NL, Williams WT, Howington R, Fong Y, Morris DE, Soderberg KA, Irene C, Reichman C, Pinter A, Parks R, Pitisuttithum P, Kaewkungwal J, Rerks-Ngarm S, Nitayaphan S, Andrews C, O'Connell RJ, Yang ZY, Nabel GJ, Kim JH, Michael NL, Montefiori DC, Liao HX, Haynes BF, Tomaras GD. 2014. Vaccine-induced IgG antibodies to V1V2 regions of multiple HIV-1 subtypes correlate with decreased risk of HIV-1 infection. *PLoS One* 9:e87572. doi:10.1371/journal.pone.0087572.

27. Yates NL, Liao HX, Fong Y, deCamp A, Vandergrift NA, Williams WT, Alam SM, Ferrari G, Yang ZY, Seaton KE, Berman PW, Alpert MD, Evans DT, O'Connell RJ, Francis D, Sinangil F, Lee C, Nitayaphan S, Rerks-Ngarm S, Kaewkungwal J, Pitisuttithum P, Tartaglia J, Pinter A, Zolla-Pazner S, Gilbert PB, Nabel GJ, Michael NL, Kim JH, Montefiori DC, Haynes BF, Tomaras GD. 2014. Vaccine-induced Env V1-V2 IgG3 correlates with lower HIV-1 infection risk and declines soon after vaccination. *Science Trans Med* 6:228–239.

28. Gottardo R, Bailer RT, Korber BT, Gnanakaran S, Phillips J, Shen X, Tomaras GD, Turk E, Imholte G, Eckler L, Wenschuh H, Zerweck J, Greene K, Gao H, Berman PW, Francis D, Sinangil F, Lee C, Nitayaphan S, Rerks-Ngarm S, Kaewkungwal J, Pitisuttithum P, Tartaglia J, Robb ML, Michael NL, Kim JH, Zolla-Pazner S, Haynes BF, Mascola JR, Self S, Gilbert P, Montefiori DC. 2013. Plasma IgG to linear epitopes in the V2 and V3 regions of HIV-1 gp120 correlate with a reduced risk of infection in the RV144 vaccine efficacy trial. *PLoS One* 8:e75665. doi:10.1371/journal.pone.0075665.

29. Montefiori DC, Karnasuta C, Huang Y, Ahmed H, Gilbert P, de Souza MS, McLinden R, Tovanabutra S, Laurence-Chenine A, Sanders-Buell E, Moody MA, Bonsignori M, Ochsenbauer C, Kappes J, Tang H, Greene K,

Gao H, LaBranche CC, Andrews C, Polonis VR, Rerks-Ngarm S, Pitisuttithum P, Nitayaphan S, Kaewkungwal J, Self SG, Berman PW, Francis D, Sinangil F, Lee C, Tartaglia J, Robb ML, Haynes BF, Michael NL, Kim JH. 2012. Magnitude and breadth of the neutralizing antibody response in the RV144 and Vax003 HIV-1 vaccine efficacy trials. *J Infect Dis* **206**:431–441.

30. Liao HX, Bonsignori M, Alam SM, McLellan JS, Tomaras GD, Moody MA, Kozink DM, Hwang KK, Chen X, Tsao CY, Liu P, Lu X, Parks RJ, Montefiori DC, Ferrari G, Pollara J, Rao M, Peachman KK, Santra S, Letvin NL, Karasavvas N, Yang ZY, Dai K, Pancera M, Gorman J, Wiehe K, Nicely NI, Rerks-Ngarm S, Nitayaphan S, Kaewkungwal J, Pitisuttithum P, Tartaglia J, Sinangil F, Kim JH, Michael NL, Kepler TB, Kwong PD, Mascola JR, Nabel GJ, Pinter A, Zolla-Pazner S, Haynes BF. 2013. Vaccine induction of antibodies against a structurally heterogeneous site of immune pressure within HIV-1 envelope protein variable regions 1 and 2. *Immunity* **38**:176–186.

31. Moody MA, Zhang R, Walter EB, Woods CW, Ginsburg GS, McClain MT, Denny TN, Chen X, Munshaw S, Marshall DJ, Whitesides JF, Drinker MS, Amos JD, Gurley TC, Eudailey JA, Foulger A, DeRosa KR, Parks R, Meyerhoff RR, Yu JS, Kozink DM, Barefoot BE, Ramsburg EA, Khurana S, Golding H, Vandergrift NA, Alam SM, Tomaras GD, Kepler TB, Kelsoe G, Liao HX, Haynes BF. 2011. H3N2 influenza infection elicits more cross-reactive and less clonally expanded anti-hemagglutinin antibodies than influenza vaccination. *PloS One* **6**:e25797. doi:10.1371/journal.pone.0025797.

32. Seaman MS, Janes H, Hawkins N, Grandpre LE, Devoy C, Giri A, Coffey RT, Harris L, Wood B, Daniels MG, Bhattacharya T, Lapedes A, Polonis VR, McCutchan FE, Gilbert PB, Self SG, Korber BT, Montefiori DC, Mascola JR. 2010. Tiered categorization of a diverse panel of HIV-1 Env pseudoviruses for assessment of neutralizing antibodies. *J Virol* **84**:1439–1452.

33. Zolla-Pazner S, Kong XP, Jiang X, Cardozo T, Nadas A, Cohen S, Totrov M, Seaman MS, Wang S, Lu S. 2011. Cross-clade HIV-1 neutralizing antibodies induced with V3-scaffold protein immunogens following priming with gp120 DNA. *J Virol* **85**:9887–9898.

34. Cardozo T, Wang S, Jiang X, Kong XP, Hioe C, Krachmarov C. 2014. Vaccine focusing to cross-subtype HIV-1 gp120 variable loop epitopes. *Vaccine* **32**:4916–4924.

35. Sather DN, Armann J, Ching LK, Mavrantoni A, Sellhorn G, Caldwell Z, Yu X, Wood B, Self S, Kalams S, Stamatatos L. 2009. Factors associated with the development of cross-reactive neutralizing antibodies during human immunodeficiency virus type 1 infection. *J Virol* **83**:757–769.

36. Simek MD, Rida W, Priddy FH, Pung P, Carrow E, Laufer DS, Lehrman JK, Boaz M, Tarragona-Fiol T, Miiro G, Birungi J, Pozniak A, McPhee DA, Manigart O, Karita E, Inwoley A, Jaoko W, Dehovitz J, Bekker LG, Pitisuttithum P, Paris R, Walker LM, Poignard P, Wrin T, Fast PE, Burton DR, Koff WC. 2009. Human immunodeficiency virus type 1 elite neutralizers: individuals with broad and potent neutralizing activity identified by using a high-throughput neutralization assay together with an analytical selection algorithm. *J Virol* **83**:7337–7348.

37. Walker LM, Phogat SK, Chan-Hui PY, Wagner D, Phung P, Goss JL, Wrin T, Simek MD, Fling S, Mitcham JL, Lehrman JK, Priddy FH, Olsen OA, Frey SM, Hammond PW, Kaminsky S, Zamb T, Moyle M, Koff WC, Poignard P, Burton DR. 2009. Broad and potent neutralizing antibodies from an African donor reveal a new HIV-1 vaccine target. *Science* **326**:285–289.

38. Walker LM, Huber M, Doores KJ, Falkowska E, Pejchal R, Julien JP, Wang SK, Ramos A, Chan-Hui PY, Moyle M, Mitcham JL, Hammond PW, Olsen OA, Phung P, Fling S, Wong CH, Phogat S, Wrin T, Simek MD, Koff WC, Wilson IA, Burton DR, Poignard P. 2011. Broad neutralization coverage of HIV by multiple highly potent antibodies. *Nature* **477**:466–470.

39. Wu X, Yang ZY, Li Y, Hogerkorp CM, Schief WR, Seaman MS, Zhou T, Schmidt SD, Wu L, Xu L, Longo NS, McKee K, O'Dell S, Louder MK, Wycuff DL, Feng Y, Nason M, Doria-Rose N, Connors M, Kwong PD, Roederer M, Wyatt RT, Nabel GJ, Mascola JR. 2010. Rational design of envelope identifies broadly neutralizing human monoclonal antibodies to HIV-1. *Science* **329**:856–861.

40. Huang J, Ofek G, Laub L, Louder MK, Doria-Rose NA, Longo NS, Imamichi H, Bailer RT, Chakrabarti B, Sharma SK, Alam SM, Wang T, Yang Y, Zhang B, Migueles SA, Wyatt R, Haynes BF, Kwong PD, Mascola JR, Connors M. 2012. Broad and potent neutralization of HIV-1 by a gp41-specific human antibody. *Nature* **491**:406–412.

41. Morris L, Chen X, Alam M, Tomaras G, Zhang R, Marshall DJ, Chen B, Parks R,

Foulger A, Jaeger F, Donathan M, Bilska M, Gray ES, Abdool Karim SS, Kepler TB, Whitesides J, Montefiori D, Moody MA, Liao HX, Haynes BF. 2011. Isolation of a human anti-HIV gp41 membrane proximal region neutralizing antibody by antigen-specific single B cell sorting. *PLoS One* **6:**e23532. doi:10.1371/journal.pone.0023532.

42. Klein F, Diskin R, Scheid JF, Gaebler C, Mouquet H, Georgiev IS, Pancera M, Zhou T, Incesu RB, Fu BZ, Gnanapragasam PN, Oliveira TY, Seaman MS, Kwong PD, Bjorkman PJ, Nussenzweig MC. 2013. Somatic mutations of the immunoglobulin framework are generally required for broad and potent HIV-1 neutralization. *Cell* **153:**126–138.

43. Sok D, Laserson U, Laserson J, Liu Y, Vigneault F, Julien JP, Briney B, Ramos A, Saye KF, Le K, Mahan A, Wang S, Kardar M, Yaari G, Walker LM, Simen BB, St John EP, Chan-Hui PY, Swiderek K, Kleinstein SH, Alter G, Seaman MS, Chakraborty AK, Koller D, Wilson IA, Church GM, Burton DR, Poignard P. 2013. The effects of somatic hypermutation on neutralization and binding in the PGT121 family of broadly neutralizing HIV antibodies. *PLoS Pathog* **9:**e1003754. doi:10.1371/journal.ppat.1003754.

44. Mascola JR, Haynes BF. 2013. HIV-1 neutralizing antibodies: understanding nature's pathways. *Immunol Rev* **254:**225–244.

45. Yu L, Guan Y. 2014. Immunologic basis for long HCDR3s in broadly neutralizing antibodies against HIV-1. *Front Immunol* **5:**250.

46. Verkoczy L, Diaz M. 2014. Autoreactivity in HIV-1 broadly neutralizing antibodies: implications for their function and induction by vaccination. *Curr Opin HIV AIDS* **9:**224–234.

47. Haynes BF, Fleming J, St Clair EW, Katinger H, Stiegler G, Kunert R, Robinson J, Scearce RM, Plonk K, Staats HF, Ortel TL, Liao HX, Alam SM. 2005. Cardiolipin polyspecific autoreactivity in two broadly neutralizing HIV-1 antibodies. *Science* **308:**1906–1908.

48. Moldt B, Rakasz EG, Schultz N, Chan-Hui PY, Swiderek K, Weisgrau KL, Piaskowski SM, Bergman Z, Watkins DI, Poignard P, Burton DR. 2012. Highly potent HIV-specific antibody neutralization *in vitro* translates into effective protection against mucosal SHIV challenge *in vivo. Proc Natl Acad Sci USA* **109:**18921–18925.

49. Parren PW, Marx PA, Hessell AJ, Luckay A, Harouse J, Cheng-Mayer C, Moore JP, Burton DR. 2001. Antibody protects macaques against vaginal challenge with a pathogenic R5 simian/human immunodeficiency virus at serum levels giving complete neutralization *in vitro. J Virol* **75:**8340–8347.

50. Hessell AJ, Rakasz EG, Poignard P, Hangartner L, Landucci G, Forthal DN, Koff WC, Watkins DI, Burton DR. 2009. Broadly neutralizing human anti-HIV antibody 2G12 is effective in protection against mucosal SHIV challenge even at low serum neutralizing titers. *PLoS Pathog* **5:**e1000433. doi:10.1371/journal.ppat.1000433.

51. Hessell AJ, Rakasz EG, Tehrani DM, Huber M, Weisgrau KL, Landucci G, Forthal DN, Koff WC, Poignard P, Watkins DI, Burton DR. 2010. Broadly neutralizing monoclonal antibodies 2F5 and 4E10 directed against the human immunodeficiency virus type 1 gp41 membrane-proximal external region protect against mucosal challenge by simian-human immunodeficiency virus SHIVBa-L. *J Virol* **84:**1302–1313.

52. Haynes BF, Verkoczy L. 2014. AIDS/HIV. Host controls of HIV neutralizing antibodies. *Science* **344:**588–589.

53. Pegu A, Yang ZY, Boyington JC, Wu L, Ko SY, Schmidt SD, McKee K, Kong WP, Shi W, Chen X, Todd JP, Letvin NL, Huang J, Nason MC, Hoxie JA, Kwong PD, Connors M, Rao SS, Mascola JR, Nabel GJ. 2014. Neutralizing antibodies to HIV-1 envelope protect more effectively *in vivo* than those to the CD4 receptor. *Sci Trans Med* **6:**243–288.

54. Shingai M, Donau OK, Plishka RJ, Buckler-White A, Mascola JR, Nabel GJ, Nason MC, Montefiori D, Moldt B, Poignard P, Diskin R, Bjorkman PJ, Eckhaus MA, Klein F, Mouquet H, Cetrulo Lorenzi JC, Gazumyan A, Burton DR, Nussenzweig MC, Martin MA, Nishimura Y. 2014. Passive transfer of modest titers of potent and broadly neutralizing anti-HIV monoclonal antibodies block SHIV infection in macaques. *J Exp Med* **211:**2061–2074.

55. Watkins JD, Siddappa NB, Lakhashe SK, Humbert M, Sholukh A, Hemashettar G, Wong YL, Yoon JK, Wang W, Novembre FJ, Villinger F, Ibegbu C, Patel K, Corti D, Agatic G, Vanzetta F, Bianchi S, Heeney JL, Sallusto F, Lanzavecchia A, Ruprecht RM. 2011. An anti-HIV-1 V3 loop antibody fully protects cross-clade and elicits T-cell immunity in macaques mucosally challenged with an R5 clade C SHIV. *PLoS One* **6:**e18207. doi:10.1371/journal.pone.0018207.

56. Halper-Stromberg A, Lu CL, Klein F, Horwitz JA, Bournazos S, Nogueira L, Eisenreich TR, Liu C, Gazumyan A, Schaefer U, Furze RC, Seaman MS, Prinjha R, Tarakhovsky A, Ravetch JV, Nussenzweig MC. 2014. Broadly neutralizing antibodies and

viral inducers decrease rebound from HIV-1 latent reservoirs in humanized mice. *Cell* **158:**989–999.

57. Barouch DH, Whitney JB, Moldt B, Klein F, Oliveira TY, Liu J, Stephenson KE, Chang HW, Shekhar K, Gupta S, Nkolola JP, Seaman MS, Smith KM, Borducchi EN, Cabral C, Smith JY, Blackmore S, Sanisetty S, Perry JR, Beck M, Lewis MG, Rinaldi W, Chakraborty AK, Poignard P, Nussenzweig MC, Burton DR. 2013. Therapeutic efficacy of potent neutralizing HIV-1-specific monoclonal antibodies in SHIV-infected rhesus monkeys. *Nature* **503:**224–228.

58. Klein F, Nogueira L, Nishimura Y, Phad G, West AP Jr, Halper-Stromberg A, Horwitz JA, Gazumyan A, Liu C, Eisenreich TR, Lehmann C, Fatkenheuer G, Shingai M, Martin M, Bjorkman PJ, Seaman MS, Zolla-Pazner S, Hedestam G, Nussenzweig MC. 2014. Enhanced HIV-1 immunotherapy by naturally arising antibodies targeting resistant variants. *J Exp Med* **211:**2361–2372.

59. Wu X, Parast AB, Richardson BA, Nduati R, John-Stewart G, Mbori-Ngacha D, Rainwater SM, Overbaugh J. 2006. Neutralization escape variants of human immunodeficiency virus type 1 are transmitted from mother to infant. *J Virol* **80:**835–844.

60. Mabuka J, Goo L, Omenda MM, Nduati R, Overbaugh J. 2013. HIV-1 maternal and infant variants show similar sensitivity to broadly neutralizing antibodies, but sensitivity varies by subtype. *AIDS* **27:**1535–1544.

61. Flynn NM, Forthal DN, Harro CD, Judson FN, Mayer KH, Para MF. 2005. Placebo-controlled phase 3 trial of a recombinant glycoprotein 120 vaccine to prevent HIV-1 infection. *J Infect Dis* **191:**654–665.

62. Pitisuttithum P, Gilbert P, Gurwith M, Heyward W, Martin M, van Griensven F, Hu D, Tappero JW, Choopanya K. 2006. Randomized, double-blind, placebo-controlled efficacy trial of a bivalent recombinant glycoprotein 120 HIV-1 vaccine among injection drug users in Bangkok, Thailand. *J Infect Dis* **194:**1661–1671.

63. Rerks-Ngarm S, Pitisuttithum P, Nitayaphan S, Kaewkungwal J, Chiu J, Paris R, Premsri N, Namwat C, de Souza M, Adams E, Benenson M, Gurunathan S, Tartaglia J, McNeil JG, Francis DP, Stablein D, Birx DL, Chunsuttiwat S, Khamboonruang C, Thongcharoen P, Robb ML, Michael NL, Kunasol P, Kim JH. 2009. Vaccination with ALVAC and AIDSVAX to prevent HIV-1 infection in Thailand. *N Engl J Med* **361:**2209–2220.

64. Burton DR, Desrosiers RC, Doms RW, Koff WC, Kwong PD, Moore JP, Nabel GJ, Sodroski J, Wilson IA, Wyatt RT. 2004. HIV vaccine design and the neutralizing antibody problem. *Nat Immunol* **5:**233–236.

65. Sanders RW, Vesanen M, Schuelke N, Master A, Schiffner L, Kalyanaraman R, Paluch M, Berkhout B, Maddon PJ, Olson WC, Lu M, Moore JP. 2002. Stabilization of the soluble, cleaved, trimeric form of the envelope glycoprotein complex of human immunodeficiency virus type 1. *J Virol* **76:**8875–8889.

66. Binley JM, Sanders RW, Clas B, Schuelke N, Master A, Guo Y, Kajumo F, Anselma DJ, Maddon PJ, Olson WC, Moore JP. 2000. A recombinant human immunodeficiency virus type 1 envelope glycoprotein complex stabilized by an intermolecular disulfide bond between the gp120 and gp41 subunits is an antigenic mimic of the trimeric virion-associated structure. *J Virol* **74:**627–643.

67. Yang X, Lee J, Mahony EM, Kwong PD, Wyatt R, Sodroski J. 2002. Highly stable trimers formed by human immunodeficiency virus type 1 envelope glycoproteins fused with the trimeric motif of T4 bacteriophage fibritin. *J Virol* **76:**4634–4642.

68. Spearman P, Lally MA, Elizaga M, Montefiori D, Tomaras GD, McElrath MJ, Hural J, De Rosa SC, Sato A, Huang Y, Frey SE, Sato P, Donnelly J, Barnett S, Corey LJ. 2011. A trimeric, V2-deleted HIV-1 envelope glycoprotein vaccine elicits potent neutralizing antibodies but limited breadth of neutralization in human volunteers. *J Infect Dis* **203:**1165–1173.

69. Forsell MN, Schief WR, Wyatt RT. 2009. Immunogenicity of HIV-1 envelope glycoprotein oligomers. *Curr Opin HIV AIDS* **4:**380–387.

70. Sather DN, Carbonetti S, Malherbe D, Pissani F, Stuart AB, Hessell AJ, Gray MD, Mikell I, Kalams SA, Haigwood NL, Stamatatos L. 2014. Emergence of broadly neutralizing antibodies and viral co-evolution in two subjects during the early stages of infection with the human immunodeficiency virus type 1. *J Virol* **88:**12968–12981.

71. Doria-Rose NA, Schramm CA, Gorman J, Moore PL, Bhiman JN, DeKosky BJ, Ernandes MJ, Georgiev IS, Kim HJ, Pancera M, Staupe RP, Altae-Tran HR, Bailer RT, Crooks ET, Cupo A, Druz A, Garrett NJ, Hoi KH, Kong R, Louder MK, Longo NS, McKee K, Nonyane M, O'Dell S, Roark RS, Rudicell RS, Schmidt SD, Sheward DJ, Soto C, Wibmer CK, Yang Y, Zhang Z, Mullikin JC, Binley JM, Sanders RW, Wilson IA, Moore JP, Ward AB, Georgiou G, Williamson C,

Abdool Karim SS, Morris L, Kwong PD, Shapiro L, Mascola JR. 2014. Developmental pathway for potent V1V2-directed HIV-neutralizing antibodies. *Nature* **509**:55–62.

72. **Correia BE, Bates JT, Loomis RJ, Baneyx G, Carrico C, Jardine JG, Rupert P, Correnti C, Kalyuzhniy O, Vittal V, Connell MJ, Stevens E, Schroeter A, Chen M, Macpherson S, Serra AM, Adachi Y, Holmes MA, Li Y, Klevit RE, Graham BS, Wyatt RT, Baker D, Strong RK, Crowe JE Jr, Johnson PR, Schief WR.** 2014. Proof of principle for epitope-focused vaccine design. *Nature* **507**:201–206.

73. **Delany I, Rappuoli R, Seib KL.** 2013. Vaccines, reverse vaccinology, and bacterial pathogenesis. *Cold Spring Harbor Perspect Med* **3**:a012476.

74. **Zhou T, Xu L, Dey B, Hessell AJ, Van Ryk D, Xiang SH, Yang X, Zhang MY, Zwick MB, Arthos J, Burton DR, Dimitrov DS, Sodroski J, Wyatt R, Nabel GJ, Kwong PD.** 2007. Structural definition of a conserved neutralization epitope on HIV-1 gp120. *Nature* **445**:732–737.

75. **Cimbro R, Gallant TR, Dolan MA, Guzzo C, Zhang P, Lin Y, Miao H, Van Ryk D, Arthos J, Gorshkova I, Brown PH, Hurt DE, Lusso P.** 2014. Tyrosine sulfation in the second variable loop (V2) of HIV-1 gp120 stabilizes V2-V3 interaction and modulates neutralization sensitivity. *Proc Natl Acad Sci USA* **111**:3152–3157.

76. **White TA, Bartesaghi A, Borgnia MJ, Meyerson JR, de la Cruz MJ, Bess JW, Nandwani R, Hoxie JA, Lifson JD, Milne JL, Subramaniam S.** 2010. Molecular architectures of trimeric SIV and HIV-1 envelope glycoproteins on intact viruses: strain-dependent variation in quaternary structure. *PLoS Pathog* **6**:e1001249. doi:10.1371/journal.ppat.1001249.

77. **Zolla-Pazner S, Cardozo T.** 2011. Structure-function relationships of HIV-1 envelope sequence-variable regions refocus vaccine design. *Nat Rev* **10**:527–535.

78. **McLellan JS, Pancera M, Carrico C, Gorman J, Julien JP, Khayat R, Louder R, Pejchal R, Sastry M, Dai K, O'Dell S, Patel N, Shahzad-ul-Hussan S, Yang Y, Zhang B, Zhou T, Zhu J, Boyington JC, Chuang GY, Diwanji D, Georgiev I, Kwon YD, Lee D, Louder MK, Moquin S, Schmidt SD, Yang ZY, Bonsignori M, Crump JA, Kapiga SH, Sam NE, Haynes BF, Burton DR, Koff WC, Walker LM, Phogat S, Wyatt R, Orwenyo J, Wang LX, Arthos J, Bewley CA, Mascola JR, Nabel GJ, Schief WR, Ward AB, Wilson IA, Kwong PD.** 2011. Structure of HIV-1 gp120 V1/V2 domain with broadly neutralizing antibody PG9. *Nature* **480**:336–343.

79. **Arthos J, Cicala C, Martinelli E, Macleod K, Van Ryk D, Wei D, Xiao Z, Veenstra TD, Conrad TP, Lempicki RA, McLaughlin S, Pascuccio M, Gopaul R, McNally J, Cruz CC, Censoplano N, Chung E, Reitano KN, Kottilil S, Goode DJ, Fauci AS.** 2008. HIV-1 envelope protein binds to and signals through integrin alpha4beta7, the gut mucosal homing receptor for peripheral T cells. *Nat Immunol* **9**:301–309.

80. **Gorny MK, Moore JP, Conley AJ, Karwowska S, Sodroski J, Williams C, Burda S, Boots LJ, Zolla-Pazner S.** 1994. Human anti-V2 monoclonal antibody that neutralizes primary but not laboratory isolates of human immunodeficiency virus type 1. *J Virol* **68**:8312–8320.

81. **Mayr LM, Cohen S, Spurrier B, Kong XP, Zolla-Pazner S.** 2013. Epitope mapping of conformational V2-specific anti-HIV human monoclonal antibodies reveals an immunodominant site in V2. *PLoS One* **8**:e70859. doi:10.1371/journal.pone.0070859.

82. **Bonsignori M, Pollara J, Moody MA, Alpert MD, Chen X, Hwang KK, Gilbert PB, Huang Y, Gurley TC, Kozink DM, Marshall DJ, Whitesides JF, Tsao CY, Kaewkungwal J, Nitayaphan S, Pitisuttithum P, Rerks-Ngarm S, Kim JH, Michael NL, Tomaras GD, Montefiori DC, Lewis GK, DeVico A, Evans DT, Ferrari G, Liao HX, Haynes BF.** 2012. Antibody-dependent cellular cytotoxicity-mediating antibodies from an HIV-1 vaccine efficacy trial target multiple epitopes and preferentially use the VH1 gene family. *J Virol* **86**:11521–11532.

83. **Gorny MK, Stamatatos L, Volsky B, Revesz K, Williams C, Wang XH, Cohen S, Staudinger R, Zolla-Pazner S.** 2005. Identification of a new quaternary neutralizing epitope on human immunodeficiency virus type 1 virus particles. *J Virol* **79**:5232–5237.

84. **Bonsignori M, Hwang KK, Chen X, Tsao CY, Morris L, Gray E, Marshall DJ, Crump JA, Kapiga SH, Sam NE, Sinangil F, Pancera M, Yongping Y, Zhang B, Zhu J, Kwong PD, O'Dell S, Mascola JR, Wu L, Nabel GJ, Phogat S, Seaman MS, Whitesides JF, Moody MA, Kelsoe G, Yang X, Sodroski J, Shaw GM, Montefiori DC, Kepler TB, Tomaras GD, Alam SM, Liao HX, Haynes BF.** 2011. Analysis of a clonal lineage of HIV-1 envelope V2/V3 conformational epitope-specific broadly neutralizing antibodies and their inferred unmutated common ancestors. *J Virol* **85**:9998–10009.

85. **Julien JP, Cupo A, Sok D, Stanfield RL, Lyumkis D, Deller MC, Klasse PJ, Burton DR, Sanders RW, Moore JP, Ward AB, Wilson IA.** 2013. Crystal structure of a soluble cleaved HIV-1 envelope trimer. *Science* **342**:1477–1483.

86. **Ivanoff LA, Dubay JW, Morris JF, Roberts SJ, Gutshall L, Sternberg EJ, Hunter E, Matthews TJ, Petteway SR Jr.** 1992. V3 loop region of the HIV-1 gp120 envelope protein is essential for virus infectivity. *Virology* **187:**423–432.

87. **Zolla-Pazner S.** 2004. Identifying epitopes of HIV-1 that induce protective antibodies. *Nat Rev* **4:**199–210.

88. **Zolla-Pazner S, Cardozo T.** 2010. Structure-function relationships of HIV-1 envelope sequence-variable regions refocus vaccine design. *Nat Rev* **10:**527–535.

89. **Jiang X, Burke V, Totrov M, Williams C, Cardozo T, Gorny MK, Zolla-Pazner S, Kong XP.** 2010. Conserved structural elements in the V3 crown of HIV-1 gp120. *Nat Struct Mol Biol* **17:**955–961.

90. **Huang CC, Tang M, Zhang MY, Majeed S, Montabana E, Stanfield RL, Dimitrov DS, Korber B, Sodroski J, Wilson IA, Wyatt R, Kwong PD.** 2005. Structure of a V3-containing HIV-1 gp120 core. *Science* **310:**1025–1028.

91. **Zolla-Pazner S.** 2005. Improving on nature: focusing the immune response on the V3 loop. *Hum Antibodies* **14:**69–72.

92. **Crooks ET, Moore PL, Franti M, Cayanan CS, Zhu P, Jiang P, de Vries RP, Wiley C, Zharkikh I, Schulke N, Roux KH, Montefiori DC, Burton DR, Binley JM.** 2007. A comparative immunogenicity study of HIV-1 virus-like particles bearing various forms of envelope proteins, particles bearing no envelope and soluble monomeric gp120. *Virology* **366:**245–262.

93. **Visciano ML, Tagliamonte M, Stewart-Jones G, Heyndrickx L, Vanham G, Jansson M, Fomsgaard A, Grevstad B, Ramaswamy M, Buonaguro FM, Tornesello ML, Biswas P, Scarlatti G, Buonaguro L.** 2013. Characterization of humoral responses to soluble trimeric HIV gp140 from a clade A Ugandan field isolate. *J Transl Med* **11:**165.

94. **Totrov M, Jiang X, Kong XP, Cohen S, Krachmarov C, Salomon A, Williams C, Seaman MS, Abagyan R, Cardozo T, Gorny MK, Wang S, Lu S, Pinter A, Zolla-Pazner S.** 2010. Structure-guided design and immunological characterization of immunogens presenting the HIV-1 gp120 V3 loop on a CTB scaffold. *Virology* **405:**513–523.

95. **Zolla-Pazner S, Cohen S, Pinter A, Krachmarov C, Wrin T, Wang S, Lu S.** 2009. Cross-clade neutralizing antibodies against HIV-1 induced in rabbits by focusing the immune response on a neutralizing epitope. *Virology* **392:**82–93.

96. **Pan R, Sampson JM, Chen Y, Vaine M, Wang S, Lu S, Kong XP.** 2013. Rabbit anti-HIV-1 monoclonal antibodies raised by immunization can mimic the antigen-binding modes of antibodies derived from HIV-1-infected humans. *J Virol* **87:**10221–10231.

97. **Burke V, Williams C, Sukumaran M, Kim SS, Li H, Wang XH, Gorny MK, Zolla-Pazner S, Kong XP.** 2009. Structural basis of the cross-reactivity of genetically related human anti-HIV-1 mAbs: implications for design of V3-based immunogens. *Structure* **17:**1538–1546.

98. **Mouquet H, Klein F, Scheid JF, Warncke M, Pietzsch J, Oliveira TY, Velinzon K, Seaman MS, Nussenzweig MC.** 2011. Memory B cell antibodies to HIV-1 gp140 cloned from individuals infected with clade A and B viruses. *PloS One* **6:**e24078. doi:10.1371/journal.pone.0024078.

99. **Corti D, Langedijk JP, Hinz A, Seaman MS, Vanzetta F, Fernandez-Rodriguez BM, Silacci C, Pinna D, Jarrossay D, Balla-Jhagjhoorsingh S, Willems B, Zekveld MJ, Dreja H, O'Sullivan E, Pade C, Orkin C, Jeffs SA, Montefiori DC, Davis D, Weissenhorn W, McKnight A, Heeney JL, Sallusto F, Sattentau QJ, Weiss RA, Lanzavecchia A.** 2010. Analysis of memory B cell responses and isolation of novel monoclonal antibodies with neutralizing breadth from HIV-1-infected individuals. *PloS One* **5:**e8805. doi:10.1371/journal.pone.0008805.

100. **McCaffrey RA, Saunders C, Hensel M, Stamatatos L.** 2004. N-linked glycosylation of the V3 loop and the immunologically silent face of gp120 protects human immunodeficiency virus type 1 SF162 from neutralization by anti-gp120 and anti-gp41 antibodies. *J Virol* **78:**3279–3295.

101. **Wyatt R, Moore J, Accola M, Desjardin E, Robinson J, Sodroski J.** 1995. Involvement of the V1/V2 variable loop structure in the exposure of human immunodeficiency virus type 1 gp120 epitopes induced by receptor binding. *J Virol* **69:**5723–5733.

102. **Gzyl J, Bolesta E, Wierzbicki A, Kmieciak D, Naito T, Honda M, Komuro K, Kaneko Y, Kozbor D.** 2004. Effect of partial and complete variable loop deletions of the human immunodeficiency virus type 1 envelope glycoprotein on the breadth of gp160-specific immune responses. *Virology* **318:**493–506.

103. **Upadhyay C, Mayr LM, Zhang J, Kumar R, Gorny MK, Nadas A, Zolla-Pazner S, Hioe CE.** 2014. Distinct mechanisms regulate exposure of neutralizing epitopes in the V2 and V3 loops of HIV-1 envelope. *J Virol* **88:**12853–12865.

104. **Pejchal R, Doores KJ, Walker LM, Khayat R, Huang PS, Wang SK, Stanfield RL, Julien JP, Ramos A, Crispin M, Depetris R, Katpally U, Marozsan A, Cupo A, Maloveste S, Liu Y, McBride R, Ito Y, Sanders RW, Ogohara C,**

Paulson JC, Feizi T, Scanlan CN, Wong CH, Moore JP, Olson WC, Ward AB, Poignard P, Schief WR, Burton DR, Wilson IA. 2011. A potent and broad neutralizing antibody recognizes and penetrates the HIV glycan shield. *Science* **334:**1097–1103.

105. Julien JP, Sok D, Khayat R, Lee JH, Doores KJ, Walker LM, Ramos A, Diwanji DC, Pejchal R, Cupo A, Katpally U, Depetris RS, Stanfield RL, McBride R, Marozsan AJ, Paulson JC, Sanders RW, Moore JP, Burton DR, Poignard P, Ward AB, Wilson IA. 2013. Broadly neutralizing antibody PGT121 allosterically modulates CD4 binding via recognition of the HIV-1 gp120 V3 base and multiple surrounding glycans. *PLoS Pathog* **9:**e1003342. doi:10.1371/journal.ppat.1003342.

106. Wu X, Zhou T, O'Dell S, Wyatt RT, Kwong PD, Mascola JR. 2009. Mechanism of human immunodeficiency virus type 1 resistance to monoclonal antibody B12 that effectively targets the site of CD4 attachment. *J Virol* **83:**10892–10907.

107. Chen L, Kwon YD, Zhou T, Wu X, O'Dell S, Cavacini L, Hessell AJ, Pancera M, Tang M, Xu L, Yang ZY, Zhang MY, Arthos J, Burton DR, Dimitrov DS, Nabel GJ, Posner MR, Sodroski J, Wyatt R, Mascola JR, Kwong PD. 2009. Structural basis of immune evasion at the site of CD4 attachment on HIV-1 gp120. *Science* **326:**1123–1127.

108. Selvarajah S, Puffer B, Pantophlet R, Law M, Doms RW, Burton DR. 2005. Comparing antigenicity and immunogenicity of engineered gp120. *J Virol* **79:**12148–12163.

109. Ahmed FK, Clark BE, Burton DR, Pantophlet R. 2012. An engineered mutant of HIV-1 gp120 formulated with adjuvant Quil A promotes elicitation of antibody responses overlapping the CD4-binding site. *Vaccine* **30:**922–930.

110. Yasmeen A, Ringe R, Derking R, Cupo A, Julien JP, Burton DR, Ward AB, Wilson IA, Sanders RW, Moore JP, Klasse PJ. 2014. Differential binding of neutralizing and non-neutralizing antibodies to native-like soluble HIV-1 Env trimers, uncleaved Env proteins, and monomeric subunits. *Retrovirology* **11:**41.

111. Bhattacharyya S, Singh P, Rathore U, Purwar M, Wagner D, Arendt H, DeStefano J, LaBranche CC, Montefiori DC, Phogat S, Varadarajan R. 2013. Design of an *Escherichia coli* expressed HIV-1 gp120 fragment immunogen that binds to b12 and induces broad and potent neutralizing antibodies. *J Biol Chem* **288:**9815–9825.

112. Montero M, van Houten NE, Wang X, Scott JK. 2008. The membrane-proximal external region of the human immunodeficiency virus type 1 envelope: dominant site of antibody neutralization and target for vaccine design. *Microbiol Mol Biol Rev* **72:**54–84.

113. Kim M, Sun ZY, Rand KD, Shi X, Song L, Cheng Y, Fahmy AF, Majumdar S, Ofek G, Yang Y, Kwong PD, Wang JH, Engen JR, Wagner G, Reinherz EL. 2011. Antibody mechanics on a membrane-bound HIV segment essential for GP41-targeted viral neutralization. *Nat Struct Mol Biol* **18:**1235–1243.

114. Song L, Sun ZY, Coleman KE, Zwick MB, Gach JS, Wang JH, Reinherz EL, Wagner G, Kim M. 2009. Broadly neutralizing anti-HIV-1 antibodies disrupt a hinge-related function of gp41 at the membrane interface. *Proc Natl Acad Sci USA* **106:**9057–9062.

115. Dennison SM, Sutherland LL, Jaeger FH, Anasti KM, Parks R, Stewart S, Bowman C, Xia SM, Zhang R, Shen X, Scearce RM, Ofek G, Yang Y, Kwong PD, Santra S, Liao HX, Tomaras G, Letvin NL, Chen B, Alam SM, Haynes BF. 2011. Induction of antibodies in rhesus macaques that recognize a fusion-intermediate conformation of HIV-1 gp41. *PLoS One* **6:**e27824. doi:10.1371/journal.pone.0027824.

116. Shen X, Parks RJ, Montefiori DC, Kirchherr JL, Keele BF, Decker JM, Blattner WA, Gao F, Weinhold KJ, Hicks CB, Greenberg ML, Hahn BH, Shaw GM, Haynes BF, Tomaras GD. 2009. *In vivo* gp41 antibodies targeting the 2F5 monoclonal antibody epitope mediate human immunodeficiency virus type 1 neutralization breadth. *J Virol* **83:**3617–3625.

Committing the Oldest Sins in the Newest Kind of Ways—Antibodies Targeting the Influenza Virus Type A Hemagglutinin Globular Head

12

JENS C. KRAUSE[1] and JAMES E. CROWE, JR.[2]

INFLUENZA HEMAGGLUTININ IS A TRIMERIC GLYCOPROTEIN OF THREE IDENTICAL SUBUNITS AND THE MAJOR PROTECTIVE ANTIGEN OF THE VIRUS

Influenza hemagglutinin (HA) is the major glycoprotein on the surface of influenza virions. It mediates receptor binding and fusion. The surface glycoprotein neuraminidase (NA) is a receptor-destroying enzyme. Even though humoral immunity to NA and other proteins and cellular immunity to several viral proteins contribute to protection against influenza infection, neutralizing antibodies directed against influenza HA are sufficient to protect against disease. The H3 HA crystal structure was solved in 1981 at 3-Å resolution (1). Since then, the crystal structures of HA molecules from H2, H5, H7, and several different H1 strains including the pandemic 1918 H1 and the pandemic 2009 H1 (2) have been determined. In brief, HA is a trimeric type I membrane glycoprotein made of three identical subunits (Fig. 1). Each subunit is synthesized as an HA0 precursor and cleaved proteolytically into an HA1 subunit that composes the membrane-distal globular head and part of the membrane-proximal stem region, and an HA2 subunit that only contributes to the stem region (Fig. 1).

[1]Children's Hospital, University of Freiburg Medical Center, 79106 Freiburg, Germany; [2]Vanderbilt Vaccine Center, Vanderbilt University Medical Center, Nashville, TN 37232-0417.
Antibodies for Infectious Diseases
Edited by James E. Crowe, Jr., Diana Boraschi, and Rino Rappuoli
© 2015 American Society for Microbiology, Washington, DC
doi:10.1128/microbiolspec.AID-0021-2014

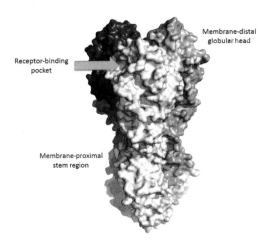

Membrane-distal globular head

Receptor-binding pocket

Membrane-proximal stem region

FIGURE 1 Space-filling model of influenza hemagglutinin HA based on PDB 1RD8 (38). The three protomers of the HA trimer are colored white, gray, or black. doi:10.1128/microbiolspec.AID-0021-2014.f1

The receptor-binding domain (RBD) of HA forms a conserved pocket on the globular head (Fig. 1). Antibodies that target the RBD or adjacent hypervariable loops can inhibit hemagglutination of red blood cells *in vitro* and binding to sialic acid of respiratory epithelial cells (Table 1). In contrast, neutralizing antibodies against the HA stem domain can prevent the pH-induced conformational change that occurs in the endosome after binding to and internalization into the host cell or by interfering with the maturation of HA0 to HA1 and HA2 (3, 4). After the discovery of the murine HA stem-specific monoclonal antibody (mAb) C179 in 1993 (5) that neutralizes H1, H2, and H5 viruses, several groups have reported that humans can generate mAbs against the influenza HA stem as well, many of which are encoded by the V_H1-69 germ line gene that specifies amino acids that seem ideally configured to reach into a hydrophobic pocket on the stem. The frequency of antibodies to the conserved HA stem region may have been increased in infected individuals after the 2009 H1N1 pandemic (6). This observation may represent a special case of original antigenic sin (7, 8, 9, 10), much talked about in the influenza field, although one might

argue that, in fact, the boosting of antibodies to conserved epitopes is consistent with the conventional understanding of B-cell memory. The original antigenic sin theory suggests that, after repeated antigenic exposure, the antibody response is biased toward epitopes that were present in the original antigenic exposure and *against* new related antigens that cause subsequent exposures. Some people have hypothesized that such cross-reactive stem antibodies lead to prepandemic influenza strains becoming extinct (11). However, the frequency of antibodies to conserved epitopes on the globular head of HA also appeared to be increased after the 2009 H1N1 pandemic (12, 13, 14, 15). Such antibodies also could have limited the circulation of prepandemic H1N1 strains. We have cloned mAbs to the H2N2 virus that circulated in humans from 1957 until 1968 from the peripheral blood of healthy donors of an appropriate age to have had exposure to H2 viruses (16). These mAbs were directed against highly conserved epitopes on the head of HA (16, 17). If such antibodies were present on a population level, they probably would limit the circulation of H2 viruses in the human population even more so than stem antibodies

TABLE 1 Characteristics of globular head versus stem HA antibodies

Characteristics	Globular head antibodies	Stem antibodies
Mechanism of action	Inhibition of receptor binding, inhibition of pH-induced conformational change (some)	Inhibition of pH-induced conformational change, interference of HA0 maturation (some)
Inhibition of hemagglutination	+++	–
Neutralization activity	++ / +++	+ / ++
Cross-reactive potential	+ / ++ (RBD)	+++
Frequency	+++	+ (higher after heterologous challenge)
In vivo activity	+++	+ / ++

because of their vastly superior potency. In general, HA globular head antibodies seem to be more frequent than stem antibodies probably because their epitope is more readily accessible on the surface of the virus and can be targeted by a wide diversity of antibodies encoded by a broad variety of antibody germ line genes (Table 1).

A lot of interest has been devoted recently toward presenting this conserved HA stem region as part of a universal vaccine against influenza because of the exciting isolation of cross-neutralizing antibodies directed against the conserved HA stem region (18). With the recent discovery of several cross-neutralizing HA globular head antibodies, the HA globular head also appears as an attractive target for vaccine design. This finding seems particularly important because the access of antibodies to the globular head is not hindered by steric constraints and because the most potent HA globular head antibodies neutralize more strongly than HA stem antibodies. Furthermore, the cocrystal structures of HA globular head antibodies in complex with HA may further serve as starting points for the design of inhibitors against the RBD. Therefore, it seems timely to review the literature on HA globular head antibodies.

THE FIRST ANTIGENIC MAPPING

The first mouse monoclonal antibodies against influenza A HA were generated by hybridoma technology in the early 1980s. By testing these mAbs in competition assays and/or through the selection and sequencing of escape mutants in embryonated egg cells, an antigenic mapping of the HA globular head could be performed for H1, H2, and H3 viruses. For the H1 antibodies, antigenic sites designated Sa, Sb, Ca$_1$, Ca$_2$, and Cb were proposed—the "S" standing for strain-specific and the "C" for cross-reactive (19). Somewhat ironically, the preservation of the supposedly strain-specific Sa antigenic site of the 1918 H1N1 HA in the pandemic 2009 virus was a major reason for antibody cross-

reactivity between those two strains (2, 20, 21). Antibodies that recognized multiple antigenic sites of the globular head of HA had already been identified in the 1980s (19). More recent X-ray cocrystallization experiments have shown subsequently that antibodies, such as 2D1 that is oriented above the center of the Sa site with its large surface area, recognize residues outside the Sa epitope and even residues within neighboring antigenic sites (2). Human antibodies that bind a single, discrete antigenic loop of a conventionally defined site on the HA head domain are probably the exception rather than the rule. The antigenic mapping of murine antibodies may not translate directly to that of human antibodies, since the antibody repertoires of different species use entirely different germ line genes. Still, it can helpful to use the antigenic mapping terms in some instances to orient influenza scientists to features on the HA globular head. One could easily use terms such as "190-helix" instead of "Sb antigenic site," but even epitopes such as the Sb antigenic site that was supposed to be a linear epitope (22) seem like a rather complex epitope of multiple loops (23). Even antibodies that target the conserved receptor-binding sites often touch this 190-helix or Sb site (Table 2).

For H3, antigenic sites designated A to D were established (24). Around the year 2000, three cocrystal structures of mouse H3 globular head antibodies were solved in complex with their HA (25, 26, 27, 28) in work reviewed in detail by Knossow and Skehel (29). The antigenic structure of each HA subtype is slightly different, and one should exercise caution when using the antigenic mapping from the HA of one subtype to describe the topography of the HA from an entirely different subtype. A case in point is the H2 HA. In the initial antigenic mapping, the authors were unable to establish discrete antigenic sites on H2 HA, since most epitopes overlapped (30). Also, about half of the antibodies cloned were influenced by receptor specificity (30).

TABLE 2 Select cross-reactive globular head HA antibodies

Characteristics	2D1	1F1	5J8	CH65/CH67	2G1, 8M2	S139/1	C05
Origin	Human hybridoma	Human hybridoma	Human hybridoma	Human plasmablast	Human hybridoma	Mouse hybridoma	Human phage display
V_H gene assignment	V_H2-70	V_H3-30	V_H4-b	V_H1-2	V_H1-69	Not described	V_H3-23
Bind(s)	Sites Sa, Sb, Ca_1	Sb, site Ca_2	RBD, sites Sb, Ca_2	RBD, site Sb	RBD	RBD, sites A, B, D	RBD, site Sb
Mimics sialic acid	n/a	–	+	+	+	+	–
Binds and/or neutralizes	Pandemic H1	1918 H1 and select 20th century strains	Most H1N1, including pandemic H1	Most H1N1 since 1977	Most H2N2	Select H1, H2, H3, and H13	Select H1, H2, H3, H9, H12
Breadth extended by avidity	Not tested	Not tested	+	+	Not tested	+	+
Note	Lead mAb for 1918/2009 cross-reactivity	Binds residues mediating receptor specificity	Three escape mutations, all outside conventional antigenic sites	Rigidified heavy chain interactions increase affinity	Lead mAbs for V_H1-69 globular head HA recognition	Fab by itself protects against H3 viruses	Cross-reactivity mediated by single antibody loop
PDB(s) of crystal structure	3LZF, 3QHZ, 3QHF	4GXU, 4GXV	4M5Y, 4M5Z	3SM5, 4HKB, 4KH3, 4KH0	4HG4, 4HFU	4GMS, 4GMT	4FQR, 4FP8, 4FNL
References	2, 20, 32, 33	20, 23, 33	13, 45	15	16, 17	47, 48	49

We now know that receptor specificity of H2 viruses is mediated by residues 226 and 228 (31), two residues that lie on the edge of the RBD. Why the murine immune response to H2 HA is so focused on the conserved RBD is not clear (16). However, human monoclonal antibodies against H2 HA also seem to be focused on this very same pocket (16, 17). Thus, such antibodies, if present on a population level, may have limited the duration of H2N2 circulation in humans to 1957 to 1968, a relatively brief period in comparison with that of other subtypes, for example, H1N1 that has been in human circulation from 1918 until 1957 and again from 1977 through the present time.

CROSS-REACTIVITY OF GLOBULAR HEAD HA ANTIBODIES

Since the HA stem is conserved within group 1 HA viruses (which includes several subtypes that have infected humans: H1, H2, H5) and group 2 HA viruses (which includes additional subtypes that have infected humans: H3, H7), respectively, some stem antibodies can neutralize multiple strains across subtypes. However, because of hypervariability of loops surrounding the RBD, the cross-reactive potential of globular head antibodies is generally thought to be more limited. Cross-reactive antibodies to the globular head HA can bind outside of the conserved RBD. Some particularly well-studied examples are the human pandemic H1N1 mAbs 2D1 (2, 20, 32, 33) (Table 2), 2B12 (20, 33), and related Sa site-specific antibodies (14). Such antibodies neutralize the pandemic 1918 and 2009 H1N1 viruses and swine H1N1 viruses, because residues in the Sa site epitope of the 1918 H1N1 are almost unchanged in the 2009 H1N1 virus (2, 20). Richard Shope discovered in the 1930s that variants of the pandemic 1918 H1N1 virus continued to circulate in pigs (34), probably because antigenic pressure in those short-lived animals is very low. Parts of those viruses were reintroduced in 2009 into human circulation through a triple reassortant virus event, so elderly people that had immunity to the 1918 H1N1 virus or swine viruses such as the New Jersey/1976 vaccine strain in the United States may have been partially protected against the 2009 H1N1 virus through Sa site-specific antibodies. There was nothing inherently cross-reactive about these antibodies; the supposedly hypervariable epitope of such antibodies was simply conserved between the two H1 viruses 1918 and 2009. MAb 2D1 did have an interesting feature, a 3-amino-acid insertion, that reconfigures that antibody-combining site by distorting and removing the CDR-H1 loop away from the antigen-antibody interface (32).

Sa site-specific antibodies such as 2D1 or 2B12 do not recognize seasonal H1N1 strains that circulated between the H1N1 pandemics (33). Strains such as A/USSR/1977 H1N1 possess three predicted N-linked glycosylation sites within its Sa antigenic site (20). It is generally believed that glycosylation at these sites shields HA from neutralization (20, 35). However, we were able to clone a panel of neutralizing antibodies that bound the Sa site based on escape mutations of the Sa site residue K166, but that were still able to neutralize A/USSR/1977 H1N1 despite the presence of said glycosylation sites (14). We presently do not understand the structural basis for the fact that glycosylation within the Sa site does not always confer escape from Sa-specific mAbs. Unexpectedly, this panel of independent antibody clones that was derived of the V_H3-7/J_H6 germ line heavy chain genes converged toward similar mutations (14). Interestingly, even essentially unmutated states of those antibodies were found in the peripheral blood (14). Persistent low-affinity memory populations may aid in the immunologic response toward a related HA that the individual subsequently encounters (8, 14, 36).

ANTIBODIES THAT TARGET RESIDUES THAT MEDIATE RECEPTOR SPECIFICITY

We cloned both mAbs 1F1 and 1I20 from one survivor of the 1918 H1N1 pandemic (33). The heavy chains of those antibodies are genetically related, but clonally independent. MAb 1I20 is strain specific, but mAb 1F1 is able to neutralize select H1N1 strains across the 20th century (33), including 1943, 1947, and 1977 viruses, but not the pandemic 2009 H1N1 virus (20). These antibodies selected for escape mutations in position P186 adjacent to the Sb antigenic site (33). The cocrystal structure of 1F1 in complex with 1918 HA shows that 1F1 does indeed make multiple contacts within the 190-helix of the Sb antigenic site, but also touches on the Ca_2 antigenic site, and reaches into the RBD (23) (Table 2). This finding supports our hypothesis that most human antibodies contact multiple conventional antigenic sites, although the number of influenza antibody cocrystal structures is too limited so far to state that this is a universal characteristic of human neutralizing antibodies to HA head domain. In addition to those conventionally defined antigenic sites, 1F1 contacts several HA residues that typically interact with the sialoglycan receptor, including 135, 153, 183, 190, 194, 222, and 225 (23). Residues D190 and D225 mediate H1 HA receptor specificity (31, 37, 38, 39, 40, 41, 42). Reverting these residues to D190E and D225G of avian H1N1 viruses significantly reduces binding for both 1F1 and 1I20 (23). While it is not surprising that two antibodies with similar genetic backgrounds recognize the same epitope (as was seen also for the V_H3-7/J_H6 germ line antibodies mentioned above [14]), we were surprised to see that the epitope of 1F1 on H1 HA is similar to the murine mAb HC63 epitope on H3 HA (28, 43), despite a rotation of the heavy chains by 20°, resulting in completely different interactions for the light chains of 1F1 and HC63. There may be only a limited number of preferred antibody-binding modes even across subtypes (23). HC63 can not only inhibit receptor binding, but also inhibits the pH-induced conformational change that happens upon receptor binding, because HC63 binds multiple HA monomers (28, 43); 1F1 Fab does not share these features (23).

ANTIBODIES THAT MIMIC SIALIC ACID, THE INFLUENZA RECEPTOR

Whittle et al. crystallized the human mAb CH65 that was cloned by plasmablast technology from the peripheral blood of a seasonal influenza vaccine recipient in complex with Λ/Solomon Islands/3/2006 HA (15). CH65 neutralized a broad range of seasonal H1N1 viruses from 1977 until 2006 (15) (Table 2). The CH65 CDR-H3 inserts into the RBD on HA1 where it mimics the physiologic receptor, sialic acid (15). CH65-resistant H1N1 strains seemed to have an insertion in position 133A of the HA, either an arginine or a lysine (15), but Schmidt et al. later found exceptions to this assumption (44). Similarly, we reported the H1N1 cross-reactive mAb 5J8 that neutralizes a broad range of H1N1 strains of the 20th century and the pandemic strains of H1N1, a spectrum of activity that seemed complementary to the mAb CH65 (13). Indeed, mAb 5J8-resistant H1N1 strains did not have an insertion in position 133A of the HA (13). Also, a cocrystal structure of 5J8 in complex with the globular HA1 head domain of A/California/07/2009 HA revealed that 5J8 also uses receptor mimicry, but both antibodies have distinct footprints and different angles of approach (45). Antibodies such as 5J8 may have also contributed to the preexisting immunity toward the pandemic 2009 virus (13), although we speculate that such antibodies were less frequent than Sa site-specific antibodies such as 2D1 (14, 20, 32, 33). MAb 5J8 elicited escape mutations in position 133A, 137, and 222, none of which is part of a conventionally defined H1N1 antigenic site and all of which are relatively well-conserved

(13). It seems likely that H1N1 cannot easily change such residues without the loss of replicative capacity (13).

The human H2N2 mAbs 8M2, 2G1, and 8F8 are also directed against the RBD (16, 17). 8M2 and 2G1 are encoded by the V_H1-69 germ line gene that was conventionally thought of as being stem specific, but it is also ideally suited for recognition of another structurally conserved influenza hydrophobic pocket, the HA RBD (17). Even though 8M2 and 2G1 were cloned from two different individuals, they both insert germ line Phe54 of CDR-H2 into the RBD, and thus provide further evidence of sequence convergence across antibodies (14). In the H2-antibody complexes, the aromatic rings of Phe54 are situated for optimal π-π interaction with the universally conserved HA Trp153 and are surrounded by further highly conserved influenza A residues (17). MAb 8F8, a V_H3-33-encoded antibody, interacts with HA Trp153 through the insertion of aromatic residue Tyr100 of CDR-H3. Escape is mediated through residues that are on the edge of the RBD (16).

MAb 2G1 showed hemagglutination-inhibition (HAI) activity against H2N2 viruses, but also against the pandemic H3N2 virus from 1968 (16). The human V_H1-69 encoded mAb F045-092 that was derived of phage display technology has been reported to cross-neutralize select strains from an even broader spectrum of influenza subtypes (H1, H2, H3, and H13) (46). S139/1 was the first head-specific mAb to be described to neutralize select strains from different influenza subtypes (H1, H2, H3, and H13; Table 2) (47). The crystal structure of the S139/1 Fab in complex with the HA from the A/Victoria/3/1975 (H3N2) virus reveals that the mAb targets residues within the RBD and contacts antigenic sites A, B, and D (48). Although S139/1 Fab is sufficient for neutralization of most H3N2 viruses, it depends on the avidity mediated by the bivalent IgG for its heterosubtypic neutralization (48). The extension of breadth through avidity is also a feature for other mAbs that target the RBD (45, 49).

The footprint of an antibody on HA is larger than the RBD, so an antibody will have to bind to at least some hypervariable residues and can compensate for this fact by avoiding high-affinity interactions dependent on these positions (48). An antibody features three hypervariable loops each on the heavy and light chain, but not all of those loops typically participate in the antigen-antibody interaction. An antibody with a very long CDR-H3 can minimize its footprint on the antigen (49). Ekiert et al. reported such an antibody, designated mAb C05; it binds and/or neutralizes selected strains from H1, H2, H3, H9, and H12 subtypes (Table 2). Apart from CDR-H3, only CDR-H1 makes additional minor interactions with HA, and only 550 Å^2 of surface area is buried on the HA by C05 (49). As with other RBD antibodies, insertions at position 133A seem to abrogate binding (49). And unlike other RBD antibodies, C05 interaction with the RBD differs considerably from sialic acid binding to HA (49). Insertions and deletions at other positions explain why other HA subtypes are not bound and/or neutralized (49).

CONCLUSIONS AND AREAS FOR FUTURE STUDIES

The antibodies described here have important potential diagnostic and therapeutic applications. Antibodies such as 1F1 or 8M2 that recognize viruses with human-receptor specificity only, but not avian-receptor specificity, could be used to screen for viruses with supposedly greater human infectivity. A collection of broadly neutralizing monoclonal antibodies can be used for comparative studies, for example, to facilitate the development of universal vaccines directed against the RBD. Passive administration of such antibodies to humans could provide protective immunity, for example, for immunocompromised individuals that would not be expected to mount a protective immune response after active immunization. Antibodies against res-

piratory-droplet-transmissible avian H5N1 viruses could be used as postexposure prophylaxis (50). Computational designs of proteins against the stem region of HA have yielded novel proteins inhibitors (51) that can be further optimized by creating comprehensive sequence-function maps obtained by deep sequencing (52). The wealth of cross-reactive antibodies against the RBD could serve as templates to design novel influenza therapeutics directed against the RBD of HA by using similar approaches. Because only few residues are universally conserved across all HAs, and such residues will likely not be the only contact residues of novel therapeutics, escape mutations will invariably occur. Based on existing structures and naturally occurring variability in those residues, it seems possible to rationally predict such escape mutations (49). One single protein or small molecule might not be sufficient to neutralize all influenza strains. It might be possible to develop multiple different inhibitors that could be tailored toward specific strains or used in conjunction with other inhibitors (including neuraminidase inhibitors) as an inhibitor cocktail.

The challenge remains how to elicit reliably broadly cross-neutralizing human mAb through vaccination. Studies suggest that individuals may have a greater chance of mounting a robust cross-neutralizing antibody response if primed with DNA vaccines (53) or immunized with adjuvants (54). The conserved stem epitopes seem to be predominantly encoded by the V_H1-69 germ line gene. Given that there is variability in V_H1-69 alleles and the number of V_H1-69 alleles a person carries, some individuals may mount a more robust immune response toward the stem than others. Even though we (16, 17) and others (46) have shown that the V_H1-69 gene element plays an important role for antibodies against the RBD as well, the still limited number of globular head antibodies suggests a more diverse genetic heritage of RBD mAbs. Although antibodies such as C05 with its 24-amino-acid CDR-H3 and 5-amino-acid insertion in CDR-H1 stand out (49), unlike HIV antibodies, most cross-reactive human influenza antibodies analyzed so far do not seem to need unusual structural features or an extraordinarily high number of somatic mutations to achieve cross-reactivity. This observation suggests that it may be easier to induce influenza cross-reactive antibodies than cross-reactive HIV antibodies. It has been proposed to design immunogens to guide precursors of mature B cells in multiple steps toward a desired response (55). We believe that H2 influenza may be a key for the design of a universal vaccine against influenza since its RBD seems to be particularly immunogenic. The molecular or structural basis for this phenomenon is not immediately apparent from structures of H2 HA by itself or in complex with antibodies (17), although the mechanism may be related to the paucity of glycosylation sites on the globular head of H2 HA. Glycosylation can modulate the ability of HA to induce cross-reactive antibodies (56). Increasing the immunogenicity of the RBD in influenza vaccines by modifying select residues of the HA globular head would be major step toward developing an additional component of a universal vaccine.

ACKNOWLEDGMENT

Conflicts of interest: We declare no conflicts.

CITATION

Krause JC, Crowe JE, Jr. 2014. Committing the oldest sins in the newest kind of ways—antibodies targeting the influenza virus type A hemagglutinin globular head. Microbiol Spectrum 2(5):AID-0021-2014.

REFERENCES

1. **Wilson IA, Skehel JJ, Wiley DC.** 1981. Structure of the haemagglutinin membrane glycoprotein of influenza virus at 3 A resolution. *Nature* **289:**366–373.
2. **Xu R, Ekiert DC, Krause JC, Hai R, Crowe JEJ, Wilson IA.** 2010. Structural basis of preexisting immunity to the 2009 H1N1 pandemic influenza virus. *Science* **328:**357–360.
3. **Corti D, Voss J, Gamblin SJ, Codoni G, Macagno A, Jarrossay D, Vachieri SG, Pinna D, Minola A, Vanzetta F, Silacci C, Fernandez-Rodriguez BM, Agatic G, Bianchi S, Giacchetto-Sasselli I, Calder L, Sallusto F, Collins P, Haire LF, Temperton N, Langedijk JP, Skehel JJ, Lanzavecchia A.** 2011. A neutralizing antibody selected from plasma cells that binds to group 1 and group 2 influenza A hemagglutinins. *Science* **333:**850–856.
4. **Ekiert DC, Friesen RH, Bhabha G, Kwaks T, Jongeneelen M, Yu W, Ophorst C, Cox F, Korse HJ, Brandenburg B, Vogels R, Brakenhoff JP, Kompier R, Koldijk MH, Cornelissen LA, Poon LL, Peiris M, Koudstaal W, Wilson IA, Goudsmit J.** 2011. A highly conserved neutralizing epitope on group 2 influenza A viruses. *Science* **333:**843–850.
5. **Okuno Y, Isegawa Y, Sasao F, Ueda S.** 1993. A common neutralizing epitope conserved between the hemagglutinins of influenza A virus H1 and H2 strains. *J Virol* **67:**2552–2558.
6. **Wrammert J, Koutsonanos D, Li GM, Edupuganti S, Sui J, Morrissey M, McCausland M, Skountzou I, Hornig M, Lipkin WI, Mehta A, Razavi B, Del Rio C, Zheng NY, Lee JH, Huang M, Ali Z, Kaur K, Andrews S, Amara RR, Wang Y, Das SR, O'Donnell CD, Yewdell JW, Subbarao K, Marasco WA, Mulligan MJ, Compans R, Ahmed R, Wilson PC.** 2011. Broadly cross-reactive antibodies dominate the human B cell response against 2009 pandemic H1N1 influenza virus infection. *J Exp Med* **208:**181–193.
7. **Davenport FM, Hennessy AV, Francis T, Jr.** 1953. Epidemiologic and immunologic significance of age distribution of antibody to antigenic variants of influenza virus. *J Exp Med* **98:**641–656.
8. **Fish S, Zenowich E, Fleming M, Manser T.** 1989. Molecular analysis of original antigenic sin. I. Clonal selection, somatic mutation, and isotype switching during a memory B cell response. *J Exp Med* **170:**1191–1209.
9. **Krause R.** 2006. The swine flu episode and the fog of epidemics. *Emerg Infect Dis* **12:**40–43.
10. **Wrammert J, Smith K, Miller J, Langley WA, Kokko K, Larsen C, Zheng NY, Mays I, Garman L, Helms C, James J, Air GM, Capra JD, Ahmed R, Wilson PC.** 2008. Rapid cloning of high-affinity human monoclonal antibodies against influenza virus. *Nature* **453:**667–671.
11. **Palese P, Wang TT.** 2011. Why do influenza virus subtypes die out? A hypothesis. *MBio* doi:10.1128/mBio.00150-11.
12. **Wrammert J, Onlamoon N, Akondy RS, Perng GC, Polsrila K, Chandele A, Kwissa M,**

Pulendran B, Wilson PC, Wittawatmongkol O, Yoksan S, Angkasekwinai N, Pattanapanyasat K, Chokephaibulkit K, Ahmed R. 2012. Rapid and massive virus-specific plasmablast responses during acute dengue virus infection in humans. *J Virol* **86:**2911–2918.

13. Krause JC, Tsibane T, Tumpey TM, Huffman CJ, Basler CF, Crowe JE. 2011. A broadly neutralizing human monoclonal antibody that recognizes a conserved, novel epitope on the globular head of the influenza H1N1 virus hemagglutinin. *J Virol* **85:**10905–10908.

14. Krause JC, Tsibane T, Tumpey TM, Huffman CJ, Briney BS, Smith SA, Basler CF, Crowe JE, Jr. 2011. Epitope-specific human influenza antibody repertoires diversify by B cell intraclonal sequence divergence and interclonal convergence. *J Immunol* **187:**3704–3711.

15. Whittle JR, Zhang R, Khurana S, King LR, Manischewitz J, Golding H, Dormitzer PR, Haynes BF, Walter EB, Moody MA, Kepler TB, Liao HX, Harrison SC. 2011. Broadly neutralizing human antibody that recognizes the receptor-binding pocket of influenza virus hemagglutinin. *Proc Natl Acad Sci USA* **108:**14216–14221.

16. Krause JC, Tsibane T, Tumpey TM, Huffman CJ, Albrecht R, Blum DL, Ramos I, Fernandez-Sesma A, Edwards KM, García-Sastre A, Basler CF, Crowe JE. 2012. Human monoclonal antibodies to pandemic 1957 H2N2 and pandemic 1968 H3N2 influenza viruses. *J Virol* **86:**6334–6340.

17. Xu R, Krause JC, McBride R, Paulson JC, Crowe JE, Wilson IA. 2013. A recurring motif for antibody recognition of the receptor-binding site of influenza hemagglutinin. *Nat Struct Mol Biol* **20:**363–370.

18. National Institute of Allergy and Infectious Diseases, National Institutes of Health, US Food and Drug Administration. 2012. Universal Influenza Vaccines Meeting Summary. 19 to 20 June 2012.

19. Caton AJ, Brownlee GG, Yewdell JW, Gerhard W. 1982. The antigenic structure of the influenza virus A/PR/8/34 hemagglutinin (H1 subtype). *Cell* **31:**417–427.

20. Krause JC, Tumpey TM, Huffman CJ, McGraw PA, Pearce MB, Tsibane T, Hai R, Basler CF, Crowe JE. 2010. Naturally occurring human monoclonal antibodies neutralize both 1918 and 2009 pandemic influenza A (H1N1) viruses. *J Virol* **84:**3127–3130.

21. Manicassamy B, Medina RA, Hai R, Tsibane T, Stertz S, Nistal-Villan E, Palese P, Basler CF, Garcia-Sastre A. 2010. Protection of mice against lethal challenge with 2009 H1N1 influenza A virus by 1918-like and classical swine H1N1 based vaccines. *PLoS Pathog* **6:**e1000745. doi: 10.1371/journal.ppat.1000745.

22. Brownlee GG, Fodor E. 2001. The predicted antigenicity of the haemagglutinin of the 1918 Spanish influenza pandemic suggests an avian origin. *Philos Trans R Soc Lond B Biol Sci* **356:**1871–1876.

23. Tsibane T, Ekiert DC, Krause JC, Martinez O, Crowe JE, Wilson IA, Basler CF. 2012. Influenza human monoclonal antibody 1F1 interacts with three major antigenic sites and residues mediating human receptor specificity in H1N1 viruses. *PLoS Pathog* **8:**e1003067. doi:10.1371/journal.ppat.1003067.

24. Wiley DC, Wilson IA, Skehel JJ. 1981. Structural identification of the antibody-binding sites of Hong Kong influenza haemagglutinin and their involvement in antigenic variation. *Nature* **289:**373–378.

25. Fleury D, Wharton SA, Skehel JJ, Knossow M, Bizebard T. 1998. Antigen distortion allows influenza virus to escape neutralization. *Nat Struct Biol* **5:**119–123.

26. Fleury D, Barrere B, Bizebard T, Daniels RS, Skehel JJ, Knossow M. 1999. A complex of influenza hemagglutinin with a neutralizing antibody that binds outside the virus receptor binding site. *Nat Struct Biol* **6:**530–534.

27. Fleury D, Daniels RS, Skehel JJ, Knossow M, Bizebard T. 2000. Structural evidence for recognition of a single epitope by two distinct antibodies. *Proteins* **40:**572–578.

28. Barbey-Martin C, Gigant B, Bizebard T, Calder LJ, Wharton SA, Skehel JJ, Knossow M. 2002. An antibody that prevents the hemagglutinin low pH fusogenic transition. *Virology* **294:**70–74.

29. Knossow M, Skehel JJ. 2006. Variation and infectivity neutralization in influenza. *Immunology* **119:**1–7.

30. Yamada A, Brown LE, Webster RG. 1984. Characterization of H2 influenza virus hemagglutinin with monoclonal antibodies: influence of receptor specificity. *Virology* **138:**276–286.

31. Connor RJ, Kawaoka Y, Webster RG, Paulson JC. 1994. Receptor specificity in human, avian, and equine H2 and H3 influenza virus isolates. *Virology* **205:**17–23.

32. Krause JC, Ekiert DC, Tumpey TM, Smith PB, Wilson IA, Crowe JE Jr. 2011. An insertion mutation that distorts antibody binding site architecture enhances function of a human antibody. *MBio* **2:**e00345-10. doi:10.1128/mBio.00345-10.

33. Yu X, Tsibane T, McGraw PA, House FS, Keefer CJ, Hicar MD, Tumpey TM, Pappas C, Perrone LA, Martinez O, Stevens J, Wilson

IA, Aguilar PV, Altschuler EL, Basler CF, Crowe JE, Jr. 2008. Neutralizing antibodies derived from the B cells of 1918 influenza pandemic survivors. *Nature* **455:**532–536.

34. **Shope RE.** 1931. Swine influenza. I. Experimental transmission and pathology. *J Exp Med* **54:**349–359.

35. **Wei CJ, Boyington JC, Dai K, Houser KV, Pearce MB, Kong WP, Yang ZY, Tumpey TM, Nabel GJ.** 2010. Cross-neutralization of 1918 and 2009 influenza viruses: role of glycans in viral evolution and vaccine design. *Sci Transl Med* **2:**24ra21. doi:10.1126/scitranslmed.3000799.

36. **Herzenberg LA, Black SJ, Tokuhisa T.** 1980. Memory B cells at successive stages of differentiation. Affinity maturation and the role of IgD receptors. *J Exp Med* **151:**1071–1087.

37. **Gamblin SJ, Haire LF, Russell RJ, Stevens DJ, Xiao B, Ha Y, Vasisht N, Steinhauer DA, Daniels RS, Elliot A, Wiley DC, Skehel JJ.** 2004. The structure and receptor binding properties of the 1918 influenza hemagglutinin. *Science* **303:**1838–1842.

38. **Stevens J, Corper AL, Basler CF, Taubenberger JK, Palese P, Wilson IA.** 2004. Structure of the uncleaved human H1 hemagglutinin from the extinct 1918 influenza virus. *Science* **303:**1866–1870.

39. **Glaser L, Stevens J, Zamarin D, Wilson IA, Garcia-Sastre A, Tumpey TM, Basler CF, Taubenberger JK, Palese P.** 2005. A single amino acid substitution in 1918 influenza virus hemagglutinin changes receptor binding specificity. *J Virol* **79:**11533–11536.

40. **Stevens J, Blixt O, Glaser L, Taubenberger JK, Palese P, Paulson JC, Wilson IA.** 2006. Glycan microarray analysis of the hemagglutinins from modern and pandemic influenza viruses reveals different receptor specificities. *J Mol Biol* **355:**1143–1155.

41. **Colman PM, Tulip WR, Varghese JN, Tulloch PA, Baker AT, Laver WG, Air GM, Webster RG.** 1989. Three-dimensional structures of influenza virus neuraminidase-antibody complexes. *Philos Trans R Soc Lond B Biol Sci* **323:**511–518.

42. **Naeve CW, Hinshaw VS, Webster RG.** 1984. Mutations in the hemagglutinin receptor-binding site can change the biological properties of an influenza virus. *J Virol* **51:**567–569.

43. **Daniels PS, Jeffries S, Yates P, Schild GC, Rogers GN, Paulson JC, Wharton SA, Douglas AR, Skehel JJ, Wiley DC.** 1987. The receptor-binding and membrane-fusion properties of influenza virus variants selected using anti-haemagglutinin monoclonal antibodies. *EMBO J* **6:**1459–1465.

44. **Schmidt AG, Xu H, Khan AR, O'Donnell T, Khurana S, King LR, Manischewitz J, Golding**

H, Suphaphiphat P, Carfi A, Settembre EC, Dormitzer PR, Kepler TB, Zhang R, Moody MA, Haynes BF, Liao H-X, Shaw DE, Harrison SC. 2013. Preconfiguration of the antigen-binding site during affinity maturation of a broadly neutralizing influenza virus antibody. *Proc Natl Acad Sci USA* **110:**264–269.

45. **Hong M, Lee PS, Hoffman RMB, Zhu X, Krause JC, Laursen NS, Yoon S-I, Song L, Tussey L, Crowe JE, Ward AB, Wilson IA.** 2013. Antibody recognition of the pandemic H1N1 Influenza virus hemagglutinin receptor binding site. *J Virol* **87:**12471–12480.

46. **Ohshima N, Iba Y, Kubota-Koketsu R, Asano Y, Okuno Y, Kurosawa Y.** 2011. Naturally occurring antibodies in humans can neutralize a variety of influenza virus strains, including H3, H1, H2, and H5. *J Virol* **85:**11048–11057.

47. **Yoshida R, Igarashi M, Ozaki H, Kishida N, Tomabechi D, Kida H, Ito K, Takada A.** 2009. Cross-protective potential of a novel monoclonal antibody directed against antigenic site B of the hemagglutinin of influenza A viruses. *PLoS Pathog* **5:**e1000350. doi:10.1371/journal.ppat.1000350.

48. **Lee PS, Yoshida R, Ekiert DC, Sakai N, Suzuki Y, Takada A, Wilson IA.** 2012. Heterosubtypic antibody recognition of the influenza virus hemagglutinin receptor binding site enhanced by avidity. *Proc Natl Acad Sci USA* **109:**17040–17045.

49. **Ekiert DC, Kashyap AK, Steel J, Rubrum A, Bhabha G, Khayat R, Lee JH, Dillon MA, O'Neil RE, Faynboym AM, Horowitz M, Horowitz L, Ward AB, Palese P, Webby R, Lerner RA, Bhatt RR, Wilson IA.** 2012. Cross-neutralization of influenza A viruses mediated by a single antibody loop. *Nature* **489:**526–532.

50. **Thornburg NJ, Nannemann DP, Blum DL, Belser JA, Tumpey TM, Desphande S, Fritz GA, Sapparapu G, Krause JC, Lee JH, Warm AB, Lee DE, Li S, Winarski KL, Spiller BW, Meiler J, Crowe JE, Jr.** 2013. Human antibodies that neutralize respiratory droplet transmissible H5N1 influenza viruses. *J Clin Invest* **123:**4405–4409.

51. **Fleishman SJ, Whitehead TA, Ekiert DC, Dreyfus C, Corn JE, Strauch EM, Wilson IA, Baker D.** 2011. Computational design of proteins targeting the conserved stem region of influenza hemagglutinin. *Science* **332:**816–821.

52. **Whitehead TA, Chevalier A, Song Y, Dreyfus C, Fleishman SJ, De Mattos C, Myers CA, Kamisetty H, Blair P, Wilson IA, Baker D.** 2012. Optimization of affinity, specificity and function of designed influenza inhibitors using deep sequencing. *Nat Biotechnol* **30:**543–548.

53. **Wei C-J, Yassine HM, McTamney PM, Gall JG, Whittle JR, Boyington JC, Nabel GJ.**

2012. Elicitation of broadly neutralizing influenza antibodies in animals with previous influenza exposure. *Sci Transl Med* **4:**147ra114. doi:10.1126/scitranslmed.3004273.

54. **Khurana S, Chearwae W, Castellino F, Manischewitz J, King LR, Honorkiewicz A, Rock MT, Edwards KM, Del Giudice G, Rappuoli R, Golding H.** 2010. Vaccines with MF59 adjuvant expand the antibody repertoire to target protective sites of pandemic avian H5N1 influenza virus. *Sci Transl Med* **2:**15ra5. doi:10.1126/scitranslmed.3000624.

55. **Haynes BF, Kelsoe G, Harrison SC, Kepler TB.** 2012. B-cell-lineage immunogen design in vaccine development with HIV-1 as a case study. *Nat Biotechnol* **30:**423–433.

56. **Medina RA, Stertz S, Manicassamy B, Zimmermann P, Sun X, Albrecht RA, Uusi-Kerttula H, Zagordi O, Belshe RB, Frey SE, Tumpey TM, Garcia-Sastre A.** 2013. Glycosylations in the globular head of the hemagglutinin protein modulate the virulence and antigenic properties of the H1N1 influenza viruses. *Sci Transl Med* **5:**187ra70. doi:10.1126/scitranslmed.3005996.

Prevention of Respiratory Syncytial Virus Infection: From Vaccine to Antibody

13

KELLY HUANG[1] and HERREN WU[2]

RESPIRATORY SYNCYTIAL VIRUS

Respiratory syncytial virus (RSV) poses a serious and significant health problem. RSV was discovered in 1956 and quickly became recognized as the leading cause of lower respiratory tract disease in infants and young children (1, 2). Preterm infants and young children with bronchopulmonary dysplasia (BPD) or congenital heart disease (CHD) are at high risk of serious RSV infection and may require hospitalizations and stays in the pediatric intensive care unit (3, 4). Although these high-risk groups experience an increased incidence of RSV disease, it is important to note that the majority of infants hospitalized for RSV are previously healthy, nonpremature children (5). In children less than 5 years of age, RSV infections account for 50 to 80% of winter bronchiolitis hospitalizations and 30 to 60% of pneumonia hospitalizations (6, 7). RSV bronchiolitis is reported as the leading cause of hospitalization for infants less than 12 months of age (8, 9, 10, 11). Hospitalization for RSV can reach rates of 1 to 20 per 1,000 infants less than 1 year of age in developed countries (12). Although not common, RSV can be fatal, as 140 to 500 infant deaths are attributed to RSV each year in the United States (13, 14). In addition to infants and young children,

[1]Department of Infectious Disease, MedImmune, LLC., Gaithersburg, MD 20878; [2]Department of Antibody Discovery and Protein Engineering, MedImmune, LLC., Gaithersburg, MD 20878.
Antibodies for Infectious Diseases
Edited by James E. Crowe, Jr., Diana Boraschi, and Rino Rappuoli
© 2015 American Society for Microbiology, Washington, DC
doi:10.1128/microbiolspec.AID-0014-2014

another risk group for RSV disease is the elderly. In fact, while mortality in children due to RSV disease has decreased over the years, mortality due to RSV disease among the elderly is still a significant problem (15, 16, 17, 18, 19, 20). Also, immunosuppressed leukemia patients or patients receiving stem cell transplant therapy experience as much as 80 to 100% mortality upon RSV infection and are therefore a high-risk group for RSV disease (21).

RSV is highly infectious and thus highly prevalent; however, RSV disease does not occur in most cases of infection. Two-thirds of infants are seropositive for RSV by their first birthday, and nearly all children have been infected by their second birthday (22). Outbreaks of RSV are seasonal, occurring during the colder months of the year and varying from year to year in peak months. In certain settings during seasonal RSV outbreaks, such as daycare centers, the attack rate of RSV approaches 100% (23). In addition, RSV is considered a major nosocomial problem for already hospitalized infants (24). Reinfection is quite common throughout life; however, it is typically less severe than the primary infection (22, 23, 25, 26). It is reported that reinfection can occur even with a highly similar virus strain (26, 27), which raises questions about the adaptive immunological response to RSV and about RSV seasonality in that acquisition of herd immunity typically slows the rate of infection until a new strain emerges and starts the next seasonal outbreak, as is observed for influenza. However, the two subtypes of RSV tend to alternate in circulation by 1- to 2-year intervals, which suggests that there is at least some lasting herd immunity (28, 29, 30, 31).

Respiratory syncytial virus is classified as part of the *Pneumovirinae* subfamily of the *Paramyxoviridae* family of viruses. RSV is an enveloped virus with a single-stranded, nonsegmented, and negative sense RNA genome. By electron microscopy, RSV is a pleomorphic virus that adopts both spheroid and long filamentous structures (32, 33,

34, 35). These spheroid and filamentous structures are decorated with three envelope glycoproteins including G (glycosylated) protein, F (fusion) protein, and SH (small hydrophobic) protein. There is one serotype of RSV and two antigenic subtypes designated as A and B. The sequence diversity of the G protein defines the A and B subtypes, with 53% sequence identity between A and B subtypes; whereas, F-protein sequence identity between subtypes is as high as 89% (36). The G protein and F protein are the major targets for antibody-mediated virus neutralization.

The first steps of virus replication include attachment to the target cell followed by viral and cellular membrane fusion. The G protein mediates the majority of the attachment process to target cells, and the F protein mediates the process of fusion. Recombinant viruses with ablated G-protein and SH-protein expression are still infectious *in vitro* (in some cell lines), suggesting that the F protein alone can mediate both attachment and fusion; however, viruses with ablated G protein are highly attenuated *in vivo* (37). The contribution of the SH protein to virus replication is unclear. Upon fusion, the ribonucleoprotein (RNP) complex, consisting of the viral genome coated by the viral N (nucleocapsid) protein along with the P (phosphoprotein) protein, L (RNA-dependent RNA polymerase) protein, and M2-1 protein (transcription factor), are released into the cytoplasm where viral genome replication, transcription, and translation occur (36). Viral genomes and proteins associate at the cell surface to form new virus particles that bud from the plasma membrane (36). *In vitro*, the F protein can mediate cell-to-cell fusion, called syncytium formation, which is the major cytopathic effect of RSV and can be easily observed by light microscopy. However, the observation of syncytium formation *in vivo* is minimal and does not appear to play a major role in viral spread. A general RSV infection process of epithelial cells is shown in Fig. 1.

The pathogenesis of RSV begins with infection of the epithelial layer of the upper respiratory tract, resulting in rhinorrhea, possibly fever and otitis media 4 to 5 days later, which generally lasts 4 to 6 days (38). Viral shedding typically lasts 3 to 8 days, but can be longer in immune-compromised individuals (38). In 25 to 40% of infections, the lower respiratory tract becomes infected, which can result in bronchiolitis or pneumonia (22). RSV infection causes necrosis of the epithelial layer of the respiratory tract, infiltration of leukocytes, edema, and excessive mucous, all of which lead to bronchial obstruction (39, 40). To make matters worse, RSV infection impairs cilia function leading to a reduced ability to clear the necrotic debris (41). Infant bronchioles have a more restricted airway resistance, resulting in greater difficulty dealing with the debris and mucous brought on by an RSV infection of the lower respiratory tract. This might explain, at least in part, why prematurity and young age are risk factors for RSV disease (42). The abnormalities in pulmonary function from RSV disease can persist for 10 years and longer (43), although it is unclear if the patients with persistent pulmonary dysfunction had an underlying condition that predisposed them to RSV disease.

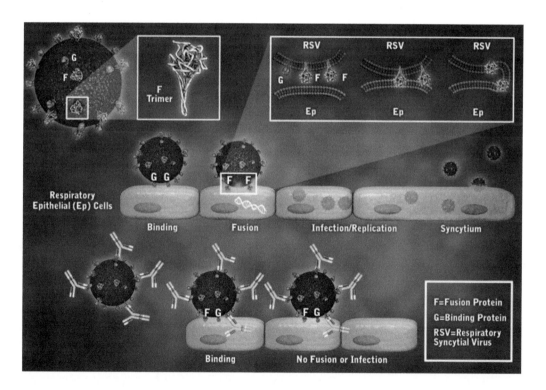

FIGURE 1 The illustration depicts the mechanism of action of RSV-neutralizing mAbs, palivizumab and motavizumab. An RSV virion is illustrated at the top left corner showing that the F and G proteins are located on the surface of the virion and the drawing below depicts G-protein-mediated attachment to cells followed by F protein mediated virus-cell fusion. The steps of fusion are shown on the top right. F protein also mediates cell-to-cell fusion resulting in syncytium formation, depicted in the middle drawing. In the final drawing on the bottom, an RSV-neutralizing antibody, either palivizumab or motavizumab, binds to F protein and blocks virus replication. It was determined that palivizumab and motavizumab do not inhibit RSV attachment, but rather F-protein-mediated virus-cell fusion and syncytia formation as reported recently (99). doi:10.1128/microbiolspec.AID-0014-2014.f1

The standard of care or treatment of RSV disease is an evolving paradigm. One goal in treatment is to reduce viral load. To this end, ribavirin, a nonspecific antiviral was used historically as a treatment for RSV. However, ribavirin is no longer recommended since it does not appear to provide a clinical benefit (44, and American Academy of Pediatrics). Another approach to treating RSV infection is to treat the pathological results of RSV, particularly inflammation. However, treatment with corticosteroids alone has proven to be ineffective (45). Because of the clinical similarity between RSV disease and asthma, bronchial dilators were explored as a treatment strategy for RSV infection, but were not efficacious (46). One success story in the treatment of RSV disease is the use of cysteinyl leukotrienes that effectively treat persistent wheezing that can follow bronchiolitis (47).

RSV is unique in its ability to cause reinfections in persons of all ages (22, 23, 25, 26, 27). This observation has led to the hypothesis that RSV infection does not induce a durable immune response. There is evidence that supports the role of both cell-mediated and humoral immunity in clearing an RSV infection. In terms of cell-mediated immunity, most RSV proteins will stimulate a cytotoxic T lymphocyte (CTL) response in seropositive individuals (48). The observation that RSV tetramer$^+$CD8$^+$ cells are reduced in the elderly population (49), a high-risk group for RSV disease, and that these cells do not have a robust proliferation response in RSV recall assays in comparison with young patients, suggests the importance of cell-mediated immunity in clearing RSV (50). The role of humoral immunity is supported by evidence from numerous studies that show antibodies restrict RSV replication and aid faster clearance by cell-mediated immunity (reviewed in reference 36). One supportive example of this is the observation that maternal antibodies acquired via transplacental passive immunization provide a protective role for neonates (12).

Another example, as discussed in detail later in this article, is that high-titer anti-RSV intravenous immunoglobulin (IVIG) and anti-RSV monoclonal antibody administration provides sterilizing immunity to RSV. Finally, there is a direct correlation between the level of neutralizing antibody in the serum and reduced risk and severity of RSV disease (25, 26, 51, 52, 53, 54, 55, 56, 57, 58).

RSV VACCINE

Despite advances in understanding the immunological correlates to protection, a vaccine for RSV is not available. RSV vaccine efforts were greatly stifled by the use of a formalin-inactivated RSV vaccine that resulted in a greater number of vaccinees hospitalized upon infection with RSV in comparison with the placebo control group (80% versus 5%, respectively) due to serious pulmonary dysfunction, and this resulted in some fatalities (59). Upon RSV infection, vaccinees experienced exaggerated lymphocyte proliferation that resulted in a high Th2 response, which is speculated to have contributed to the high degree of lung inflammation (59). The formalin-inactivated RSV vaccine results were recapitulated in animal models with vaccines consisting of recombinant viral proteins (60, 61, 62), which may guide current vaccine development. For instance, the use of recombinant RSV viral protein vaccines might be safer for the elderly population to prevent reinfection, but may not be preferred for the pediatric population to prevent primary RSV infection out of concern for provoking a high Th2 response. Strategies for pediatric vaccine include attenuated RSV or virus vectors expressing RSV antigens. Attenuated virus vaccines will need to be sufficiently attenuated to greatly minimize the chance of reversion to wild-type virus. Virus vectored antigens typically possess low immunogenicity and will need to be engineered to improve the ability to provoke cell-mediated immune responses. All pediatric vaccine strategies will need to address the challenges of immunological immaturity and maternal antibodies that hamper vaccine efforts (63, 64, 65, 66). Further understanding of the correlates of protection against RSV infection and the correlates of risk will greatly benefit vaccine development efforts.

Since the identification of RSV, the need for a vaccine has long been recognized (1). However, the efforts to develop a safe and effective vaccine against RSV have been met with great challenges. This has steered researchers to seek alternative approaches. Early evidence suggested that passive immunization with antibodies may be a viable alternative for the prophylaxis of RSV infection. It was found that the severity of RSV-induced pneumonia was inversely related to the titer of maternal neutralizing antibody in infants (53). Moreover, the level of serum IgG to RSV F (fusion) protein has correlated with the protective effect against RSV reinfection and illness severity (51). However, there was controversial view about antibodies in the early days, since vaccine results seemed to imply that serum antibodies confer little protection and might even exacerbate disease (67). In addition, the incidence of RSV-induced bronchiolitis peaks in infants between 1 and 6 months of age when maternal antibodies are still present (68). Further studies in animal models using monoclonal or polyclonal antibodies have helped delineate the protection role of antibodies and enhanced confidence in the antibody-mediated prophylaxis approach. Two research teams showed that animals (mice and cotton rats) are protected against lung infection by the administration of mouse anti-RSV monoclonal antibodies prior to RSV challenge (69, 70). In addition, it was found that human convalescent antiserum to RSV administered intraperitoneally to cotton rats provided near-complete pulmonary protection upon RSV challenge (71). Furthermore, human IVIG was shown to reduce RSV replication in the lungs of the RSV-infected monkeys (72). Evidence of enhanced pathology due to the administration

of anti-RSV antibodies in the presence of RSV was not observed in any of these animal studies, which is in contrast to the results of the formalin-inactivated vaccine administered to humans.

IMMUNOPROPHYLAXIS OF RSV INFECTION: FROM DISCOVERY TO MARKET APPROVAL

Intravenous Immunoglobulin

Since IVIG was shown to protect animals against RSV infection (71, 72), it seemed likely that passive immunization with human IVIG would prevent RSV infection in high-risk children. Human clinical trials were conducted to test this hypothesis (73, 74). It was concluded that monthly infusions of standard immune globulin containing RSV-neutralizing antibodies could be safely administered to high-risk pediatric patients. There was a trend toward less severe RSV illness in IVIG-treated patients compared with the control group, as measured by the length of hospitalization. However, standard IVIG lacked sufficient RSV-neutralizing antibody titer to confer full protection against severe RSV illness (74). To improve on efficacy, an effective screening assay to identify plasma-yielding immunoglobulin with high RSV-neutralizing and animal-protective activities was developed (75). Among seven assays tested to identify such RSV antibody activity, a microneutralization assay was found to be most useful. Microneutralization-screened IVIG, so called RSV-IVIG, has 5-fold better activity to neutralize RSV than standard IVIG.

Two major clinical trials were conducted using RSV-IVIG (76, 77). The results from these randomized, controlled trials were very promising; they demonstrated the safety and efficacy of RSV-IVIG in preventing RSV infection in pediatric patients. In the National Institute of Allergy and Infectious Diseases (NIAID) study, 249 children with prematurity, BPD, or CHD were enrolled (76). Monthly infusions at 750 mg/kg resulted in a 63% reduction in RSV hospitalizations and in a 97% reduction in the number of days in the intensive care unit. The adverse events were generally mild. The PREVENT study sponsored by MedImmune, Inc. (Gaithersburg, MD) was a larger trial, which enrolled 510 children with BPD and/or a history of prematurity (77). In this study, it was demonstrated that monthly administration of 750 mg of RSV-IVIG per kg reduced RSV hospitalization by 41%. The PREVENT study reported a 53% reduction in the total number of RSV hospitalization days, a 60% reduction in the number of RSV days with increased oxygen requirement, and a 54% reduction in the number of RSV hospital days with a moderate or severe lower respiratory track illness upon RSV-IVIG administration. Similar to the NIAID study results, RSV-IVIG was shown to be safe and well tolerated in the PREVENT study, as well, with only 1 to 3% of treated children experiencing medically significant adverse events related to RSV-IVIG administration. The safety profile was similar to other IVIG treatments. Based on these trial results, the U.S. Food and Drug Administration (FDA) approved MedImmune's RSV-IVIG (RespiGam) on 18 January 1996 for the prevention of serious lower respiratory tract infection caused by RSV in children <24 months of age with BPD or a history of premature birth (≤35 weeks gestation). This was a major milestone in the development of effective medicine against severe RSV disease. It validated the hypothesis of passive immunization with antibodies as an effective approach for the prophylaxis of RSV infection in humans. In separate trials, RSV-IVIG was tested to treat RSV-infected infants and young children. Unfortunately, despite giving the very high dose of 1,500 mg/kg, there was no significant therapeutic effect (78, 79).

Monoclonal Antibody

Although RSV-IVIG is a safe and effective immunoprophylaxis against RSV infection, there are some drawbacks. RSV-IVIG is derived from human donors screened for a high titer of RSV-neutralizing activity. Despite the fact that the production of RSV-IVIG utilizes modern viral inactivation methods, concerns about transmission of unsuspected blood-borne pathogens have remained. RSV-IVIG requires monthly intravenous infusion and is time consuming, typically lasting several hours with the administration of a total fluid volume of 15 ml/kg. This could cause fluid overload in some children (76, 77). In addition, RSV-IVIG, similar to other IVIGs, may potentially interfere with routine administration schedules of certain vaccines, like measles, mumps, and rubella (80). Furthermore, in a trial in children with CHD, RSV-IVIG did not show a statistically significant decrease in RSV hospitalization for all children with CHD (although there was a trend). Also, there was a significantly higher frequency of unanticipated cyanotic episodes and poor outcomes after surgery among children with cyanotic CHD in the RSV-IVIG group than in the control group (81). The hyperviscosity caused by 750 mg of RSV-IVIG per kg was speculated to be one of the potential causes.

To improve upon RSV-IVIG, researchers turned toward recombinant monoclonal antibodies (mAbs) as a second-generation product. There were great technology advancements in the antibody field from 1975 to 1990. Several key technologies were invented, including hybridoma, chimeric antibody, antibody humanization, and recombinant antibody expression in mammalian cell cultures. These technologies allowed researchers to produce highly specific mAbs against RSV with high affinity. The humanization approach was a key component in the development of the second-generation RSV product. This approach was used to reshape hybridoma-derived murine monoclonal antibodies to be human-like, and enabled evasion of the human immune system to reduce unwanted immunogenicity. Advances in mammalian expressing technologies enabled high-quantity production of RSV mAbs in a defined medium without the concerns of potential blood-borne pathogens.

During the same period of time, basic knowledge about RSV also greatly accumulated, allowing researchers to identify appropriate RSV antigens as antibody targets. In animal studies (69, 70), researchers found that mAbs against two RSV glycoproteins, F and G, confer protection; however, antibodies against other RSV proteins, such as N protein and P protein, have no significant effect. The substantially conserved sequence identity of F protein between subtypes, in comparison with G protein (36), suggests that F protein is likely a more ideal target than G protein for developing broad neutralizing mAbs among different RSV strains. Further study by the use of a large panel of neutralizing mAbs against the F protein of RSV A2 strain was conducted to construct a detailed topological and operational map of epitopes involved in neutralization and fusion (82). In this study, researchers immunized mice by sequential infection with RSV A2 and recombinant vaccinia virus expressing RSV F.

In the 1990s, there were three recombinant anti-RSV F-protein mAbs, two IgG1, and one IgA tested in humans. One of the antibodies, a humanized IgG1/κ RSHZ19 (SB 209763) was developed by GlaxoSmithKline. RSHZ19 had demonstrated RSV-neutralization ability in mice (83). In an early trial in healthy men at single ascending doses of 0.025 to 10 mg/kg, RSHZ19 was shown to be safe and well tolerated, and immunogenicity against RSHZ19 was not detected (84). However, RSHZ19 administered at repeat doses (two intramuscular doses, 8 weeks apart) up to 10 mg/kg failed in a pediatric trial to protect infants born prematurely or with BPD against RSV lower respiratory tract infection (85). The trial showed that RSHZ19 had a mean half-life of 32.5 days and did not induce detectable antidrug immunogenicity. The authors suggested that higher doses should be considered in additional trials. However, no further study was reported, and RSHZ19 was never licensed in any worldwide market.

The second antibody HNK20 is a mouse IgA secreted by hybridomas derived from lung lymphocytes of RSV-immunized mice (86) and was developed by OraVax. The rationale of using IgA is that it is the dominant antibody isotype in the upper airway secretions. It is also less likely to induce inflammatory responses at the mucosal surface since it cannot fix complement factors efficiently. HNK20 was developed as a nose-drop treatment with the intent of protecting the site of initial infection, thus preventing infection from spreading to the lungs. HNK20 was shown to protect the upper and lower respiratory tract from RSV infections in mice (86) and in rhesus monkeys (87). In rhesus monkeys, HNK20 administered at ~0.5 mg/kg intranasally once daily for 2 days before RSV challenge and for 4 days after challenge reduced viral load in the nose, throat, and lungs by 3 to 4 $\log_{10}$/ml. After treatment, HNK20 remained at viral neutralization levels in nasal secretions for >24 h. Encouraged by these results, human clinical trials were conducted (88). However, HNK20 did not reduce the RSV hospitalization rate significantly in a phase III trial during which >600 high-risk infants received intranasal prophylaxis treatment. In a subgroup analysis, a trend with reduced RSV hospitalization was observed for infants younger than 4 months at study entry. The overall results were not encouraging, and there was no additional clinical development of HNK20 (88).

The third antibody, palivizumab (also named MEDI-493 and Synagis) was developed by MedImmune, Inc., as described in the following section.

Palivizumab: the Only Approved mAb for Preventing RSV Infection

The antibody, mAb 1129, is one from a panel of antibodies derived from hybridomas used to characterize the neutralization epitopes of RSV F protein in a study described earlier (82), and it showed neutralization of a broad spectrum of RSV isolates. This antibody was licensed to and further developed by MedImmune, Inc. for potential applications in humans.

Murine mAb 1129 was humanized by a complementarity-determining region (CDR)-grafting approach (Fig. 2) (89). The light-chain CDRs were transplanted onto the human K102 VL/Jκ4 framework regions. The heavy-chain CDRs were transplanted onto the human Cor/CE-1 VH framework regions. Several murine residues on framework 4 regions of VH and VL were retained to potentially maintain the structural integrity of the binding site. In addition, because of an unintended frameshift during the humanization process, the first four residues of the light chain CDR1, SASS, were substituted by four random, nonhuman, nonmouse residues, KCQL. The humanized antibody (IgG1/κ), palivizumab, recognizes a conserved neutralizing epitope on the RSV F protein with a binding affinity ~1 to 2 nM in K_d, which is similar to that of the chimeric derivative of the parental antibody (Fig. 1).

Palivizumab was tested against a panel of 57 clinical isolates of RSV consisting of 34 A and 23 B subtypes, and was shown to have broad neutralization activity against all test isolates. When compared with RSV-IVIG in the microneutralization and fusion-inhibition assays, palivizumab demonstrated a 20- to 30-fold enhanced potency. In a cotton rat prophylaxis study, palivizumab was able to reduce RSV titers in the lung by more than 99% at a dose of 2.5 mg/kg. Furthermore, the administration of palivizumab did not induce increased RSV infection or pathology (89). Supported by the *in vitro* and *in vivo* results, palivizumab was further evaluated as an immunoprophylaxis agent against RSV infection in high-risk human infants.

Several clinical trials were conducted to evaluate the safety and efficacy of palivizumab. The most notable trial was the multicenter Phase III IMpact study (90). In this study, 1,502 children with prematurity (≤35 weeks) or BPD were randomly assigned to receive either five monthly intramuscular injections of palivizumab (15 mg/kg) or an equivalent volume of placebo. Palivizumab was shown to reduce RSV hospitalization incidence by 55% (hospitalization occurrence was 10.6% for placebo treated versus 4.8% for palivizumab treated). In addition, palivizumab treatment resulted in fewer days spent in the hospital, less time on oxygen support, reduced moderate/severe lower respiratory tract illness, and a lower incidence of intensive care unit admission due to RSV infection. It was concluded that palivizumab is safe and effective for the prevention of serious RSV illness in premature children and those with BPD. Based on these clinical results, palivizumab was approved by the FDA in 1998 for immunoprophylaxis of serious RSV respiratory disease in premature infants and children with BPD. Subsequently, an additional study was conducted to demonstrate the efficacy of palivizumab in young children with CHD (n = 1,287) (91), and this resulted in FDA approval to use palivizumab as immunoprophylaxis in this patient population. Palivizumab was also approved in Europe in 1999, and in Japan in 2002. Currently, it is licensed in over 60 countries and has been administered to more than one million high-risk infants and children.

Motavizumab and Motavizumab-YTE

The approval of palivizumab validates the approach for targeting RSV F protein. However, despite the use of palivizumab, there still existed an unmet medical need regarding RSV infection. For example, some infants treated with palivizumab still become infected by RSV and require hospitalization. In addition, there are no adequate preventative or treatment measures available for adult immunocompromised patients. A second-generation antibody, motavizumab, was generated (92, 93) and tested in human clinical trials by MedImmune. It is an affinity-optimized, humanized mAb derived from palivizumab. A direct-evolution approach was used to substantially improve the binding kinetics, both k_{on} and k_{off}, of the antibody to F protein which is mediated by only 13 amino acid substitutions. Motavizumab binds to RSV F protein with 70-fold higher affinity than palivizumab, and exhibits a ~20-fold improvement in the viral neutralization potency *in vitro*. In a cotton rat prophylaxis model, motavizumab was found to be more potent in reducing nasal and lung RSV titers than palivizumab.

Multiple clinical trials of motavizumab were conducted. In a pivotal phase III, noninferiority trial, 6,635 high-risk infants and children were enrolled and received 15 mg/kg motavizumab or palivizumab monthly for 5 months (94). Recognizing that it may be challenging to show superiority against an effective agent, this trial was designed to evaluate whether motavizumab was noninferior and potentially superior to palivizumab in reducing the RSV hospitalization rate and other RSV-associated endpoints. The trial results showed that the motavizumab group had a 26% lower RSV hospitalization rate than the palivizumab group, which achieved the noninferiority primary endpoint. In addition, motavizumab was shown to be superior to palivizumab in one of the secondary endpoints for reducing RSV-specific outpatient medically attended lower respiratory tract infection (MALRI) by 50% compared with palivizumab ($P = 0.005$). Overall, adverse events were not significantly different between these two groups. However, the incidence of cutaneous reactions were higher in the motavizumab group (7.2% versus 5.1% with palivizumab; $P < 0.001$). The overall results suggest motavizumab may provide an improved alternative in preventing serious RSV infection in high-risk infants and children. In a separate trial that compared motavizumab with palivizumab in children with CHD ($n = 1,236$) for safety and tolerability, both molecules were shown to have similar safety profiles with the exception of cutaneous reactions, which occurred more frequently in motavizumab recipients (95). In 2008, MedImmune submitted a Biologics License Application (BLA) for motavizumab to the FDA for the prevention of serious RSV respiratory disease in high-risk pediatric patients.

In 2010, The Antiviral Drugs Advisory Committee to the FDA voted not to recommend approval of motavizumab, citing a concern on the risk/benefit profile. The FDA requested additional safety and efficacy data before considering motavizumab for approval. Subsequently, MedImmune withdrew the BLA and discontinued further development of motavizumab for the prophylaxis of serious RSV respiratory disease.

Both palivizumab and motavizumab have a serum half-life of up to ~3 weeks and require monthly dosing during the RSV season. With the intent to reduce the dosing frequency, the antibody constant region (Fc) of motavizumab was engineered to enhance its binding affinity to neonatal Fc receptor (FcRn). Studies have shown that FcRn plays a key role in maintaining the serum IgG concentration. IgG binds to FcRn in a pH-dependent manner, as it binds tightly at acidic pH and has almost no binding at neutral pH. This differential binding mechanism allows efficient recycling of IgG back to circulation during the pinocytosis event. Three mutations (M252**Y**/S254**T**/T256**E**) were introduced to the Fc region of motavizumab, resulting in a new molecule named motavizumab-YTE (also named MEDI-557). These mutations, termed YTE, increase the binding of antibody to human FcRn at pH 6 by ~10-fold while maintaining its very low or no binding ability to FcRn at pH 7.4. In pharmacokinetic studies in cynomolgus monkeys, the serum half-life and lung bioavailability of motavizumab-YTE were increased by 4-fold compared with motavizumab (96). A randomized dose-escalation phase I human trial in healthy adults ($n = 31$) was conducted to evaluate the pharmacokinetics, tolerability, and safety of motavizumab-YTE (97). A single dose of motavizumab-YTE or motavizumab (0.3, 3, 15, or 30 mg/kg) was administered intravenously, and the data were collected for 240 days. It was found that the half-life of motavizumab-YTE was 2- to 4-fold longer than that of motavizumab. In addition, motavizumab-YTE remains fully functional during the course of 240 days in circulation,

(A)

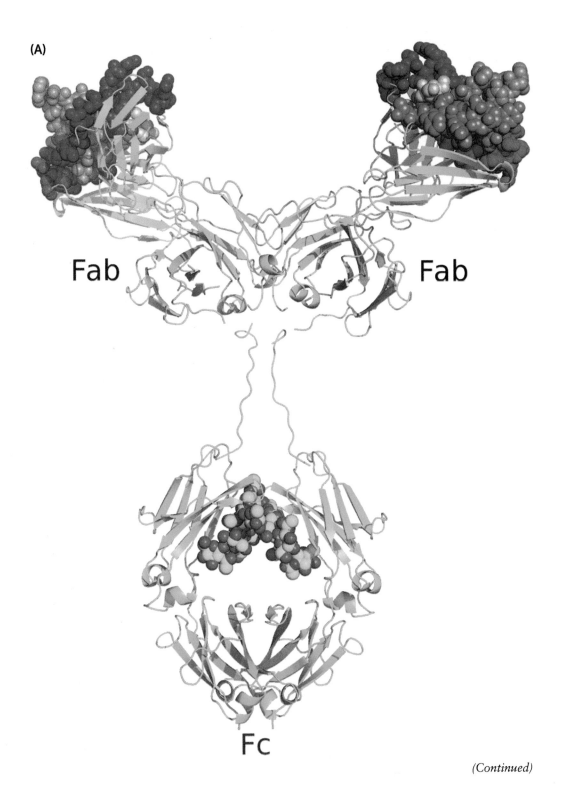

Fab

Fab

Fc

(Continued)

(B)

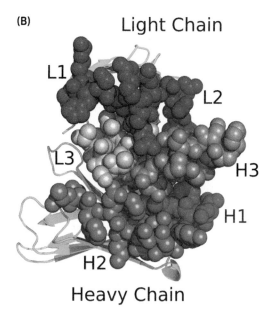

FIGURE 2 **(A) Palivizumab was generated by CDR-grafting humanization of murine mAb 1129. Murine CDR regions are depicted in ball structure. The remaining regions are human origin. (B) Top view of the six murine CDRs that were grafted to human frameworks. doi:10.1128/microbiolspec. AID-0014-2014.f2**

as determined by RSV neutralization activity. Motavizumab-YTE was well tolerated and had an extended half-life of up to 100 days.

FUTURE OPPORTUNITIES FOR TREATMENT AND PREVENTION OF RSV INFECTION

There are continued efforts in searching for new approaches to treat or prevent RSV infection. Recently, several very potent anti-RSV antibodies were isolated from peripheral blood memory B cells by genetic programming (98). In microneutralization assay, these human antibodies were ~2 log more potent than palivizumab. One of the most potent antibodies, D25, was tested in a cotton rat prophylaxis model and achieved full prevention of lung viral replication at a dose of 0.6 mg/kg compared with the required 2 mg/kg of palivizumab to achieve

same protection. These potent anti-RSV antibodies are currently licensed to MedImmune for further development. MedImmune is applying its half-life extension YTE technology to these antibodies. The goal is to provide patients with a very potent long-lasting antibody that can be administered less frequently, perhaps once per quarter or once per RSV season. In addition to mAbs, other emerging drug modalities are being explored. Ablynx is currently developing an anti-RSV F protein Nanobody (ALX-0141) to treat RSV infections. Nanobody is a technology based on the camelid VHH domain, about one-tenth the size of mAb. ALX-0141 is a trivalent Nanobody and is developed for delivery directly into the lungs by inhalation; it is currently in phase I human trial. In addition, Symphogen had once developed a recombinant oligoclonal antibody approach to prevent RSV infection, Sym003. Sym003 is a mixture of six unique antibodies against RSV and was in preclinical development. However, there are no new reports in recent years, and the program is no longer shown on the Symphogen website. It is likely that this project was suspended for further development. Alnylam has developed an RNAi approach (ALN-RSV01) for the treatment of RSV infection. Its RNAi therapeutic was designed to target the nucleocapsid "N" gene, which is required for RSV replication. The molecule was tested in a phase IIb trial against progressive bronchiolitis syndrome (BOS) in lung transplant patients. A dose of 0.6 mg/kg or placebo was administered by inhalation once daily for 5 days. In all analyses, inhaled ALN-RSV01 was associated with a clinically meaningful reduction in the incidence of BOS, and the drug was safe and well tolerated. However, the study narrowly missed its primary endpoint of reduction in BOS in an intent-to-treat analysis of confirmed RSV-infected patients. There are no new reports on the status of this program.

Palivizumab continues to remain the only approved prophylaxis drug against RSV. Despite the challenges in developing vaccines or new drugs against RSV, these new approaches offer promises for RSV intervention in the future.

ACKNOWLEDGMENTS

We thank Vaheh Oganesyan for providing the antibody model structures used in Fig. 2.

We declare a conflict of interest: Both authors are employees of MedImmune, which developed and markets palivizumab.

CITATION

Wu H, Huang K. 2014. Prevention of respiratory syncytial virus infection: from vaccine to antibody. Microbiol Spectrum 2(4):AID 0014-2014.

REFERENCES

1. **Chanock R, Roizman B, Myers R.** 1957. Recovery from infants with respiratory illness of a virus related to chimpanzee coryza agent (CCA). I. Isolation, properties and characterization. *Am J Hyg* **66:**281–290.
2. **Beem M, Wright FH, Hamre D, Egerer R, Oehme M.** 1960. Association of the chimpanzee coryza agent with acute respiratory disease in children. *N Engl J Med* **263:**523–530.
3. **Boyce TG, Mellen BG, Mitchel EF, Jr, Wright PF, Griffin MR.** 2000. Rates of hospitalization for respiratory syncytial virus infection among children in Medicaid. *J Pediatr* **137:**865–870.
4. **Hall CB, Weinberg GA, Iwane MK, Blumkin AK, Edwards KM, Staat MA, Auinger P, Griffin MR, Poehling KA, Erdman D, Grijalva CG, Zhu Y, Szilagyi P.** 2009. The burden of respiratory syncytial virus infection in young children. *N Engl J Med* **360:**588–598.
5. **Wang EE, Law BJ, Boucher FD, Stephens D, Robinson JL, Dobson S, Langley JM, McDonald J, MacDonald NE, Mitchell I.** 1996. Pediatric Investigators Collaborative Network on Infections in Canada (PICNIC) study of admission and management variation in patients hospitalized with respiratory syncytial viral lower respiratory tract infection. *J Pediatr* **129:**390–395.
6. **Flaherman V, Li S, Ragins A, Masaquel A, Kipnis P, Escobar GJ.** 2010. Respiratory syncytial virus testing during bronchiolitis episodes of care in an integrated health care delivery system: a retrospective cohort study. *Clin Ther* **32:**2220–2229.
7. **Shay DK, Holman RC, Newman RD, Liu LL, Stout JW, Anderson LJ.** 1999. Bronchiolitis-associated hospitalizations among US children, 1980–1996. *JAMA* **282:**1440–1446.
8. **Fryzek JP, Martone WJ, Groothuis JR.** 2011. Trends in chronologic age and infant respiratory syncytial virus hospitalization: an 8-year cohort study. *Adv Ther* **28:**195–201.
9. **Leader S, Kohlhase K.** 2002. Respiratory syncytial virus-coded pediatric hospitalizations, 1997 to 1999. *Pediatr Infect Dis J* **21:**629–632.
10. **Leader S, Kohlhase K.** 2003. Recent trends in severe respiratory syncytial virus (RSV) among US infants, 1997 to 2000. *J Pediatr* **143:**S127–S132.
11. **Stockman LJ, Curns AT, Anderson LJ, Fischer-Langley G.** 2012. Respiratory syncytial virus-associated hospitalizations among infants and young children in the United States, 1997–2006. *Pediatr Infect Dis J* **31:**5–9.
12. **Glezen WP, Paredes A, Allison JE, Taber LH, Frank AL.** 1981. Risk of respiratory syncytial virus infection for infants from low-income families in relationship to age, sex, ethnic group, and maternal antibody level. *J Pediatr* **98:**708–715.
13. **Shay DK, Holman RC, Roosevelt GE, Clarke MJ, Anderson LJ.** 2001. Bronchiolitis-associated mortality and estimates of respiratory syncytial virus-associated deaths among US children, 1979–1997. *J Infect Dis* **183:**16–22.
14. **Thompson WW, Shay DK, Weintraub E, Brammer L, Cox N, Anderson LJ, Fukuda K.** 2003. Mortality associated with influenza and respiratory syncytial virus in the United States. *JAMA* **289:**179–186.
15. **Falsey AR, Walsh EE.** 2005. Respiratory syncytial virus infection in elderly adults. *Drugs Aging* **22:**577–587.
16. **Walsh EE, Falsey AR, Hennessey PA.** 1999. Respiratory syncytial and other virus infections in persons with chronic cardiopulmonary disease. *Am J Respir Crit Care Med* **160:**791–795.
17. **Hall CB, Long CE, Schnabel KC.** 2001. Respiratory syncytial virus infections in previously healthy working adults. *Clin Infect Dis* **33:**792–796.
18. **Sorvillo FJ, Huie SF, Strassburg MA, Butsumyo A, Shandera WX, Fannin SL.** 1984. An outbreak of respiratory syncytial virus pneumonia in a nursing home for the elderly. *J Infect* **9:**252–256.
19. **Vikerfors T, Grandien M, Olcen P.** 1987. Respiratory syncytial virus infections in adults. *Am Rev Respir Dis* **136:**561–564.
20. **Dowell SF, Anderson LJ, Gary HE, Jr, Erdman DD, Plouffe JF, File TM, Jr, Marston BJ, Breiman RF.** 1996. Respiratory syncytial

virus is an important cause of community-acquired lower respiratory infection among hospitalized adults. *J Infect Dis* **174:**456–462.

21. **Whimbey E, Champlin RE, Couch RB, Englund JA, Goodrich JM, Raad I, Przepiorka D, Lewis VA, Mirza N, Yousuf H, Tarrand JJ, Bodey GP.** 1996. Community respiratory virus infections among hospitalized adult bone marrow transplant recipients. *Clin Infect Dis* **22:**778–782.

22. **Glezen WP, Taber LH, Frank AL, Kasel JA.** 1986. Risk of primary infection and reinfection with respiratory syncytial virus. *Am J Dis Child* **140:**543–546.

23. **Henderson FW, Collier AM, Clyde WA Jr, Denny FW.** 1979. Respiratory-syncytial-virus infections, reinfections and immunity. A prospective, longitudinal study in young children. *N Engl J Med* **300:**530–534.

24. **Groothuis J, Bauman J, Malinoski F, Eggleston M.** 2008. Strategies for prevention of RSV nosocomial infection. *J Perinatol* **28:**319–323.

25. **Beem M.** 1967. Repeated infections with respiratory syncytial virus. *J Immunol* **98:**1115–1122.

26. **Hall CB, Walsh EE, Long CE, Schnabel KC.** 1991. Immunity to and frequency of reinfection with respiratory syncytial virus. *J Infect Dis* **163:**693–698.

27. **Hall CB, Douglas RG Jr, Geiman JM, Messner MK.** 1975. Nosocomial respiratory syncytial virus infections. *N Engl J Med* **293:**1343–1346.

28. **Hall CB, Walsh EE, Schnabel KC, Long CE, McConnochie KM, Hildreth SW, Anderson LJ.** 1990. Occurrence of groups A and B of respiratory syncytial virus over 15 years: associated epidemiologic and clinical characteristics in hospitalized and ambulatory children. *J Infect Dis* **162:**1283–1290.

29. **Peret TC, Hall CB, Schnabel KC, Golub JA, Anderson LJ.** 1998. Circulation patterns of genetically distinct group A and B strains of human respiratory syncytial virus in a community. *J Gen Virol* **79**(Pt 9)**:**2221–2229.

30. **Waris M.** 1991. Pattern of respiratory syncytial virus epidemics in Finland: two-year cycles with alternating prevalence of groups A and B. *J Infect Dis* **163:**464–469.

31. **White LJ, Waris M, Cane PA, Nokes DJ, Medley GF.** 2005. The transmission dynamics of groups A and B human respiratory syncytial virus (hRSV) in England & Wales and Finland: seasonality and cross-protection. *Epidemiol Infect* **133:**279–289.

32. **Bachi T, Howe C.** 1973. Morphogenesis and ultrastructure of respiratory syncytial virus. *J Virol* **12:**1173–1180.

33. **Jeffree CE, Rixon HW, Brown G, Aitken J, Sugrue RJ.** 2003. Distribution of the attach-ment (G) glycoprotein and GM1 within the envelope of mature respiratory syncytial virus filaments revealed using field emission scanning electron microscopy. *Virology* **306:**254–267.

34. **Okamoto Y, Kudo K, Ishikawa K, Ito E, Togawa K, Saito I, Moro I, Patel JA, Ogra PL.** 1993. Presence of respiratory syncytial virus genomic sequences in middle ear fluid and its relationship to expression of cytokines and cell adhesion molecules. *J Infect Dis* **168:**1277–1281.

35. **Roberts SR, Compans RW, Wertz GW.** 1995. Respiratory syncytial virus matures at the apical surfaces of polarized epithelial cells. *J Virol* **69:**2667–2673.

36. **Collins PL, Crowe JE.** 2007. Respiratory syncytial virus and metapneumovirus, p 1601. *In* Knipe DM, Howley PM (ed), *Fields Virology*, 5th ed. Lippincott Williams & Wilkins, Philadelphia, PA.

37. **Teng MN, Whitehead SS, Collins PL.** 2001. Contribution of the respiratory syncytial virus G glycoprotein and its secreted and membrane-bound forms to virus replication in vitro and in vivo. *Virology* **289:**283–296.

38. **Black CP.** 2003. Systematic review of the biology and medical management of respiratory syncytial virus infection. *Respir Care* **48:**209–233.

39. **Aherne W, Bird T, Court SD, Gardner PS, McQuillin J.** 1970. Pathological changes in virus infections of the lower respiratory tract in children. *J Clin Pathol* **23:**7–18.

40. **Neilson KA, Yunis EJ.** 1990. Demonstration of respiratory syncytial virus in an autopsy series. *Pediatr Pathol* **10:**491–502.

41. **Tristram DA, Hicks W, Jr, Hard R.** 1998. Respiratory syncytial virus and human bronchial epithelium. *Arch Otolaryngol Head Neck Surg* **124:**777–783.

42. **Hogg JC, Williams J, Richardson JB, Macklem PT, Thurlbeck WM.** 1970. Age as a factor in the distribution of lower-airway conductance and in the pathologic anatomy of obstructive lung disease. *N Engl J Med* **282:**1283–1287.

43. **Johnston ID.** 1999. Effect of pneumonia in childhood on adult lung function. *J Pediatr* **135:**33–37.

44. **Leyssen P, De Clercq E, Neyts J.** 2008. Molecular strategies to inhibit the replication of RNA viruses. *Antiviral Res* **78:**9–25.

45. **Patel H, Platt R, Lozano JM, Wang EE.** 2004. Glucocorticoids for acute viral bronchiolitis in infants and young children. *Cochrane Database Syst Rev* **3:**CD004878. doi:10.1002/14651858. CD004878.

46. **Kellner JD, Ohlsson A, Gadomski AM, Wang EE.** 2000. Bronchodilators for bronchiolitis.

Cochrane Database Syst Rev **2**:CD001266. doi:10.1002/14651858.CD001266.

47. **Bisgaard H, Study Group on Montelukast and Respiratory Syncytial Virus.** 2003. A randomized trial of montelukast in respiratory syncytial virus postbronchiolitis. *Am J Respir Crit Care Med* **167**:379–383.

48. **Cherrie AH, Anderson K, Wertz GW, Openshaw PJ.** 1992. Human cytotoxic T cells stimulated by antigen on dendritic cells recognize the N, SH, F, M, 22K, and 1b proteins of respiratory syncytial virus. *J Virol* **66**:2102–2110.

49. **de Bree GJ, Heidema J, van Leeuwen EM, van Bleek GM, Jonkers RE, Jansen HM, van Lier RA, Out TA.** 2005. Respiratory syncytial virus-specific CD8+ memory T cell responses in elderly persons. *J Infect Dis* **191**:1710–1718.

50. **Cusi MG, Martorelli B, Di Genova G, Terrosi C, Campoccia G, Correale P.** 2010. Age related changes in T cell mediated immune response and effector memory to Respiratory Syncytial Virus (RSV) in healthy subjects. *Immun Ageing* **7**:14. doi:10.1186/1742-4933-7-14.

51. **Kasel JA, Walsh EE, Frank AL, Baxter BD, Taber LH, Glezen WP.** 1987. Relation of serum antibody to glycoproteins of respiratory syncytial virus with immunity to infection in children. *Viral Immunol* **1**:199–205.

52. **Bruhn FW, Yeager AS.** 1977. Respiratory syncytial virus in early infancy. Circulating antibody and the severity of infection. *Am J Dis Child* **131**:145–148.

53. **Lamprecht CL, Krause HE, Mufson MA.** 1976. Role of maternal antibody in pneumonia and bronchiolitis due to respiratory syncytial virus. *J Infect Dis* **134**:211–217.

54. **Ogilvie MM, Vathenen AS, Radford M, Codd J, Key S.** 1981. Maternal antibody and respiratory syncytial virus infection in infancy. *J Med Virol* **7**:263–271.

55. **Parrott RH, Kim HW, Arrobio JO, Hodes DS, Murphy BR, Brandt CD, Camargo E, Chanock RM.** 1973. Epidemiology of respiratory syncytial virus infection in Washington, D.C. II. Infection and disease with respect to age, immunologic status, race and sex. *Am J Epidemiol* **98**:289–300.

56. **Stensballe LG, Ravn H, Kristensen K, Agerskov K, Meakins T, Aaby P, Simoes EA.** 2009. Respiratory syncytial virus neutralizing antibodies in cord blood, respiratory syncytial virus hospitalization, and recurrent wheeze. *J Allergy Clin Immunol* **123**:398–403.

57. **Falsey AR, Walsh EE.** 1998. Relationship of serum antibody to risk of respiratory syncytial virus infection in elderly adults. *J Infect Dis* **177**:463–466.

58. **Piedra PA, Jewell AM, Cron SG, Atmar RL, Glezen WP.** 2003. Correlates of immunity to respiratory syncytial virus (RSV) associated-hospitalization: establishment of minimum protective threshold levels of serum neutralizing antibodies. *Vaccine* **21**:3479–3482.

59. **Kim HW, Canchola JG, Brandt CD, Pyles G, Chanock RM, Jensen K, Parrott RH.** 1969. Respiratory syncytial virus disease in infants despite prior administration of antigenic inactivated vaccine. *Am J Epidemiol* **89**:422–434.

60. **Connors M, Collins PL, Firestone CY, Sotnikov AV, Waitze A, Davis AR, Hung PP, Chanock RM, Murphy BR.** 1992. Cotton rats previously immunized with a chimeric RSV FG glycoprotein develop enhanced pulmonary pathology when infected with RSV, a phenomenon not encountered following immunization with vaccinia–RSV recombinants or RSV. *Vaccine* **10**:175 484.

61. **Hancock GE, Speelman DJ, Heers K, Bortell E, Smith J, Cosco C.** 1996. Generation of atypical pulmonary inflammatory responses in BALB/c mice after immunization with the native attachment (G) glycoprotein of respiratory syncytial virus. *J Virol* **70**:7783–7791.

62. **Murphy BR, Sotnikov AV, Lawrence LA, Banks SM, Prince GA.** 1990. Enhanced pulmonary histopathology is observed in cotton rats immunized with formalin-inactivated respiratory syncytial virus (RSV) or purified F glycoprotein and challenged with RSV 3-6 months after immunization. *Vaccine* **8**:497–502.

63. **Karron RA, Wright PF, Belshe RB, Thumar B, Casey R, Newman F, Polack FP, Randolph VB, Deatly A, Hackell J, Gruber W, Murphy BR, Collins PL.** 2005. Identification of a recombinant live attenuated respiratory syncytial virus vaccine candidate that is highly attenuated in infants. *J Infect Dis* **191**:1093–1104.

64. **Murphy BR, Alling DW, Snyder MH, Walsh EE, Prince GA, Chanock RM, Hemming VG, Rodriguez WJ, Kim HW, Graham BS.** 1986. Effect of age and preexisting antibody on serum antibody response of infants and children to the F and G glycoproteins during respiratory syncytial virus infection. *J Clin Microbiol* **24**:894–898.

65. **Shinoff JJ, O'Brien KL, Thumar B, Shaw JB, Reid R, Hua W, Santosham M, Karron RA.** 2008. Young infants can develop protective levels of neutralizing antibody after infection with respiratory syncytial virus. *J Infect Dis* **198**:1007–1015.

66. **Yamazaki H, Tsutsumi H, Matsuda K, Nagai K, Ogra PL, Chiba S.** 1994. Effect of maternal antibody on IgA antibody response in nasopharyngeal secretion in infants and children

during primary respiratory syncytial virus infection. *J Gen Virol* **75**(Pt 8):2115–2119.

67. **Kapikian AZ, Mitchell RH, Chanock RM, Shvedoff RA, Stewart CE.** 1969. An epidemiologic study of altered clinical reactivity to respiratory syncytial (RS) virus infection in children previously vaccinated with an inactivated RS virus vaccine. *Am J Epidemiol* **89:**405–421.

68. **Chanock RM, Parrott RH, Vargosko AJ, Kapikian AZ, Knight V, Johnson KM.** 1962. Acute respiratory diseases of viral etiology. IV. Respiratory syncytial virus. *Am J Public Health* **52:**918–925.

69. **Walsh EE, Schlesinger JJ, Brandriss MW.** 1984. Protection from respiratory syncytial virus infection in cotton rats by passive transfer of monoclonal antibodies. *Infect Immun* **43:**756–758.

70. **Taylor G, Stott EJ, Bew M, Fernie BF, Cote PJ, Collins AP, Hughes M, Jebbett J.** 1984. Monoclonal antibodies protect against respiratory syncytial virus infection in mice. *Immunology* **52:**137–142.

71. **Prince GA, Hemming VG, Horswood RL, Chanock RM.** 1985. Immunoprophylaxis and immunotherapy of respiratory syncytial virus infection in the cotton rat. *Virus Res* **3:**193–206.

72. **Hemming VG, Prince GA, Horswood RL, London WJ, Murphy BR, Walsh EE, Fischer GW, Weisman LE, Baron PA, Chanock RM.** 1985. Studies of passive immunotherapy for infections of respiratory syncytial virus in the respiratory tract of a primate model. *J Infect Dis* **152:**1083–1087.

73. **Groothuis JR, Levin MJ, Rodriguez W, Hall CB, Long CE, Kim HW, Lauer BA, Hemming VG.** 1991. Use of intravenous gamma globulin to passively immunize high-risk children against respiratory syncytial virus: safety and pharmacokinetics. The RSVIG Study Group. *Antimicrob Agents Chemother* **35:**1469–1473.

74. **Meissner HC, Fulton DR, Groothuis JR, Geggel RL, Marx GR, Hemming VG, Hougen T, Snydman DR.** 1993. Controlled trial to evaluate protection of high-risk infants against respiratory syncytial virus disease by using standard intravenous immune globulin. *Antimicrob Agents Chemother* **37:**1655–1658.

75. **Siber GR, Leszcynski J, Pena-Cruz V, Ferren-Gardner C, Anderson R, Hemming VG, Walsh EE, Burns J, McIntosh K, Gonin R.** 1992. Protective activity of a human respiratory syncytial virus immune globulin prepared from donors screened by microneutralization assay. *J Infect Dis* **165:**456–463.

76. **Groothuis JR, Simoes EA, Levin MJ, Hall CB, Long CE, Rodriguez WJ, Arrobio J, Meissner HC, Fulton DR, Welliver RC.** 1993. Prophylactic administration of respiratory syncytial virus immune globulin to high-risk infants and young children. The Respiratory Syncytial Virus Immune Globulin Study Group. *N Engl J Med* **329:**1524–1530.

77. **The PREVENT Study Group.** 1997. Reduction of respiratory syncytial virus hospitalization among premature infants and infants with bronchopulmonary dysplasia using respiratory syncytial virus immune globulin prophylaxis. *Pediatrics* **99:**93–99.

78. **Rodriguez WJ, Gruber WC, Welliver RC, Groothuis JR, Simoes EA, Meissner HC, Hemming VG, Hall CB, Lepow ML, Rosas AJ, Robertsen C, Kramer AA.** 1997. Respiratory syncytial virus (RSV) immune globulin intravenous therapy for RSV lower respiratory tract infection in infants and young children at high risk for severe RSV infections: Respiratory Syncytial Virus Immune Globulin Study Group. *Pediatrics* **99:**454–461.

79. **Rodriguez WJ, Gruber WC, Groothuis JR, Simoes EA, Rosas AJ, Lepow M, Kramer A, Hemming V.** 1997. Respiratory syncytial virus immune globulin treatment of RSV lower respiratory tract infection in previously healthy children. *Pediatrics* **100:**937–942.

80. **American Academy of Pediatrics.** 1997. Measles, p 353. *In* Peter G (ed), *Red Book: Report of the Committee on Infectious Diseases,* 24th ed. American Academy of Pediatrics, Elk Grove Village, IL.

81. **Simoes EA, Sondheimer HM, Top FH, Jr, Meissner HC, Welliver RC, Kramer AA, Groothuis JR.** 1998. Respiratory syncytial virus immune globulin for prophylaxis against respiratory syncytial virus disease in infants and children with congenital heart disease. The Cardiac Study Group. *J Pediatr* **133:**492–499.

82. **Beeler JA, van Wyke Coelingh K.** 1989. Neutralization epitopes of the F glycoprotein of respiratory syncytial virus: effect of mutation upon fusion function. *J Virol* **63:**2941–2950.

83. **Tempest PR, Bremner P, Lambert M, Taylor G, Furze JM, Carr FJ, Harris WJ.** 1991. Reshaping a human monoclonal antibody to inhibit human respiratory syncytial virus infection in vivo. *Biotechnology (N Y)* **9:**266–271.

84. **Everitt DE, Davis CB, Thompson K, DiCicco R, Ilson B, Demuth SG, Herzyk DJ, Jorkasky DK.** 1996. The pharmacokinetics, antigenicity, and fusion-inhibition activity of RSHZ19, a humanized monoclonal antibody to respiratory syncytial virus, in healthy volunteers. *J Infect Dis* **174:**463–469.

85. **Meissner HC, Groothuis JR, Rodriguez WJ, Welliver RC, Hogg G, Gray PH, Loh R,**

Simoes EA, Sly P, Miller AK, Nichols AI, Jorkasky DK, Everitt DE, Thompson KA. 1999. Safety and pharmacokinetics of an intramuscular monoclonal antibody (SB 209763) against respiratory syncytial virus (RSV) in infants and young children at risk for severe RSV disease. *Antimicrob Agents Chemother* **43**:1183–1188.

86. Weltzin R, Hsu SA, Mittler ES, Georgakopoulos K, Monath TP. 1994. Intranasal monoclonal immunoglobulin A against respiratory syncytial virus protects against upper and lower respiratory tract infections in mice. *Antimicrob Agents Chemother* **38**:2785–2791.

87. Weltzin R, Traina-Dorge V, Soike K, Zhang JY, Mack P, Soman G, Drabik G, Monath TP. 1996. Intranasal monoclonal IgA antibody to respiratory syncytial virus protects rhesus monkeys against upper and lower respiratory tract infection. *J Infect Dis* **174**:256–261.

88. Weltzin R, Monath TP. 1999. Intranasal antibody prophylaxis for protection against viral disease. *Clin Microbiol Rev* **12**:383–393.

89. Johnson S, Oliver C, Prince GA, Hemming VG, Pfarr DS, Wang SC, Dormitzer M, O'Grady J, Koenig S, Tamura JK, Woods R, Bansal G, Couchenour D, Tsao E, Hall WC, Young JF. 1997. Development of a humanized monoclonal antibody (MEDI-493) with potent in vitro and in vivo activity against respiratory syncytial virus. *J Infect Dis* **176**:1215–1224.

90. The IMpact-RSV Study Group. 1998. Palivizumab, a humanized respiratory syncytial virus monoclonal antibody, reduces hospitalization from respiratory syncytial virus infection in high-risk infants. *Pediatrics* **102**:531–537.

91. Feltes TF, Cabalka AK, Meissner HC, Piazza FM, Carlin DA, Top FH, Jr, Connor EM, Sondheimer HM, Cardiac Synagis Study Group. 2003. Palivizumab prophylaxis reduces hospitalization due to respiratory syncytial virus in young children with hemodynamically significant congenital heart disease. *J Pediatr* **143**:532–540.

92. Wu H, Pfarr DS, Tang Y, An LL, Patel NK, Watkins JD, Huse WD, Kiener PA, Young JF. 2005. Ultra-potent antibodies against respiratory syncytial virus: effects of binding kinetics and binding valence on viral neutralization. *J Mol Biol* **350**:126–144.

93. Wu H, Pfarr DS, Johnson S, Brewah YA, Woods RM, Patel NK, White WI, Young JF, Kiener PA. 2007. Development of motavizumab, an ultra-potent antibody for the prevention of respiratory syncytial virus infection in the upper and lower respiratory tract. *J Mol Biol* **368**:652–665.

94. Carbonell-Estrany X, Simoes EA, Dagan R, Hall CB, Harris B, Hultquist M, Connor EM, Losonsky GA, Motavizumab Study Group. 2010. Motavizumab for prophylaxis of respiratory syncytial virus in high-risk children: a noninferiority trial. *Pediatrics* **125**:e35–e51. doi:10.1542/peds.2008-1036.

95. Feltes TF, Sondheimer HM, Tulloh RM, Harris BS, Jensen KM, Losonsky GA, Griffin MP, Motavizumab Cardiac Study Group. 2011. A randomized controlled trial of motavizumab versus palivizumab for the prophylaxis of serious respiratory syncytial virus disease in children with hemodynamically significant congenital heart disease. *Pediatr Res* **70**:186–191.

96. Dall'acqua WF, Kiener PA, Wu H. 2006. Properties of human IgG1s engineered for enhanced binding to the neonatal Fc receptor (FcRn). *J Biol Chem* **281**:23514–23524.

97. Robbie GJ, Criste R, Dall'acqua WF, Jensen K, Patel NK, Losonsky GA, Griffin MP. 2013. A novel investigational Fc-modified humanized monoclonal antibody, motavizumab-YTE, Has an extended half-life in healthy adults. *Antimicrob Agents Chemother* **57**:6147–6153.

98. Kwakkenbos MJ, Diehl SA, Yasuda E, Bakker AQ, van Geelen CM, Lukens MV, van Bleek GM, Widjojoatmodjo MN, Bogers WM, Mei H, Radbruch A, Scheeren FA, Spits H, Beaumont T. 2010. Generation of stable monoclonal antibody-producing B cell receptor-positive human memory B cells by genetic programming. *Nat Med* **16**:123–128.

99. Huang K, Incognito L, Cheng X, Ulbrandt ND, Wu H. 2010. Respiratory syncytial virus-neutralizing monoclonal antibodies motavizumab and palivizumab inhibit fusion. *J Virol* **84**:8132–8140.

Human Metapneumovirus

14

JENNIFER E. SCHUSTER[1] and JOHN V. WILLIAMS[2,3]

INTRODUCTION

Human metapneumovirus (HMPV), a paramyxovirus first discovered in 2001, is a significant cause of respiratory tract disease in children and adults (1). Humoral immunity plays an important role in HMPV infection, and the study of HMPV antibodies provides important clinical information including the seroprevalence of HMPV, age of primary infection, serological cross-protection between HMPV subgroups, evaluation of vaccine immunogenicity, and strategies for prophylaxis and therapy using monoclonal antibodies (mAbs).

SEROPREVALENCE OF HMPV INFECTION

Primary HMPV infection in children can be determined by seroconversion, which typically occurs within the first 1 to 2 years of life. In an Israeli cohort, 80% of children 2 months of age had evidence of HMPV antibodies, reflective of the broad adult seroprevalence and maternal transmission of

[1]Department of Pediatrics, Children's Mercy Hospital, Kansas City, MO 64108-4619; [2]Department of Pediatrics, Vanderbilt University School of Medicine, Nashville, TN 37232-2581; [3]Department of Pathology, Microbiology, and Immunology, Vanderbilt University School of Medicine, Nashville, TN 37232-2581.
Antibodies for Infectious Diseases
Edited by James E. Crowe, Jr., Diana Boraschi, and Rino Rappuoli
© 2015 American Society for Microbiology, Washington, DC
doi:10.1128/microbiolspec.AID-0020-2014

immunity. Consistent with waning maternally derived antibodies, only 30% of children at 13 months were seropositive. However, 52% of children had HMPV antibodies at 24 months, suggesting that primary infection had occurred (2). By school age, nearly all children have been infected with HMPV. In a Japanese cohort, 77% of children 2 to 5 years of age were seropositive and 100% of children >10 years of age had HMPV antibodies (3). Reinfection occurs throughout childhood and can be assessed by repeated measurements of serology. In one cohort, HMPV-infected children had both a positive IgM and IgG at the time of acute infection, indicating a history of previous infection. These children had a 4-fold IgG rise in convalescent serology, suggesting that a positive IgG is not entirely protective (4). In a cohort of Thai children, 99.7% had positive HMPV serology. As they were followed longitudinally, 5% had evidence of reinfection, as defined by a 4-fold serology rise, during the 4-year study period (5). HMPV seroconversion typically occurs later than respiratory syncytial virus (RSV). In children aged 4 to 11 months, 48% had positive RSV antibody titers, but only 11% had anti-HMPV antibodies. In children over the age of 2 years, seroprevalence is similar (6, 7).

Almost all adults have serologic evidence of prior HMPV infection. Older adults are at increased risk of severe disease, which some researchers postulate is due to waning immunity (8). However, in a German cohort, >90% of people 60 to 89 years of age had neutralizing antibodies (9). Similarly, Japanese adults were followed longitudinally to determine whether the presence of HMPV antibody was protective. Nine subjects with baseline positive titers by enzyme-linked immunosorbent assay (ELISA) and neutralization assay became infected with HMPV during the study period. Infection was associated with a rise in antibody titer by both methods, demonstrating that a positive antibody titer is not fully protective (10).

Last, seroconversion can be used to detect asymptomatic HMPV infection in adults. In one study, young adults had the highest rates of asymptomatic infection at 4% (8).

ANTIBODY SPECIFICITY

Avian pneumovirus (APV) is the other member of the *Metapneumovirus* genus, and researchers postulate that HMPV diverged from APV type C 200 to 400 years ago (11, 12, 13). The N protein is 80% conserved between APV/A, B, and C, and 100% conserved between APV/C and HMPV. An N-protein polyclonal antibody, which targets a conserved peptide, cross-reacted with all members of APV and HMPV, while an anti-N mAb cross-reacted with both APV/C and HMPV (14). Sera from animals infected with APV/C cross-reacted with HMPV fusion (F) protein, and sera from HMPV-infected animals cross-reacted with APV/C F protein. However, HMPV polyclonal sera did not cross-react with APV/A or B (15), consistent with the closer relationship of HMPV to APV/C. Sera from animals infected with RSV, a member of the same subfamily as HMPV, do not neutralize HMPV *in vitro* and vice versa (16). Thus, HMPV is serologically distinct from other related pneumoviruses.

ANTIBODY CROSS-PROTECTION

Four genetic subgroups of HMPV (A1, A2, B1, and B2) circulate with year-to-year variability (17) (Fig. 1). The subgroups are antigenically related with some evidence of cross-neutralization (18). In hamsters, serum neutralization titers showed a 48% antigenic relatedness between subgroups A and B, and, in nonhuman primates, titers were 64 to 99% related (19). HMPV-infected hamsters were protected against subsequent challenge with a heterologous subgroup virus. Sera from infected hamsters neutralized both homologous and heterologous subgroups *in vitro*; however, the neutralizing capacity against the heterologous subgroup was reduced by 16-fold. African green monkeys and macaques displayed similar cross-protection (20, 21). In humans, sera from HMPV-infected children cross-neutralized other subgroups with varying degrees of efficacy. For example, sera from an HMPV A2-infected child neutralized A2 and B2 viruses, but had no activity against B1 *in vitro* (22).

The F protein is highly conserved and immunogenic (13, 18, 23). Antigenic mapping studies using mAbs defined a number of antigenic regions on HMPV F analogous to sites described on RSV F (Fig. 2) (24, 25). Sera from hamsters infected with recombinant parainfluenza 1 (rPIV1) expressing HMPV F neutralized both homologous and heterologous HMPV viruses *in vitro*. Thus, the F protein is a mediator of antibody cross-protection, and it likely mediates some, although not full, protection against reinfection (19).

Unlike F, the glycoprotein (G) is highly variable and contains only 31 to 35% similarity between the A and B subgroups (12, 26). Convalescent sera from HMPV-infected children reacted with only one G protein, presumably the infecting subgroup. This specificity would suggest that the different HMPV subgroups could be considered serotypes if only categorized by the G protein (27); however, F is thought to be the primary target of neutralizing and protective antibodies. Several different approaches have shown that G antibodies are not neutralizing *in vitro* or protective *in vivo* (28, 29, 30).

ANTIBODY RESPONSE TO INFECTION

Twenty-one days postinfection, HMPV-infected cotton rats developed a neutralizing antibody response. The average serum-neutralizing titer was 1:180, which correlated with lung protection (31). In macaques infected with wild-type (WT) HMPV, antibody titer and efficacy waned over time, leading to symptomatic reinfection. Repeat inoculations of HMPV boosted neutralizing antibodies, but, despite boosting, antibody titer waned 18 weeks after initial infection.

Antibody titers at 58 weeks after the initial infection were much lower, animals were completely unprotected against heterologous reinfection, and 2 of 3 animals were not protected against homologous reinfection. The remaining animal had partial, but not full, protection against infection. Interestingly, infection with NL/1/00, a subgroup A virus, induced higher neutralizing titers than NL/1/99, a subgroup B virus (21). Thus, animal studies suggest that, while antibodies can mediate protection, titers wane over time. This phenomenon likely contributes to the capacity of HMPV to reinfect humans throughout life.

AGE-RELATED ANTIBODY DEVELOPMENT

Older adults are an at-risk population for severe respiratory viral infections, including HMPV. One contributing factor is thought to be waning humoral immunity. In a mouse model, both virus-specific and neutralizing antibody responses were higher in younger mice infected with HMPV than in older mice (32). However, in a cohort of nonhospitalized adults infected with HMPV, older adults had a significantly higher acute HMPV titer compared with young adults. Older adults also had a significantly higher convalescent titer contributing to a significantly higher overall rise in titer compared with young adults. Older adults had a trend toward a higher rise in neutralizing antibody, although this was not significant (33).

IMMUNOGLOBULIN CLASSES

IgG and IgA are produced after HMPV infection. In a BALB/c mouse model, IgG1 and IgG2a were detectable 5 days after HMPV infection, and antibody titer peaked at day 8. No IgA or IgE was detected (34). IgG2a antibodies were the dominant immune response in mice immunized with viruslike particles (VLPs) (35).

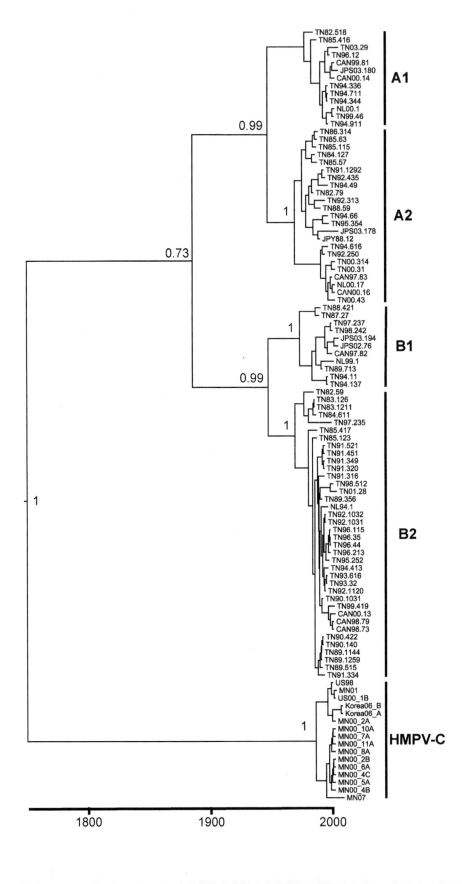

In an adult cohort, HMPV titers in patients with acute infection were compared with HMPV titers in uninfected patients. Serum IgG titer, but not nasal IgA, was associated with the likelihood of developing HMPV reinfection ($11.93 \pm 1.25 \log_2$ in infected individuals vs 12.86 ± 1.23 in uninfected individuals, $P = 0.001$). Although infected adults had lower HMPV IgG titers, the protective level of IgG remains unclear. HMPV-infected adults had significantly lower neutralizing titers compared with uninfected adults. In a longitudinal study, 71% of adults with a baseline microneutralization assay (MNA) titer of $\leq 10.5 \log_2$ were infected compared with 36% infected among adults with a baseline MNA titer $>10.5 \log_2$ (33). These data suggest that there may be a minimum protective threshold of serum-neutralizing antibody titer.

INDUCTION OF ANTIBODIES BY IMMUNIZATION

An effective HMPV vaccine will need to induce an antibody response, and the goal is a high neutralizing antibody titer. Potential types of immunizations include live attenuated HMPV strains, inactivated virus, DNA and protein vaccines, and VLPs. DNA and protein vaccines and VLPs will be discussed separately under antigenic proteins.

Live attenuated HMPV vaccines include strains containing gene deletions or other attenuating mutations. Golden Syrian hamsters infected with HMPVΔSH (deleted short hydrophobic protein) mounted a similar neutralizing antibody response to rHMPV; however, the deletion mutant was not attenuated. Hamsters infected with the attenuated viruses HMPVΔG and HMPVΔSH/G mounted a neutralizing antibody response, but at 6-fold lower titer than rHMPV, and the animals were not fully protected from challenge (36). Therefore, the SH protein is not immunogenic and the G protein is weakly immunogenic. Other immunogenic, attenuated viruses include temperature-sensitive HMPV, which was immunogenic and protective in hamsters (37); a virus lacking an N-linked carbohydrate in the F protein, which was immunogenic and protective in mice (38); and viruses with the F protein RGD-binding sequence mutated, which was immunogenic and protective in cotton rats (39). The conserved RGD motif of the F protein serves to bind integrins as receptors for HMPV (40, 41).

In a phase 1 clinical trial, humans with negative HMPV serology were infected with rHMPV-SH (containing a stabilization mutation in the SH protein). Only 15% had a ≥ 4-fold increase in IgG to HMPV F, 20% had a ≥ 4-fold increase in serum HMPV F IgA, and 30% had a ≥ 4-fold rise in nasal wash IgA (42). Thus, the development of a live attenuated vaccine that will produce an effective neutralizing antibody response in previously infected adults may be difficult.

Formalin-inactivated (FI) HMPV is immunogenic in cotton rats. The vaccine induced neutralizing antibodies, and animals were protected against HMPV challenge (43). However, the vaccine was less effective in macaques. One dose of FI-HMPV induced binding antibodies, but 2 doses were needed to yield neutralizing antibodies. Antibody titer rapidly declined 4 weeks later, and animals were not

FIGURE 1 **Maximum clade credibility tree of HMPV and avian metapneumovirus (AMPV) F nucleotide diversity. Phylogenetic analysis of 85 full-length HMPV F nucleotide sequences from Canada (CAN), Japan (JPS or JPY), Tennessee (TN), or the Netherlands (NL) and 16 AMPV F sequences. The first two digits of the HMPV sequence names indicate the year of the isolate. The names of the AMPV sequences indicate geographic origin (US, United States; UK, United Kingdom; MN, Minnesota) and year. The posterior probability of divergence is indicated at each node. Scale bar represents time in years. Reprinted from reference 13 with permission of the publisher http://creativecommons.org/licenses/by/2.0/legalcode. doi:10.1128/microbiolspec.AID-0020-2014.f1**

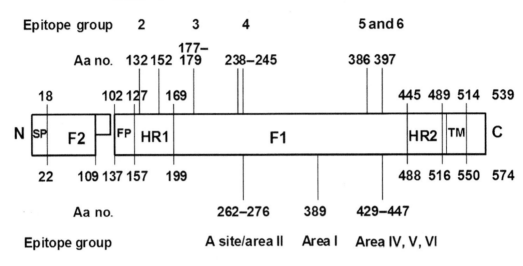

FIGURE 2 Schematic of HMPV and RSV F protein domain structures and relative location of MARM mutation sites. Indicated are the N terminus (N), signal peptide (SP), fusion peptide (FP), heptad repeat 1 (HR1), heptad repeat 2 (HR2), transmembrane domain (TM), and C terminus (C), as well as the F1 and F2 segments of the F protein. The amino acid positions that border domains (predicted) or cleavage sites and C termini (known) are indicated. Also depicted are the relative positions of the HMPV epitope group MARM mutations and corresponding MARM mutation sites on the RSV F protein. Reprinted with permission from Ulbrandt ND, Ji H, Patel NK, Barnes AS, Wilson S, Kiener PA, Suzich J, McCarthy MP. 2008. *J Gen Virol* 89:3113–3118. Copyright 2008 Society for General Microbiology. Permission conveyed through Copyright Clearance Center, Inc. doi:10.1128/microbiolspec.AID-0020-2014.f2

protected against challenge 15 weeks after a third immunization (44). Furthermore, FI-HMPV was associated with enhanced disease upon HMPV challenge in cotton rats and macaques, similar to that observed with FI-RSV vaccine in the 1960s (43, 44).

ANTIGENIC PROTEINS

The HMPV genome contains 8 genes that encode 9 proteins (1). The F, G, and SH protein are outer membrane proteins and likely targets for antibodies. To identify antigenic determinants, each of these 3 proteins was inserted into rPIV-1, a model vaccine system. In hamsters, immunization with PIV-1/HMPV F induced an antibody titer similar to WT HMPV and a high level of neutralizing

antibodies, which conferred lower airway protection. The G protein, expressed by rPIV-1, was less immunogenic than WT HMPV and did not induce neutralizing antibodies. Last, the SH protein did not induce any binding or neutralizing antibodies. Neither rPIV-1/G nor rPIV-1/SH were associated with significant protection against viral replication upon HMPV challenge. Therefore, the F protein is the main antigenic determinant (28).

In Syrian golden hamsters, chimeric bovine/human PIV3 containing HMPV F induced a neutralizing antibody response equivalent to WT HMPV infection (45). This chimeric virus also was immunogenic in African green monkeys, but neutralizing antibody titers were lower compared with animals infected with WT HMPV (46).

Similarly, soluble F-protein vaccines, generated from both A and B subgroup lineage, are protective in hamsters, and F-specific antibodies were present in all animals. Animals immunized with the A-lineage F protein had higher titers compared with B-lineage F, and an adjuvanted F protein was more immunogenic than an unadjuvanted F protein. Adjuvanted F induced a high neutralizing antibody titer (47). F-protein vaccines were more immunogenic than DNA vaccines in a cotton rat model, and the protein vaccine yielded high neutralizing antibody titers (mean 1:570) (23). VLPs containing the F and matrix (M) proteins are immunogenic and protective in a mouse model. After two immunizations, animals had an F-specific antibody response similar to WT HMPV and were protected against challenge (48).

Although the F protein appears to be the primary driver of humoral immunity, the G protein does induce an antibody response. In a cotton rat model, soluble G protein was immunogenic, but it was not protective (30). Mice immunized with the G protein in a vaccinia virus system developed a G-specific antibody response that neutralized homologous but not heterologous virus (49). However, VLPs expressing the G protein were not immunogenic, unlike VLPs containing both the F and G proteins (35). Although SH is generally not immunogenic, a truncated version of the protein expressed by vaccinia virus induced a modest neutralizing antibody response (49).

In humans, the antibody response is much more diverse. In an Irish cohort, antibodies to HMPV M, nucleoprotein (N), and phosphoprotein (P) were identified (50). Antibody responses to N and M typically occurred only in sera with high neutralizing titers (generally >1:160) (51). Other groups have postulated that many F and G antibodies may be conformation dependent, whereas antibodies to N and P may recognize polypeptides (52). Thus, an effective vaccine strategy might include whole outer membrane proteins in conjunction with immunogenic areas of internal proteins.

MONOCLONAL ANTIBODIES

Since the HMPV F protein is highly immunogenic and protective, F-specific mAbs could have clinical use in high-risk hosts, similar to the respiratory syncytial virus anti-F protein mAb, palivizumab (53). Murine mAbs generated against the F protein of HMPV neutralized both A and B subgroups of the virus. Two of these mAbs were effective prophylactically in a hamster model. Although viral replication was minimally decreased in the nasal turbinates, hamsters did not have replicating virus in the lungs at doses of 3 mg/kg. These two mAbs, 234 and 338, bound to the F protein of both the A and B subgroups with nanomolar affinity (54). Mice prophylaxed or treated postinfection with mAb 338 had decreased lung histopathology and airway obstruction compared with mock treated mice (55). DS7, a fully human mAb, neutralized all four subgroups of HMPV *in vitro*, and intranasal DS7 had therapeutic efficacy against HMPV infection in a cotton rat model. The DS7 mAb also had subnanomolar affinity for the F protein (24).

Monoclonal antibody resistant mutants (MARMs) have identified 5 epitopes on the F protein. Two of these epitopes have analogous epitopes on the RSV F protein (Fig. 2) (25). Crystallization of DS7 with the F protein identified a novel antigenic site on the protein, which is a highly conserved area among HMPV subgroups (56).

The F protein is only 33% conserved between RSV and HMPV, and polyclonal sera against one does not cross-react with the other (1, 16). However, one human mAb isolated from screening 114,000 B cells neutralized both viruses. This mAb, MPE8, is an anti-RSV F mAb in its germ line configuration, but it contains light chain mutations in the variable region, affording it activity against HMPV. MPE8 had prophylactic efficacy against HMPV and RSV and prevented death in a mouse model of pneumonia virus of mice, another paramyxovirus. The epitope is distinct from, but in close proximity to, the epitope recognized by palivizumab (57). Another group reported a human mAb isolated by screening B cells against HMPV F protein by ELISA (58). This mAb, 54G10, exhibited broadly neutralizing activity *in vitro* against all 4 subgroups of HMPV and bound to recombinant HMPV F protein with subnanomolar affinity. 54G10 provided potent prophylactic efficacy against all 4 HMPV subgroups in a mouse model, as well as therapeutic efficacy (tested only against A2). The generation of MARMs identified the 54G10 epitope as a region relatively conserved in RSV F and other paramyxoviruses (59). Consistent with a shared epitope, 54G10 neutralized RSV *in vitro* and exhibited both prophylactic and therapeutic efficacy in a mouse model (58). The discovery of mAbs with activity against both HMPV and RSV raises the possibility of not only clinical antibodies that target both viruses, but also epitope-based vaccines that elicit neutralizing antibodies against two distinct viruses.

CONCLUSIONS

Humoral immunity is important in HMPV infection. Further studies are needed to elucidate the level of protective antibody, both after infection and after immunization, as well as to explore the utility of monoclonal antibodies for prophylaxis and therapy against HMPV.

ACKNOWLEDGMENT

Conflicts of interest: We disclose no conflicts.

CITATION

Schuster JE, Williams JV. 2014. Human metapneumovirus. Microbiol Spectrum 2(5):AID-0020-2014.

REFERENCES

1. van den Hoogen BG, de Jong JC, Groen J, Kuiken T, de Groot R, Fouchier RA, Osterhaus AD. 2001. A newly discovered human pneumovirus isolated from young children with respiratory tract disease. *Nat Med* 7:719–724.

2. **Wolf DG, Zakay-Rones Z, Fadeela A, Greenberg D, Dagan R.** 2003. High seroprevalence of human metapneumovirus among young children in Israel. *J Infect Dis* 188:1865–1867.

3. **Ebihara T, Endo R, Kikuta H, Ishiguro N, Yoshioka M, Ma X, Kobayashi K.** 2003. Seroprevalence of human metapneumovirus in Japan. *J Med Virol* 70:281–283.

4. **Ebihara T, Endo R, Kikuta H, Ishiguro N, Ishiko H, Hara M, Takahashi Y, Kobayashi K.** 2004. Human metapneumovirus infection in Japanese children. *J Clin Microbiol* 42:126–132.

5. **Pavlin JA, Hickey AC, Ulbrandt N, Chan YP, Endy TP, Boukhvalova MS, Chunsuttiwat S, Nisalak A, Libraty DH, Green S, Rothman AL, Ennis FA, Jarman R, Gibbons RV, Broder CC.** 2008. Human metapneumovirus reinfection among children in Thailand determined by ELISA using purified soluble fusion protein. *J Infect Dis* 198:836–842.

6. **Ebihara T, Endo R, Kikuta H, Ishiguro N, Ishiko H, Kobayashi K.** 2004. Comparison of the seroprevalence of human metapneumovirus and human respiratory syncytial virus. *J Med Virol* 72:304–306.

7. **Dunn SR, Ryder AB, Tollefson SJ, Xu M, Saville BR, Williams JV.** 2013. Seroepidemiologies of human metapneumovirus and respiratory syncytial virus in young children, determined with a new recombinant fusion protein enzyme-linked immunosorbent assay. *Clin Vaccine Immunol* 20:1654–1656.

8. **Falsey AR, Erdman D, Anderson LJ, Walsh EE.** 2003. Human metapneumovirus infections in young and elderly adults. *J Infect Dis* 187:785–790.

9. **Lusebrink J, Wiese C, Thiel A, Tillmann RL, Ditt V, Muller A, Schildgen O, Schildgen V.** 2010. High seroprevalence of neutralizing capacity against human metapneumovirus in all age groups studied in Bonn, Germany. *Clin Vaccine Immunol* 17:481–484.

10. **Okamoto M, Sugawara K, Takashita E, Muraki Y, Hongo S, Nishimura H, Matsuzaki Y.** 2010. Longitudinal course of human metapneumovirus antibody titers and reinfection in healthy adults. *J Med Virol* 82:2092–2096.

11. **de Graaf M, Osterhaus AD, Fouchier RA, Holmes EC.** 2008. Evolutionary dynamics of human and avian metapneumoviruses. *J Gen Virol* 89:2933–2942.

12. **Yang CF, Wang CK, Tollefson SJ, Lintao LD, Liem A, Chu M, Williams JV.** 2013. Human metapneumovirus G protein is highly conserved

within but not between genetic lineages. *Arch Virol* **158**:1245–1252.

13. **Yang CF, Wang CK, Tollefson SJ, Piyaratna R, Lintao LD, Chu M, Liem A, Mark M, Spaete RR, Crowe JE, Jr, Williams JV.** 2009. Genetic diversity and evolution of human metapneumovirus fusion protein over twenty years. *Virol J* **6**:138. doi:10.1186/1743-422X-6-138.

14. **Alvarez R, Jones LP, Seal BS, Kapczynski DR, Tripp RA.** 2004. Serological cross-reactivity of members of the Metapneumovirus genus. *Virus Res* **105**:67–73.

15. **Luo L, Sabara MI, Li Y.** 2009. Analysis of antigenic cross-reactivity between subgroup C avian pneumovirus and human metapneumovirus by using recombinant fusion proteins. *Transbound Emerg Dis* **56**:303–310.

16. **Wyde PR, Chetty SN, Jewell AM, Boivin G, Piedra PA.** 2003. Comparison of the inhibition of human metapneumovirus and respiratory syncytial virus by ribavirin and immune serum globulin in vitro. *Antiviral Res* **60**:51–59.

17. **Williams JV, Wang CK, Yang CF, Tollefson SJ, House FS, Heck JM, Chu M, Brown JB, Lintao LD, Quinto JD, Chu D, Spaete RR, Edwards KM, Wright PF, Crowe JE, Jr.** 2006. The role of human metapneumovirus in upper respiratory tract infections in children: a 20-year experience. *J Infect Dis* **193**:387–395.

18. **Peret TC, Boivin G, Li Y, Couillard M, Humphrey C, Osterhaus AD, Erdman DD, Anderson LJ.** 2002. Characterization of human metapneumoviruses isolated from patients in North America. *J Infect Dis* **185**:1660–1663.

19. **Skiadopoulos MH, Biacchesi S, Buchholz UJ, Riggs JM, Surman SR, Amaro-Carambot E, McAuliffe JM, Elkins WR, St Claire M, Collins PL, Murphy BR.** 2004. The two major human metapneumovirus genetic lineages are highly related antigenically, and the fusion (F) protein is a major contributor to this antigenic relatedness. *J Virol* **78**:6927–6937.

20. **MacPhail M, Schickli JH, Tang RS, Kaur J, Robinson C, Fouchier RA, Osterhaus AD, Spaete RR, Haller AA.** 2004. Identification of small-animal and primate models for evaluation of vaccine candidates for human metapneumovirus (hMPV) and implications for hMPV vaccine design. *J Gen Virol* **85**:1655–1663.

21. **van den Hoogen BG, Herfst S, de Graaf M, Sprong L, van Lavieren R, van Amerongen G, Yuksel S, Fouchier RA, Osterhaus AD, de Swart RL.** 2007. Experimental infection of macaques with human metapneumovirus induces transient protective immunity. *J Gen Virol* **88**:1251–1259.

22. **Matsuzaki Y, Itagaki T, Abiko C, Aoki Y, Suto A, Mizuta K.** 2008. Clinical impact of human metapneumovirus genotypes and genotype-specific seroprevalence in Yamagata, Japan. *J Med Virol* **80**:1084–1089.

23. **Cseke G, Wright DW, Tollefson SJ, Johnson JE, Crowe JE, Jr, Williams JV.** 2007. Human metapneumovirus fusion protein vaccines that are immunogenic and protective in cotton rats. *J Virol* **81**:698–707.

24. **Williams JV, Chen Z, Cseke G, Wright DW, Keefer CJ, Tollefson SJ, Hessell A, Podsiad A, Shepherd BE, Sanna PP, Burton DR, Crowe JE, Jr, Williamson RA.** 2007. A recombinant human monoclonal antibody to human metapneumovirus fusion protein that neutralizes virus in vitro and is effective therapeutically in vivo. *J Virol* **81**:8315–8324.

25. **Ulbrandt ND, Ji H, Patel NK, Barnes AS, Wilson S, Kiener PA, Suzich J, McCarthy MP.** 2008. Identification of antibody neutralization epitopes on the fusion protein of human metapneumovirus. *J Gen Virol* **89**:3113–3118.

26. **Ishiguro N, Ebihara T, Endo R, Ma X, Kikuta H, Ishiko H, Kobayashi K.** 2004. High genetic diversity of the attachment (G) protein of human metapneumovirus. *J Clin Microbiol* **42**:3406–3414.

27. **Endo R, Ebihara T, Ishiguro N, Teramoto S, Ariga T, Sakata C, Hayashi A, Ishiko H, Kikuta H.** 2008. Detection of four genetic subgroup-specific antibodies to human metapneumovirus attachment (G) protein in human serum. *J Gen Virol* **89**:1970–1977.

28. **Skiadopoulos MH, Biacchesi S, Buchholz UJ, Amaro-Carambot E, Surman SR, Collins PL, Murphy BR.** 2006. Individual contributions of the human metapneumovirus F, G, and SH surface glycoproteins to the induction of neutralizing antibodies and protective immunity. *Virology* **345**:492–501.

29. **Mok H, Tollefson SJ, Podsiad AB, Shepherd BE, Polosukhin VV, Johnston RE, Williams JV, Crowe JE, Jr.** 2008. An alphavirus replicon-based human metapneumovirus vaccine is immunogenic and protective in mice and cotton rats. *J Virol* **82**:11410–11418.

30. **Ryder AB, Tollefson SJ, Podsiad AB, Johnson JE, Williams JV.** 2010. Soluble recombinant human metapneumovirus G protein is immunogenic but not protective. *Vaccine* **28**:4145–4152.

31. **Williams JV, Tollefson SJ, Johnson JE, Crowe JE, Jr.** 2005. The cotton rat (Sigmodon hispidus) is a permissive small animal model of human metapneumovirus infection, pathogenesis, and protective immunity. *J Virol* **79**:10944–10951.

32. **Darniot M, Pitoiset C, Petrella T, Aho S, Pothier P, Manoha C.** 2009. Age-associated aggravation of clinical disease after primary metapneumovirus infection of BALB/c mice. *J Virol* **83**:3323–3332.

33. **Falsey AR, Hennessey PA, Formica MA, Criddle MM, Biear JM, Walsh EE.** 2010. Humoral immunity to human metapneumovirus infection in adults. *Vaccine* **28:**1477–1480.

34. **Darniot M, Petrella T, Aho S, Pothier P, Manoha C.** 2005. Immune response and alteration of pulmonary function after primary human metapneumovirus (hMPV) infection of BALB/c mice. *Vaccine* **23:**4473–4480.

35. **Levy C, Aerts L, Hamelin ME, Granier C, Szecsi J, Lavillette D, Boivin G, Cosset FL.** 2013. Virus-like particle vaccine induces cross-protection against human metapneumovirus infections in mice. *Vaccine* **31:**2778–2785.

36. **Biacchesi S, Skiadopoulos MH, Yang L, Lamirande EW, Tran KC, Murphy BR, Collins PL, Buchholz UJ.** 2004. Recombinant human Metapneumovirus lacking the small hydrophobic SH and/or attachment G glycoprotein: deletion of G yields a promising vaccine candidate. *J Virol* **78:**12877–12887.

37. **Herfst S, de Graaf M, Schrauwen EJ, Sprong L, Hussain K, van den Hoogen BG, Osterhaus AD, Fouchier RA.** 2008. Generation of temperature-sensitive human metapneumovirus strains that provide protective immunity in hamsters. *J Gen Virol* **89:**1553–1562.

38. **Liu P, Shu Z, Qin X, Dou Y, Zhao Y, Zhao X.** 2013. A live attenuated human metapneumovirus vaccine strain provides complete protection against homologous viral infection and cross-protection against heterologous viral infection in BALB/c mice. *Clin Vaccine Immunol* **20:**1246–1254.

39. **Wei Y, Zhang Y, Cai H, Mirza AM, Iorio RM, Peeples ME, Niewiesk S, Li J.** 2014. Roles of the putative integrin-binding motif of the human metapneumovirus fusion (f) protein in cell-cell fusion, viral infectivity, and pathogenesis. *J Virol* **88:**4338–4352.

40. **Cox RG, Livesay SB, Johnson M, Ohi MD, Williams JV.** 2012. The human metapneumovirus fusion protein mediates entry via an interaction with RGD-binding integrins. *J Virol* **86:**12148–12160.

41. **Cseke G, Maginnis MS, Cox RG, Tollefson SJ, Podsiad AB, Wright DW, Dermody TS, Williams JV.** 2009. Integrin alphavbeta1 promotes infection by human metapneumovirus. *Proc Natl Acad Sci USA* **106:**1566–1571.

42. **Talaat KR, Karron RA, Thumar B, McMahon BA, Schmidt AC, Collins PL, Buchholz UJ.** 2013. Experimental infection of adults with recombinant wild-type human metapneumovirus. *J Infect Dis* **208:**1669–1678.

43. **Yim KC, Cragin RP, Boukhvalova MS, Blanco JC, Hamlin ME, Boivin G, Porter DD, Prince GA.** 2007. Human metapneumovirus: enhanced pulmonary disease in cotton rats immunized with formalin-inactivated virus vaccine and challenged. *Vaccine* **25:**5034–5040.

44. **de Swart RL, van den Hoogen BG, Kuiken T, Herfst S, van Amerongen G, Yuksel S, Sprong L, Osterhaus AD.** 2007. Immunization of macaques with formalin-inactivated human metapneumovirus induces hypersensitivity to hMPV infection. *Vaccine* **25:**8518–8528.

45. **Tang RS, Schickli JH, MacPhail M, Fernandes F, Bicha L, Spaete J, Fouchier RA, Osterhaus AD, Spaete R, Haller AA.** 2003. Effects of human metapneumovirus and respiratory syncytial virus antigen insertion in two 3' proximal genome positions of bovine/human parainfluenza virus type 3 on virus replication and immunogenicity. *J Virol* **77:**10819–10828.

46. **Tang RS, Mahmood K, Macphail M, Guzzetta JM, Haller AA, Liu H, Kaur J, Lawlor HA, Stillman EA, Schickli JH, Fouchier RA, Osterhaus AD, Spaete RR.** 2005. A host-range restricted parainfluenza virus type 3 (PIV3) expressing the human metapneumovirus (hMPV) fusion protein elicits protective immunity in African green monkeys. *Vaccine* **23:**1657–1667.

47. **Herfst S, de Graaf M, Schrauwen EJ, Ulbrandt ND, Barnes AS, Senthil K, Osterhaus AD, Fouchier RA, van den Hoogen BG.** 2007. Immunization of Syrian golden hamsters with F subunit vaccine of human metapneumovirus induces protection against challenge with homologous or heterologous strains. *J Gen Virol* **88:**2702–2709.

48. **Cox RG, Erickson JJ, Hastings AK, Becker JC, Johnson M, Craven RE, Tollefson SJ, Boyd KL, Williams JV.** 2014. Human metapneumovirus virus-like particles induce protective B and T cell responses in a mouse model. *J Virol* **88:**6368–6379.

49. **Tedcastle AB, Fenwick F, Robinson MJ, Toms GL.** 2014. Immunogenicity in mice of human metapneumovirus with a truncated SH glycoprotein. *J Med Virol* **86:**547–557.

50. **O'Shaughnessy L, Carr M, Crowley B, Carberry S, Doyle S.** 2011. Recombinant expression and immunological characterisation of proteins derived from human metapneumovirus. *J Clin Virol* **52:**236–243.

51. **Ishiguro N, Ebihara T, Endo R, Ma X, Kawai E, Ishiko H, Kikuta H.** 2006. Detection of antibodies against human metapneumovirus by Western blot using recombinant nucleocapsid and matrix proteins. *J Med Virol* **78:**1091–1095.

52. **Tedcastle AB, Fenwick F, Ingram RE, King BJ, Robinson MJ, Toms GL.** 2012. The characterization of monoclonal antibodies to human metapneumovirus and the detection of multiple forms of the virus nucleoprotein and phosphoprotein. *J Med Virol* **84:**1061–1070.

53. **Pediatrics.** 1998. Palivizumab, a humanized respiratory syncytial virus monoclonal antibody, reduces hospitalization from respiratory syncytial virus infection in high-risk infants. The IMpact-RSV Study Group. *Pediatrics* **102**:531–537.

54. **Ulbrandt ND, Ji H, Patel NK, Riggs JM, Brewah YA, Ready S, Donacki NE, Folliot K, Barnes AS, Senthil K, Wilson S, Chen M, Clarke L, MacPhail M, Li J, Woods RM, Coelingh K, Reed JL, McCarthy MP, Pfarr DS, Osterhaus AD, Fouchier RA, Kiener PA, Suzich JA.** 2006. Isolation and characterization of monoclonal antibodies which neutralize human metapneumovirus in vitro and in vivo. *J Virol* **80**:7799–7806.

55. **Hamelin ME, Gagnon C, Prince GA, Kiener P, Suzich J, Ulbrandt N, Boivin G.** 2010. Prophylactic and therapeutic benefits of a monoclonal antibody against the fusion protein of human metapneumovirus in a mouse model. *Antiviral Res* **88**:31–37.

56. **Wen X, Krause JC, Leser GP, Cox RG, Lamb RA, Williams JV, Crowe JE, Jr, Jardetzky TS.** 2012. Structure of the human metapneumovirus fusion protein with neutralizing antibody identifies a pneumovirus antigenic site. *Nat Struct Mol Biol* **19**:461–463.

57. **Corti D, Bianchi S, Vanzetta F, Minola A, Perez L, Agatic G, Guarino B, Silacci C, Marcandalli J, Marsland BJ, Piralla A, Percivalle E, Sallusto F, Baldanti F, Lanzavecchia A.** 2013. Cross-neutralization of four paramyxoviruses by a human monoclonal antibody. *Nature* **501**:439–443.

58. **Schuster JE, Cox RG, Hastings AK, Boyd KL, Wadia J, Chen Z, Burton DR, Williamson RA, Williams JV.** 2014. A broadly neutralizing human monoclonal antibody exhibits in vivo efficacy against both human metapneumovirus and respiratory syncytial virus. *J Infect Dis* doi:10.1093/infdis/jiu307.

59. **McLellan JS, Chen M, Chang JS, Yang Y, Kim A, Graham BS, Kwong PD.** 2010. Structure of a major antigenic site on the respiratory syncytial virus fusion glycoprotein in complex with neutralizing antibody 101F. *J Virol* **84**:12236–12244.

Dengue Antibody-Dependent Enhancement: Knowns and Unknowns

15

SCOTT B. HALSTEAD[1]

Antibody-dependent enhancement (ADE) is a phenomenon involving infectious IgG antibody immune complexes that mediate the worsening of diseases involving a wide spectrum of microbes and vertebrates. ADE is a new type of Gell-Coombs immunopathology: type I, IgE-mediated immediate hypersensitivity; type II, antibody-mediated acute immune complex disease; type III, IgG-mediated complement-dependent foreign antigen immune complex disease; type IV, cell-mediated immune and autoimmune diseases; and type V, IgG immune complex enhancement of microbial infection in Fc-receptor (FcR)-bearing cells. Three of these immunopathologies are mediated by IgG antibodies. Type V immuno-pathology differs in function from type II and III immunopathologies in that immune complexes are not directly cytotoxic but serve to increase disease severity by regulating the productivity of intracellular microbial infection. In type II immunopathologies, IgG antibodies are often directed at autoantigens and include acute rheumatic fever where microbial antigens mimic antigens in various human tissues, generating an immune response that breaks down immune tolerance. In type III immunopathologies foreign antigen-antibody complexes are often trapped in the basement membranes of endothelial linings. Examples include acute serum sickness, glomerular nephritis, and postimmunization diseases such as break-through measles and respiratory syncytial virus infections in vaccine recipients

[1]Department of Preventive Medicine and Biometrics, Uniformed Services University of the Health Sciences, Bethesda, MD 20814.
Antibodies for Infectious Diseases
Edited by James E. Crowe, Jr., Diana Boraschi, and Rino Rappuoli
© 2015 American Society for Microbiology, Washington, DC
doi:10.1128/microbiolspec.AID-0022-2014

that result in destructive complement-fixing virus-IgG immune complexes predominantly in the lung (1).

An early report of the ADE phenomenon, *in vitro*, was by Hawkes, who observed a greater number of plaques in chick embryo fibroblast monolayers infected with Murray Valley encephalitis virus (MVEV) preincubated with high dilutions of chicken antisera than in virus-only controls (2). In further studies the authors concluded that this phenomenon was the result of antibodies stabilizing the spontaneous degradation of MVEV (3). A different explanation emerged when enhanced infection of dengue virus (DENV) was observed in cultures of peripheral blood mononuclear cells from dengue immune compared with nonimmune subhuman primates (4). This phenomenon was subsequently attributed to enhanced growth of DENV infection in primary monocytes and macrophages in the presence of nonneutralizing enhancing dengue antibodies (5–7). It was shown subsequently that MVEV infection enhancement occurred in functional chicken macrophages that comprise 2% of chick embryo fibroblast monolayers (8). Because of the conformational requirement that Fcγ receptors and IgG Fcγ termini be of the same vertebrate phylogenetic class, ADE in chick embryo fibroblasts was observed only when MVEV antibodies were raised in chickens, not in mammals (9). Because monocytes and macrophages were identified as the principal hosts of *in vivo* DENV infection, the phenomenon of ADE was suggested as an immunopathologic mechanism (10–16).

Different lines of scientific inquiry over the past four decades have sharpened our understanding of microbial antibody-mediated pathogenesis mechanisms in vertebrate hosts. During initial studies of ADE it was assumed that the observed increased growth of virus, which in some cases was 100- to 1,000-fold, was the result of phenomena extrinsic to mononuclear phagocytes such as an increase in rates of attachment or internalization of immune complexes to target cells resulting in an increased number of infected cells compared with controls (6, 7, 17). These mechanisms were studied in mouse macrophage-like cells when West Nile immune complexes attached to FcR-bearing cell surfaces more rapidly compared with naked virus particles (18, 19). With feline infectious peritonitis virus an increased number of peritoneal macrophages were infected *in vitro* in the presence compared with the absence of antibodies (20). It is also possible that immune complexes were internalized more rapidly than was naked virus as observed in an HIV-1 model (21).

These mechanical explanations of ADE changed radically when human macrophages were infected *in vitro* using Ross River virus (RRV) immune complexes, or in mouse models *in vivo*. In humans, acute infections with RRV often evolve to a postinfection arthritis of many months' duration. It was observed that arthritis patients' synovial cells stained for RRV antigens and synovial fluids contained interferon-γ (IFNγ). In an attempt to model this phenomenon, chronic RRV infections were established in mouse macrophage cell lines and in primary human monocytes/macrophages (22). Unexpectedly, the incubation of RRV with diluted RRV antiserum resulted in enhanced infection in these cells through a complex intracellular process involving the suppression of innate cellular immunity by immune complexes. This involved a reduction of the production of reactive nitrogen radicals via NOS2 and the downregulation of INF-α and IFN-β production by abolishing IRF-1 and nuclear factor-ΚB gene expression. Also, there was a marked increase in IL-10 gene transcription and protein production (23, 24). This immune complex suppressive phenomenon required an infectious agent since the ligation of FcγR by zymosan-antibody complexes in the presence of RRV did not ablate antiviral transcription (24). Thus, rather than simply involving an increase in the number of infected cells, ADE in RRV is a complex intracellular phenomenon involving increased intracellular production of virus as a result of immune complex suppression of innate cellular immunity.

These observations were quickly expanded to dengue. The DENVs are a group of four closely related members of the *Flavivirus* genus. DENV-1 through -4 share 60 to 70% genetic homology and are inoculated by the bite of infected *Aedes aegypti*. Initial infections with any of the four DENVs raise protective type-specific antibodies, but the dominant population of antibodies are cross-reactive and nonneutralizing. These efficiently enhance infection by a different DENV type (5, 25–29). *In vitro* studies of FcR-bearing cells show that monoclonal dengue antibodies of many specificities may form infectious immune complexes, the major requirement being attachment to a virion surface antigen at a subneutralizing antibody concentration (30, 31). In practice, antibodies directed at surface epitopes that are not involved in virus entry efficiently produce ADE (32). Indeed, the high rate at which infants acquire severe dengue disease during their first dengue infection when maternal polyclonal dengue antibodies have degraded below protective levels is a unique illustration of the ADE phenomenon in human medicine (10, 33–39). Studies of the pathogenesis of innate and acquired host immune responses to many acute and chronic human and animal infectious diseases show evidence that cross-linking of IgG immune complexes with Fcγ receptors increases intracellular infection, thus contributing to disease severity by a mechanism labeled intrinsic ADE-(iADE) (40, 41). iADE distinguishes intracellular mechanisms from the extrinsic mechanisms of ADE—an increase in infectivity, infection rate, or the number of infected cells by immune complexes compared with infection with the microorganism only. Extrinsic and intrinsic ADE have been measured as contributing a 3-fold or a 100-fold increase in virus production, respectively (42).

The ADE phenomenon has attracted wide interest in viral pathogenesis research because many viruses replicate in macrophages *in vivo*, and this phenomenon is correlated with enhanced disease in many partially immune vertebrate hosts (43–45). Here, the focus will be on iADE in dengue infections as the mechanism that controls the conversion of a mild self-limited acute illness to the dengue vascular permeability syndrome (DVPS). DVPS is the underlying pathophysiological mechanism of dengue hemorrhagic fever/dengue shock syndrome (DHF/DSS) as defined by the 1997 WHO Technical Guidelines (Dengue Haemorrhagic Fever: Diagnosis, Prevention, Treatment and Control. 1997. World Health Organization, Geneva, Switzerland, p. 1–84).

ADE as a pathogenesis mechanism should lead ultimately to a coherent explanation for all the phenomena that comprise DVPS. The basic physiological disturbances and the critical timing of DVPS during the course of a dengue illness are described in Table 1. DVPS usually presents in individuals immune to a single DENV who experience a heterotypic dengue infection (46). A small fraction of cases occurs during a second heterotypic (third) DENV infection (47). DVPS also occurs during primary dengue infections in individuals circulating passively acquired dengue antibodies. In animal models the simple passive transfer of dengue antibodies sensitizes hosts to DVPS during a subsequent DENV infection. Based on these observations, it is conceivable that DVPS might occur during dengue infections in individuals who had previously received blood transfusions from dengue-immune donors. This phenomenon has not yet been reported. But whatever the case, DVPS regularly occurs during primary

TABLE 1 Dengue vascular permeability syndrome

A dengue syndrome that occurs late in the course (on or near defervescence) of an acute dengue illness consisting of:

(a) Thrombocytopenia

(b) Altered hemostasis: most commonly prolonged bleeding time and/or elevated aPTT (activated partial thromboplastin time) and/or elevated prothrombin time

(c) Activated complement, by classical and alternative pathways

(d) Elevated liver transaminase enzymes

(e) Vascular permeability. Clinically significant loss of fluid and small macromolecules (e.g., albumin) into interstitial spaces, most commonly to serosal cavities dengue infections in infants born to women who previously had acquired multiple dengue infections (33, 34, 48). While in dengue-endemic countries this phenomenon contributes 5% of all hospitalized cases, in general, it is poorly studied and vastly under-reported.

As in all infectious diseases, dengue infections progress through phases during which afferent and efferent phenomena predominate. Afferent phenomena are those that improve or potentiate the infection process and pathogenicity of the infecting microorganism. Efferent phenomena are those that counter the pathogenic potential of the infecting microorganism and that lead to the elimination of the infection. For most infections, researchers studying afferent phenomena focus on microbial offensive and defensive weapons, but in dengue, enhancing antibodies and the specific immune complexes that are made contribute powerfully to potentiate infection and disease outcome in dengue. It is my contention that DVPS is the result either of pathogenic factors released directly by infected tissues and/or as an outcome of normal host efferent efforts to control and end infection. In either of these cases, disease severity is directly related to the mass of dengue-infected tissues. Because DVPS in individuals experiencing second dengue infections is essentially identical to that occurring in infants, it is crucial that pathogenesis hypotheses and research efforts focus on unitary mechanisms of DVPS that explain passively as well as actively acquired dengue immunity. The known and unknown afferent and efferent factors contributing to ADE regulation of dengue disease severity will be identified and discussed below according to the outline in Table 2.

KNOWNS

Afferent

Host Genetic Factors Contributing to Susceptibility to DVPS

Many human genetic factors have been identified as being significantly associated with increased or decreased incidence of DVPS during secondary dengue infections. These have been described in recent reviews (49). These factors will not be further considered or discussed here.

Enhancing Antibodies

The sensitizing infection

Human experimentation has established that there is a DENV-2 infection refractory period of three months following an initial DENV-1 infection (50). Possibly related to this protective phenomenon, sera obtained shortly after a primary DENV infection were found to have abundant heterotypic antibodies that formed large immune aggregates on the surface of primary human macrophages that were neutralized in solution but not eliminated via phagocytic clearance (51). After this refractory period, second dengue infections occur, and a portion are expressed as clinical illness. Varying amounts of heterotypic neutralizing antibodies are raised following a primary dengue infection. The natural histories of antibody responses following infection by DENV-1, -2, -3, or -4 including heterotypic antibodies are often unknown.

Infection-enhancing antibodies are an observed risk factor for enhanced dengue disease (52), and an enhanced peak viremia (measured before antibody response starts) has been shown to be an anticipatory correlate of severe disease (53, 54). Recent pathology studies of human autopsies and tissues from mouse models have firmly established the central role of monocytes, macrophages, and immature and mature dendritic cells as infected target cells (13–16, 55).

In dengue-endemic countries monotypic infections with DENV-1, -2, -3, or -4 sensitize individuals to disease accompanying a first heterotypic (second) dengue infection. This phenomenon accounts for around 95% of hospitalized and carefully defined DVPS (47). The clinical outcomes of first heterotypic dengue infection are time dependent. First heterotypic infections occurring at less than a

TABLE 2 Context for understanding "known" and studying "unknown" factors that contribute to the pathogenesis of the dengue vascular permeability syndrome via ADE

Knowns

1. Afferent:
   a. Host genetic factors enhancing susceptibility to DVPS
   b. "Enhancing" antibodies
      i. Sensitizing infections
      ii. Attributes of iADE
      iii. Role of infection sequence
      iv. Role of different myeloid cells
      v. Role of different FcγRs in iADE
   c. Role of DENV in ADE
      i. Enhanced growth of DENV-2 in primary human monocytes
      ii. Differences in ability of DENV-2 strains to be neutralized by DENV-1 antibodies
      iii. DENV-2 genetic differences associated with rapid enhancement of the severity of DENV-2 infection 20 years after infection with DENV-1
      iv. Genetic differences in DENV-2 isolates recovered from disease of enhanced severity 4 years after DENV-1 and 8 years after DENV-3
2. Efferent:
   Overview

Unknowns

1. Afferent:
   a. Host genetic factors enhancing susceptibility to DVPS
   b. "Enhancing" antibodies
      i. Sensitizing infections
      ii. Attributes of iADE
      iii. Role of infection sequence
      iv. Role of different myeloid cells
      v. Role of different FcγRs in iADE
   c. Role of DENV in ADE
      i. Enhanced growth of DENV-2 in primary human monocytes
      ii. Differences in ability of DENV-2 strains to be neutralized by DENV-1 antibodies
      iii. DENV-2 genetic differences associated with rapid enhancement of the severity of DENV-2 infection 20 years after infection with DENV-1
      iv. Genetic differences in DENV-2 isolates recovered from disease of enhanced severity 4 years after DENV-1 and 8 years after DENV-3
2. Efferent:
   Overview

two-year interval are partially protected, resulting in inapparent infections or mild disease (56–59). After that time, DVPS has been observed in 2 to 4% of all second dengue infections combined (for a discussion of the pathogenicity of different sequences of heterotypic dengue infection, see below) (30). The frequency and severity of DVPS increases as the interval between the first and second infections lengthens. This phenomenon was observed when hospitalization and case fatality rates were compared among individuals who were 15 to 39 years old when they experienced first heterotypic DENV-2 infections either 4 or 20 years after a DENV-1 infection.

In 1977 to 1979, around 45% of the population of Cuba (at that time, age groups <1 to 40 were dengue naïve) was infected with DENV-1, a virus introduced into Cuba only once. DENV-2 circulated on the island in 1981, 4 years after DENV-1, and DENV-2, at an interval of 20 years. Hospitalization rates per 10,000 secondary DENV-2 infections at the 20-year interval were 8.2 times higher than at those at a 4-year interval. The case fatality rate was 4.7 times higher when second heterotypic DENV-2 infections occurred at a 20-year compared with a 4-year interval (60). This observation was subsequently correlated with a sustained decline in heterotypic DENV-2 neutralizing antibody titers over a period of 20 years following DENV-1 infections in 1977 to 1979 (61). Heterotypic antibodies have been observed to be important in the modulation of second DENV infections in cultures of primary human monocytes (52). Low dilutions of preinfection sera from children who had inapparent secondary DENV-2 infections almost invariably reduced or neutralized DENV-2 infections in primary human monocytes, while preinfection sera from children who developed an illness requiring hospitalization had little or no detectable heterotypic neutralizing antibodies (52). This observation suggests that low levels of heterotypic neutralizing antibodies (most were anti-DENV-1) did not prevent DENV-2 infection but downregulated DENV-2 clinical responses. In this study, around one-fifth of monotypically dengue-immune school children lacked heterotypic DENV-2 antibodies measured in primary human monocyte cultures and developed DHF when infected by DENV-2. This is virtually the same ratio as for the occurrence of shock during sequential DENV-1 then DENV-2 in Rayong, Thailand (62). Prior infection with two different DENVs (second heterotypic dengue infection) also sensitizes to DVPS, but at a frequency about 50-fold lower than a single DENV infection (47).

In the *in vitro* ADE literature antibodies to many flaviviruses enhance DENV infection in FcR-bearing cells (63). Should this be true for *in vivo* infections, opportunities abound for flavivirus group virus infections to sensitize to enhanced dengue infections. In Southeast Asia the DENVs cocirculate with Japanese encephalitis (JE), in India with JE and West Nile, in Pakistan with West Nile, in Australia with the Kunjin strain of West Nile, and in most of the American region with yellow fever or yellow fever 17D vaccine. Importantly, in Thailand it was observed that children with previous wild-type JE infections or who were immunized with killed JE vaccine developed mild overt dengue illness at a higher frequency than did flavivirus-susceptible patients infected with the same DENV (64). Dengue infections in JE-immune patients not only increased the rate of mild overt dengue disease, but the ensuing illness lasted 2 times longer than dengue illnesses in nonimmune patients. This establishes the ability of JE antibodies to mildly enhance human dengue infections. The *in vitro* correlates of this observation have not been described. Prior to this observation, based upon data trends in a large vaccine study, it was thought that JE vaccination reduced the severity of DHF accompanying a second dengue infection (65).

A large amount of literature has emerged on the role of nonneutralizing antibodies in enhancing DENV infections. It has been observed that a considerable fraction of all antibodies circulating after a first heterotypic dengue infection are directed at prM (32, 66). prM antibodies target immature or partially immature DENV via the pr peptide. A significant fraction of all DENVs produced *in vitro* are immature or partially immature, as are an unknown fraction of DENVs circulating during natural human infections (67). Immature DENVs cannot be processed in the endosome to result in infection. prM antibodies were found to be highly cross-reactive with all DENV serotypes and generally to have poor neutralizing capacity (32, 68). Recent studies showed that prM antibodies enhance the infectivity of noninfectious immature DENV particles (32, 69, 70). Monoclonal DENV antibodies directed at several E domains have been found to interact with immature particles, resulting in infection enhancement in FcR-bearing cells (71, 72).

The attributes of iADE

This is a remarkably complex phenomenon, triggered by attachment of IgG-microbial pathogen complexes to FcRs of many classes, resulting in messages being passaged and expressed via the cytoplasmic tail. Much of what we know about FcR signaling comes from other pathogens—*Leishmania* amastigotes, for instance. The importance of macrophage receptors in the generation of cytokines in *Leishmania*-infected macrophages was recognized when interleukin (IL)-12 production in BALB/c mouse bone marrow macrophages in response to lipopolysaccharide was suppressed after ligation of FcR, complement, or scavenger receptors (73). Both mRNA synthesis and protein secretion were diminished to near undetectable levels following receptor ligation. Suppression was specific to IL-12 since TNFα production was not inhibited. Also, the ligation of mouse FcγR with immune complexes was shown to enhance the production of IL-10 (74). Stimulation of mouse bone marrow macrophages by lipopolysaccharide resulted in some IL-10 production, but the addition of red blood cell (RBC) opsonized with IgG antibodies dramatically enhanced IL-10 production. Immune complexes not only induce activated macrophages to produce IL-10, but they also induce both macrophages and dendritic cells to switch off their production of IL-12 (73, 75). The IL-10 induction by IgG-amastigotes did not occur in macrophages from mice lacking the common gamma chain that signals through FcγR 1, 3, and 4, indicating that one or all of these three receptors were involved. Subsequent studies using defined immune complexes demonstrated that all three of the FcγRs that signal through gamma were capable of signaling for IL-10 production in macrophages (76). The implication from these studies is that in some settings, IgG itself biases the immune response toward a Th2-type response. Indeed, for some species of *Leishmania*, chronicity of infection requires that amastigotes be coated with IgG (77). This phenomenon is now very well established (78–80).

That IL-10 induction by ligation of FcγR was a generic process was demonstrated with a nonmicrobial antigen (81). Lipopolysaccharide-treated BALB/c mouse macrophages when exposed to ovalbumin alone developed T cell responses driven to Th-1 and characterized by the production of IFNγ. When the same antigen was complexed with IgG anti-ovalbumin, T cell responses were driven to Th2 and produced IL-4. This Th2-like phenotype was stable and was retained when the T cells were subsequently restimulated under nonbiasing conditions. Mice vaccinated with IgG-opsonized ovalbumin made high levels of IgG Ab of the IgG1 isotype. The T cell biasing and its reversal via FcγR ligation was also observed *in vivo*. Using macrophages from gene knockout mice, the production of IFNγ and IL-4 by T cells was shown to be controlled by the macrophage cytokines IL-12 and IL-10, respectively. These and other studies demonstrate that the ligation of FcγR on activated macrophages reverses the Th1 biasing that accompanies innate immune responses to microbial products.

How do antibody-coated amastigotes result in the production of IL-10 by macrophages? Ligation of macrophage FcγR produces a rapid and enhanced activation of two mitogen-activated protein kinases: ERK and p38 (82). The activation of ERK leads to the phosphorylation of serine 10 on histone H3 at the *il-10* gene, making the promoter more accessible to transcription factors generated in response to p38 activation (83). Activation of both mitogen-activated protein kinases was required for IL-10 synthesis. In addition to ERK activation, an inflammatory stimulus, such as low-molecular-weight hyaluronic acid from the extracellular matrix, must also be present. The combination of these two signals resulted in the superinduction of IL-10 (84). Macrophages lacking FcγR, or macrophages treated with an inhibitor of spleen tyrosine kinase that is activated following FcγR ligation, failed to activate ERK and consequently failed to produce IL-10 following infection with *Leishmania* amastigotes.

During *in vitro* ADE DENV-2 infection in the THP-1 cell model (human monocytic Fcγ receptor-bearing continuous cell line) intracellular DENV production was increased as a result of idiosyncratic Fcγ-receptor signaling (85). When immune complexes ligate FcγRI and FcγRIIA, at least two of the following types of suppression pathways are expressed: DAK, Atg5-Atg12, SARM, and TANK plus the positive Th2 cytokine regulator, IL10. Collectively, these phenomena downregulate antiviral responses in ADE-infected target cells. DAK and Atg5-Atg12 of RIG-I/MDA5 abolish expression of RIG-I/MDA5 and weaken the RIG-I/MDA5 signaling pathway as monitored through levels of downstream signaling molecules: IPS-1, IKKi, TRAF-3, TBK-I, etc. One outcome is decreased production of type-I IFN as well as IFN-activated antiviral molecules (86). Activation of SARM and TANK results in expression blockage of Toll-like receptors (TLR) 3, 4, and 7 (87). This inhibits MyD88-dependent and MyD88-independent signaling pathways, resulting in another route for type I IFN suppression. As a result of at least these two suppression pathways, ADE-infected THP-1 cells secreted reduced levels of type I IFN and at the same time suppressed the transcription and translation of IL-12, IFN-γ, and TNF-α, facilitating the expression and synthesis of the anti-inflammatory cytokines. ADE infection also suppressed the innate anti-DENV mediator, nitric oxide radicals, by disrupting the transcription of the inducible nitric oxide synthase (iNOS) gene transcription factor, IRF-1(85). This suppressive mode is believed to be mediated by IL-10 activity. IL-10 is synthesized at an early phase of ADE infection in THP-1 cells. In this experimental setting, IL-10 not only induces Th2 biasing but operates via the suppressors of cytokine signalling (SOCS) system to suppress the JAK/STAT signaling pathway, resulting in suppression of iNOS gene expression and reduction of nitric oxide radical production. The viral enhancement effect of IL-10 is abolished with small interfering RNA specific to the IL-10 gene (86). It can be concluded that *in vitro*, iADE infection not only facilitates viral entry but also modifies innate and adaptive intracellular antiviral mechanisms, resulting in enhanced DENV replication.

Critically, the same responses are observed *in vivo*. Genome-wide transcriptomes from peripheral blood mononuclear cells collected during the acute phase from children with dengue fever (DF) or DHF were compared using microarray analysis (88). Patients with DHF had decreased levels of NO, reduced IFN transcript in peripheral blood mononuclear cells, and increased IL-10 blood levels compared with patients with milder illness. IFN gene upregulation and IFN-α production were significantly elevated in patients with mild compared with severe dengue illness. In other studies, during the acute stage of severe disease increased production of IL-10 and downregulation of multiple IFN regulatory genes were noted (89–91). The protective role of IFN in moderating dengue infection has been demonstrated in a mouse model and suggested for humans with DF (92–94). The precise role of immune-complex-elicited IL-10 production on the clinical evolution of severe dengue infections is not well understood but may be responsible for the observed Th1 to Th2 shift in DHF (95).

Pathologic studies of human tissues have established monocytes, macrophages, and immature and mature dendritic cells as significant targets for DENV infection (13–16, 96, 97). In humans, secondary dengue infections follow a stereotypical course with severe outcomes, shock or gastrointestinal hemorrhage, accompanying vascular collapse that results from capillary permeability occurring around the time of defervescence (98). Indirect evidence suggests that cytokines mediate dengue vascular permeability. Much work has been directed at the measurement of cytokine blood levels in patients late in the acute phase, just prior to onset of shock (99, 100). High levels of viremia early in the disease and high levels of pro-inflammatory and immunomodulatory cytokines including IL-10 late in the disease are associated with severe outcomes (101).

However, during ADE-infection of primary monocytes, IL-10 synthesis peaked at the same serum dilution that produced peak virus yield (42). In addition, point mutations at the IL-10 promoter, positions -1082 A/G, -819 C/T, and -592 C/A, result in polymorphism that differentiates monocytes into high, intermediate, and low IL-10 producers. How these phenotypes correlate with disease severity requires more investigation.

Role of infection sequence

Second DENV infections can occur in 12 combinations, at least 10 of which have been documented to result in hospitalized disease (47). The sequence of infection may be highly determinative of disease severity. Secondary DENV-2 infections resulted in shock syndrome patients, while secondary DENV-1, -3, and -4 did not in the 1980 cohort study in Rayong, Thailand (62). The specific infection sequences associated with DSS cases were known from virus isolations in acute phase sera and antibodies in pre-illness sera or by applying the original antigenic sin phenomenon to paired sera (102). Although secondary DENV-1 infections were most common that year, DSS occurred only during secondary DENV-2 infections. Burmese workers came to a similar conclusion in their 1984 to 1988 longitudinal seroepidemiological study in Yangon, Myanmar (103). By contrast, in an Indonesian study DSS was associated with sequences ending in DENV-1, -3, and -4, but not DENV-2, even though secondary DENV-2 infections occurred (104). DENV-3 was associated with an outbreak of DHF/DSS in Tahiti in a population that had prior infection experience with DENV-1 and DENV-2 (105). Also in Tahiti, DENV-1 circulating in 2001 was enhanced to produce severe clinical disease by antibodies to DENV-2 that had circulated 4 to 5 years earlier (106).

Role of different myeloid cells

Much early published work on dengue and Ross River virus (RRV) used primary human mononuclear phagocytes to study iADE. To date, virtually all research has been carried out using DENV-2. When dengue iADE was tested in four different primary human myeloid cells derived from the same peripheral blood leukocyte (PBL) donors, viral infection and cytokine responses differed significantly (42).

Human monocytes, activated macrophages, and mature dendritic cells supported ADE, while immature dendritic cells did not. Infection of macrophages by DENV-2 alone or as fully neutralized immune complexes stimulated high levels of α and β IFN, and these were downmodulated under ADE conditions and replaced by secretion of IL-6 and TNFα. Type I IFNs were not produced or suppressed by iADE infection of monocytes with DENV-2 (42, 107). However, during ADE infection of primary monocytes, IL-10 synthesis peaked at the same serum dilution that produced peak virus yield (42). In addition, point mutations at the IL-10 promoter, positions -1082 A/G, -819 C/T, and -592 C/A, result in polymorphisms that differentiate monocytes into high, intermediate, and low IL-10 producers.

It should be noted that FcR-bearing continuous cell lines that are incapable of producing interferon have been used to detect extrinsic ADE but do not detect or produce iADE. A prime example is K562 cells, widely used to measure enhancing properties of dengue antibodies (108). Published research results using K-562 cells are often at odds with results obtained using primary human myeloid cells—the one group measuring extrinsic ADE and the other iADE (52, 109).

Role of different FcγRs in iADE

When the ability of DENV immune complexes to be internalized following interactions with human FcγRIA and FcγRIIA was studied in a model system, the FcγRIIA mediated both iADE and immune phagocytosis, while FcγRIA mediated uptake of immune complexes via phagocytosis (110). Genes for human FcγRIIA have been transfected into continuous monkey kidney cells, transforming them into cells capable of detecting and expressing the capacity of DENV immune complexes to be neutralized or to enhance infections. These systems, employing Fcγ RIIA have been used to assay *in vivo* viremia and to measure the protective versus enhancing properties of sera containing mixtures of DENV and antibodies (111–115).

In the *Leishmania* mouse model, it was observed that mouse IgG1and IgG2a/c induce IL-10 from mouse macrophages *in vitro* equally well but through different FcγR subtypes: IgG1 through FcγRIII, and IgG2a/c primarily through FcγRI but also through FcγRIII. In sharp contrast, mice lacking IgG1 develop earlier and stronger IgG2a/c, IgG3, and IgM responses to *Leishmania mexicana* infection and yet are more resistant to the infection (116). Thus, IgG1, but not IgG2a/c or IgG3, is pathogenic *in vivo*, in agreement with prior studies indicating that FcγRIII is required for chronic disease. This calls into question the assumption that mouse macrophages, which should secrete IL-10 in response to both IgG1 and IgG2a/c immune complexes, are the most important source of IL-10 generated by IgG-FcγR engagement in *L. mexicana* infection.

Role of DENVs

Enhanced growth of DENV-2 in primary human monocytes

A single study suggests that DENVs isolated from patients with differing degrees of disease severity may themselves be biologically different. The biological behavior of wild-type DENV-2 isolated from children with mild secondary dengue infections was compared with DENV-2s from children with grade I-III dengue hemorrhagic fever. All isolates were made in C6-36 cells from children presenting to Children's Hospital during the 1980 DENV-2 outbreak in Bangkok, Thailand (117). DENV-2 that had been passaged in C6-36 cells only once or twice from mild illnesses replicated to lower titers in cultures of human primary monocytes either with or without enhancing concentrations of polyclonal dengue antibodies than did DENV-2 strains isolated from DHF patients. The small number of subjects with mild illness jeopardizes the statistical significance of these observations. Nonetheless, these preliminary observations suggest the possibility that viral factors, whether surface antigens, attachment sites for entry into leukocytes, or intrinsic replica-

tion properties in human mononuclear phagocytes, might contribute to enhanced DENV infection and to the severity of the disease.

Differences in ability of DENV-2 strains to be neutralized by DENV-1 antibodies

Differences in genetic and viral structure among DENV-2 viruses that are associated with disease outcome during a first heterotypic dengue infection are well established, and the impact of these differences has been well studied (118). The actual sites on the virion that mediate these differences in human disease expression are still unknown. The first DENV to be recovered in the northern hemisphere was DENV-2 TR 1751 (119). Dengue outbreaks prior to World War II have been attributed to DENV-2 by serological studies in Panama and Cuba (120, 121). In 1963, DENV-3 was introduced into the northern hemisphere, first recognized in Puerto Rico (122). The geographic extent and intensity of transmission of these viruses was never measured, but conditions for sequential infection existed and no DHF/DSS outbreaks were reported. In 1977, DENV-1 was introduced into the Caribbean and quickly spread throughout the region (153). Again, sequential infections—DENV-2 then DENV-1 or DENV-3, then DENV-1—were possible, but there are no reports of DHF/DSS.

However, when an Asian DENV-2 was introduced into Cuba in 1981 following the 1977 to 1979 virgin soil introduction of DENV-1, a major DHF/DSS epidemic ensued (123, 124). But similar sequential introductions of the American genotype DENV-2 in 1995, five years after introduction of DENV-1 in 1990, failed to produce any DHF/DSS at all (125). Fortunately, this event occurred in the Amazonian city of Iquitos, population 344,686, where an ongoing longitudinal serological cohort permitted reconstruction of past events. It was estimated that 49,000 secondary DENV-2 infections occurred in 1995 and that these should have produced about 10,000 cases of DHF/DSS. Careful study of hospital records found no DHF/DSS-like disease. In fact, secondary infections were accompanied by mild disease at attack rates far below observed dengue infections.

Full-length sequences of the Asian and American DENV-2 genomes from viremic sera revealed a total of six encoded amino acid charge differences in the prM, E, NS4b, and NS5 genes along with structural changes in the 5′ and 3′ nontranslated regions (126). Stored Peruvian anti-DENV-1 human sera from 1990 were found to highly neutralize American genotype DENV-2 strains but not to neutralize Asian genotype DENV-2 strains (127). This suggests the existence of American genotype DENV-2 strains of envelope structure(s) analogous to structure(s) on DENV-1 strains. The loss or modification of this structure on Asian genotype DENV-2 strains suggests that American DENV-2 strains are more closely related to an ancestral DENV-2, while the Asian genotype DENV-2 strains have emerged more recently, possibly due to positive selective pressure exerted by ADE (128). Most people who read the dengue literature must assume, based upon citations, that American genotype DENV-2 strains are intrinsically incapable of producing severe dengue disease. That any DENV possesses the intrinsic property of producing an enhanced dengue disease is simply wrong. It is when viral attributes come into play at any stage of a heterotypic infection that "virulence" is an outcome. In Iquitos, it appears that American genotype DENV-2 infections were down-modulated rather than enhanced in those individuals circulating highly cross-reactive DENV-1 antibodies.

DENV-2 genetic differences associated with rapid enhancement of the severity of DENV-2 infection 20 years after infection with DENV-1

A dramatic increase, month to month, in case fatality rates and the severity of dengue disease was observed in humans of all ages who, in 1981 and 1997, experienced a DENV-2 infection 4 and 20 years after a DENV-1 infection

(129). During a 2001 to 2002 Havana outbreak a similar rapid increase in disease pathogenicity was observed in individuals who experienced a DENV-3 infection 24 years after infection with DENV-1 (130–132). Initially, it was hypothesized that this phenomenon might be caused by the emergence of neutralization escape mutants, as DENV-2 was serially passaged in individuals circulating DENV-1 antibodies (129). As discussed above, DENV-1 infections produce heterotypic antibodies that partially neutralize DENV-2. These might be expected to generate neutralization escape mutants that are no longer neutralized and that could produce enhanced infections and disease. It was suggested that the proportion of individuals infected with escape mutants might increase with time, producing the observed month-to-month increases in pathogenicity.

In January 1997, the sensitive Cuban surveillance system detected dengue cases in Santiago de Cuba just two months after illness in the index case (identified retrospectively). Acute phase sera were sent to the Havana laboratory for serological testing and virus isolation. The DENV-2 strains that circulated in 1981 and 1997 in Cuba both belonged to the American/Asian genotype circulating in the Americas since 1981. Twenty-nine DENV-2 isolates were obtained during the early (low pathogenicity) and the late (high pathogenicity) stages of the 1997 epidemic. The 1997 Cuban DENV-2 strain amino acid alignment showed a substitution methionine/threonine at position E340 specific for viruses isolated from Cuba, Venezuela, and Martinique (133). This nonconserved substitution is located in an antigenic region containing multiple T- and B-cell epitopes. Another nonconservative change leucine/glutamine at E 131 was observed in Jamaica/83 and Cuba/97 isolates. Remarkably, only two nonconserved substitutions in the E gene were found between the Jamaica 1983 and the 1997 Cuban strains, indicating that there has been very little *in situ* evolution of DENV-2 following its introduction from Asia. Of interest, the Cuban

DENV-2 isolates maintain the presence of N at position 390 of Asian DENV-2 strains, a site predicted to be a determinant of the American genotype DENV-2 that causes only mild disease (126). As the E gene sequences from these isolates were found to be conserved over the period of the outbreak, the hypothesis that envelope gene escape mutants contributed to the observed increased disease severity is negated (133).

The complete genes of six of the 1997 DENV-2 isolates were sequenced. A strong conservation of structural genes and proteins and of the noncoding regions was again noted. However, nucleotide substitutions were observed in NS genes, notably in NS1 and NS5 (134). Most synonymous mutations generally correlated with the time of sampling. It was possible to divide the isolates into two groups based upon five substitutions —those from the beginning of the 1997 epidemic (January to February) and from the latter parts of the epidemic (June to July). One of these five nucleotide substitutions produced a functionally significant amino acid replacement, threonine (thr) to serine (ser), at residue 164 in the NS1 protein. An alignment of this NS1 protein sequence in GenBank revealed that amino acids in this region are highly conserved. DENV-2 strains usually have Thr at this position, with the exception of the Thailand strain PUO-280 of the Asian I genotype, which has Ser, like the latest Cuban isolates (135). Strains of DENV-2 may differ significantly in the structure of genomic viral RNA 3′ nontranslated region (NTR), and these structural differences have also been correlated with mild disease (126). However, the DENV strains from the 1997 epidemic had no difference in their 3′ NTR or 5′ NTR compared with other Asian/American strains.

In further work, nucleotides 379 to 601 were sequenced from 15 viruses from different periods of the outbreak. Data from six DENV-2 strains sequenced previously were included (133). Two additional complete DENV-2 strains were sequenced directly from serum samples (130). Of 23 DENV-2 strains obtained during the course of the epidemic, five viruses from the first part of the epidemic had thr at position 164, while the isolates on and after 25 February had ser at this position (130, 136). By July, mosquito control efforts were well established and cases began to decline, with a marked reduction in cases in August. The switch from threonine to serine at NS1 position 164 appears to have been fixed within a few months of the virus having been introduced into Cuba.

Genetic differences in DENV-2 isolates recovered from disease of enhanced severity 4 years after DENV-1 and 8 years after DENV-3

Similar dengue disease phenomena were observed among pediatric patients in Managua, Nicaragua, and adults in Taiwan (137, 138). Further information has been published (136). In Nicaragua, a prospective seroepidemiological cohort study made possible a complex dissection of the contributing host and viral factors involved (138). In the dengue season of 2005–2006, 34 patients with DENV-2 infections were admitted to Hospital Infantil Manuel de Jesus Rivera in Managua, 10 with the diagnosis of DHF/DSS (30%). During 2006–2007 and 2008–2009, the severity of DENV-2 disease increased dramatically (85% of cases were secondary infections). Of 102 children with DENV-2 infections admitted to the hospital during these nonconsecutive transmission seasons 64% had DHF/DSS, an unparalleled increase in this hospital's 20-year experience with dengue admissions. Differing from the situation in Cuba, where DENV-2 introductions in 1981 and 1997 were rapidly controlled by effective vector control, dengue transmission in Nicaragua was continuous.

In Cuba, introductions of DENV-2 in 1981 and 1997 and DENV-3 in 2001 were preceded by DENV-1 infections in 1977-1978, whereas in Nicaragua DENV-3 had circulated in Managua in 1994 to 1998, DENV-2 had circulated in 1999 to 2002, and DENV-1 in 2002 to 2005, with DENV-2 again in 2005 to 2009. During this latter period a large number of DENV-2 strains were collected from children with dengue diseases of all degrees of severity. Over 200 of these viruses were subjected to full-length or partial sequencing, and as had been observed in Cuba, a stable clade shift was noted: NI-1 to NI-2B in 2008–2009. This replacement event was associated with nine nonsynonymous amino acid mutations (R97K in capsid [C], K94R in nonstructural protein 1 [NS1], and P245T in nonstructural protein 3 [NS3], N245S in NS4B, M492V in envelope [E], L279F in NS1, and K200Q, T290I, and R401K in nonstructural protein 5 [NS5]) and four mutations in the viral NTR. Clade NI-2B peak viremia titers were higher than viremias with clade NI-1 viruses in children with the diagnosis of dengue fever. By analyzing the age distribution of cases, it was concluded that NI-1 DENV-2 produced disease with an apparent increase in pathogenicity in children who were immune to DENV-1 because there was cross-protection when infections occurred at short intervals, while more severe disease was observed at longer intervals. By contrast, clade NI-2B DENV-2 infections produced disease of increased pathogenicity in children of all ages who had been infected by DENV-3 during 1994 to 1998. The authors noted that clade NI-2B DENV-2 strains grew to higher titers than clade NI-1 viruses in C6/36, primary human dendritic cells, U937 DC-SIGN, and K-562 cells, but ADE was not studied using DENV-3 antibodies. This group made no attempt to grow clade NI-1 or NI-2B DENV-2 strains in the presence of human DENV-1 or DENV-3 antibodies *in vitro* in primary human monocytes or macrophages to model ADE infections.

Efferent

The incubation period of disease ending in DVPS is unknown but is presumed to be the same as that of dengue fever. In children, progression of the illness is characteristic. A relatively mild first phase with an abrupt onset of fever, malaise, vomiting, headache, anorexia, and cough may be followed after 2 to 5 days by rapid deterioration and physical collapse (139). In Thailand, the median day of admission to the hospital after the onset of fever is day 4. In this second phase, the patient usually has cold and clammy extremities, a warm trunk, a flushed face, and diaphoresis. Patients are restless and irritable and complain of midepigastric pain. Frequently, scattered petechiae appear on the forehead and extremities, spontaneous ecchymoses may develop, and easy bruisability and bleeding at sites of venipuncture are common findings. Circumoral and peripheral cyanosis may occur. Respirations are rapid and often labored. The pulse is weak, rapid, and thready, and the heart sounds are faint. The pulse pressure frequently is narrow (<20 mm Hg); systolic and diastolic pressure may be low or unobtainable. The liver may become palpable two or three finger breadths below the costal margin and usually is firm and nontender. Early sonograms show thickening of the gallbladder duct and after initiation of intravenous resuscitation may show thickening of the gall bladder duct, perivesicular edema, ascites, and pleural effusions. At this same time chest radiographs may show unilateral (right) or bilateral pleural effusions. Approximately 2 to 5% of patients have gross ecchymosis or gastrointestinal bleeding. After a 24- or 36-hour period of crisis, convalescence is fairly rapid in children who recover. The temperature may return to normal before or during the stage of shock.

There is evidence of an important human dengue resistance gene. Epidemiologic studies of the 1981 Cuban outbreak demonstrated a higher risk for DHF/DSS in white than in black individuals (121). A search for DHF/DSS in black children in Haiti revealed no cases, despite the presence of high dengue type 1, 2, and 4 infection rates and circulation of the Southeast Asian genotype dengue 2 viruses (140). Several HLA antigens have shown differing frequencies in DHF/DSS cases and controls (141). Early in the acute vascular permeability stage of secondary DENV infection, rapid activation of the complement system occurs (142, 143). During shock, blood levels of C1q, C3, C4, C5, C6, C7, C8, and C3 proactivator are depressed, and C3 catabolic rates are elevated. The blood clotting and fibrinolytic systems are activated (139, 144). As yet, neither the mediator of vascular permeability nor the complete mechanism of altered hemostasis has been identified unequivocally. The kinin system apparently is not involved. Studies show that levels of tumor necrosis factor, interleukin-2, and interferon-γ are elevated at the time of vascular permeability (144). The strongest correlates to vascular permeability are inverse levels of platelet counts and reductions in accelerated partial thromboplastin time (145). Capillary damage allows fluid, electrolytes, protein, and, in some instances, red blood cells to leak into intravascular spaces. This internal redistribution of fluid, together with deficits caused by fasting, thirsting, and vomiting, results in hemoconcentration, hypovolemia, increased cardiac work, tissue hypoxia, metabolic acidosis, and hyponatremia. A mild degree of disseminated intravascular coagulation, plus liver damage and thrombocytopenia, could contribute additively to produce hemorrhage.

In serial blood samples taken early in the illness of individuals experiencing secondary dengue infections it is possible to identify peak viremia or dengue NS1 concentrations that can be measured. These were used successfully to observe enhanced dengue infections and to predict subsequent disease severity (53, 54, 146). It is critical that viremia be measured in the absence of antibodies—a very difficult task.

Because of the delay of onset of serious vascular permeability to around defervescence, there is a widespread hypothesis that vascular permeability is somehow related to T cell activity—specifically, the result of dengue-infected cells being attacked by activated T lymphocytes. Cytokine production should be quantitatively related to the number of infected target cells. The reduced risk for DHF/DSS in protein-calorie malnourished children and the increased risk for DHF/DSS in girls versus boys are consistent with the

hypothesis that a competent immune elimination system is available to generate the cytokines that produce DHF/DSS (147–149).

It is widely held that the process of eliminating DENV-infected cells generates a cascade of chemokines and cytokines that contribute to the pathophysiology of dengue disease syndromes. This has been termed "a perfect cytokine storm" (150). Given the evidence of increased infected cell mass in severe dengue infections, the cytokines generated by interactions between virus-infected cells and the host immune response would appear to be quantitatively proportional to viral load and not exaggerated or "abnormal." Since dengue is not a cytophilic virus, cellular infection proceeds until the infected cell is eliminated. A wide misconception is that peak viremia that occurs early in infection represents peak "viral load." In fact, the quantity of virus in the blood during the course of infection only describes the kinetics of extracellular virus clearance. As discussed above, it is likely that elimination of DENV-infected cells continues well after onset of antibody production, resulting in peak cellular infection (viral load) at around the time of defervescence, and cellular infection is not eliminated until well after the end of viremia. Of interest, a major effort failed to detect circulating CD8+ T cells during the late acute illness phase of DHF patients (151). This suggested to the authors that CD8+ T cells might be located only in the tissues where DENV replication had occurred. Alternatively, as in a Japanese encephalitis model, the antibody component of the adaptive immune response may play a much more important role in terminating dengue infections than previously thought (152).

UNKNOWNS

The elements of the preceding section are briefly reprised here. Ideally, these are accompanied by the identification of research questions and provision of detailed research protocols. The state of dengue research on the intracellular ADE is very primitive. The best I can do is to suggest a research approach. In almost all instances the approach involves the direct investigation of primary human myeloid cells with infectious DENV immune complexes. It is crucial that researchers use cells from flavivirus-naïve donors. Long ago, it was shown that dengue-immune individuals circulate mononuclear phagocytes that act as if a dengue antibody was strongly attached (6). Thus, when DENV is added, the iADE and extrinsic ADE phenomena ensue. Many of the most complex problems in iADE can only be approached by investigating primary human myeloid cells.

Afferent

Host Genetic Factors Enhancing Susceptibility to DVPS

Human genetic factors promoting dengue disease severity are not discussed in this article. The contribution of human genetic variables will be better understood when they can be placed into a rational understanding of how extrinsic phenomena and normal human biology control ADE.

"Enhancing" Antibodies

Sensitizing infections

As described above, the initial single dengue infection is known as the "sensitizing infection." The immune response to this infection participates in ADE accompanying infection with a heterotypic dengue virus.

- Studies of iADE have almost exclusively focused on DENV-2. A high priority is to extend studies as quickly as possible to the complete range of DENV. ADE should be tested using type-specific polyclonal human antibodies and not mouse or even human monoclonal antibodies. ADE is complex. The test systems should retain essential complexity.
- DVPS in infants occurs under completely different immunological circumstances than during first heterotypic dengue in-

fections. The failure of anyone in the past four decades to seriously study this very important and biologically unique phenomenon is simply mind-boggling. I am sorry to say I do not regard the published studies of Libraty and Simmons as having asked serious research questions (35, 36). Kliks led the way (34). Why not use maternal serum as a surrogate of cord blood for each individual infant and test it along with the virus isolated? This unique clinical phenomenon not only illustrates the role played by dengue antibodies in modulating disease expression but, also, the bifurcated role of dengue antibodies— protection for several months after birth at high concentrations and enhancing infections some months later at subneutralizing concentrations.

- The contribution of immature DENV particles to iADE is of interest. Immature DEN virions are not infectious for human myeloid cells, but in the presence of enhancing dengue antibodies, ADE infection occurs readily (32, 69). It has been surmised that immature DENVs are released into circulation during human infections, as antibodies to prM (immature DENV antigen) frequently are observed (32).

Attributes of iADE

The precise mechanisms fueling enhanced production of DENV in monocytes and macrophages require further study, as neither the production of IL-10 nor suppression of type I interferon are critical to the iADE phenomenon.

Role of infection sequence

There are at least 12 sequences of infection that make 12 unique immune complexes. We already have preliminary data that suggest that the outcome of infection differs according to the specific immune complexes (e.g., JE antibody-DENV immune complexes). One of the most critical absent studies is the characterization of infection, cytokine, and innate immune responses of different immune complexes in primary human myeloid cells (which cells to use is an important question and is addressed below). Antibodies to JE complexed with DENV result in mild ADE. Thus, this immune complex sends messages down the tail of the FcR that are very different from a complex formed by a DENV and antibodies from a primary dengue infection. What is the exact effect on iADE, and what is the molecular mechanism that controls response differences, if any?

Role of different myeloid cells
How myeloid cell phenotypes correlate with disease severity and iADE requires more investigation. We must start by going back to human autopsies and identifying macrophage targets for DENV infection using comprehensive cell markers. These investigations are currently in their infancy (16). All human myeloid cells should be studied separately.

Role of different FcγRs in iADE
This is another huge field for research. It should be remembered the DVPS occurs in individuals who circulate myeloid cells that express various FcRs, often on the same cell. Ultimately, iADE needs to be studied using this inherent complexity.

Role of DENV in ADE

Enhanced growth of DENV-2 recovered from severe compared with mild disease in primary human monocytes
The simple experiment as designed in the published paper should be repeated (117).

Differences in ability of DENV-2 strains to be neutralized by DENV-1 antibodies
The actual sites on the virion that mediate these differences in human disease expression are still unknown. Differences in genetic and viral structure between DENV-2 viruses that are and are not associated with epidemic DHF/DSS during a first heterotypic dengue infection are well established. Viral contri-

butions to these differences have not been studied in the appropriate *in vitro* system, e.g., primary human myeloid cells from flavirus-naïve individuals.

DENV-2 genetic differences associated with a major increase in disease severity of DENV-2 infection 20 years after infection with DENV-1
What are the kinetics of growth of DENV-2 in the primary human myeloid cell assay system with and without the NS1 amino acid changes?

Genetic differences in DENV-2 isolates recovered from disease of enhanced severity 4 years after DENV-1 and 8 years after DENV-3
The authors have a surfeit of research materials (138). The only sensible approach to studying these phenomena is to test the reagents in the ADE primary human myeloid cell system. This will have to be done on a large scale. Differences in the viral productivity of cells infected using infectious immune complexes should provide outcomes that can be related to any of a number of viral, antibody, or cellular differences.

Efferent

The final scenario that results in DVPS has been amazingly difficult to learn about. Complement split products and key cytokines have been thought to mediate vascular permeability at the same time these factors were thought to produce thrombocytopenia and altered hemostasis. The failure of cortisone administered early to suppress cytokine production or reduce the incidence of vascular permeability was a wake-up call. An alternative mechanism is needed. I suggest that DVPS is a dengue toxemia. Dengue NS1 directly causes all of the elements of DVPS—activated complement, thrombocytopenia, altered hemostasis, and vascular damage. As a direct toxin, NS1 should produce its damage in proportion to the concentration of NS1 presented to key systems and tissues. ADE functions directly to increase the concentration of NS1 proportionate to infected cell mass. But why doesn't DVPS occur earlier in the disease when peak NS1 blood levels are achieved? Why does DVPS suddenly worsen at defervescence? I posit that this is related to the onset of killer T cell activity. T cells damage dengue-infected cells, resulting in a final bolus release of NS1. When this exceeds a threshold, DVPS reaches its critical level of damage. This hypothesis also includes the possibility that NS1-antibody complexes may retain significant toxicity. I challenge the dengue research community to prove me wrong.

ACKNOWLEDGMENT

Conflict of interest: I disclose no conflicts.

CITATION

Halstead SB. 2014. Dengue antibody-dependent enhancement: knowns and unknowns. Microbiol Spectrum 2(6):AID-0022-2014.

REFERENCES

1. **Delgado MF, Coviello S, Monsalvo AC, Melendi GA, Hernandez JZ, Batalle JP, Diaz L, Trento A, Chang HY, Mitzner W, Ravetch J, Melero JA, Irusta PM, Polack FP.** 2009. Lack of antibody affinity maturation due to poor Toll-like receptor stimulation leads to enhanced respiratory syncytial virus disease. *Nat Med* **15:**34–41.
2. **Hawkes RA.** 1964. Enhancement of the infectivity of arboviruses by specific antisera produced in domestic fowls. *Aust J Exp Biol Med Sci* **42:**465–482.
3. **Hawkes RA, Lafferty KJ.** 1967. The enhancement of virus infectivity by antibody. *Virology* **33:**250–261.
4. **Halstead SB, Chow J, Marchette NJ.** 1973. Immunologic enhancement of dengue virus replication. *Nat New Biol* **243:**24–26.
5. **Halstead SB, O'Rourke EJ.** 1977. Antibody-enhanced dengue virus infection in primate leukocytes. *Nature* **265:**739–741.
6. **Halstead SB, O'Rourke EJ.** 1977. Dengue viruses and mononuclear phagocytes. I. Infection enhancement by non-neutralizing antibody. *J Exp Med* **146:**201–217.
7. **Halstead SB, O'Rourke EJ, Allison AC.** 1977. Dengue viruses and mononuclear phagocytes. II. Identity of blood and tissue leukocytes supporting *in vitro* infection. *J Exp Med* **146:**218–228.
8. **Kliks S, Halstead SB.** 1980. An explanation for enhanced virus plaque formation in chick embryo cells. *Nature* **285:**504–505.
9. **Kliks S, Halstead SB.** 1983. Role of antibodies and host cells in plaque enhancement of Murray Valley encephalitis virus. *J Virol* **46:**394–404.
10. **Halstead SB.** 1980. Immunological parameters of Togavirus disease syndromes, p 107–173. *In* Schlesinger RW (ed), *The Togaviruses, Biology, Structure, Replication.* Academic Press, New York, NY.
11. **Boonpucknavig S, Boonpucknavig V, Bhamarapravati N, Nimmannitya S.** 1979. Immunofluorescence study of skin rash in patients with dengue hemorrhagic fever. *Arch Pathol Lab Med* **103:**463–466.
12. **Hall WC, Crowell TP, Watts DM, Barros VL, Kruger H, Pinheiro F, Peters CJ.** 1991. Demonstration of yellow fever and dengue antigens in formalin-fixed paraffin-embedded human liver by immunohistochemical analysis. *Am J Trop Med Hyg* **45:**408–417.
13. **Durbin AP, Vargas MJ, Wanionek K, Hammond SN, Gordon A, Rocha C, Balmaseda A, Harris E.** 2008. Phenotyping of peripheral blood mononuclear cells during acute dengue illness demonstrates infection and increased activation of monocytes in severe cases compared to classic dengue fever. *Virology* **376:**429–435.
14. **Balsitis SJ, Coloma J, Castro G, Alava A, Flores D, McKerrow JH, Beatty PR, Harris E.** 2009. Tropism of dengue virus in mice and humans defined by viral nonstructural protein 3-specific immunostaining. *Am J Trop Med Hyg* **80:**416–424.
15. **Jessie K, Fong MY, Devi S, Lam SK, Wong KT.** 2004. Localization of dengue virus in naturally infected human tissues, by immunohistochemistry and *in situ* hybridization. *J Infect Dis* **189:**1411–1418.
16. **Aye KS, Charngkaew K, Win N, Wai KZ, Moe K, Punyadee N, Thiemmeca S, Suttitheptumrong A, Sukpanichnant S, Malasit P, Halstead SB.** 2014. Pathologic highlights of dengue hemorrhagic fever in 13 autopsy cases from Myanmar. *Hum Pathol* **45:**1221–1233.
17. **Halstead SB.** 1982. Immune enhancement of viral infection. *Prog Allergy* **31:**301–364.
18. **Gollins SW, Porterfield JS.** 1984. Flavivirus infection enhancement in macrophages: radioactive and biological studies on the effect of antibody on virus fate. *J Gen Virol* **65:**1261–1272.
19. **Gollins SW, Porterfield JS.** 1985. Flavivirus infection enhancement in macrophages: an electron microscopic study of viral cellular entry. *J Gen Virol* **66:**1969–1982.

20. **Olsen C, Scott F.** 1993. Evaluation of antibody-dependent enhancement of feline infectious peritonitis virus infectivity using *in situ* hybridization. *Microb Pathog* **14:**275–285.

21. **Robinson WE Jr, Montefiori DC, Gillespie DH, Mitchell WM.** 1989. Complement-mediated, antibody-dependent enhancement of HIV-1 infection *in vitro* is characterized by increased protein and RNA syntheses and infectious virus release. *J Acquir Immune Defic Syndr* **2:**33–42.

22. **Linn ML, Aaskov JG, Suhrbier A.** 1996. Antibody-dependent enhancement and persistence in macrophages of an arbovirus associated with arthritis. *J Gen Virol* **77:**407–411.

23. **Lidbury BA, Mahalingam S.** 2000. Specific ablation of antiviral gene expression in macrophages by antibody-dependent enhancement of Ross River virus infection. *J Virol* **74:**8376–8381.

24. **Suhrbier A, La Linn M.** 2003. Suppression of antiviral responses by antibody-dependent enhancement of macrophage infection. *Trends Immunol* **24:**165–168.

25. **Halstead SB.** 2009. Antibodies determine virulence in dengue. *Ann NY Acad Sci* **1171**(Suppl 1): E48–E56.

26. **Smith SA, Zhou Y, Olivarez NP, Broadwater AH, de Silva AM, Crowe JE Jr.** 2012. Persistence of circulating B memory cell clones with potential for dengue virus disease enhancement for decades following infection. *J Virol* **86:**2665–2675.

27. **de Alwis R, Beltramello M, Messer WB, Sukupolvi-Petty S, Wahala WM, Kraus A, Olivarez NP, Pham Q, Brian J, Tsai WY, Wang WK, Halstead S, Kliks S, Diamond MS, Baric R, Lanzavecchia A, Sallusto F, de Silva AM.** 2011. In-depth analysis of the antibody response of individuals exposed to primary dengue virus infection. *PLoS Negl Trop Dis* **5:**e1188. doi:10.1371/journal.pntd.0001188.

28. **Beltramello M, Williams KL, Simmons CP, Macagno A, Simonelli L, Quyen NT, Sukupolvi-Petty S, Navarro-Sanchez E, Young PR, de Silva AM, Rey FA, Varani L, Whitehead SS, Diamond MS, Harris E, Lanzavecchia A, Sallusto F.** 2010. The human immune response to dengue virus is dominated by highly cross-reactive antibodies endowed with neutralizing and enhancing activity. *Cell Host Microbe* **8:**271–283.

29. **Wahala WM, Kraus AA, Haymore LB, Accavitti-Loper MA, de Silva AM.** 2009. Dengue virus neutralization by human immune sera: role of envelope protein domain III-reactive antibody. *Virology* **392:**103–113.

30. **Halstead SB.** 2003. Neutralization and antibody dependent enhancement of dengue viruses. *Adv Virus Res* **60:**421–467.

31. **Halstead SB, Venkateshan CN, Gentry MK, Larsen LK.** 1984. Heterogeneity of infection enhancement of dengue 2 strains by monoclonal antibodies. *J Immunol* **132:**1529–1532.

32. **Dejnirattisai W, Jumnainsong A, Onsirisakul N, Fitton P, Vasanawathana S, Limpitikul W, Puttikhunt C, Edwards C, Duangchinda T, Supasa S, Chawansuntati K, Malasit P, Mongkolsapaya J, Screaton G.** 2010. Cross-reacting antibodies enhance dengue virus infection in humans. *Science* **328:**745–748.

33. **Halstead SB, Nimmannitya S, Cohen SN.** 1970. Observations related to pathogenesis of dengue hemorrhagic fever. IV. Relation of disease severity to antibody response and virus recovered. *Yale J Biol Med* **42:**311–328.

34. **Kliks SC, Nimmannitya S, Nisalak A, Burke DS.** 1988. Evidence that maternal dengue antibodies are important in the development of dengue hemorrhagic fever in infants. *Am J Trop Med Hyg* **38:**411–419.

35. **Libraty DH, Acosta LP, Tallo V, Segubre-Mercado E, Bautista A, Potts JA, Jarman RG, Yoon IK, Gibbons RV, Brion JD, Capeding RZ.** 2009. A prospective nested case-control study of dengue in infants: rethinking and refining the antibody-dependent enhancement dengue hemorrhagic fever model. *PLoS Med* **6:**e1000171. doi:10.1371/journal.pmed.1000171.

36. **Simmons CP, Chau TN, Thuy TT, Tuan NM, Hoang DM, Thien NT, Lien le B, Quy NT, Hieu NT, Hien TT, McElnea C, Young P, Whitehead S, Hung NT, Farrar J.** 2007. Maternal antibody and viral factors in the pathogenesis of dengue virus in infants. *J Infect Dis* **196:**416–424.

37. **Chau TN, Anders KL, Lien le B, Hung NT, Hieu LT, Tuan NM, Thuy TT, Phuong le T, Tham NT, Lanh MN, Farrar JJ, Whitehead SS, Simmons CP.** 2010. Clinical and virological features of dengue in Vietnamese infants. *PLoS Negl Trop Dis* **4:**e657. doi:10.1371/journal.pntd.0000657.

38. **Chau TN, Hieu NT, Anders KL, Wolbers M, Lien le B, Hieu LT, Hien TT, Hung NT, Farrar J, Whitehead S, Simmons CP.** 2009. Dengue virus infections and maternal antibody decay in a prospective birth cohort study of Vietnamese infants. *J Infect Dis* **200:**1893–1900.

39. **Chau TN, Quyen NT, Thuy TT, Tuan NM, Hoang DM, Dung NT, Lien le B, Quy NT, Hieu NT, Hieu LT, Hien TT, Hung NT, Farrar J, Simmons CP.** 2008. Dengue in Vietnamese infants: results of infection-enhancement assays correlate with age-related disease epidemiology, and cellular immune responses correlate with disease severity. *J Infect Dis* **198:**516–524.

40. **Halstead SB, Mahalingam S, Marovich MA, Ubol S, Mosser DM.** 2010. Intrinsic antibody-

dependent enhancement of microbial infection in macrophages: disease regulation by immune complexes. *Lancet Infect Dis* **10:**712–722.

41. **Ubol S, Halstead SB.** 2010. How innate immune mechanisms contribute to antibody-enhanced viral infections. *Clin Vaccine Immunol* **17:**1829–1835.

42. **Boonnak K, Dambach KM, Donofrio GC, Marovich MA.** 2011. Cell type specificity and host genetic polymorphisms influence antibody dependent enhancement of dengue virus infection. *J Virol* **85:**1671–1683.

43. **Sullivan NJ.** 2001. Antibody-mediated enhancement of viral disease. *Curr Top Microbiol Immunol* **260:**145–169.

44. **Tirado SM, Yoon KJ.** 2003. Antibody-dependent enhancement of virus infection and disease. *Viral Immunol* **16:**69–86.

45. **Huisman W, Martina BE, Rimmelzwaan GF, Gruters RA, Osterhaus AD.** 2009. Vaccine-induced enhancement of viral infections. *Vaccine* **27:**505–512.

46. **Halstead SB.** 1970. Observations related to pathogenesis of dengue hemorrhagic fever. VI. Hypotheses and discussion. *Yale J Biol Med* **42:**350–362.

47. **Gibbons RV, Kalanarooj S, Jarman RG, Nisalak A, Vaughn DW, Endy TP, Mammen MP Jr, Srikiatkhachorn A.** 2007. Analysis of repeat hospital admissions for dengue to estimate the frequency of third or fourth dengue infections resulting in admissions and dengue hemorrhagic fever, and serotype sequences. *Am J Trop Med Hyg* **77:**910–913.

48. **Halstead SB, Lan NT, Myint TT, Shwe TN, Nisalak A, Soegijanto S, Vaughn DW, Endy T.** 2002. Infant dengue hemorrhagic fever: research opportunities ignored. *Emerg Infect Dis* **12:**1474–1479.

49. **Coffey LL, Mertens E, Brehin AC, Fernandez-Garcia MD, Amara A, Despres P, Sakuntabhai A.** 2009. Human genetic determinants of dengue virus susceptibility. *Microbes Infect* **11:**143–156.

50. **Sabin AB.** 1952. Research on dengue during World War II. *Am J Trop Med Hyg* **1:**30–50.

51. **Chan KR, Zhang SL, Tan HC, Chan YK, Chow A, Lim AP, Vasudevan SG, Hanson BJ, Ooi EE.** 2011. Ligation of Fc gamma receptor IIB inhibits antibody-dependent enhancement of dengue virus infection. *Proc Natl Acad Sci USA* **108:**12479–12484.

52. **Kliks SC, Nisalak A, Brandt WE, Wahl L, Burke DS.** 1989. Antibody-dependent enhancement of dengue virus growth in human monocytes as a risk factor for dengue hemorrhagic fever. *Am J Trop Med Hyg* **40:**444–451.

53. **Vaughn DW, Green S, Kalayanarooj S, Innis BL, Nimmannitya S, Suntayakorn S, Endy TP, Raengsakulrach B, Rothman AL, Ennis FA,** Nisalak A. 2000. Dengue viremia titer, antibody response pattern, and virus serotype correlate with disease severity. *J Infect Dis* **181:**2–9.

54. **Libraty DH, Endy TP, Houng HS, Green S, Kalayanarooj S, Suntayakorn S, Chansiriwongs W, Vaughn DW, Nisalak A, Ennis FA, Rothman AL.** 2002. Differing influences of virus burden and immune activation on disease severity in secondary dengue-3 virus infections. *J Infect Dis* **185:** 1213–1221.

55. **Wu SJ, Grouard-Vogel G, Sun W, Mascola JR, Brachtel E, Putvatana R, Louder MK, Filgueira L, Marovich MA, Wong HK, Blauvelt A, Murphy GS, Robb ML, Innes BL, Birx DL, Hayes CG, Frankel SS.** 2000. Human skin Langerhans cells are targets of dengue virus infection [see comments]. *Nat Med* **6:**816–820.

56. **Montoya M, Gresh L, Mercado JC, Williams KL, Vargas MJ, Gutierrez G, Kuan G, Gordon A, Balmaseda A, Harris E.** 2013. Symptomatic versus inapparent outcome in repeat dengue virus infections is influenced by the time interval between infections and study year. *PLoS Negl Trop Dis* **7:** e2357. doi:10.1371/journal.pntd.0002357.

57. **Gordon A, Kuan G, Mercado JC, Gresh L, Aviles W, Balmaseda A, Harris E.** 2013. The Nicaraguan pediatric dengue cohort study: incidence of inapparent and symptomatic dengue virus infections, 2004–2010. *PLoS Negl Trop Dis* **7:**e2462. doi:10.1093/aje/kwp092.

58. **Anderson KB, Gibbons RV, Cummings DA, Nisalak A, Green S, Libraty DH, Jarman RG, Srikiatkhachorn A, Mammen MP, Darunee B, Yoon IK, Endy TP.** 2013. A shorter time interval between first and second dengue infections is associated with protection from clinical illness in a school-based cohort in Thailand. *J Infect Dis* **209:**360–368.

59. **Grange L, Simon-Loriere E, Sakuntabhai A, Gresh L, Paul R, Harris E.** 2014. Epidemiological risk factors associated with high global frequency of inapparent dengue virus infections. *Front Immunol* **5:**280.

60. **Guzman MG, Kouri G, Valdes L, Bravo J, Vazquez S, Halstead SB.** 2002. Enhanced severity of secondary dengue-2 infections: death rates in 1981 and 1997 Cuban outbreaks. *Rev Panam Salud Publica* **11:**223–227.

61. **Guzman MG, Alvarez M, Rodriguez-Roche R, Bernardo L, Montes T, Vazquez S, Morier L, Alvarez A, Gould EA, Kouri G, Halstead SB.** 2007. Neutralizing antibodies after infection with dengue 1 virus. *Emerg Infect Dis* **13:**282–286.

62. **Sangkawibha N, Rojanasuphot S, Ahandrik S, Viriyapongse S, Jatanasen S, Salitul V, Phanthumachinda B, Halstead SB.** 1984. Risk factors in dengue shock syndrome: a prospective

epidemiologic study in Rayong, Thailand. I. The 1980 outbreak. *Am J Epidemiol* **120:**653–669.

63. **Halstead SB, Porterfield JS, O'Rourke EJ.** 1980. Enhancement of dengue virus infection in monocytes by flavivirus antisera. *Am J Trop Med Hyg* **29:**638–642.

64. **Anderson KB, Gibbons RV, Thomas SJ, Rothman AL, Nisalak A, Berkelman RL, Libraty DH, Endy TP.** 2011. Preexisting Japanese encephalitis virus neutralizing antibodies and increased symptomatic dengue illness in a school-based cohort in Thailand. *PLoS Negl Trop Dis* **5:**e1311. doi:10.1371/journal.pntd.0001311.

65. **Hoke CH Jr, Nisalak A, Sangawhipa N, Jatanasen S, Laorakpongse T, Innis BL, Kotchasenee S, Gingrich JB, Latendresse J, Fukai K, et al.** 1988. Protection against Japanese encephalitis by inactivated vaccines. *N Engl J Med* **319:**608–614.

66. **Lai CY, Tsai WY, Lin SR, Kao CL, Hu HP, King CC, Wu HC, Chang GJ, Wang WK.** 2008. Antibodies to envelope glycoprotein of dengue virus during the natural course of infection are predominantly cross-reactive and recognize epitopes containing highly conserved residues at the fusion loop of domain II. *J Virol* **82:**6631–6643.

67. **Yu IM, Zhang W, Holdaway HA, Li L, Kostyuchenko VA, Chipman PR, Kuhn RJ, Rossmann MG, Chen J.** 2008. Structure of the immature dengue virus at low pH primes proteolytic maturation. *Science* **319:**1834–1837.

68. **Rodenhuis-Zybert IA, Wilschut J, Smit JM.** 2011. Partial maturation: an immune-evasion strategy of dengue virus? *Trends Microbiol* **19:**248–254.

69. **Rodenhuis-Zybert IA, van der Schaar HM, Voorham JMD, van der Ende-Metselaar H, Lei HY, Wilschut J, Smit JM.** 2010. Immature dengue virus: a veiled pathogen? *PLoS Pathog* **6:**e1000718. doi:10.1371/journal.ppat.1000718.

70. **Rodenhuis-Zybert IA, Moesker B, da Silva Voorham JM, van der Ende-Metselaar H, Diamond MS, Wilschut J, Smit JM.** 2011. A fusion-loop antibody enhances the infectious properties of immature flavivirus particles. *J Virol* **85:**11800–11808.

71. **da Silva Voorham JM, Rodenhuis-Zybert IA, Ayala Nunez NV, Colpitts TM, van der Ende-Metselaar H, Fikrig E, Diamond MS, Wilschut J, Smit JM.** 2012. Antibodies against the envelope glycoprotein promote infectivity of immature dengue virus serotype 2. *PLoS One* **7:**e29957. doi:10.1371/journal.pone.0029957.

72. **Cherrier MV, Kaufmann B, Nybakken GE, Lok SM, Warren JT, Chen BR, Nelson CA, Kostyuchenko VA, Holdaway HA, Chipman PR, Kuhn RJ, Diamond MS, Rossmann MG, Fremont DH.** 2009. Structural basis for the preferential recognition of immature flaviviruses by a fusion-loop antibody. *EMBO J* **28:**3269–3276.

73. **Sutterwala FS, Noel GJ, Clynes R, Mosser DM.** 1997. Selective suppression of interleukin-12 induction after macrophage receptor ligation. *J Exp Med* **185:**1977–1985.

74. **Sutterwala FS, Noel GJ, Salgame P, Mosser DM.** 1998. Reversal of proinflammatory responses by ligating the macrophage Fcgamma receptor type I. *J Exp Med* **188:**217–222.

75. **Anderson CF, Lucas M, Gutierrez-Kobeh L, Field AE, Mosser DM.** 2004. T cell biasing by activated dendritic cells. *J Immunol* **173:**955–961.

76. **Ioan-Facsinay A, de Kimpe SJ, Hellwig SM, van Lent PL, Hofhuis FM, van Ojik HH, Sedlik C, da Silveira SA, Gerber J, de Jong YF, Roozendaal R, Aarden LA, van den Berg WB, Saito T, Mosser D, Amigorena S, Izui S, van Ommen GJ, van Vugt M, van de Winkel JG, Verbeek JS.** 2002. FcgammaRI (CD64) contributes substantially to severity of arthritis, hypersensitivity responses, and protection from bacterial infection. *Immunity* **16:**391–402.

77. **Kima PE, Constant SL, Hannum L, Colmenares M, Lee KS, Haberman AM, Shlomchik MJ, McMahon-Pratt D.** 2000. Internalization of *Leishmania mexicana* complex amastigotes via the Fc receptor is required to sustain infection in murine cutaneous leishmaniasis. *J Exp Med* **191:**1063–1068.

78. **Padigel UM, Farrell JP.** 2005. Control of infection with *Leishmania major* in susceptible BALB/c mice lacking the common gamma-chain for FcR is associated with reduced production of IL-10 and TGF-beta by parasitized cells. *J Immunol* **174:**6340–6345.

79. **Mosser DM.** 2003. The many faces of macrophage activation. *J Leukoc Biol* **73:**209–212.

80. **Miles SA, Conrad SM, Alves RG, Jeronimo SM, Mosser DM.** 2005. A role for IgG immune complexes during infection with the intracellular pathogen *Leishmania. J Exp Med* **201:**747–754.

81. **Anderson CF, Gerber JS, Mosser DM.** 2002. Modulating macrophage function with IgG immune complexes. *J Endotoxin Res* **8:**477–481.

82. **Lucas M, Zhang X, Prasanna V, Mosser DM.** 2005. ERK activation following macrophage FcgammaR ligation leads to chromatin modifications at the IL-10 locus. *J Immunol* **175:**469–477.

83. **Murray HW, Masur H, Keithly JS.** 1982. Cell-mediated immune response in experimental visceral leishmaniasis. I. Correlation between resistance to *Leishmania donovani* and lymphokine-generating capacity. *J Immunol* **129:**344–350.

84. **Yang Z, Mosser DM, Zhang X.** 2007. Activation of the MAPK, ERK, following *Leishmania amazonensis* infection of macrophages. *J Immunol* **178:**1077–1085.

85. **Chareonsirisuthigul T, Kalayanarooj S, Ubol S.** 2007. Dengue virus (DENV) antibody-dependent enhancement of infection upregulates the production of anti-inflammatory cytokines, but suppresses anti-DENV free radical and pro-inflammatory cytokine production, in THP-1 cells. *J Gen Virol* **88:**365–375.

86. **Ubol S, Phuklia W, Kalayanarooj S, Modhiran N.** 2010. Mechanisms of immune evasion induced by a complex of dengue virus and pre-existing enhancing antibodies. *J Infect Dis* **201:** 923–935.

87. **Modhiran N, Kalayanarooj S, Ubol S.** 2010. Subversion of innate defenses by the interplay between DENV and pre-existing enhancing antibodies: TLRs signaling collapse. *PLoS Negl Trop Dis* 4:e924. doi:10.1371/journal.pntd.0000924.

88. **Ubol S, Masrinoul P, Chaijaruwanich J, Kalayanarooj S, Charoensuthikul T, Kasisith J.** 2008. Differences in global gene expression in peripheral blood mononuclear cells indicate a significant role of the innate responses in progression of dengue fever but not dengue hemorrhagic fever. *J Infect Dis* **197:**1459–1467.

89. **Chen LC, Lei HY, Liu CC, Shiesh SC, Chen SH, Liu HS, Lin YS, Wang ST, Shyu HW, Yeh TM.** 2006. Correlation of serum levels of macrophage migration inhibitory factor with disease severity and clinical outcome in dengue patients. *Am J Trop Med Hyg* **74:**142–147.

90. **Simmons CP, Popper S, Dolocek C, Chau TN, Griffiths M, Dung NT, Long TH, Hoang DM, Chau NV, Thao le TT, Hien TT, Relman DA, Farrar J.** 2007. Patterns of host genome-wide gene transcript abundance in the peripheral blood of patients with acute dengue hemorrhagic fever. *J Infect Dis* **195:**1097–1107.

91. **Nguyen TH, Lei HY, Nguyen TL, Lin YS, Huang KJ, Le BL, Lin CF, Yeh TM, Do QH, Vu TQ, Chen LC, Huang JH, Lam TM, Liu CC, Halstead SB.** 2004. Dengue hemorrhagic fever in infants: a study of clinical and cytokine profiles. *J Infect Dis* **189:**221–232.

92. **Shresta S, Kyle JL, Snider HM, Basavapatna M, Beatty PR, Harris E.** 2004. Interferon-dependent immunity is essential for resistance to primary dengue virus infection in mice, whereas T- and B-cell-dependent immunity are less critical. *J Virol* **78:**2701–2710.

93. **Shresta S, Sharar KL, Prigozhin DM, Snider HM, Beatty PR, Harris E.** 2005. Critical roles for both STAT1-dependent and STAT1-independent pathways in the control of primary dengue virus infection in mice. *J Immunol* **175:**3946–3954.

94. **Navarro-Sanchez E, Despres P, Cedillo-Barron L.** 2005. Innate immune responses to dengue virus. *Arch Med Res* **36:**425–435.

95. **Chaturvedi UC, Raghupathy R, Pasca AS, Elbishbishi EA, Agarwal R, Nagar R, Misra A, Kapoor S, Mathur A, Khan M, Azizieh F.** 1999. Shift from a Th1-type response to Th1-type in dengue haemorrhagic fever. *Curr Sci* **76:**63–69.

96. **Kou Z, Quinn M, Chen H, Rodrigo WW, Rose RC, Schlesinger JJ, Jin X.** 2008. Monocytes, but not T or B cells, are the principal target cells for dengue virus (DV) infection among human peripheral blood mononuclear cells. *J Med Virol* **80:**134–146.

97. **Blackley S, Kou Z, Chen H, Quinn M, Rose RC, Schlesinger JJ, Coppage M, Jin X.** 2007. Primary human splenic macrophages, but not T or B cells, are the principal target cells for dengue virus infection *in vitro*. *J Virol* **81:**13325–13334.

98. **Cohen SN, Halstead SB.** 1966. Shock associated with dengue infection. I. Clinical and physiologic manifestations of dengue hemorrhagic fever in Thailand, 1964. *J Pediatrics* **68:**448–456.

99. **Rothman AL.** 2010. Cellular immunology of sequential dengue virus infection and its role in disease pathogenesis. *Curr Top Microbiol Immunol* **338:**83–98.

100. **Bethell DB, Flobbe K, Cao XT, Day NP, Pham TP, Buurman WA, Cardosa MJ, White NJ, Kwiatkowski D.** 1998. Pathophysiologic and prognostic role of cytokines in dengue hemorrhagic fever. *J Infect Dis* **177:**778–782.

101. **Green S, Vaughn DW, Kalayanarooj S, Suntayakorn S, Nisalak A, Nimmannitya S, Innis BL, Kurane I, Rothman AL, Ennis FA.** 1997. 46th Meeting of the American Society of Tropical Medicine and Hygiene, Orlando, FL. *AJTMH* **57:**113.

102. **Halstead SB, Rojanasuphot S, Sangkawibha N.** 1983. Original antigenic sin in dengue. *Am J Trop Med Hyg* **32:**154–156.

103. **Thein S, Aung MM, Shwe TN, Aye M, Zaw A, Aye K, Aye KM, Aaskov J.** 1997. Risk factors in dengue shock syndrome. *Am J Trop Med Hyg* **56:**566–572.

104. **Graham RR, Juffrie M, Tan R, Hayes CG, Laksono I, Ma'roef C, Erlin, Sutaryo,Porter KR, Halstead SB.** 1999. A prospective sero-epidemiologic study on dengue in children four to nine years of age in Yogyakarta, Indonesia I. Studies in 1995–1996. *Am J Trop Med Hyg* **61:**412–419.

105. **Chungue E, Spiegel A, Roux J, Laudon F, Cardines R.** 1990. Dengue-3 in French Polynesia: preliminary data. *Med J Aust* **152:**557–558.

106. **Hubert B, Halstead SB.** 2009. Dengue 1 virus and dengue hemorrhagic fever, French Polynesia, 2001. *Emerg Infect Dis* **15:**1265–1270.

107. **Kou Z, Lim JY, Beltramello M, Quinn M, Chen H, Liu SN, Martinez-Sobrido L, Diamond MS, Schlesinger JJ, de Silva A, Sallusto F, Jin X.** 2011.

Human antibodies against dengue enhance dengue viral infectivity without suppressing type I interferon secretion in primary human monocytes. *Virology* **410**:240–247.

108. **Chotiwan N, Roehrig JT, Schlesinger JJ, Blair CD, Huang CY.** 2014. Molecular determinants of dengue virus 2 envelope protein important for virus entry in FcgammaRIIA-mediated antibody-dependent enhancement of infection. *Virology* **456–457**:238–246.

109. **Laoprasopwattana K, Libraty D, Endy T, Nisalak A, Chunsittiwat S, Vaughn DW, Reed G, Ennis FA, Rothman A, Green S.** 2005. Dengue virus (DV) enhancing antibody activity in preillness plasma does not predict subsequent disease severity or viremia in secondary DV infection. *J Infect Dis* **192**:510–519.

110. **Rodrigo WW, Jin X, Blackley SD, Rose RC, Schlesinger JJ.** 2006. Differential enhancement of dengue virus immune complex infectivity mediated by signaling-competent and signaling-incompetent human Fcgamma RIA (CD64) or FcgammaRIIA (CD32). *J Virol* **80**:10128–10138.

111. **Moi ML, Lim CK, Takasaki T, Kurane I.** 2010. Involvement of the Fc{gamma} receptor IIA cytoplasmic domain in antibody-dependent enhancement of dengue virus infection. *J Gen Virol* **91**:103–111.

112. **Moi ML, Lim CK, Kotaki A, Takasaki T, Kurane I.** 2010. Development of an antibody-dependent enhancement assay for dengue virus using stable BHK-21 cell lines expressing FcgammaRIIA. *J Virol Methods* **163**:205–209.

113. **Moi ML, Lim CK, Kotaki A, Takasaki T, Kurane I.** 2010. Discrepancy in dengue virus neutralizing antibody titers between plaque reduction neutralizing tests with Fcgamma receptor (FcgammaR)-negative and FcgammaR-expressing BHK-21 cells. *Clin Vaccine Immunol* **17**:402–407.

114. **Moi ML, Lim CK, Kotaki A, Takasaki T, Kurane I.** 2011. Detection of higher levels of dengue viremia using FcgammaR-expressing BHK-21 cells than FcgammaR-negative cells in secondary infection but not in primary infection. *J Infect Dis* **203**:1405–1414.

115. **Moi ML, Takasaki T, Saijo M, Kurane I.** 2014. Determination of antibody concentration as the main parameter in a dengue virus antibody-dependent enhancement assay using FcgammaR-expressing BHK cells. *Arch Virol* **159**:103–116.

116. **Buxbaum LU.** 2011. Type I IFNs promote the early IFN-gamma response and the IL-10 response in *Leishmania mexicana* infection. *Parasite Immunol* **32**:153–160.

117. **Morens DM, Marchette NJ, Chu MC, Halstead SB.** 1991. Growth of dengue type 2 virus isolates in human peripheral blood leukocytes correlates with severe and mild dengue disease. *Am J Trop Med Hyg* **45**:644–651.

118. **Rico-Hesse R.** 2003. Microevolution and virulence of dengue viruses. *Adv Virus Res* **59**:315–341.

119. **Anderson CR, Downs WG.** 1956. Isolation of dengue virus from a human being in Trinidad. *Science* **124**:224–225.

120. **Rosen L.** 1958. Observations on the epidemiology of dengue in Panama. *Am J Hyg* **68**:45–58.

121. **Guzman MG, Kouri GP, Bravo J, Soler M, Vazquez S, Morier L.** 1990. Dengue hemorrhagic fever in Cuba, 1981: a retrospective seroepidemiologic study. *Am J Trop Med Hyg* **42**:179–184.

122. **Neff JM, Morris L, Gonzalez-Alcover R, Coleman PH, Lyss SB, Negron H.** 1967. Dengue fever in a Puerto Rican community. *Am J Epidemiol* **86**:162–184.

123. **Kouri GP, Guzman MG, Bravo JR, Triana C.** 1989. Dengue haemorrhagic fever/dengue shock syndrome: lessons from the Cuban epidemic, 1981. *Bull World Health Organ* **67**:375–380.

124. **Guzman MG, Deubel V, Pelegrino JL, Rosario D, Marrero M, Sariol C, Kouri G.** 1995. Partial nucleotide and amino acid sequences of the envelope and the envelope/nonstructural protein-1 gene junction of four dengue-2 virus strains isolated during the 1981 Cuban epidemic. *Am J Trop Med Hyg* **52**:241–246.

125. **Watts DM, Porter KR, Putvatana P, Vasquez B, Calampa C, Hayes CG, Halstead SB.** 1999. Failure of secondary infection with American genotype dengue 2 to cause dengue haemorrhagic fever [see comments]. *Lancet* **354**:1431–1434.

126. **Leitmeyer KC, Vaughn DW, Watts DM, Salas R, Villalobos I, de Chacon, Ramos C, Rico-Hesse R.** 1999. Dengue virus structural differences that correlate with pathogenesis. *J Virol* **73**:4738–4747.

127. **Kochel TJ, Watts DM, Halstead SB, Hayes CG, Espinosa A, Felices V, Caceda R, Bautista T, Montoya Y, Douglas S, Russell KL.** 2002. Effect of dengue-1 antibodies on American dengue-2 viral infection and dengue haemorrhagic fever. *Lancet* **360**:310–312.

128. **Vasilakis N, Weaver SC.** 2008. The history and evolution of human dengue emergence. *Adv Virus Res* **72**:1–76.

129. **Guzman MG, Kouri G, Halstead SB.** 2000. Do escape mutants explain rapid increases in dengue case-fatality rates within epidemics? *Lancet* **355**:1902–1903.

130. **Rodriguez-Roche R, Sanchez L, Burgher Y, Rosario D, Alvarez M, Kouri G, Halstead SB, Gould EA, Guzman MG.** 2011. Virus role during intraepidemic increase in dengue disease severity. *Vector Borne Zoonotic Dis* **11**:675–681.

131. **Alvarez M, Rodriguez R, Bernardo L, Vasquez S, Morier L, Gonzalez D, Castro O, Kouri G,**

Halstead SB, Guzman MG. 2006. Dengue hemorrhagic fever caused by sequential dengue 1 - 3 infections at a long interval: Havana epidemic, 2001–2002. *Am J Trop Med Hyg* **75:**1113–1117.

132. **Gonzalez D, Castro OE, Kouri G, Perez JM, Martinez E, Vazquez S, Rosario D, Cancio R, Guzman MG.** 2005. Classical dengue hemorrhagic fever resulting from two dengue infections spaced 20 years or more apart: Havana, dengue 3 epidemic, 2001–2. *Int J Infect Dis* **9:**280–285.

133. **Rodriguez-Roche R, Alvarez M, Gritsun T, Rosario D, Halstead SB, Kouri G, Guzman MG.** 2005. Dengue virus type 2 in Cuba, 1997: conservation of E gene sequence in isolates obtained at different times during the epidemic. *Arch Virol* **150:**415–425.

134. **Rodriguez-Roche R, Alvarez M, Gritsun T, Halstead SB, Kouri G, Gould EA, Guzman MG.** 2005. Virus evolution during a severe dengue epidemic in Cuba, 1997. *Virology* **334:**154–159.

135. **Blok J, Gibbs AJ, McWilliam SM, Vitarana UT.** 1991. NS 1 gene sequences from eight dengue-2 viruses and their evolutionary relationships with other dengue-2 viruses. *Arch Virol* **118:**209–223.

136. **Halstead SB.** 2014. Intraepidemic increases in dengue disease severity: applying lessons on surveillance and transmission, p 84–101. *In* Whitehorn J, Farrar J (ed), *Clinical Insights: Dengue Fever: Transmission, Diagnosis and Surveillance.* Future Medicine, London, United Kingdom.

137. **Chen HL, Lin SR, Liu HF, King CC, Hsieh SC, Wang WK.** 2008. Evolution of dengue virus type 2 during two consecutive outbreaks with an increase in severity in southern Taiwan in 2001–2002. *Am J Trop Med Hyg* **79:**495–505.

138. **OhAinle M, Balmaseda A, Macalalad AR, Tellez Y, Zody MC, Saborio S, Nunez A, Lennon NJ, Birren BW, Gordon A, Henn MR, Harris E.** 2011. Dynamics of dengue disease severity determined by the interplay between viral genetics and serotype-specific immunity. *Sci Transl Med* **3:**114ra128.

139. **Farrar J.** 2008. Clinical features, p 121–191. *In* Halstead SB (ed), *Dengue,* vol. 1. Imperial College Press, London, United Kingdom.

140. **Halstead SB, Streit TG, Lafontant JG, Putvatana R, Russell K, Sun W, Kanesa-Thasan N, Hayes CG, Watts DM.** 2001. Haiti: absence of dengue hemorrhagic fever despite hyperendemic dengue virus transmission. *Am J Trop Med Hyg* **65:**180–183.

141. **Halstead SB.** 2008. Pathogenesis: risk factors prior to infection, p 219–256. *In* Halstead SB (ed), *Dengue,* vol. 5. Imperial College Press, London, United Kingdom.

142. **Bokisch VA, Top FH Jr, Russell PK, Dixon FJ, Muller-Eberhard HJ.** 1973. The potential pathogenic role of complement in dengue hemorrhagic shock syndrome. *N Engl J Med* **289:**996–1000.

143. **Memoranda.** 1973. Pathogenic mechanisms in dengue hemorrhagic fever. Report of an international collaborative study. *Bull. WHO* **48:**117–132.

144. **Halstead SB.** 2008. Pathophysiology, p 285–326. *In* Halstead SB (ed), *Dengue,* vol. 5. Imperial College Press, London, United Kingdom.

145. **Wills B, Tran VN, Nguyen TH, Truong TT, Tran TN, Nguyen MD, Tran VD, Nguyen VV, Dinh TT, Farrar J.** 2009. Hemostatic changes in Vietnamese children with mild dengue correlate with the severity of vascular leakage rather than bleeding. *Am J Trop Med Hyg* **81:**638–644.

146. **Libraty DH, Young PR, Pickering D, Endy TP, Kalayanarooj S, Green S, Vaughn DW, Nisalak A, Ennis FA, Rothman AL.** 2002. High circulating levels of the dengue virus nonstructural protein NS1 early in dengue illness correlate with the development of dengue hemorrhagic fever. *J Infect Dis* **186:**1165–1168.

147. **Kalayanarooj S, Nimmannitya S.** 2005. Is dengue severity related to nutritional status? *Southeast Asian J Trop Med Public Health* **36:**378–384.

148. **Nimmannitya S, Halstead SB, Cohen S, Margiotta MR.** 1969. Dengue and chikungunya virus infection in man in Thailand, 1962–1964. I. Observations on hospitalized patients with hemorrhagic fever. *Am J Trop Med Hyg* **18:**954–971.

149. **Anders KL, Nguyet NM, Chau NV, Hung NT, Thuy TT, Lien le B, Farrar J, Wills B, Hien TT, Simmons CP.** 2011. Epidemiological factors associated with dengue shock syndrome and mortality in hospitalized dengue patients in Ho Chi Minh City, Vietnam. *Am J Trop Med Hyg* **84:**127–134.

150. **Pang T, Cardosa MJ, Guzman MG.** 2007. Of cascades and perfect storms: the immunopathogenesis of dengue haemorrhagic fever-dengue shock syndrome (DHF/DSS). *Immunol Cell Biol* **85:**43–45.

151. **Dung NT, Duyen HT, Thuy NT, Ngoc TV, Chau NV, Hien TT, Rowland-Jones SL, Dong T, Farrar J, Wills B, Simmons CP.** 2010. Timing of CD8+ T cell responses in relation to commencement of capillary leakage in children with dengue. *J Immunol* **184:**7281–7287.

152. **Larena M, Regner M, Lee E, Lobigs M.** 2011. Pivotal role of antibody and subsidiary contribution of CD8+ T cells to recovery from infection in a murine model of Japanese encephalitis. *J Virol* **85:**5446–5455.

153. **Pan American Health Organization.** 1978. Dengue in the Caribbean, 1977. Proceedings of a workshop held in Montego Bay, Jamaica, 8 to 11 May 1978. Scientific Publication 375. Pan American Health Organization, Washington, DC.

Immunotherapeutic Approaches To Prevent Cytomegalovirus- Mediated Disease

16

EDITH ACQUAYE-SEEDAH,[1] ZACHARY P. FRYE,[2] and JENNIFER A. MAYNARD[2]

INTRODUCTION

First visualized in 1904 as large inclusions in tissue sections from luetic infants and isolated in 1957 (1), the human cytomegalovirus (CMV) is a remarkably successful pathogen. Worldwide, there is a 50 to 90% probability of infection by age 50 without any clear markers of genetic susceptibility. Primary infection results in life-long latency, requiring continuous vigilance by the host immune system and characterized by serum antibody titers and a strong cytotoxic T-cell response. While most individuals will be infected with at least one strain of CMV, infection rarely leads to disease in immunocompetent individuals. However, CMV is a primary cause of congenital neurological defects and causes disease in those with compromised immune systems, such as transplant patients, with only limited therapies available.

Symptomatic CMV disease is often observed in infants who received the virus from an infected mother in utero, patients receiving hematopoietic stem cell or solid organ transplants, and patients with immunosuppressive diseases such as human immunodeficiency virus (HIV) and AIDS (Table 1). Primary maternal infection during gestation represents an ~40% risk of intrauterine transmission to

[1]Department of Biochemistry, University of Texas at Austin, Austin, TX 78712; [2]Department of Chemical Engineering, University of Texas at Austin, Austin, TX 78712.
Antibodies for Infectious Diseases
Edited by James E. Crowe, Jr., Diana Boraschi, and Rino Rappuoli
© 2015 American Society for Microbiology, Washington, DC
doi:10.1128/microbiolspec.AID-0009-2013

TABLE 1 Treatment spectrum for high-risk CMV demographic groups

Demographic	Infection risk	Treatment
Healthy individual	Primary infection, followed by latency; occasionally mononucleosis syndrome similar to that caused by Epstein-Barr virus	None; typically asymptomatic
Fetus of CMV⁻ mother, newborn	Primary infection with high risk of serious neurological effects (e.g., hearing loss, retardation, microcephaly, seizures in 10–17%); high mortality rate of those with symptomatic disease (~30% reported)	Antiviral therapy or IVIG provided to mother during gestation to prevent primary infection
CMV⁻ solid organ transplant patient	Primary infection risk if the donor is CMV⁺; historically, 10–50% develop symptomatic disease including leukopenia, retinitis, tissue-invasive disease (e.g., nephritis, pancreatitis); increased graft rejection; "early" disease during the first 3 months has been reduced significantly due to prophylactic antiviral therapy	IVIG to prevent primary infection Cellular immunotherapy with genetically modified T cells expressing CMV-specific TCRs
CMV⁺ solid organ transplant patient	Lower risk of secondary infection due to reactivation of latent infection while immunosuppressed; risk of acquiring a different CMV strain if the donor is CMV⁺; increased graft rejection	Antiviral therapy
CMV⁺ and CMV⁻ stem cell transplant patient	Primary infection (~30% CMV⁻ recipients) and secondary infection (~70% CMV⁺ recipients) due to reactivation of latent infection while immunosuppressed; most common form of disease is CMV pneumonia with a 30–60% mortality rate	Antiviral therapy for first 100 days posttransplant; high mortality rate if CMV disease appears after the first 100 days (~50%) Adoptive transfer of CMV-specific T cells isolated from donor material to prevent infection Some evidence to support IVIG
HIV/AIDS patient	Primary or secondary infection when CD4⁺ T cell count is <50/μl; retinitis, pneumonitis	Antiviral therapy

the fetus, with congenital viral infection affecting 0.5 to 3% of all births (~40,000 per year in the United States)—more children than are affected with Down syndrome, fetal alcohol syndrome, and spina bifida (2). The consequences of congenital disease are severe: vision and hearing loss, mental retardation, and even death, amounting to an estimated $4 billion per year in the United States alone. The rate of vertical transmission is reduced to ~2% in pregnant women who have previously been infected with CMV and have circulating anti-CMV antibodies (3), suggesting a protective role for antibodies against primary infection. Solid organ transplantation, particularly of a CMV seropositive (CMV⁺) organ into a CMV seronegative (CMV⁻) recipient, with the associated immunosuppressive regimen, greatly increases patient susceptibility to primary CMV infection and transplant failure, while secondary infection may result due to reactivation of latent CMV in a CMV⁺ recipient. Similar risks are observed for HIV and AIDS patients with T-cell counts of <50/μl and high-risk elderly with reduced naive T-cell receptor (TCR) diversity (4) but are less common given the prevalence of antiretroviral therapies.

For these reasons, when the Institute of Medicine was commissioned in 1999 to prioritize vaccine development based upon quality-adjusted life years, a vaccine to prevent CMV was judged "head and shoulders" above all other potential vaccines with regard to cost effectiveness (estimated at $300,000 per affected child) (5). Remarkably, while a CMV vaccine has been a top priority for nearly 40 years (5, 6), none of the candidates evaluated has been licensed. One challenge has been the lack of a clear serological correlate of protection, which may be different for the different patient groups. In the meantime, antiviral therapeutics are the standard of care, with high-titer CMV immunoglobulin and adoptive T-cell transfer emerging as alternatives. Considering the success of antibody therapeutics to treat some viral diseases (7), the apparent protective role of antibodies against CMV and recent identification of neutralizing epitopes in CMV, antibody therapeutics present an attractive option until a vaccine becomes available. This review focuses on the current use and potential of antibody therapies to treat CMV disease.

THE INFECTION

Virus Structure and Life Cycle

CMV is a ubiquitous beta herpesvirus type 5, related to the herpes simplex viruses, Epstein-Barr virus, and varicella zoster, the causative agent of chicken pox. Specialized strains appear to have coevolved with and become restricted to their respective mammalian hosts. The human CMV genome is among the largest and most complex animal virus genomes, with a large 235-kb double-stranded linear DNA genome encoding ~165 open reading frames (8). The genome and some viral mRNAs are surrounded by an icosahedral nucleocapsid, enveloped by the viral tegument proteins and a lipid bilayer, which is studded with at least 20 different glycoproteins forming a number of complexes. The whole unit spans 200 to 300 nm in diameter (Fig. 1). CMV can spread directly from cell to cell but destroys infected cells by lytic replication, resulting in a high serum viral load which correlates with end-organ disease. CMV disease is monitored by quantitative PCR to detect CMV DNA in leukocytes or serum and detection of the tegument structural protein pp65 in peripheral blood leukocytes by immunostaining.

The virion contains several major glycoprotein complexes at the cell surface. (i) Two

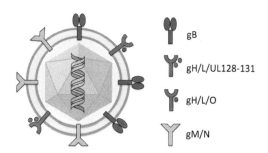

FIGURE 1 **Human CMV structure. The 235-kb double-stranded linear DNA genome is surrounded by an icosahedral nucleocapsid, enveloped by the viral tegument proteins (including pp65, which harbors a dominant cytotoxic T lymphocyte epitope) and lipid bilayer, which is studded with at least 20 glycoproteins. The fusogenic glycoprotein gB binds some cell surface receptors and appears to be immunodominant, but neutralizing antibodies recognizing this protein only block viral entry into fibroblasts. The gH/L dimer appears to bind specific receptors and potentiate gB-membrane fusion. When occurring as a gH/L/O complex, it is also involved in entry into fibroblasts, a process that appears to occur via direct membrane fusion. In contrast, the gH/L/UL128-131 pentameric complex is required for entry into epithelial and endothelial cells, a process mediated by endocytosis and low-pH fusion. The gM/N complex is the most abundant on the virion surface, initiating adsorption to cells by binding heparin sulfate proteoglycans. The gN may be heavily glycosylated to shield the virion against antibody recognition. doi:10.1128/microbiolspec.AID-0009-2013.f1**

molecules of glycoprotein B (gB), in which each 160-kDa monomer is cleaved and then joined by a disulfide bond to include a 115-kDa surface unit and a 55-kDa transmembrane component. The gB has been reported to bind epidermal growth factor receptors and integrins and is a type 3 fusogen, which initiates membrane fusion. (ii) A disulfide-linked heterodimer formed by the gM and gN proteins is the most abundant complex and may initiate adsorption to cells by binding heparin sulfate proteoglycans. (iii) The gH/gL/gO disulfide-linked trimer is notable, as all herpes viruses use a gH/gL complex to mediate fusion of the viral envelope with the cellular membrane, although the CMV gH/gL cocrystal structure does not resemble a typical fusogen (9). The gH is an 86-kDa glycoprotein, present in nuclear and cytoplasmic membranes of infected cells and in the viral envelope. While gH binds the $\alpha_v\beta_3$ integrin, the 32-kDa gL forms extensive contacts with gH and is required for gH to fold and localize properly at the cell surface. The gO does not appear to be crucial for membrane fusion but appears to chaperone gH/gL incorporation into new virions (10). (iv) A second gH/gL complex combined with the trimeric products of UL128, 130, and 131 (UL128-131) has recently been characterized in greater detail, revealing critical roles during invasion of endothelial and epithelial cells (11).

In vivo, the virus infects a broad spectrum of cells, including macrophages, fibroblasts, epithelial, neural, and muscle cells, allowing it to affect multiple organ systems and cause a wide range of diseases, including pneumonia, gastrointestinal disease, retinitis, hepatitis, and encephalitis. CMV entry into cells is a complex process initiated by adsorption onto the cell surface, followed by specialized invasion strategies for different cell types (Fig. 2). In particular, fibroblast entry is mediated by the fusogenic gB and potentiated by the gH/gL/gO complex, possibly involving β1 integrins and epidermal growth factor receptors, followed by direct fusion of the viral envelope with the cell membrane (11, 12). In contrast, infection of endothelial cells, epithelial cells, and macrophages requires the gH/gL/UL128-131 pentamer. When associated with the cell surface, this complex triggers endocytosis, followed by a gB- and gH-dependent fusion of the viral membrane with the endosomal membrane (13, 14). In addition to the gH/gL/UL128-131 pentamer, viral entry into these cells appears to require a different gB conformation to trigger fusion (12). The ability of CMV strains to invade fibroblasts has been used historically to characterize strains, vaccines, and antibodies. However, it has been recognized that during laboratory culture, strains such as AD169 and the Towne vaccine strain readily acquire mutations in the UL128-131 genes that restrict their tropism to fibroblasts, raising concerns over their clinical relevance.

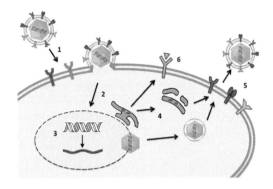

FIGURE 2 **Human CMV life cycle. (1) The virion binds to cells via the gB and gH/L/UL128-131 glycoproteins and specific cellular receptors, followed by direct membrane fusion (fibroblasts) or endocytosis and low-pH-mediated membrane fusion (endothelial and epithelial cells). (2) The virion contents are released into the cytoplasm, allowing the nucleocapsid to translocate to the nucleus for DNA replication and transcription and packaged viral transcripts to be directly translated. (3) Transcripts are translated in the cytoplasm, followed by processing in the endoplasmic reticulum and Golgi body. (4) Viral DNA and proteins are assembled and enveloped to create new virions, followed by (5) release into the extracellular surroundings or directly into another cell. (6) During this process, fragments of viral proteins are combined with host MHC class I in the endoplasmic reticulum for presentation on the cell surface. Antibodies can directly affect the cellular attachment and internalization steps to prevent primary infection, while T-cell recognition of viral pMHC complexes is crucial for identifying and lysing infected cells. doi:10.1128/microbiolspec.AID-0009-2013.f2**

Virus-Immune Détente

Primary infection of immunocompetent CMV⁻ individuals rarely leads to active disease but instead leads to a lifelong latent infection, characterized by periodic reactivation and secondary infection. During latency, multiple copies of the CMV genome appear to reside in a small number of mononuclear cells. Secondary or superinfection with a new CMV strain can be monitored by serum viral titer, a correlate for disease severity. Maintenance of latency requires continual monitoring by the host immune system, such that ~5 to 10% of all CD8⁺ and CD4⁺ T cells recognize CMV peptides, a number which increases to ~30%

in the elderly. To prevent disease in susceptible populations, current treatments include (i) antiviral agents to prevent replication (primarily ganciclovir) in the first 3 months posttransplantation, which are associated with significant toxicity and not approved for use in pregnant women; (ii) polyvalent immunoglobulin preparations enriched in antibodies against CMV (CMV-IVIG); and (iii) adoptive immunotherapy by ex vivo expansion of CMV-specific T cells, which are then reinfused into the patient. Antivirals and CMV-IVIG target viral proteins involved in replication to restrict viral dissemination and limit disease severity in CMV⁻ pregnant women and solid organ recipients, while T-cell therapy has demonstrated efficacy in maintaining latency after stem cell transplantation but has not been standardized for routine use.

While the magnitude of their role has been debated, antibodies appear to limit viral loads by inhibiting aspects of cellular invasion. An early analysis purified antibodies from the serum of seropositive individuals by immunoadsorption onto recombinant vaccinia virus expressing gB. The purified antibodies were then used to neutralize CMV strain AD169 invasion into fibroblasts, concluding that 40 to 70% of neutralizing antibodies target gB (15, 16). Three antigenic domains were later defined: AD-1, a conformational epitope located between residues 552 and 635; AD-2, a linear epitope between residues 69 and 78; and AD-3, another linear epitope at the carboxy terminus, between residues 783 and 906 (17). AD-1 is involved in gB oligomerization and is immunodominant, with antibodies binding this epitope present in all tested individuals. Interestingly, these responses are comprised of neutralizing and nonneutralizing antibodies competing for the same site, which may assist in viral immune evasion (18). Antibodies recognizing AD-2 are only present in about half of individuals but are potently neutralizing. Sequencing has revealed similar variable region usage for antibodies binding AD-2 within a single individual, suggesting that they are derived from a small

number of B cells and that the epitope may be difficult to access and/or poorly immunogenic (19). More recently, sequencing of gB-specific memory B cells isolated from seven seropositive individuals showed that >90% of the corresponding antibodies are nonneutralizing. This work also identified two additional, potently neutralizing gB epitopes: AD-4 and AD-5. Antibodies binding these epitopes do not block viral attachment but neutralize a postadsorption fusion event (20). Collectively, neutralizing anti-gB antibodies affect early events of infection and have been shown to prevent viral penetration of fibroblasts and cell-to-cell spread. However, while gB is key for viral entry, it is not essential for viral attachment, assembly, or egress, and thus, anti-gB antibodies may not represent the most critical components of the protective humoral immune response.

More recently, analysis with cell surface-expressed and purified CMV antigens suggested that the major neutralizing antibody response blocking entry into epithelial cells is directed against the gH/gL complex and not gB (21). Anti-gH/L neutralizing antibodies isolated from patient memory B cells either neutralized viral infection on all cell types tested with moderate 50% inhibitory concentration (IC_{50}) values or potently protected epithelial, endothelial, and myeloid cells with low IC_{50} values, between 20 and 200 pM, but did not protect fibroblasts. Competition assays showed that antibodies in the first group recognized at least three distinct neutralizing sites on gB and two on gH, while antibodies in the second group recognized at least seven distinct sites on the gH/L/UL128-131 complex, some of which span the interfaces between adjacent proteins (21, 22). Even short peptides from UL128 and UL130 elicit high neutralizing titers in rabbits which are able to block viral entry into epithelial cells from the mucosa (23). This is consistent with other reports that anti-gH antibodies, which are present at high levels during acute infection, block cell-to-cell spread (24) while those against UL128 and UL130 specifically inhibit endothelial cell invasion (14, 23, 25). Less potently neutralizing human monoclonal antibodies recognizing other viral glycoproteins (gB, gH, or gM/gN complex) have been isolated which neutralized infection of epithelial/endothelial cells as well as fibroblasts (22), although their epitopes are less well characterized. It has been suggested that the extensive glycosylation on gN may serve to shield these glycoproteins from neutralizing antibodies (26).

Cellular immune responses to CMV are mediated primarily by the cytolytic activity of $CD8^+$ cells, but these require $CD4^+$ help to persist (27). After a primary infection, latency is maintained by an array of immune evasion tactics, including down-regulation and degradation of antigen-presenting major histocompatibility complex (MHC) molecules to avoid recognition by cytotoxic T cells (28). The role of cellular immunity has been demonstrated convincingly by adoptive transfer studies in which donor-derived, CMV-specific $CD8^+$-T-cell lines or clones were first isolated by coculture with virus or antigen-pulsed dendritic cells, expanded in vitro, and finally, infused into HLA-matched hematopoietic stem cell transfer patients. This procedure restored antigen-specific immunity and prevented CMV-associated clinical outcomes (29, 30); however, it is time-intensive and laborious, requiring a total of 4 to 6 weeks for cell line expansion (31). Recent efforts to streamline the process have included direct isolation of CMV-specific T cells via HLA tetramers prior to in vitro expansion and T-cell transfection with genes encoding CMV-specific TCRs (32). Several T-cell lines recognizing pp65 peptides in complex with multiple HLA restrictions have been shown to be effective in vitro, in terms of cytokine secretion and target cell lysis (33), but it remains to be seen whether these can be transferred to the clinic.

As these procedures evolve, a key question becomes "what T-cell specificities are required for protection?" Careful analysis of the molecular details of this recognition event requires identification of the peptides and corresponding TCRs involved in protection. Several immunodominant T-cell epitopes have been identified, including the tegument phosphoproteins 65 (pp65, the most abundant protein in the tegument) and 150 (pp150) and the immediate-early protein 1 (IE-1) which are conserved across strains (34, 35). Transcripts of pp65 are packaged within virions and translated directly after cellular invasion; thus their display provides an early marker for infection. The dominant effector cells in adoptive immunotherapy respond to these three peptides (29, 30). One clinical study adoptively transferred pp65 or IE-1-specific $CD8^+$ T cells, observing a dramatic reduction of viral load in all 9 patients (36). In contrast, in vitro experiments using peptides derived from 213 open reading frames demonstrated T-cell responses to more than 70% of expressed genes (37). This raises the question "are the dominant epitopes we observe in vivo actually critical for CMV suppression or an artifact of viral immune evasion tactics?"

Looking at the other half of the interaction, analyses of the $\alpha\beta$ $CD8^+$ TCR sequence diversity has identified a large number of public TCRs, comprised of the same germ line variable regions and used by different individuals to recognize these dominant CMV peptides when presented by HLA (38). The cells displaying public TCRs recognize virally infected cells with greater avidity and exhibit a more terminally differentiated phenotype (39). Recently, tetramers comprised of the $pp65_{495-503}$ peptide in complex with the human HLA A*0201 were used to isolate human $CD8^+$ T cells, which were then subjected to single-cell sequencing of the TCR alpha and beta chains. Public and nonpublic TCR sequences were observed, and TCR sequence diversity was correlated with serum antibody titers as an indirect measure of viral titer and disease propensity. The primary conclusion of this study was that the diversity, but not the magnitude, of the cellular response inversely correlated with the serum anti-CMV titer, which is itself a marker for increased viral load (40). These data suggest that immunotherapeutic approaches based on a few immunodominant peptides or public TCRs will be less effective than one based on a larger set of interactions.

Vaccine Development

A vaccine to prevent CMV disease has been a top priority since 1999, and despite considerable effort, none are likely to receive regulatory approval soon (5, 6). Challenges have included the lack of a clear serological correlate of protection, appropriate animal models, and target population. To maximize the clinical benefit, it has been suggested that all seronegative young women, CMV⁻ stem cell donors, and solid organ transplant recipients be immunized to protect future children and transplant recipients, respectively. Over the last 50 years, two vaccine approaches have been extensively evaluated in clinical trials: live attenuated vaccine and gB-based subunit vaccines, with numerous other DNA, vectored virus, and peptide formulations in development (for a review, see reference 41).

Two live attenuated strains have been developed and evaluated in vaccine trials, the laboratory-adapted AD169 and Towne's strains. The first clinical trials with Towne's, originally a neonatal clinical isolate, demonstrated that it could elicit both neutralizing antibodies and T-cell responses lasting up to 10 years, with a good safety profile. It was subsequently shown to reduce viral load and mitigate CMV disease, but not to prevent primary or secondary infection, when administered to kidney transplant patients at least 8 weeks prior to transplantation (42, 43, 44). When administered to seronegative mothers, Towne's showed no efficacy in reducing transmission from children shedding CMV virions (45). In a challenge study with healthy volunteers, vaccinated individuals were protected more than seronegative individuals but were still 5 to 10 times more likely to become ill than naturally seropositive individuals. This may be a result of Towne's deletions in the UL128-131 region, meaning that the vaccine can induce antibodies blocking fibro-

blast but not epithelial cell invasion. More-recent efforts to improve live attenuated vaccines include coadministration with interleukin-12 as an adjuvant (46) and chimerization with the unattenuated Toledo strain. The moderate protective effects observed in live attenuated CMV vaccine trials, coupled with concerns that heavily attenuated strains are less relevant (47) and pose regulatory concerns, have slowed development of these vaccines.

The second most developed vaccine strategy is a subunit vaccine, based on the observation that gB dominates the humoral immune response. While prior trials focused on safety and immunogenicity, in 2009, a subunit vaccine was shown for the first time to be effective against primary maternal CMV infection and, later, in transplant recipients. This vaccine is comprised of a squalene-water emulsion of an engineered gB with the novel proprietary adjuvant MF59. The gB protein is modified to remove the internal cleavage site and introduce a stop codon before the transmembrane region, resulting in a soluble product expressed in CHO cells. In a phase II placebo-controlled efficacy trial, 18 of 225 women receiving the vaccine versus 31 of 216 receiving placebo acquired primary CMV infection during a 1-year period, for overall vaccine efficacy of ≈50%. Peak levels of anti-gB were about fivefold higher than in naturally seropositive individuals but did not induce antibodies preventing endothelial/epithelial cell invasion (48). A subsequent phase II randomized study with kidney and liver transplant patients showed that anti-gB titers correlated inversely with the duration of viremia (49). This adjuvanted gB subunit vaccine remains the most promising candidate, but additional trials are required for licensure. A variety of additional vaccine designs have been evaluated, including recombinant canary pox and peptide vaccines designed to elicit strong cellular responses against known immunodominant peptides (50).

While still in early stages, new approaches based on the pentameric gH/L/128-131 complex—notably absent from the AD169 and Towne's vaccine strains—appear promising. This complex is essential for viral invasion of endothelial/epithelial cells, and clinical studies have determined that antibodies recognizing the UL128-131 complex appear within 2 to 4 weeks after infection, last for at least a year, and are stronger than responses to gH (25). Moreover, the bulk of the neutralizing response in CMV-IVIG is now thought to be mediated by antibodies binding gH/L/UL128-131 (21), and these have been proposed as a correlate of protection (51, 52). When the complex is restored to the AD169 vaccine strain, it induced 10-fold-higher neutralizing antibody titers than AD169 or the gB subunit vaccine in rabbits and monkeys (53). This effect has been shown consistently across several animal models, as a modified vaccinia Ankara virus expressing all five rhesus homologs developed neutralizing antibody titers similar to natural infection and exhibited reduced plasma loads after postvaccination challenge in monkeys (54). Finally, an alphavirus replicon particle coexpressing only gH/gL produced broadly cross-reactive complement-independent neutralizing antibodies in mice at higher titers than those with gB (55).

THERAPEUTIC ANTIBODIES

Polyclonal CMV-IVIG

The available antibody-based anti-CMV therapies are polyvalent immunoglobulin preparations enriched in antibodies against CMV (CMV-IVIG) (Table 2) and were of particular interest before antivirals became widely available. The CMV-IG is made by pooling serum from ~1,000 donors screened for high anti-CMV serum titers and purifying the antibodies by cold ethanol precipitation, followed by a low-pH or solvent-detergent virus inactivation step. This process results in a product with ~50 mg of immunoglobulin G (IgG)/ml and anti-gB titers of ~1:400,000, two- to fourfold higher than in seropositive individuals, although lot-to-lot variability is observed (56). While the enzyme-linked immunosorbent assay titer is a primary characteristic, it does not always track with the neutralization titer and in some cases, standard IVIG can have a higher neutralizing titer than CMV-IVIG (57). This activity typically protects endothelial and epithelial cells more potently than fibroblasts. A recent report suggested that the bulk of the neutralizing response in CMV-IVIG (Cytogam) is due to antibodies recognizing the gH/L/128-131 pentamer with little role for anti-gB antibodies (21). Antibody isotype may also be a key criterion, as IgG3 antibodies have been found to be 10-fold more potently neutralizing than the IgG1 isotype (58). Collectively, the antibodies in CMV-IVIG are thought to act by neutralizing the virus' ability to infect both fibroblast and endothelial/epithelial cells (59), reducing inflammation, and/or reducing cytokine-mediated immune responses, although these latter mechanisms have not been well characterized (60).

CMV-IVIG was first licensed in 1991 and is well tolerated with no severe side effects. It has been used for prophylaxis of CMV disease associated with at-risk patients receiving solid organ and stem cell transplants, typically, CMV$^-$ recipients with CMV$^+$ donors. To improve efficacy, it is often combined with antiviral therapy. However, the results of clinical trials evaluating its use have been variable, most likely due to lot-to-lot variability, various doses and schedules, and mixed patient populations with different risk profiles. While early studies suggested that prophylactic CMV-IVIG could reduce the severity of CMV infection in liver transplant patients (61), others have suggested that it is less effective than combinations of antivirals (62) and that IVIG-antiviral combination therapy could actually increase both survival and rejection risk (63). With high-risk kidney transplant recipients, IVIG is associated with an excellent 1-year survival rate (64) and combination therapy with low-dose valaciclovir was efficacious in preventing CMV disease (65). A meta-analysis pooling 11 trials with almost 700 solid

TABLE 2 Antibody-based CMV therapeutics

Therapeutic	Target	Indication	Development stage	Source or reference
Human immune sera; polyclonal (Cytogam; CSL/Behring, MedImmune)	CMV envelope glycoproteins (block virus entry)	Transplant recipients, congenital CMV	Approved	www.cytogam.com/
Human immune sera; polyclonal (Cytotect; Biotests AG)	CMV envelope glycoproteins (block virus entry)	Transplant recipients, congenital CMV	Approved	http://paviour.org/cytotect.htm
Human monoclonal antibody (MSL109; PDL)	CMV envelope glycoprotein H (block virus entry)	CMV retinitis; stem cell transplant recipients	Phase I/II trials completed; no further progress	85, 87
Human monoclonal antibody MSL109 in combination with ganciclovir	CMV envelope glycoprotein H (block virus entry)	CMV retinitis	Phase I/II	83, 92
Human IgG1 monoclonal antibody C23/regavirumab (Teijin Ltd.)	gB epitope	CMV retinitis in HIV[+] individuals, bone marrow recipients	Phase II	81; US5043281 (1990)
Human neutralizing monoclonal antibodies (Humabs, LLC)	CMV gUL131A-128 trimer		Preclinical	22, 88; US7947274 (2011)
TCR-like antibody	CMV peptide p64 or p65 displayed by MHC		Preclinical	90
TCR anti CD3-bispecific antibody	CMV-infected cells		Preclinical	91
Humanized antibodies (Scotgen Biopharm)	gB, gH epitopes	CMV infection in immunocompromised patients	Preclinical	24, 80
Combination of monoclonal antibodies (Children's Hospital, Inc.)	Human CMV glycoprotein A		Preclinical	US5126130 (1987)

organ transplant recipients found a positive effect of prophylactic CMV-IVIG on recipients: improved total survival and moderately reduced CMV disease and CMV-associated deaths (66). CMV-IVIG use in stem cell transplant patients is less promising. A multicenter, randomized, double-blind, dose-effect, placebo-controlled study of 200 stem cell transplants concluded that the use of immunoglobulin therapy did not significantly reduce CMV infection and disease (67). A second meta-analysis combining 30 trials with 4,223 stem cell transplant patients observed no differences in mortality, infections of any kind, CMV infections, or graft-versus-host disease (68). As a result of this variability, IVIG therapy is approved, but is not standard treatment, for transplant patients.

The presence of maternal antibodies to CMV reduces the risk of fetal infection (3), indicating the potential for antibodies to prevent and/or treat congenital CMV infection. Passive immunization studies with pregnant guinea pigs have demonstrated that antibodies to the virus or gB reduce the fetal infection rate and enhance fetal survival (69, 70). Furthermore, adoptive transfer of B memory cells was protective in T- and B-cell-deficient mice (71). Subsequently, several nonrandomized human trials using CMV-IVIG to prevent CMV infection in utero have been performed. In one, 181 pregnant women with confirmed primary CMV infection were divided into a treatment group (women who had amniocentesis to confirm fetal infection) and a prevention group (those who did not undergo amniocentesis) (72). The treatment group included 55 women, 31 who received Cytotect IVIG, resulting in one infected newborn (3%), and 14 who received no treatment, resulting in seven infected newborns (50%). The prevention group included 37 women receiving Cytotect IVIG, resulting in 6 infected newborns (16%), and 47 who did not receive treatment, resulting in 19 infected newborns (40%). More recently, a case-controlled study compared 32 children with hearing and/or psychomotor deficits with 32 healthy, age- and gestation-matched control children. The mothers of both groups had confirmed or probable primary CMV infection at <20 weeks of gestation. The only risk factor for these children was whether the mother had received CMV-IVIG after infection: of the case patients, 4/32 received IVIG, while 27/32 control mothers received IVIG (73). While promising, larger studies are needed to draw a clear conclusion, especially for an expensive intervention that requires screening for serologic confirmation of infection followed by monthly CMV-IVIG administration (74).

Monoclonal Antibodies

The apparent protective role of antibodies against congenital CMV suggests that these polyclonal immune responses could be deconvoluted to a discrete number of highly protective epitopes. These could, in principle, be targeted with high efficacy by a monoclonal or oligoclonal antibody preparation (75, 76). This perspective is supported by the early characterization of human monoclonal antibody C23 which neutralized the ability of AD169 and clinical CMV isolates to infect lung fibroblasts 1,000 times more potently than human IVIG (77). Monoclonal antibodies have the additional benefits of being very well characterized, with epitopes, binding affinities, and neutralizing mechanisms described;

their biochemical and biophysical properties engineered to meet specific design targets; and since they are purified from monoclonal cultures, minimal lot-to-lot variability (78).

Most efforts in developing CMV-neutralizing monoclonal antibodies have targeted the gH viral glycoprotein, as low anti-gH titer is a risk factor for CMV disease (79) (Table 2). Phase I clinical trials of several anti-gB and anti-gH human monoclonal antibodies have demonstrated a pharmacokinetic profile similar to that of human IgG1 and lack of immunogenicity, supporting their safe use in passive immunotherapy applications (80, 81, 82). One anti-gH IgG1 human monoclonal antibody isolated from the spleen of a CMV-seropositive individual was able to block in vitro infection of multiple cell types by laboratory and clinical strains of CMV, with IC_{50} values between 0.03 and 1.02 µg/ml (83, 84). As this antibody also effectively treated CMV retinitis when combined with ganciclovir in rat models, it was evaluated in a series of clinical trials as MSL-109 (Sevirumab/ Protovir; Protein Design Labs), but unfortunately, it has not shown sufficient efficacy.

A randomized placebo-controlled human trial to assess the efficacy of MSL-109 to delay progression of CMV retinitis in AIDS patients was halted after it failed to slow progression of the blinding eye disease (85). Indeed, the MSL-109 treatment group had a higher mortality rate than the placebo group. Subsequently, serum CMV titers were associated with a higher risk of mortality in AIDS patients with CMV retinitis, implying that MSL-109 was ineffective in clearing plasma CMV (86). Similarly, stem cell transplant recipients with CMV^+ donors or recipients received MSL-109 biweekly in a randomized, double-blind study. The MSL-109 treatment group showed no difference in survival or pp65 antigenemia versus the placebo groups (87). Recently, it has been suggested that the MSL-109 failure may have been due to the rapid generation of nongenetic escape variants. It appears that infected cells present gH on their surface during viral replication. The gH is available to bind and endocytose circulating MSL-109, and the gH/MSL-109 complex is then incorporated into the viral envelope with the MSL-109 Fc domain exposed. The gH/L complex is no longer available to bind epithelial/endothelial receptors, but the Fc domain of MSL-109 is available to bind Fc receptors, altering the cellular trophism of the virus (84).

Recently, a novel method was used to characterize the repertoire of CMV-reactive antibodies in CMV-immune donors. Human B lymphocytes from CMV-seropositive donors were immortalized with Epstein-Barr virus, followed by screening for CMV neutralization. Of the 1,664 clones screened, 29 neutralized CMV infectivity. Of the four further characterized, two bound gB AD-2, two bound gH, and all were able to neutralize lab strain AD169 or a clinical isolate in both fibroblast and endothelial invasion assays. Importantly, these monoclonal antibodies were ~20-fold more potent than the Cytotect IVIG, supporting development of antibody cocktails over IVIG (88). As described above, it appears that additional potently neutralizing epitopes are present on the pentameric gH/gL/UL128-131 complex and may present promising targets for passive immunotherapy (21, 22). Other less potently neutralizing human monoclonal antibodies isolated from memory B cells recognized viral glycoprotein gB, gH, or gM/gN and were shown to neutralize infection of both epithelial/endothelial cells and fibroblasts (22).

Apart from traditional passive immunotherapies relying on a single antibody to sequester a single epitope, new paradigms are emerging which could be applied to prevent CMV replication or lyse CMV-infected cells. For instance, adoptive immunotherapy has also shown that T cells recognizing the pp65, pp150, and I-E1 peptides form the dominant population of effector cells and uniquely identify CMV$^+$ cells early in infection (34, 35). Antibodies mimicking the specificity of public TCRs recognizing these peptides could deliver a cytotoxic payload or direct cytotoxic lymphocytes to these cells, approaches which have

been explored for HIV and cancer treatment (89). An antibody that could be used for this approach has been isolated from a large human Fab phage display library that recognizes HLA A2/pp65$_{495-503}$ with a 300-nM affinity and is able to specifically detect peptide on the surface of fibroblasts in vitro (90). A similar approach formed a bispecific antibody by chemically linking OKT3 (an FDA-approved anti-CD3 antibody which binds and activates T cells) to CMV-IVIG polyclonal anti-CMV antibodies. After incubation with CMV-infected fibroblasts, specific lysis of CMV-infected cells was demonstrated in vitro (80% for the test versus <20% for the control) (91). Additional reports documenting CMV-neutralizing human monoclonal antibodies (Table 2) reflect the breadth of efforts to development of human/humanized monoclonal antibodies to neutralization CMV.

FUTURE CHALLENGES

Based on the high rates of CMV infection in adults and the large percentage of CMV-specific T cells in seropositive individuals, preventing infection appears to be an unattainable goal. In the absence of a vaccine, antibody therapies to prevent or control disease in susceptible populations may be the best solution. Here, there is strong evidence that adoptive transfer of cytotoxic T cells with CMV specificity is able to control secondary disease in stem cell transplant patients, while administration of hyperimmune IVIG appears effective in some solid organ transplant patients and is promising in seronegative pregnant women. In conjunction with recent insights into the function of CMV glycoprotein complexes, further elucidation of protective B- and T-cell epitopes present in the UL128-131 trimer and associated gH/gL pentamer is expected to contribute to design of immunotherapeutics with greater specificity and potency. Ultimately, potent cocktails of high-affinity monoclonal antibodies binding neutralizing epitopes on the virus and TCR-like antibodies to target infected cells may prove effective at suppressing CMV replication.

ACKNOWLEDGMENTS

This work was supported by generous grants from NSF (DBI-0964137) and NIH (NIGMS R01GM095638) to J.A.M.

Conflicts of interest: We declare no conflict.

CITATION

Acquaye-Seedah E, Frye ZP, Maynard JA. 2013. Immunotherapeutic approaches to prevent cytomegalovirus-mediated disease. Microbiol Spectrum 2(1):AID-0009-2013.

REFERENCES

1. **Craig JM, Macauley JC, Weller TH, Wirth P.** 1957. Isolation of intranuclear inclusion producing agents from infants with illnesses resembling cytomegalic inclusion disease. *Proc Soc Exp Biol Med* **94**:4–12.

2. **Johnson J, Anderson B, Pass RF.** 2012. Prevention of maternal and congenital cytomegalovirus infection. *Clin Obstet Gynecol* **55**:521–530.

3. **Fowler KB, Stagno S, Pass RF.** 2003. Maternal immunity and prevention of congenital cytomegalovirus infection. *JAMA* **289**:1008–1011.

4. **Smithey MJ, Li G, Venturi V, Davenport MP, Nikolich-Zugich J.** 2012. Lifelong persistent viral infection alters the naive T cell pool, impairing CD8 T cell immunity in late life. *J Immunol* **189**: 5356–5366.

5. **Arvin AM, Fast P, Myers M, Plotkin S, Rabinovich R.** 2004. Vaccine development to prevent cytomegalovirus disease: report from the National Vaccine Advisory Committee. *Clin Infect Dis* **39**:233–239.

6. **Khanna R, Diamond DJ.** 2006. Human cytomegalovirus vaccine: time to look for alternative options. *Trends Mol Med* **12**:26–33.

7. **Marasco WA, Sui J.** 2007. The growth and potential of human antiviral monoclonal antibody therapeutics. *Nat Biotechnol* **25**:1421–1434.

8. **Dolan A, Cunningham C, Hector RD, Hassan-Walker AF, Lee L, Addison C, Dargan DJ, McGeoch DJ, Gatherer D, Emery VC, Griffiths PD, Sinzger C, McSharry BP, Wilkinson GW, Davison AJ.** 2004. Genetic content of wild-type human cytomegalovirus. *J Gen Virol* **85**:1301–1312.

9. **Vanarsdall AL, Ryckman BJ, Chase MC, Johnson DC.** 2008. Human cytomegalovirus glycoproteins gB and gH/gL mediate epithelial cell-cell fusion when expressed either in *cis* or in *trans*. *J Virol* **82**:11837–11850.

10. **Ryckman BJ, Chase MC, Johnson DC.** 2010. Human cytomegalovirus TR strain glycoprotein O acts as a chaperone promoting gH/gL incorporation into virions but is not present in virions. *J Virol* **84**:2597–2609.

11. **Ryckman BJ, Chase MC, Johnson DC.** 2008. HCMV gH/gL/UL128-131 interferes with virus entry into epithelial cells: evidence for cell type-specific receptors. *Proc Natl Acad Sci USA* **105**: 14118–14123.

12. **Vanarsdall AL, Chase MC, Johnson DC.** 2011. Human cytomegalovirus glycoprotein gO complexes with gH/gL, promoting interference with viral entry into human fibroblasts but not entry into epithelial cells. *J Virol* **85**:11638–11645.

13. **Wang D, Shenk T.** 2005. Human cytomegalovirus virion protein complex required for epithelial and endothelial cell tropism. *Proc Natl Acad Sci USA* **102**:18153–18158.

14. **Wang D, Yu QC, Schroer J, Murphy E, Shenk T.** 2007. Human cytomegalovirus uses two distinct pathways to enter retinal pigmented epithelial cells. *Proc Natl Acad Sci USA* **104**:20037–20042.

15. **Britt WJ, Vugler L, Butfiloski EJ, Stephens EB.** 1990. Cell surface expression of human cytomegalovirus (HCMV) gp55-116 (gB): use of HCMV-recombinant vaccinia virus-infected cells in analysis of the human neutralizing antibody response. *J Virol* **64**:1079–1085.

16. **Marshall GS, Rabalais GP, Stout GG, Waldeyer SL.** 1992. Antibodies to recombinant-derived glycoprotein B after natural human cytomegalovirus infection correlate with neutralizing activity. *J Infect Dis* **165**:381–384.

17. **Navarro D, Lennette E, Tugizov S, Pereira L.** 1997. Humoral immune response to functional regions of human cytomegalovirus glycoprotein B. *J Med Virol* **52**:451–459.

18. **Speckner A, Glykofrydes D, Ohlin M, Mach M.** 1999. Antigenic domain 1 of human cytomegalovirus glycoprotein B induces a multitude of different antibodies which, when combined, results in incomplete virus neutralization. *J Gen Virol* **80**(Pt 8):2183–2191.

19. **Schrader JW, McLean GR.** 2007. Location, location, timing: analysis of cytomegalovirus epitopes for neutralizing antibodies. *Immunol Lett* **112**:58–60.

20. **Potzsch S, Spindler N, Wiegers AK, Fisch T, Rucker P, Sticht H, Grieb N, Baroti T, Weisel F, Stamminger T, Martin-Parras L, Mach M, Winkler TH.** 2011. B cell repertoire analysis

identifies new antigenic domains on glycoprotein B of human cytomegalovirus which are target of neutralizing antibodies. *PLoS Pathog* 7:e1002172.

21. **Fouts AE, Chan P, Stephan JP, Vandlen R, Feierbach B.** 2012. Antibodies against the gH/gL/UL128/UL130/UL131 complex comprise the majority of the anti-cytomegalovirus (anti-CMV) neutralizing antibody response in CMV hyperimmune globulin. *J Virol* 86:7444–7447.

22. **Macagno A, Bernasconi NL, Vanzetta F, Dander E, Sarasini A, Revello MG, Gerna G, Sallusto F, Lanzavecchia A.** 2010. Isolation of human monoclonal antibodies that potently neutralize human cytomegalovirus infection by targeting different epitopes on the gH/gL/UL128-131A complex. *J Virol* 84:1005–1013.

23. **Saccoccio FM, Sauer AL, Cui X, Armstrong AE, el Habib SE, Johnson DC, Ryckman BJ, Klingelhutz AJ, Adler SP, McVoy MA.** 2011. Peptides from cytomegalovirus UL130 and UL131 proteins induce high titer antibodies that block viral entry into mucosal epithelial cells. *Vaccine* 29:2705–2711.

24. **Hamilton AA, Manuel DM, Grundy JE, Turner AJ, King SI, Adair JR, White P, Carr FJ, Harris WJ.** 1997. A humanized antibody against human cytomegalovirus (CMV) gpUL75 (gH) for prophylaxis or treatment of CMV infections. *J Infect Dis* 176:59–68.

25. **Genini E, Percivalle E, Sarasini A, Revello MG, Baldanti F, Gerna G.** 2011. Serum antibody response to the gH/gL/pUL128-131 five-protein complex of human cytomegalovirus (HCMV) in primary and reactivated HCMV infections. *J Clin Virol* 52:113–118.

26. **Kropff B, Burkhardt C, Schott J, Nentwich J, Fisch T, Britt W, Mach M.** 2012. Glycoprotein N of human cytomegalovirus protects the virus from neutralizing antibodies. *PLoS Pathog* 8:e1002999.

27. **Schmueck M, Fischer AM, Hammoud B, Brestrich G, Fuehrer H, Luu SH, Mueller K, Babel N, Volk HD, Reinke P.** 2012. Preferential expansion of human virus-specific multifunctional central memory T cells by partial targeting of the IL-2 receptor signaling pathway: the key role of CD4$^+$ T cells. *J Immunol* 188:5189–5198.

28. **Reddehase MJ.** 2000. The immunogenicity of human and murine cytomegaloviruses. *Curr Opin Immunol* 12:390–396.

29. **Riddell SR, Watanabe KS, Goodrich JM, Li CR, Agha ME, Greenberg PD.** 1992. Restoration of viral immunity in immunodeficient humans by the adoptive transfer of T cell clones. *Science* 257:238–241.

30. **Walter EA, Greenberg PD, Gilbert MJ, Finch RJ, Watanabe KS, Thomas ED, Riddell SR.** 1995. Reconstitution of cellular immunity against cytomegalovirus in recipients of allogeneic bone marrow by transfer of T-cell clones from the donor. *N Engl J Med* 333:1038–1044.

31. **Sellar RS, Peggs KS.** 2012. Therapeutic strategies for the prevention and treatment of cytomegalovirus infection. *Expert Opin Biol Ther* 12:1161–1172.

32. **Einsele H, Hebart H.** 2004. CMV-specific immunotherapy. *Hum Immunol* 65:558–564.

33. **Schub A, Schuster IG, Hammerschmidt W, Moosmann A.** 2009. CMV-specific TCR-transgenic T cells for immunotherapy. *J Immunol* 183:6819–6830.

34. **Greenberg PD, Reusser P, Goodrich JM, Riddell SR.** 1991. Development of a treatment regimen for human cytomegalovirus (CMV) infection in bone marrow transplantation recipients by adoptive transfer of donor-derived CMV-specific T cell clones expanded in vitro. *Ann N Y Acad Sci* 636:184–195.

35. **Slezak SL, Bettinotti M, Selleri S, Adams S, Marincola FM, Stroncek DF.** 2007. CMV pp65 and IE-1 T cell epitopes recognized by healthy subjects. *J Transl Med* 5:17.

36. **Cobbold M, Khan N, Pourgheysari B, Tauro S, McDonald D, Osman H, Assenmacher M, Billingham L, Steward C, Crawley C, Olavarria E, Goldman J, Chakraverty R, Mahendra P, Craddock C, Moss PA.** 2005. Adoptive transfer of cytomegalovirus-specific CTL to stem cell transplant patients after selection by HLA-peptide tetramers. *J Exp Med* 202:379–386.

37. **Sylwester AW, Mitchell BL, Edgar JB, Taormina C, Pelte C, Ruchti F, Sleath PR, Grabstein KH, Hosken NA, Kern F, Nelson JA, Picker LJ.** 2005. Broadly targeted human cytomegalovirus-specific CD4+ and CD8+ T cells dominate the memory compartments of exposed subjects. *J Exp Med* 202:673–685.

38. **Trautmann L, Rimbert M, Echasserieau K, Saulquin X, Neveu B, Dechanet J, Cerundolo V, Bonneville M.** 2005. Selection of T cell clones expressing high-affinity public TCRs within human cytomegalovirus-specific CD8 T cell responses. *J Immunol* 175:6123–6132.

39. **Wynn KK, Fulton Z, Cooper L, Silins SL, Gras S, Archbold JK, Tynan FE, Miles JJ, McCluskey J, Burrows SR, Rossjohn J, Khanna R.** 2008. Impact of clonal competition for peptide-MHC complexes on the CD8+ T-cell repertoire selection in a persistent viral infection. *Blood* 111:4283–4292.

40. **Wang GC, Dash P, McCullers JA, Doherty PC, Thomas PG.** 2012. T cell receptor alphabeta diversity inversely correlates with pathogen-specific antibody levels in human cytomegalovirus infection. *Sci Transl Med* 4:128–142.

41. **Schleiss MR.** 2008. Cytomegalovirus vaccine development. *Curr Top Microbiol Immunol* **325:** 361–382.

42. **Plotkin SA, Higgins R, Kurtz JB, Morris PJ, Campbell DA, Jr, Shope TC, Spector SA, Dankner WM.** 1994. Multicenter trial of Towne strain attenuated virus vaccine in seronegative renal transplant recipients. *Transplantation* **58:** 1176–1178.

43. **Elek SD, Stern H.** 1974. Development of a vaccine against mental retardation caused by cytomegalovirus infection in utero. *Lancet* **i:**1–5.

44. **Yow MD, Demmler GJ.** 1992. Congenital cytomegalovirus disease—20 years is long enough. *N Engl J Med* **326:**702–703.

45. **Adler SP, Starr SE, Plotkin SA, Hempfling SH, Buis J, Manning ML, Best AM.** 1995. Immunity induced by primary human cytomegalovirus infection protects against secondary infection among women of childbearing age. *J Infect Dis* **171:**26–32.

46. **Jacobson MA, Sinclair E, Bredt B, Agrillo L, Black D, Epling CL, Carvidi A, Ho T, Bains R, Girling V, Adler SP.** 2006. Safety and immunogenicity of Towne cytomegalovirus vaccine with or without adjuvant recombinant interleukin-12. *Vaccine* **24:**5311–5319.

47. **Cui X, Meza BP, Adler SP, McVoy MA.** 2008. Cytomegalovirus vaccines fail to induce epithelial entry neutralizing antibodies comparable to natural infection. *Vaccine* **26:**5760–5766.

48. **Pass RF, Zhang C, Evans A, Simpson T, Andrews W, Huang ML, Corey L, Hill J, Davis E, Flanigan C, Cloud G.** 2009. Vaccine prevention of maternal cytomegalovirus infection. *N Engl J Med* **360:** 1191–1199.

49. **Griffiths PD, Stanton A, McCarrell E, Smith C, Osman M, Harber M, Davenport A, Jones G, Wheeler DC, O'Beirne J, Thorburn D, Patch D, Atkinson CE, Pichon S, Sweny P, Lanzman M, Woodford E, Rothwell E, Old N, Kinyanjui R, Haque T, Atabani S, Luck S, Prideaux S, Milne RS, Emery VC, Burroughs AK.** 2011. Cytomegalovirus glycoprotein-B vaccine with MF59 adjuvant in transplant recipients: a phase 2 randomised placebo-controlled trial. *Lancet* **377:**1256–1263.

50. **La Rosa C, Longmate J, Lacey SF, Kaltcheva T, Sharan R, Marsano D, Kwon P, Drake J, Williams B, Denison S, Broyer S, Couture L, Nakamura R, Kelsey MI, Krieg AM, Diamond DJ, Zaia JA.** 2012. Clinical evaluation of safety and immunogenicity of PADRE-cytomegalovirus (CMV) and tetanus-CMV fusion peptide vaccines with or without PF03512676 adjuvant. *J Infect Dis* **205:**1294–1304.

51. **Lilleri D, Kabanova A, Lanzavecchia A, Gerna G.** 2012. Antibodies against neutralization epitopes of human cytomegalovirus gH/gL/pUL128-130-131 complex and virus spreading may correlate with virus control in vivo. *J Clin Immunol* **32:**1324–1331.

52. **Lilleri D, Kabanova A, Revello MG, Percivalle E, Sarasini A, Genini E, Sallusto F, Lanzavecchia A, Corti D, Gerna G.** 2013. Fetal human cytomegalovirus transmission correlates with delayed maternal antibodies to gH/gL/pUL128-130-131 complex during primary infection. *PLoS One* **8:** e59863.

53. **Fu TM, Wang D, Freed DC, Tang A, Li F, He X, Cole S, Dubey S, Finnefrock AC, ter Meulen J, Shiver JW, Casimiro DR.** 2012. Restoration of viral epithelial tropism improves immunogenicity in rabbits and rhesus macaques for a whole virion vaccine of human cytomegalovirus. *Vaccine* **30:** 7469–7474.

54. **Wussow F, Yue Y, Martinez J, Deere JD, Longmate J, Herrmann A, Barry PA, Diamond DJ.** 2013. A vaccine based on the rhesus cytomegalovirus UL128 complex induces broadly neutralizing antibodies in rhesus macaques. *J Virol* **87:**1322–1332.

55. **Loomis RJ, Lilja AE, Monroe J, Balabanis KA, Brito LA, Palladino G, Franti M, Mandl CW, Barnett SW, Mason PW.** 2013. Vectored codelivery of human cytomegalovirus gH and gL proteins elicits potent complement-independent neutralizing antibodies. *Vaccine* **31:**919–926.

56. **Roy DM, Grundy JE.** 1992. Evaluation of neutralizing antibody titers against human cytomegalovirus in intravenous gamma globulin preparations. *Transplantation* **54:**1109–1110.

57. **Planitzer CB, Saemann MD, Gajek H, Farcet MR, Kreil TR.** 2011. Cytomegalovirus neutralization by hyperimmune and standard intravenous immunoglobulin preparations. *Transplantation* **92:**267–270.

58. **Gupta CK, Leszczynski J, Gupta RK, Siber GR.** 1996. IgG subclass antibodies to human cytomegalovirus (CMV) in normal human plasma samples and immune globulins and their neutralizing activities. *Biologicals* **24:**117–124.

59. **Adler SP, Nigro G.** 2009. Findings and conclusions from CMV hyperimmune globulin treatment trials. *J Clin Virol* **46**(Suppl 4)**:**S54–S57.

60. **Filipovich AH, Peltier MH, Bechtel MK, Dirksen CL, Strauss SA, Englund JA.** 1992. Circulating cytomegalovirus (CMV) neutralizing activity in bone marrow transplant recipients: comparison of passive immunity in a randomized study of four intravenous IgG products administered to CMV-seronegative patients. *Blood* **80:** 2656–2660.

61. **Snydman DR, Werner BG, Dougherty NN, Griffith J, Rubin RH, Dienstag JL, Rohrer RH, Freeman R, Jenkins R, Lewis WD, Hammer S,**

O'Rourke E, Grady GF, Fawaz K, Kaplan MM, Hoffman MA, Katz AT, Doran M. 1993. Cytomegalovirus immune globulin prophylaxis in liver transplantation. A randomized, double-blind, placebo-controlled trial. *Ann Intern Med* **119:** 984–991.

62. King SM, Superina R, Andrews W, Winston DJ, Dunn S, Busuttil RW, Colombani P, Paradis K. 1997. Randomized comparison of ganciclovir plus intravenous immune globulin (IVIG) with IVIG alone for prevention of primary cytomegalovirus disease in children receiving liver transplants. *Clin Infect Dis* **25:**1173–1179.

63. Fisher RA, Kistler KD, Ulsh P, Bergman GE, Morris J. 2012. The association between cytomegalovirus immune globulin and long-term recipient and graft survival following liver transplantation. *Transpl Infect Dis* **14:**121–131.

64. Leroy F, Sechet A, Abou Ayache R, Thierry A, Belmouaz S, Desport E, Bauwens M, Bridoux F, Touchard G. 2006. Cytomegalovirus prophylaxis with intravenous polyvalent immunoglobulin in high-risk renal transplant recipients. *Transplant Proc* **38:**2324–2326.

65. Toussaint ND, Tan MB, Nicholls K, Walker RG, Cohney SJ. 2011. Low-dose valaciclovir and cytomegalovirus immunoglobulin to prevent cytomegalovirus disease in high-risk renal transplant recipients. *Nephrology (Carlton)* **16:**113–117.

66. Bonaros N, Mayer B, Schachner T, Laufer G, Kocher A. 2008. CMV-hyperimmune globulin for preventing cytomegalovirus infection and disease in solid organ transplant recipients: a meta-analysis. *Clin Transplant* **22:**89–97.

67. Cordonnier C, Chevret S, Legrand M, Rafi H, Dhedin N, Lehmann B, Bassompierre F, Gluckman E. 2003. Should immunoglobulin therapy be used in allogeneic stem-cell transplantation? A randomized, double-blind, dose effect, placebo-controlled, multicenter trial. *Ann Intern Med* **139:**8–18.

68. Raanani P, Gafter-Gvili A, Paul M, Ben-Bassat I, Leibovici L, Shpilberg O. 2009. Immunoglobulin prophylaxis in hematopoietic stem cell transplantation: systematic review and meta-analysis. *J Clin Oncol* **27:**770–781.

69. Chatterjee A, Harrison CJ, Britt WJ, Bewtra C. 2001. Modification of maternal and congenital cytomegalovirus infection by anti-glycoprotein b antibody transfer in guinea pigs. *J Infect Dis* **183:**1547–1553.

70. Bratcher DF, Bourne N, Bravo FJ, Schleiss MR, Slaoui M, Myers MG, Bernstein DI. 1995. Effect of passive antibody on congenital cytomegalovirus infection in guinea pigs. *J Infect Dis* **172:**944–950.

71. Klenovsek K, Weisel F, Schneider A, Appelt U, Jonjic S, Messerle M, Bradel-Tretheway B, Winkler TH, Mach M. 2007. Protection from CMV infection in immunodeficient hosts by adoptive transfer of memory B cells. *Blood* **110:** 3472–3479.

72. Nigro G, Adler SP, La Torre R, Best AM. 2005. Passive immunization during pregnancy for congenital cytomegalovirus infection. *N Engl J Med* **353:**1350–1362.

73. Nigro G, Adler SP, Parruti G, Anceschi MM, Coclite E, Pezone I, Di Renzo GC. 2012. Immunoglobulin therapy of fetal cytomegalovirus infection occurring in the first half of pregnancy—a case-control study of the outcome in children. *J Infect Dis* **205:**215–227.

74. Cahill AG, Odibo AO, Stamilio DM, Macones GA. 2009. Screening and treating for primary cytomegalovirus infection in pregnancy: where do we stand? A decision-analytic and economic analysis. *Am J Obstet Gynecol* **201:**466, e1–7.

75. Nowakowski A, Wang C, Powers DB, Amersdorfer P, Smith TJ, Montgomery VA, Sheridan R, Blake R, Smith LA, Marks JD. 2002. Potent neutralization of botulinum neurotoxin by recombinant oligoclonal antibody. *Proc Natl Acad Sci USA* **99:**11346–11350.

76. Maynard JA, Maassen CBM, Leppla SH, Brasky K, Patterson JL, Iverson BL, Georgiou G. 2002. Protection against anthrax toxin by recombinant antibody fragments correlates with antigen affinity. *Nat Biotechnol* **20:**597–601.

77. Masuho Y, Matsumoto Y, Tomiyama T, Sugano T, Ono S. 1990. Characterization of human anticytomegalovirus monoclonal antibody as biologics. *Dev Biol Stand* **71:**127–136.

78. Maynard J, Georgiou G. 2000. Antibody engineering. *Annu Rev Biomed Eng* **2:**339–376.

79. Rasmussen L, Morris S, Wolitz R, Dowling A, Fessell J, Holodniy M, Merigan TC. 1994. Deficiency in antibody response to human cytomegalovirus glycoprotein gH in human immunodeficiency virus-infected patients at risk for cytomegalovirus retinitis. *J Infect Dis* **170:**673–677.

80. Tempest PR, White P, Buttle M, Carr FJ, Harris WJ. 1995. Identification of framework residues required to restore antigen binding during reshaping of a monoclonal antibody against the glycoprotein gB of human cytomegalovirus. *Int J Biol Macromol* **17:**37–42.

81. Arizono H, Sugano T, Kaida S, Shibusawa K, Karasawa Y, Esumi Y, Kondo S, Kiyoki M. 1994. Pharmacokinetics of a new human monoclonal antibody against cytomegalovirus. Third communication: correspondence of the idiotype activity and virus neutralization activity of the new monoclonal antibody, regavirumab in rat serum and its pharmacokinetics in rats and monkeys. *Arzneimittelforschung* **44:**909–913.

82. **Drobyski WR, Gottlieb M, Carrigan D, Ostberg L, Grebenau M, Schran H, Magid P, Ehrlich P, Nadler PI, Ash RC.** 1991. Phase I study of safety and pharmacokinetics of a human anticytomegalovirus monoclonal antibody in allogeneic bone marrow transplant recipients. *Transplantation* **51:**1190–1196.

83. **Nokta M, Tolpin MD, Nadler PI, Pollard RB.** 1994. Human monoclonal anti-cytomegalovirus (CMV) antibody (MSL 109): enhancement of in vitro foscarnet- and ganciclovir-induced inhibition of CMV replication. *Antivir Res* **24:**17–26.

84. **Manley K, Anderson J, Yang F, Szustakowski J, Oakeley EJ, Compton T, Feire AL.** 2011. Human cytomegalovirus escapes a naturally occurring neutralizing antibody by incorporating it into assembling virions. *Cell Host Microbe* **10:**197–209.

85. **Gilpin AM, Holbrook JT, Jabs DA, Meinert CL.** 2003. Data and safety monitoring board deliberations resulting in the early termination of the Monoclonal Antibody Cytomegalovirus Retinitis Trial. *Control Clin Trials* **24:**92–98.

86. **Jabs DA, Gilpin AM, Min YI, Erice A, Kempen JH, Quinn TC.** 2002. HIV and cytomegalovirus viral load and clinical outcomes in AIDS and cytomegalovirus retinitis patients: Monoclonal Antibody Cytomegalovirus Retinitis Trial. *AIDS* **16:**877–887.

87. **Boeckh M, Bowden RA, Storer B, Chao NJ, Spielberger R, Tierney DK, Gallez-Hawkins G, Cunningham T, Blume KG, Levitt D, Zaia JA.** 2001. Randomized, placebo-controlled, double-blind study of a cytomegalovirus-specific monoclonal antibody (MSL-109) for prevention of cytomegalovirus infection after allogeneic hematopoietic stem cell transplantation. *Biol Blood Marrow Transplant* **7:**343–351.

88. **Funaro A, Gribaudo G, Luganini A, Ortolan E, Lo Buono N, Vicenzi E, Cassetta L, Landolfo S,** Buick R, Falciola L, Murphy M, Garotta G, Malavasi F. 2008. Generation of potent neutralizing human monoclonal antibodies against cytomegalovirus infection from immune B cells. *BMC Biotechnol* **8:**85.

89. **Liddy N, Bossi G, Adams KJ, Lissina A, Mahon TM, Hassan NJ, Gavarret J, Bianchi FC, Pumphrey NJ, Ladell K, Gostick E, Sewell AK, Lissin NM, Harwood NE, Molloy PE, Li Y, Cameron BJ, Sami M, Baston EE, Todorov PT, Paston SJ, Dennis RE, Harper JV, Dunn SM, Ashfield R, Johnson A, McGrath Y, Plesa G, June CH, Kalos M, Price DA, Vuidepot A, Williams DD, Sutton DH, Jakobsen BK.** 2012. Monoclonal TCR-redirected tumor cell killing. *Nat Med* **18:**980–987.

90. **Makler O, Oved K, Netzer N, Wolf D, Reiter Y.** 2010. Direct visualization of the dynamics of antigen presentation in human cells infected with cytomegalovirus revealed by antibodies mimicking TCR specificity. *Eur J Immunol* **40:**1552–1565.

91. **Lum LG, Ramesh M, Thakur A, Mitra S, Deol A, Uberti JP, Pellett PE.** 2012. Targeting cytomegalovirus-infected cells using T cells armed with anti-CD3 x anti-CMV bispecific antibody. *Biol Blood Marrow Transplant* **18:**1012–1022.

92. **Borucki MJ, Spritzler J, Asmuth DM, Gnann J, Hirsch MS, Nokta M, Aweeka F, Nadler PI, Sattler F, Alston B, Nevin TT, Owens S, Waterman K, Hubbard L, Caliendo A, Pollard RB.** 2004. A phase II, double-masked, randomized, placebo-controlled evaluation of a human monoclonal anti-cytomegalovirus antibody (MSL-109) in combination with standard therapy versus standard therapy alone in the treatment of AIDS patients with cytomegalovirus retinitis. *Antivir Res* **64:**103–111.

17

Rotavirus

MANUEL A. FRANCO[1] and HARRY B. GREENBERG[2,3]

INTRODUCTION

Rotaviruses (RV) are ubiquitous highly infectious double-stranded RNA viruses of importance in public health because of the severe acute gastroenteritis (GE) they cause in young children and many other animal species. They are very well adapted to their host, causing frequent symptomatic and asymptomatic reinfections. Antibodies are the major component of the immune system that protects infants against RV reinfection. The relationship between the virus and the B cells (Bc) that produce these antibodies is complex and incompletely understood (1). In this review, the following basic aspects of RV-specific Bc (RV-Bc) will be addressed: (i) ontogeny; (ii) use of immunoglobulin (Ig) genes; (iii) differential distribution (compartmentalization) in the intestinal and systemic immune systems; (iv) specificity of RV-Ig produced and the mechanisms by which it mediates protection; and finally, (v) practical applications for the use of RV-Ig, including RV-Ig as a prophylactic or therapeutic agent and as a correlate of protection. The immune response generated against RV vaccines has been recently reviewed (2, 3) and will only be briefly discussed. The focus of this review is antibodies induced by natural RV infection in humans, but reference to studies

[1]Facultad de Ciencias y Medicina, Pontificia Universidad Javeriana, Bogotá, Colombia; [2]Departments of Medicine and Microbiology and Immunology, Stanford University School of Medicine, Stanford, CA 94305; [3]Veterans Affairs Palo Alto Health Care System, Palo Alto, CA 94304.

Antibodies for Infectious Diseases
Edited by James E. Crowe, Jr., Diana Boraschi, and Rino Rappuoli
© 2015 American Society for Microbiology, Washington, DC
doi:10.1128/microbiolspec.AID-0011-2013

of the murine and porcine animal models of RV infection will be made when necessary.

THE ANTIBODY RESPONSE AGAINST RV

(i) Ontogeny of RV-Bc and RV-Ig

A newborn receives important quantities of RV-IgG and RV-IgM transplacentally. High levels of these transplacentally transmitted Igs correlate with lower numbers of RV infections in young children and probably mediate protection against severe RV disease (4). In addition, maternal antibodies are also transferred to the infant through breast milk. It has been postulated that colostrum secretory IgA (sIgA) can be systemically absorbed to some degree (5), but most antibodies in the serum of neonates are transplacentally acquired and do not contain RV-IgA. Although breast milk antibodies are thought to have a local intestinal antiviral effect, this effect is relatively modest when it comes to preventing severe RV disease (1). In animal models, high-titered serum maternal antibodies (similar to what is observed in children from low-income countries) have some protective effect and can also inhibit the response to an RV vaccine (6). In contrast, low-titered maternal antibody in serum (as seen in children from high-income countries) did not protect against infection. The experimental conditions that induced low-titered maternal antibody in serum had a complex effect on subsequent immune response, which included an increase in the numbers of RV antibody-secreting cells (ASC) in the intestine induced upon infection in a porcine model system (7). In children, the presence of high-titered maternal antibodies in both serum and milk is thought to partially explain the lower immunogenicity of RV vaccines in low-income countries (3). The effect of maternal antibody levels and quality on RV vaccine immunogenicity in children needs to be further investigated (3).

Fortunately, RV is one of a few microbial antigens for which a flow cytometry assay to identify and characterize Bc expressing RV-Ig

at the membrane surface has been developed. Bc that bind green fluorescent protein (GFP)-containing RV virus-like particles (VLPs) made from viral core protein VP2 and intermediate capsid protein VP6 (an immunodominant antibody target) are considered RV-Bc. Figure 1 shows an example of a typical experiment using RV GFP-containing VLPs, and Table 1 gives a summary of the subsets of RV-Bc that

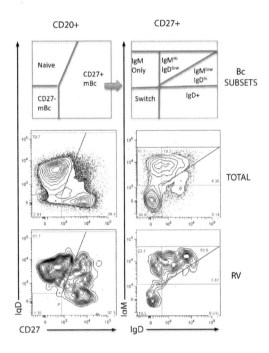

FIGURE 1 Flow cytometry experiment to characterize and compare RV-Bc to total Bc subsets (from reference 11 with modifications). Top row plots illustrate the Bc subsets considered. Middle row dot plots are gated on total CD20$^+$ Bc. Bottom row plots are gated on CD20$^+$ Bc that bind fluorescent RV VLPs (RV-Bc). As a first step in this analysis, Bc are evaluated for the expression of IgD and CD27 (left dot plots). IgD$^+$ CD27$^-$ Bc are naive cells, and IgD$^-$ CD27$^-$ (IgM, IgG, or IgA$^+$) are a low-frequency subset of mBc. The CD27$^+$ Bc of the left panels are further analyzed for the expression of IgD and IgM (right dot plots). IgM$^-$ IgD$^-$ cells are classical switched mBc; IgM$^+$ IgD$^-$ cells are called IgM-only mBc and resemble in many ways the switched mBc. IgD$^+$ IgM$^-$ cells are a poorly characterized subset of mBc. Double-positive IgM$^+$ IgD$^+$ mBc are a heterogeneous population of mBc; in the present experiment, they are further subdivided into IgM^{hi} IgD^{low} (a phenotype that resembles marginal zone Bc) and IgM^{low} IgD^{hi}. doi:10.1128/microbiolspec.AID-0011-2013.f1

TABLE 1 Blood-circulating Bc subsets in healthy adults and their enrichment or not in RV-Bc

Bc subset common name (phenotype)	Function and/or relationship of the Bc subset to disease	Enrichment in RV-Bc	Reference(s)
Naive (CD27⁻ IgD⁺ IgM⁺)	Bc that have emigrated from the bone marrow and express the preimmune repertoire of Ig	No	53
IgM mBc (CD27⁺ IgD⁺ IgM⁺)	Bc that probably represent a heterogeneous subpopulation, an important part of which has a prediversified repertoire of Ig; the CD27⁺ IgD^low IgM^hi subset resembles marginal zone Bc and are particularly enriched in RV-mBc	Yes	11, 20, 53
CD27⁻ mBc (CD27⁻ IgD⁻ IgM or IgG or IgA⁺)	Atypical mBc that do not express CD27 and that are enriched in patients with autoimmune diseases such as lupus	Yes in the IgG⁺ subset	53
IgM-only mBc (CD27⁺ IgD⁻ IgM⁺)	A minor mBc population that expresses IgM and seems to be related to switch mBc	Yes	20
Switch mBc (CD27⁺ IgD⁻ IgM⁻ IgG or IgA⁺)	Classical mBc subset that expresses IgG or IgA	Decreased frequency	11, 20, 53

have been shown to specifically bind GFP-containing VLPs using flow cytometry-based assays.

Unexpectedly, children are born with a high number (approximately 1 to 2%) of RV-Bc with a naive phenotype (8). These Bc secrete antibodies that have a low affinity to VP6 (9). Intriguingly, by 2 months of age, children will have a high number of RV-Bc that express IgM, IgD, and CD27 (generally considered a marker constellation for memory Bc [mBc]), irrespective of whether the children have had an RV infection, as evidenced by the presence of RV-IgA in serum (10). It is uncertain at present if these RV-mBc have or have not been induced by asymptomatic or symptomatic RV infections (either enteric or systemic) that, for some reason, do not induce serum RV-IgA. However, they may be playing a role in RV immunity. In experiments in which human IgM-mBc (mostly IgD⁺) are passively transferred to RV-infected immunodeficient mice, they are able to switch to IgG ASC and mediate immunity against RV antigenemia and viremia (11). Moreover, RV-mBc from adults are enriched in the IgD^low IgM^hi CD27⁺ subset of Bc (11) (Fig. 1, Table 1). This phenotype is reminiscent of spleen marginal zone Bc, a subset that has been postulated to develop (by an unknown mechanism) a prediversified Ig repertoire and to participate in "innate" Ig responses to pathogens (12).

Between 6 months (when maternal antibodies wane) and 3 years of age, almost every child will have been infected by RV, and approximately 50% of them will have had at least one symptomatic infection that consists primarily of diarrhea and vomiting (3). The primary Bc response in the peripheral blood of these children is characterized acutely by the presence of circulating RV-IgM ASC (13). Between 1 and 2 weeks after infection, the classical IgD⁻ CD27⁺ mBc appear in blood (14), and concomitantly, RV-IgA and IgM can be detected in serum (15) and stool (16). Importantly, in the serum of these children, secretory antibodies (antibodies that have been secreted to the intestinal lumen) can also be identified (17). RV sIgs present in the stool and serum originate from intestinal lamina propria RV ASCs that secrete polymeric antibodies. These antibodies are transported by the polymeric Ig receptor, present on the basolateral membrane of enterocytes, to the lumen of the intestine. In the lumen, proteases cleave the receptor, leaving part of it covalently attached to the Ig. This portion of the receptor, known as the secretory component, serves as a marker of sIg and protects the Igs from degradation in the harsh intestinal lumen. By an unknown mechanism, some of these sIg antibodies are retrotranscytosed and reach the systemic circulation (18). Four months after viral infection, RV-IgA persist in the circulation of children but the RV-sIg have disappeared (17). This finding has been associated with the fact that the production of local intestinal antibodies is short lived compared to antibodies (especially RV-IgG) present in serum (see below for discussion on the persistence of RV-Ig) (19).

Children and adults can be reinfected with RV, with the majority of reinfections being less symptomatic or asymptomatic compared to the first one or two. When caring for children with RV infections, up to 50% of parents become infected and half of them will have mild GE symptoms. Among the elderly, it is not uncommon for symptomatic RV outbreaks to reoccur, presumably due to waning immunity and or immunesenescence in this population (1).

(ii) Ig Gene Usage of RV-Bc

The relatively high number of circulating RV-Bc and the availability of a flow cytometry assay (Fig. 1) to detect them have permitted extensive studies of the Ig genes used by these cells in human peripheral blood and, to a much lesser degree, the intestine (9, 20, 21). The general strategy to perform these studies has been to clone and express the genes of single RV-Bc sorted (using the same strategy used to identify RV-Bc by flow cytometry described above and in Fig. 1) and in some cases expanded in vitro. These studies are robust because the genes amplified by PCR come from single cells and the specificity and functionality of the antibody they produce can be further tested.

Initial findings showed that, compared to non-antigen-specific Bc, RV-Bc of healthy adults have a biased usage of VH genes (21). In addition, the RV-Bc VH, D, JH, VL, and JL segment usage, extent of junctional diversity, and mean H chain complementarity-determining region 3 length of adults and infants were found to be similar (21). The genetic resemblance between cells from infants

and adults was unexpected, since it was thought that children's Bc would have similarities to Bc present during the fetal period, which have a particular repertoire of VH and VL gene usage and lack junctional diversity. These results suggested that the Bc repertoire is not a limiting determinant of the quality of antibody responses to RV in children (21). Nonetheless, a subsequent report showed that VH sequences of RV-Bc from children with acute RV GE have a lower number of mutations than those of the corresponding adult sequences (22). Besides, further studies that concentrated on VP6-specific antibodies encoded by the VH1-46 gene segment (an immunodominant gene in RV-Bc of both children and adults) showed that the mutations detected in adults conferred functional advantages to these antibodies (9). For instance, somatic mutations in the H chain CDR2 region of these antibodies generated a prolonged off-rate in VP6 binding and increased antiviral activity in an in vitro intracellular neutralization assay. Of note, using three-dimensional cryoelectron microscopy, investigators demonstrated that these antibodies bind VP6 where this protein forms viral type 1 channels, suggesting that the mechanism of intracellular neutralization could involve inhibition of viral RNA release during replication (9).

More recently, the Ig gene repertoire of VP6-Bc in circulating naive (CD19$^+$ IgD$^+$ CD27$^-$) or mBc subsets (CD19$^+$ IgD$^+$ CD27$^+$ IgM mBc or CD19$^+$ IgD$^-$ CD27$^+$ switched mBc that in these experiments include IgM-only mBc) from healthy adults has been evaluated (20). As previously stated, compared to non-antigen-specific mBc, RV-mBc had an increased frequency of IgM mBc (Table 1). Also, IgM RV-mBc had a shorter CDR3 length than naive and RV-switched mBc. This could be explained by both lower numbers of N and P nucleotide additions and shorter D segment length, due to increased exonuclease activity. A comparable finding was observed for total non-antigen-specific IgM-mBc, suggesting that IgM RV-mBc are probably selected by the same unidentified mechanism (20). In addition, the authors observed that switched RV-mBc were enriched in IgM-only mBc at the expense of IgA mBc (Table 1) and had a lower frequency of somatic mutations. These findings suggest that RV-mBc have undergone less extensive maturation in germinal centers (where switching and somatic hypermutation occur). Although the IgM mBc and switched mBc subpopulations of RV-mBc thus seem to be selected by different mechanisms, they share a very intriguing difference from naive RV-Bc. While the VH1 family is the dominant VH gene family used by naive RV-mBc, the VH3 family is dominant in both subtypes of RV-mBc. Particularly, the dominance of the VH1-46 gene segment usage is high in naive RV-Bc (28.6%) compared with IgM and switched RV-mBc (7.8 and 8.3%, respectively). In contrast, the VH3 family is the predominant VH family used by naive mBc and the two subtypes of mBc in total non-antigen-specific Bc. Altogether, these findings indicate that, unexpectedly, the dominant naive RV-VH1-expressing Bc do not have an advantage in the two selection processes that give rise to IgM and switched RV-mBc. Hence, more studies are necessary at both the ontological and functional levels to understand the relationship between the RV-specific naive and memory repertoires of Bc.

The investigations described above have been performed with blood-circulating Bc, and as previously stated, RV-Bc are probably concentrated in the intestine (see below for discussion on the compartmentalization of RV-Bc). Accordingly, two recent studies addressed the genes used by intestinal RV-Bc in healthy adult subjects (23, 24). In the first report, IgG or IgM plasma cells from the small bowel (CD138$^+$ CD27$^+$ that still express surface Ig of the corresponding isotype) capable of binding 2/6 RV-VLPs were purified by cell sorting (23). Ig genes from Bc derived from three donors were cloned, sequenced, and expressed. The VH genes of 26 Bc clones obtained (22 IgA, 4 IgM) were highly mutated and preferentially expressed the VH4 family, which is not dominant among peripheral blood RV-Bc (23). Ten of the IgA antibodies were expressed, and 8 were shown to bind RV but not a control antigen. In the second report, the genes from total non-antigen-specific IgA and IgG plasmablasts (CD38$^+$ CD27$^+$ cells still expressing the corresponding Ig isotype) from the lamina propria of the terminal ileum of healthy adult volunteers were cloned and expressed in vitro (6). Although the IgG plasmablasts were approximately 10 times less frequent than the IgA plasmablasts, the IgH, IgK, and IgL chain gene repertoire of both types of plasmablasts were similar to each other and to their blood-circulating counterparts. The reactivity profile of Ig produced by the Bc clones against a large panel of self-antigens, intestinal bacteria, and RV was characterized. Approximately 30% of intestinal IgA and IgG plasmablast antibodies were polyreactive, and the majority of these recognized RV 2/6 VLPs. Only 1 of 137 IgA and 2 of 85 IgG plasmablast clones were exclusively specific for the RV VLPs (24). Thus, the majority of intestinal plasmablasts that recognize RV (most probably VP6) are polyreactive. This observation underscores the necessity to characterize the reactivity of RV-Ig obtained from blood-circulating Bc in the studies previously described. Hence, future investigations to directly compare the blood and intestinal RV-Bc repertoires seem warranted.

(iii) Compartmentalization of RV-Bc

Although the largest amount of RV replication in both animals and humans occurs in the intestinal tract, infection is generally accompanied by antigenemia and viremia. Low levels of systemic RV replication commonly occur in animals, and many children have elevated liver enzyme levels, suggesting that mild hepatitis is a common feature of RV infection (2). With this pattern of infection, it is not surprising that the distribution of RV-Bc in animals is biased to intestinal localization but also has an important systemic component (25). For this reason, the RV model has been useful to test the hypothesis that the immune system functions in compartments (1). According to this hypothesis, an immune response will be tailored to best function at the anatomical niche where it develops, and lymphocytes specific for a specific pathogen will concentrate in the compartment of entry of that pathogen. For RV, this is clearly the case. During an acute infection, most viral reactive Bc are concentrated in the intestine (25). However, concomitant with viremia, RV-Bc also appear in the spleen and bone marrow (25). Nine months after primary RV infection in a mouse, effector ASC predominantly secrete RV-IgA (the isotype suited to survive in the harsh environment of the intestinal lumen), rather than RV-IgG, and are concentrated in the small intestinal lamina propria and, to a lesser extent, in Peyer's patches (Fig. 2, top panel). In contrast, equal numbers of IgG and IgA RV-ASC are present in the spleen and bone marrow (Fig. 2, top panel). When comparing RV-mBc (characterized by flow cytometry) at these late time points after infection, it is estimated that a mouse will have approximately the same number of RV-mBc in the spleen and in the Peyer's patches (for technical reasons, RV-mBc were not evaluated in the intestinal lamina propria) (Fig. 2, middle panel). However, the frequency of RV-mBc as a fraction of total cells in each organ is higher in the Peyer's patches (Fig. 2, bottom panel), indicating a selective accumulation in these organs. An important prediction of the compartmentalization hypothesis is that RV-Bc that have been primed in a given Peyer's patch will have the capacity to migrate to the blood and, from there, selectively to other Peyer's patches, lamina propria, and other parts of the intestinal compartment to provide a thorough protection against the pathogen. This prediction has been directly demonstrated for RV (26), and the compartmentalized migration of the RV-Bc has been shown to depend on the expression of the integrin $\alpha 4\beta 7$ (the intestinal homing receptor) and the chemokine receptor 9 (CCR9) (1). Of note, relatively high levels of $\alpha 4\beta 7$ are expressed by intestinally committed mBc/ASC compared to

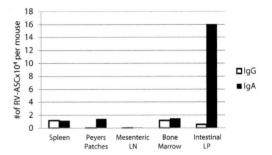

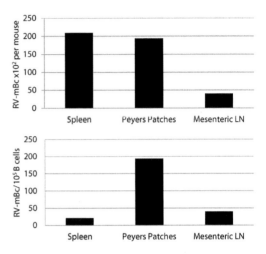

FIGURE 2 Distribution of RV-Bc 9 months after primary oral infection of mice in selected organs (data from experiments reported in reference 25). The top panel shows numbers of IgG and IgA RV ASC per mouse, in different organs, evaluated by enzyme-linked immunospot assay. The middle panel shows numbers of RV-mBc (small IgD⁻ Bc) that bind RV VLPs per mouse, in different organs, evaluated by flow cytometry. The bottom panel shows the same data as the second panel but expressed as RV-mBc per 10⁵ cells of the respective organ. LN, lymph node; LP, lamina propria. doi:10.1128/microbiolspec.AID-0011-2013.f2

naive Bc that also express this receptor (1). Since the CCR9 ligand, the chemokine TECK, is selectively expressed in the small intestine, RV-Bc that express CCR9 will home specifically to this portion of the intestine, where RV predominantly replicates. In humans, a direct relationship has been shown between circulating RV-ASCs and the presence of RV-specific ASCs in the human small intestinal lamina propria (27). Moreover, in children with an acute RV infection, the great majority of blood-circulating RV-ASC express both intestinal homing receptors (Fig. 3, left panel) (14). In the convalescent phase of viral infection, approximately one-third of RV-mBc express both receptors and are presumably targeted to the small intestine. Another third only express α4β7 (presumably targeted to other parts of the intestine and other mucosal surfaces), and the final third express neither receptor (presumably targeted to the spleen and other systemic organs) (Fig. 3, right panel) (13, 14). This result (Fig. 3) is consistent with a compartmentalized mBc response to RV in humans, as observed in animals (Fig. 2).

(iv) Mechanisms of Protection and Specificity of RV-Ig

Although in mice RV-Bc can play a contributory role in viral clearance (28), they are primarily necessary for preventing reinfection (29). The localization of RV-Bc to the intestine seems to be critical for these cells to be able to mediate their antiviral effect, since in immunodeficient mice chronically infected with RV, the transfer of α4β7⁺ mBc is associated with an antiviral response in the intestine and viral clearance, while the transfer of α4β7⁻ mBc is associated with a serum response and viral

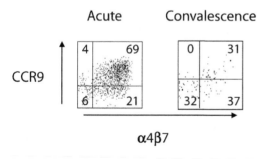

Acute   Convalescence

CCR9

| 4 | 69 | 0 | 31 |
| 6 | 21 | 32 | 37 |

α4β7

FIGURE 3 **Expression of the integrin α4β7 (the intestinal homing receptor) and CCR9 (chemokine receptor 9 whose ligand, TECK or CCL25, is selectively expressed in the small intestine) on RV-Bc (Bc that bind fluorescent RV VLPs) in children with acute (left dot plot)- or convalescent (right dot plot)-phase RV infection. The figure is from reference 14, with modifications. doi:10.1128/microbiolspec.AID-0011-2013.f3**

persistence (30). In this model, both wild-type and IgA-deficient Bc expressing the intestinal homing receptor mediated viral immunity, although the latter did so with somewhat lesser efficiency (31). This suggests that intestinal localization and, to a lesser extent, Ig isotype are critical factors in the protection mechanism. Another factor that seems critical in determining the capacity of a Bc to protect against RV is the age at which the mice are immunized. The age of immunization is, itself, related to the capacity of the mouse to develop CD4⁺ T cells. Mouse pups immunized orally with a heterologous, poorly replication-competent simian RV were less protected than adult mice and produced less RV intestinal IgA and neutralizing antibodies. This finding was associated with the immature T-cell response in the pups (32). In fact, more than 90% of the intestinal IgA in adult mice is CD4⁺ T-cell dependent (29). Although the T-cell-independent response may aid in viral clearance (28), the mechanism of how the virus stimulates it is not completely clear. In T-cell-deficient mice, RV can induce a strong Bc polyclonal activation (33), and this phenomenon has been linked, in one study, to the capacity of VP7 to stimulate Bc via Toll 4 receptor (34). In vitro, RV has been shown to induce activation and differentiation of human Bc, present in peripheral blood mononuclear cells, into ASC (35). However, this effect was not observed with purified Bc, suggesting the participation of other cells in activating the Bc; most likely dendritic cells that produce alpha interferon. In children, intestinal IgA responses are frequently short lived (16), while systemic IgG responses tend to persist (19). It has also been shown that children, like mice, have an age-related delay in the development of neutralizing Ig (54). A primary infection in young children thus develops in the context of an immature immune system, with a poor capacity to stimulate memory CD4⁺ T cells and with the development of a T-cell-independent/innate Bc response that may, in some cases, not persist.

The great majority of RV-Igs both in animals (36) and humans (1) are directed against VP6. The role played by most of these antibodies in RV immunity is incompletely understood, but it has been postulated that some of these antibodies mediate intracellular neutralization (37). It is hypothesized that during the transcytosis of polymeric IgA from the basolateral membrane of enterocytes to the gut lumen, these Ig bind virus VP6 and "expulse" it to the gut lumen. Loading of the sIgA may occur in the crypt enterocytes that express the polymeric Ig receptor. When these enterocytes reach the tip of the villi (site of RV infection), they still may have some IgA that can mediate the proposed viral expulsion. This model has been supported by in vitro experiments in which neutralization of RV can be achieved if the anti-VP6 dimeric IgA antibodies are delivered intracellularly to infected cells (38). Furthermore, in mice, protection by these antibodies is dependent on transcytosis of mucosal Igs by the polymeric Ig receptor (39) and not mediated via immune exclusion (see below) (40). Of note, several recent reports have identified llama VP6-directed monoclonal antibodies with substantial traditional neutralization activity (41, 42). The mechanistic and structural basis of these findings has not yet been determined, and numerous attempts to find comparable VP6 antibodies in mice and humans have thus far been unsuccessful.

The classical mechanism of Ig-mediated protection against RV involves viral exclusion (block of enterocyte infection) by neutralizing antibodies directed against the virus outer proteins VP4 and VP7 (1). The mechanism of neutralization for both types of antibodies has been described in detail. Based on structural studies, two main neutralizing epitopes have been described for VP7. The VP7-1 epitope lies at the three corners of VP7 trimers and involves at least two VP7 molecules. Antibodies against this epitope neutralize the virus by stabilizing the capsid and preventing viral uncoating. The VP7-2 epitope is in the center of the protein, and the mechanism of neutralization is unknown (43, 44). VP4, the virus spike protein, is cleaved in two proteins, VP5*,

which constitutes the stalk of the spike, and VP8*, localized on the tip of the stalk, which mediates initial cellular attachment. At least four structurally defined epitopes have been identified in VP8*, and antibodies against them mediate neutralization by blocking virus attachment to cells (43). Five structurally defined epitopes have been identified for VP5* (43). The VP5-1 epitope is located in the apical hydrophobic loops of the protein and seems to block the association of VP5* with membranes, probably blocking membrane penetration (44). The mechanisms of neutralization of antibodies directed to the other epitopes are not completely clear at present.

THERAPEUTIC AND PROPHYLACTIC APPLICATIONS OF RV ANTIBODIES

RV-Ig can have therapeutic/prophylactic applications and has been used as a correlate of protection for RV vaccines. The latter have been recently reviewed (3) and will only be briefly mentioned here.

Passive administration of RV-Ig can shorten the duration of RV infection in animals (1). Oral administration of commercial human Ig preparations, with high titers of neutralizing RV-Ig, have been shown to be of clinical benefit in children with RV GE (45). This type of treatment may be helpful for children with primary and acquired immunodeficiency and prolonged RV infection (1, 46). Careful kinetic studies of children suffering primary immunodeficiency, who presented with chronic diarrhea and RV excretion, confirmed that RV-Ig can survive passage in the gastrointestinal tract and temporarily reduce viral excretion (46). However, preparations of human Ig are expensive, and multiple alternatives have been investigated. Treatment with Igs extracted from colostrum from immunized bovines was shown to reduce stool frequency and to accelerate viral clearance in children with RV GE (47). An even less expensive strategy has been to treat children with Ig extracted from eggs of chickens immunized with human RV (48). Further investigation of strategies to improve the efficacy of orally administered antibodies includes studies of single-chain antibody fragments expressed from llama antibody genes (42, 49). The advantages of this approach are that the antibodies are relatively small, soluble, acid- and heat-resistant, and easy to express in multiple vectors, including lactobacilli. Surprisingly, in two such studies, antibodies directed to RV VP6 possessed broad neutralizing activity in vitro and conferred protection against diarrhea in mice (41, 42). It is possible that the small size of the VHH antibodies may enable access to VP6 on the complete triple-layered viral particle that is covered by VP4 and VP7. Testing of these VHH constructs in a clinical setting and further evaluation of the preparations mentioned before (bovine colostrum and chicken IgY) are necessary to determine their practical utility. Furthermore, testing the value of human Ig in relevant clinical settings is necessary; for example, a recent Cochrane Database systematic review concluded that no randomized controlled trials assessing the effectiveness or safety of oral immunoglobulin preparations for the treatment of RV diarrhea in hospitalized low-birth-weight infants have been published (50).

Two safe and effective RV vaccines, the monovalent G1P[8] Rotarix vaccine (RV1) and the bovine reassortant pentavalent RotaTeq vaccine (RV5) are recommended by WHO for worldwide use (3). Nonetheless, they are clearly less efficacious in the poorer countries of Africa and Asia, where they would be most useful, than in the Americas and Europe. For this and other practical reasons, these vaccines need to be improved and/or better ones developed (3). Our poor understanding of the mechanisms of protection induced by RV vaccines, and in particular the lack of good correlates of protection, hamper this process, as does our lack of insight as to why the vaccines perform less effectively in the poorest countries. Total serum RV-IgA measured shortly after vaccination is the correlate of protection currently most widely used (1). It is

very unlikely that total RV IgA is actually the effector of protection but rather a surrogate marker of other more specific immune effectors. Given this indirect measure, it should not be unexpected that some vaccinees with serum RV-IgA responses develop mild RV GE, whereas in others, the protection provided by the vaccine can exceed the levels predicted by the serum RV-IgA response (2, 3). The first incongruity can be best explained because of the induction of serum RV-IgA without intestinal RV-IgA. This occurs in mice infected with some heterologous RV, for which the viral dose that induces antigenemia is lower than the dose that induces intestinal infection. When low doses of these RV are used for infection, serum RV-IgA can be detected in the absence of intestinal RV-IgA and these mice are susceptible to infection with a homologous RV (1). In children, this has been hypothesized to occur with the vaccines based on rhesus RV (1). A similar situation may exist with the RV5 bovine reassortant vaccine, for which the level of serum RV-IgA exceeds the level of protection in several clinical studies in developing countries (2). The second incongruity, the excess actual protection observed when compared to serum RV-IgA responses (or neutralization responses), occurs most frequently with homologous vaccines, like RV1. In this case, it is possible that the excess protection is explained by an antibody response in the intestine (where the vaccine virus has been shown to replicate) that is not "strong" enough to be reflected in the circulation.

Importantly, RV1 and RV5 have similar efficacy against severe RV GE in countries where a high diversity of strains cocirculate, supporting the conclusion that immunity to RV has a substantial heterotypic component (3). For this reason, the specificity of the Bc response is probably only a secondary aspect of an ideal correlate of protection and probably explains why serum RV-IgA is a better correlate than the homotypic neutralization response. Thus, efforts to identify stronger correlates of protection may have to concentrate on strategies to better evaluate the intestinal RV-Ig responses that have the capacity to persist over time. Although stool RV-IgA has been shown to be a good correlate of protection for natural RV infection (16), this parameter may not be useful for evaluating protection induced by RV vaccines because of the interference in the measurement of vaccine-induced RV-Ig by maternal antibodies from breast-feeding (10). This is particularly true in developing countries, where the frequency of breast-feeding is high and the basal levels of preimmune stool RV-IgA mask vaccine-induced coproconversions. As an alternative, measurement of blood-circulating intestinally induced RV-Bc has been proposed (3). In a gnotobiotic pig model, for example, both systemic and intestinal RV ASCs have been shown to be a good correlate of protective immunity to human RV challenge (51). In spite of this, it is not clear if measurement of RV ASC can predict long-term persistence of immunity, and alternative efforts have concentrated on the study of RV-mBc. As previously mentioned, during an acute RV infection in children, circulating IgD⁻ RV-mBc express intestinal-homing receptors ($\alpha4\beta7^+$, $CCR9^+$) and thus probably reflect mucosal immunity (14). In agreement with this finding, a correlation between protection from disease and plasma RV-IgA and $\alpha4\beta7^+$ $CCR9^+$ IgD⁻ circulating RV-mBc was found in a trial of the attenuated human RV1 vaccine precursor. However, the correlation coefficients with protection for both parameters were low, making them of little practical use (10).

FUTURE CHALLENGES

RV-Bc have been studied at many levels, opening several fruitful areas of basic research on the interaction between Bc and an enteric human viral pathogen. Critical questions that remain to be addressed include (i) the relationship between the preimmune repertoire and the mBc repertoire, especially in the intestine. The studies described above, which take advantage of the high numbers of RV-naive Bc, make RV one of the few human pathogens in which this question has started to be addressed and need to be pursued. (ii) Currently, immunologists are puzzled by the mechanism of selection, function, and biological relevance of the IgM mBc (12). Since RV-mBc are enriched in this subset, RV antigen may be used as a tool to unravel the mystery of IgM mBc. Further studies of this mBc subset and of the innate and T-cell-independent antibody response against RV will likely expand our understanding of RV immunity. (iii) The study of RV-Bc may help clarify the extent and mechanisms that determine compartmentalization of the immune system. As discussed, limited studies of intestinal RV-Bc suggest that they use a different Ig gene repertoire than RV-Bc in circulation, and a direct comparison of both compartments would help confirm that this is the case.

From a practical point of view, ongoing clinical studies are evaluating whether llama-derived single molecule antibodies against VP6 can provide broad protection against RV, as predicted from animal studies. If this is the case, future studies should be aimed at examining the possibility that humans are also able to generate such antibodies and that this phenomenon might help explain heterotypic immunity. An alternative option for passive protection could be to design antibodies against conserved heterotypic neutralizing epitopes on VP7 and/or VP4. In this respect, antibodies against the VP5-1 epitope seem appealing because of their conserved nature and essential functional role of the VP5 domain in viral penetration.

Concerning correlates of protection for RV vaccines, it is possible that formal statistical analysis of serum RV-IgA responses from children in the large clinical trials that have been performed to date will establish this parameter as a practical surrogate marker of protection. Even if so, as discussed above, the development of better correlates seems desirable, and in this respect, two areas of further study seem promising. (i) The characterization of serum RV-sIg induced by RV vaccines may be a useful way to obtain an indirect measure of the immune response generated in the intestine. Preliminary studies have shown that this is possible (J. Angel and M. Franco, unpublished data). However, an important number (approximately one-third) of placebo recipients appear to have plasma RV-sIg in the absence of detectable RV-IgA. This can be explained because, at this age, RV-sIg is mostly composed of IgM RV-sIg (Angel and Franco, unpublished). The best (but not exclusive) explanation for these RV-sIg (presumably IgM) responses in nonvaccinated children are low-level asymptomatic infections: at the age of RV vaccination (2 to 3 months), RV RNA may be detected by a sensitive PCR in the stools of up to one-third of healthy children (52). (ii) Further studies of circulating RV-mBc (particularly those primed in the intestine) and their relationship with levels of intestinal and serum Ig (10, 53) may also be helpful to identify improved correlates of protection. Our poor understanding of IgM RV-mBc, and the fact that they are probably present in children that have not been infected with RV (defined by the absence of serum RV-IgA), hinder these studies.

ACKNOWLEDGMENTS

This work was supported by funds from the Pontificia Universidad Javeriana, Colciencias grant 1203-521-28212, by NIH grants R01 AI012362-24 and P30DK56339 to H.B.G., and by a merit review Veterans Affairs grant to H.B.G.

Conflicts of interest: We disclose no conflicts.

CITATION

Franco MA, and Greenberg HB. 2013. Rotavirus. Microbiol Spectrum 1(2):AID-0011-2013

REFERENCES

1. **Franco MA, Angel J, Greenberg HB.** 2006. Immunity and correlates of protection for rotavirus vaccines. *Vaccine* **24:**2718–2731.

2. **Angel J, Franco MA, Greenberg HB.** 2007. Rotavirus vaccines: recent developments and future considerations. *Nat Rev Microbiol* **5:**529–539.

3. **Angel J, Franco MA, Greenberg HB.** 2012. Rotavirus immune responses and correlates of protection. *Curr Opin Virol* **2:**419–425.

4. **Ray PG, Kelkar SD, Walimbe AM, Biniwale V, Mehendale S.** 2007. Rotavirus immunoglobulin levels among Indian mothers of two socioeconomic groups and occurrence of rotavirus infections among their infants up to six months. *J Med Virol* **79:**341–349.

5. **Ogra SS, Weintraub D, Ogra PL.** 1977. Immunologic aspects of human colostrum and milk. III. Fate and absorption of cellular and soluble components in the gastrointestinal tract of the newborn. *J Immunol* **119:**245–248.

6. **Nguyen TV, Yuan L, Azevedo MS, Jeong KI, Gonzalez AM, Iosef C, Lovgren-Bengtsson K, Morein B, Lewis P, Saif LJ.** 2006. High titers of circulating maternal antibodies suppress effector and memory B-cell responses induced by an attenuated rotavirus priming and rotavirus-like particle-immunostimulating complex boosting vaccine regimen. *Clin Vaccine Immunol* **13:**475–485.

7. **Nguyen TV, Yuan L, Azevedo MS, Jeong KI, Gonzalez AM, Iosef C, Lovgren-Bengtsson K, Morein B, Lewis P, Saif LJ.** 2006. Low titer maternal antibodies can both enhance and suppress B cell responses to a combined live attenuated human rotavirus and VLP-ISCOM vaccine. *Vaccine* **24:**2302–2316.

8. **Parez N, Garbarg-Chenon A, Fourgeux C, Le Deist F, Servant-Delmas A, Charpilienne A, Cohen J, Schwartz-Cornil I.** 2004. The VP6 protein of rotavirus interacts with a large fraction of human naive B cells via surface immunoglobulins. *J Virol* **78:**12489–12496.

9. **Kallewaard NL, McKinney BA, Gu Y, Chen A, Prasad BV, Crowe JE, Jr.** 2008. Functional maturation of the human antibody response to rotavirus. *J Immunol* **180:**3980–3989.

10. **Rojas OL, Caicedo L, Guzman C, Rodriguez LS, Castaneda J, Uribe L, Andrade Y, Pinzon R, Narvaez CF, Lozano JM, De Vos B, Franco MA, Angel J.** 2007. Evaluation of circulating intestinally committed memory B cells in children vaccinated with attenuated human rotavirus vaccine. *Viral Immunol* **20:**300–311.

11. **Narvaez CF, Feng N, Vasquez C, Sen A, Angel J, Greenberg HB, Franco MA.** 2012. Human rotavirus-specific IgM memory B cells have differential cloning efficiencies and switch capacities and play a role in antiviral immunity in vivo. *J Virol* **86:**10829–10840.

12. **Reynaud CA, Descatoire M, Dogan I, Huetz F, Weller S, Weill JC.** 2012. IgM memory B cells: a mouse/human paradox. *Cell Mol Life Sci* **69:**1625–1634.

13. **Gonzalez AM, Jaimes MC, Cajiao I, Rojas OL, Cohen J, Pothier P, Kohli E, Butcher EC, Greenberg HB, Angel J, Franco MA.** 2003. Rotavirus-specific B cells induced by recent infection in adults and children predominantly express the intestinal homing receptor α4β7. *Virology* **305:**93–105.

14. **Jaimes MC, Rojas OL, Kunkel EJ, Lazarus NH, Soler D, Butcher EC, Bass D, Angel J, Franco MA, Greenberg HB.** 2004. Maturation and trafficking markers on rotavirus-specific B cells during acute infection and convalescence in children. *J Virol* **78:**10967–10976.

15. **Ray PG, Kelkar SD.** 2004. Measurement of antirotavirus IgM/IgA/IgG responses in the serum samples of Indian children following rotavirus diarrhoea and their mothers. *J Med Virol* **72:**416–423.

16. **Coulson BS, Grimwood K, Hudson IL, Barnes GL, Bishop RF.** 1992. Role of coproantibody in clinical protection of children during reinfection with rotavirus. *J Clin Microbiol* **30:**1678–1684.

17. **Hjelt K, Grauballe PC, Andersen L, Schiotz PO, Howitz P, Krasilnikoff PA.** 1986. Antibody response in serum and intestine in children up to six months after a naturally acquired rotavirus gastroenteritis. *J Pediatr Gastroenterol Nutr* **5:**74–80.

18. **Mantis NJ, Forbes SJ.** 2010. Secretory IgA: arresting microbial pathogens at epithelial borders. *Immunol Investig* **39:**383–406.

19. **Bernstein DI, McNeal MM, Schiff GM, Ward RL.** 1989. Induction and persistence of local rotavirus antibodies in relation to serum antibodies. *J Med Virol* **28:**90–95.

20. **Tian C, Luskin GK, Dischert KM, Higginbotham JN, Shepherd BE, Crowe JE, Jr.** 2008. Immunodominance of the VH1-46 antibody gene segment in the primary repertoire of human rotavirus-specific B cells is reduced in the memory compartment through somatic mutation of nondominant clones. *J Immunol* **180:**3279–3288.

21. **Weitkamp JH, Kallewaard N, Kusuhara K, Bures E, Williams JV, LaFleur B, Greenberg HB, Crowe JE, Jr.** 2003. Infant and adult human B cell responses to rotavirus share common immunodominant variable gene repertoires. *J Immunol* **171:**4680–4688.

22. **Weitkamp JH, Lafleur BJ, Greenberg HB, Crowe JE Jr.** 2005. Natural evolution of a human virus-specific antibody gene repertoire by somatic hypermutation requires both hotspot-directed and randomly-directed processes. *Hum Immunol* **66:**666–676.

23. **Di Niro R, Mesin L, Raki M, Zheng NY, Lund-Johansen F, Lundin KE, Charpilienne A, Poncet D, Wilson PC, Sollid LM.** 2010. Rapid generation of rotavirus-specific human monoclonal antibodies from small-intestinal mucosa. *J Immunol* **185:**5377–5383.

24. **Benckert J, Schmolka N, Kreschel C, Zoller MJ, Sturm A, Wiedenmann B, Wardemann H.** 2011. The majority of intestinal IgA$^+$ and IgG$^+$ plasmablasts in the human gut are antigen-specific. *J Clin Investig* **121:**1946–1955.

25. **Youngman KR, Franco MA, Kuklin NA, Rott LS, Butcher EC, Greenberg HB.** 2002. Correlation of tissue distribution, developmental phenotype, and intestinal homing receptor expression of antigen-specific B cells during the murine anti-rotavirus immune response. *J Immunol* **168:**2173–2181.

26. **Bowman EP, Kuklin NA, Youngman KR, Lazarus NH, Kunkel EJ, Pan J, Greenberg HB, Butcher EC.** 2002. The intestinal chemokine thymus-expressed chemokine (CCL25) attracts IgA antibody-secreting cells. *J Exp Med* **195:**269–275.

27. **Brown KA, Kriss JA, Moser CA, Wenner WJ, Offit PA.** 2000. Circulating rotavirus-specific antibody-secreting cells (ASCs) predict the presence of rotavirus-specific ASCs in the human small intestinal lamina propria. *J Infect Dis* **182:**1039–1043.

28. **VanCott JL, McNeal MM, Flint J, Bailey SA, Choi AH, Ward RL.** 2001. Role for T cell-independent B cell activity in the resolution of primary rotavirus infection in mice. *Eur J Immunol* **31:**3380–3387.

29. **Franco MA, Greenberg HB.** 1995. Role of B cells and cytotoxic T lymphocytes in clearance of and immunity to rotavirus infection in mice. *J Virol* **69:**7800–7806.

30. **Williams MB, Rose JR, Rott LS, Franco MA, Greenberg HB, Butcher EC.** 1998. The memory B cell subset responsible for the secretory IgA response and protective humoral immunity to rotavirus expresses the intestinal homing receptor, alpha4beta7. *J Immunol* **161:**4227–4235.

31. **Kuklin NA, Rott L, Feng N, Conner ME, Wagner N, Muller W, Greenberg HB.** 2001. Protective intestinal anti-rotavirus B cell immunity is dependent on alpha 4 beta 7 integrin expression but does not require IgA antibody production. *J Immunol* **166:**1894–1902.

32. **VanCott JL, Prada AE, McNeal MM, Stone SC, Basu M, Huffer B, Jr, Smiley KL, Shao M, Bean JA, Clements JD, Choi AH, Ward RL.** 2006. Mice develop effective but delayed protective immune responses when immunized as neonates either intranasally with nonliving VP6/LT(R192G) or orally with live rhesus rotavirus vaccine candidates. *J Virol* **80:**4949–4961.

33. **Blutt SE, Warfield KL, Lewis DE, Conner ME.** 2002. Early response to rotavirus infection involves massive B cell activation. *J Immunol* **168:**5716–5721.

34. **Blutt SE, Crawford SE, Warfield KL, Lewis DE, Estes MK, Conner ME.** 2004. The VP7 outer capsid protein of rotavirus induces polyclonal B-cell activation. *J Virol* **78:**6974–6981.

35. **Narvaez CF, Franco MA, Angel J, Morton JM, Greenberg HB.** 2010. Rotavirus differentially infects and polyclonally stimulates human B cells depending on their differentiation state and tissue of origin. *J Virol* **84:**4543–4555.

36. **Ishida SI, Feng N, Gilbert JM, Tang B, Greenberg HB.** 1997. Immune responses to individual rotavirus proteins following heterologous and homologous rotavirus infection in mice. *J Infect Dis* **175:**1317–1323.

37. **Burns JW, Siadat-Pajouh M, Krishnaney AA, Greenberg HB.** 1996. Protective effect of rotavirus VP6-specific IgA monoclonal antibodies that lack neutralizing activity. *Science* **272:**104–107.

38. **Feng N, Lawton JA, Gilbert J, Kuklin N, Vo P, Prasad BV, Greenberg HB.** 2002. Inhibition of rotavirus replication by a non-neutralizing, rotavirus VP6-specific IgA mAb. *J Clin Investig* **109:**1203–1213.

39. **Schwartz-Cornil I, Benureau Y, Greenberg H, Hendrickson BA, Cohen J.** 2002. Heterologous protection induced by the inner capsid proteins of rotavirus requires transcytosis of mucosal immunoglobulins. *J Virol* **76:**8110–8117.

40. **Corthesy B, Benureau Y, Perrier C, Fourgeux C, Parez N, Greenberg H, Schwartz-Cornil I.** 2006. Rotavirus anti-VP6 secretory immunoglobulin A contributes to protection via intracellular neutralization but not via immune exclusion. *J Virol* **80:**10692–10699.

41. **Aladin F, Einerhand AW, Bouma J, Bezemer S, Hermans P, Wolvers D, Bellamy K, Frenken LG, Gray J, Iturriza-Gomara M.** 2012. In vitro neutralisation of rotavirus infection by two broadly specific recombinant monovalent llama-derived antibody fragments. *PLoS One* **7:**e32949.

42. **Garaicoechea L, Olichon A, Marcoppido G, Wigdorovitz A, Mozgovoj M, Saif L, Surrey T, Parreno V.** 2008. Llama-derived single-chain antibody fragments directed to rotavirus VP6 protein possess broad neutralizing activity in vitro and confer protection against diarrhea in mice. *J Virol* **82:**9753–9764.

43. **Aoki ST, Settembre EC, Trask SD, Greenberg HB, Harrison SC, Dormitzer PR.** 2009. Structure of rotavirus outer-layer protein VP7 bound with a neutralizing Fab. *Science* **324:**1444–1447.

44. **Trask SD, McDonald SM, Patton JT.** 2012. Structural insights into the coupling of virion assembly and rotavirus replication. *Nat Rev Microbiol* **10:**165–177.

45. **Guarino A, Canani RB, Russo S, Albano F, Canani MB, Ruggeri FM, Donelli G, Rubino A.** 1994. Oral immunoglobulins for treatment of acute rotaviral gastroenteritis. *Pediatrics* **93:**12–16.

46. **Losonsky GA, Johnson JP, Winkelstein JA, Yolken RH.** 1985. Oral administration of human serum immunoglobulin in immunodeficient patients with viral gastroenteritis. A pharmacokinetic and functional analysis. *J Clin Investig* **76:**2362–2367.

47. **Sarker SA, Casswall TH, Mahalanabis D, Alam NH, Albert MJ, Brussow H, Fuchs GJ, Hammerstrom L.** 1998. Successful treatment of rotavirus diarrhea in children with immunoglobulin from immunized bovine colostrum. *Pediatr Infect Dis J* **17:**1149–1154.

48. **Sarker SA, Casswall TH, Juneja LR, Hoq E, Hossain I, Fuchs GJ, Hammarstrom L.** 2001. Randomized, placebo-controlled, clinical trial of hyperimmunized chicken egg yolk immunoglobulin in children with rotavirus diarrhea. *J Pediatr Gastroenterol Nutr* **32:**19–25.

49. **Pant N, Hultberg A, Zhao Y, Svensson L, Pan-Hammarstrom Q, Johansen K, Pouwels PH, Ruggeri FM, Hermans P, Frenken L, Boren T, Marcotte H, Hammarstrom L.** 2006. Lactobacilli expressing variable domain of llama heavy-chain antibody fragments (lactobodies) confer protection against rotavirus-induced diarrhea. *J Infect Dis* **194:**1580–1588.

50. **Pammi M, Haque KN.** 2011. Oral immunoglobulin for the treatment of rotavirus diarrhea in low birth weight infants. *Cochrane Database Syst Rev* **2011:**CD003742.

51. **Yuan L, Ward LA, Rosen BI, To TL, Saif LJ.** 1996. Systematic and intestinal antibody-secreting cell responses and correlates of protective immunity to human rotavirus in a gnotobiotic pig model of disease. *J Virol* **70:**3075–3083.

52. **Amar CF, East CL, Gray J, Iturriza-Gomara M, Maclure EA, McLauchlin J.** 2007. Detection by PCR of eight groups of enteric pathogens in 4,627 faecal samples: re-examination of the English case-control Infectious Intestinal Disease Study (1993–1996). *Eur J Clin Microbiol Infect Dis* **26:**311–323.

53. **Rojas OL, Narvaez CF, Greenberg HB, Angel J, Franco MA.** 2008. Characterization of rotavirus specific B cells and their relation with serological memory. *Virology* **380:**234–242.

54. **Ward RL, Kirkwood CD, Sander DS, Smith VE, Shao M, Bean JA, Sack DA, Bernstein DI.** 2006. Reductions in cross-neutralizing antibody responses in infants after attenuation of the human rotavirus vaccine candidate 89-12. *J Infect Dis* **194:**1729–1736.

Bacterial Toxins—Staphylococcal Enterotoxin B

18

BETTINA C. FRIES[1] and AVANISH K. VARSHNEY[1]

INTRODUCTION

Staphylococcal Enterotoxins

Staphylococcus aureus is a nonmotile, ubiquitous, gram-positive coccus which is a major human pathogen responsible for a wide range of infections, including skin and soft tissue infections, bacteremia, pneumonia, and several toxin-mediated diseases. Among many extracellular proteins, *S. aureus* strains also secrete a variety of potent toxins which include alpha hemolysin, enterotoxins, leukocidins, and exfoliative toxins, all of which are directly associated with particular disease manifestations. To date, more than 33 enterotoxin sequences have been described in various *S. aureus* genomes. Enterotoxins are heat stable and exert their effect on the epithelium of the intestinal tract when ingested, and thus, they are a common cause of food poisoning. Several enterotoxins are potent superantigens (SAgs) that, in a non-antigen (Ag)-dependent way, predominantly activate CD4$^+$ T cells (1) but also activate other immune cells. The SAgs of *S. aureus* include toxic shock syndrome toxin 1 (TSST-1), enterotoxin serotypes A to E and I (*sea, seb, sec, sed, see,* and *sei*), and enterotoxin-like serotypes G (*selG*), H (*selH*), and J to U (*selJ* to *selU*). Of these SAgs, *sea* to *see* have the ability to induce emesis in monkeys and

[1]Department of Medicine/Infectious Diseases and Department of Microbiology and Immunology, Albert Einstein College of Medicine, Bronx, NY 10461.

Antibodies for Infectious Diseases
Edited by James E. Crowe, Jr., Diana Boraschi, and Rino Rappuoli
© 2015 American Society for Microbiology, Washington, DC
doi:10.1128/microbiolspec.AID-0002-2012

arethus referred to as classic enterotoxins. The remaining SAgs either have not been tested for emetic activity or lack emetic activity and are therefore referred to as enterotoxin-like proteins (*selG*, *selH*, and *selJ* to *selU*). For the most part, staphylococcal SAgs are encoded by mobile genetic elements, which include extrachromosomal plasmids as well as chromosomal prophages, transposons, and pathogenicity islands. It is noteworthy that a chromosomally carried enterotoxin-like gene (*selX*) was recently identified (2). The *seb* gene is carried on the pathogenicity island SaPI3. The genes of SAgs *selG*, *selI*, *selM*, *selO*, and *selU* are located in the enterotoxin gene cluster (egc) and are among the most prevalent SAgs in clinical *S. aureus* isolates. They are expressed by *S. aureus* during logarithmic growth and shut off expression once a certain bacterial density is reached. Consequently, they do not induce a humoral response in the human host. In contrast, non-egc-associated SAgs (e.g., *sea*, *seb*, *sec*, and *tsst-1*) are expressed in late-logarithmic and stationary growth, induce a specific antibody (Ab) response in the human host, and are a prominent cause of cause toxic shock (3).

SEB

Staphylococcal enterotoxin B (SEB) is the prototype of a non-egc-associated potent SAg. It is categorized as a category B select agent because it is the most potent staphylococcal enterotoxin, and much lower quantities are sufficient to produce a toxic effect than with synthetic chemicals. Furthermore, SEB is extremely stable and easily produced in large quantities. At low concentrations, SEB can cause multi-organ system failure and death. During the 1960s, when the United States had an offensive biological warfare program, SEB was studied as a biological weapon and stockpiled with various other bioweapons prior to its destruction in 1972 (4). Based on those investigations, the effective dose of SEB that would incapacitate 50% of the exposed population was estimated to be 0.0004 μg/kg of body weight, whereas the 50% lethal dose was

estimated to be 0.02 μg/kg of body weight for humans exposed by the inhalation route. A convention on the "Prohibition of the Development, Production and Stockpiling of Bacteriological (Biological) and Toxin Weapons and on Their Destruction" was signed by the United Kingdom, U.S., and U.S.S.R. governments in 1972. The U.S. government opted to reestablish research programs for vaccine and therapeutic development against biological weapons after suspicion arose that the U.S.S.R. was continuing the stockpiling and testing of biological weapons. Major NIH grant funding reinvigorated research on biological warfare agents after 11 September 2001 and especially after the anthrax attacks occurred in the U.S. mail system. Despite extensive efforts, however, there is no therapy or vaccine approved for human use against SEB to date.

THE INFECTION

Description of Agent

SEB is a well-characterized 28-kDa protein that consists of 239 amino acids and is most closely related to SEC1, with whom it shares structural as well as 67% amino acid homology (5, 6). SEB is water soluble, heat labile, and resistant to proteolytic enzymes, including pepsin, trypsin, and papain. The crystal structure of SEB was first determined in 1992 to a resolution of 2.5 Å (6) and later (7) to a resolution of 1.5 Å. The refined model contained 1,948 protein atoms and 177 water molecules and had an excellent geometry with root-mean-square (rms) deviation of 0.007 Å and 1.73° in bond lengths and bond angles, respectively. As a SAg, SEB crosslinks Ag-presenting cells (APCs) and T cells by forming a ternary complex between the immune receptors major histocompatibility complex (MHC) class II and specific Vβ chains of the T-cell receptors (TcR) (6, 8, 9, 10). SEB protein is ellipsoidal, tightly and compactly folded into two unequal-sized domains of mixed α/β structure. Although the overall fold of SEB is similar to those of other microbial

SAgs, it lacks the zinc-binding site and only possesses one MHC class II binding site. The SEB residues implicated in TcR binding are 18, 19, 20, 22, 23, 26, 60, 90, 91, 177, 178, and 210. The suggested residues involved in binding of SEB to the MHC binding site are 43 to 47, 65, 67, 89, 92, 94, 96, 98, 115, 209, 211, and 215. Furthermore, the C-terminal disulfide loop (residues 113 to 126) in SEB has high flexibility, and it has been suggested to be responsible for emetic properties (6). Additional data from native gel electrophoresis and plasmon resonance affinity measurements indicate that the SEB-TcR complex can even form in the absence of MHC class II and that SEB-TcR interaction increases the binding to the MHC class II molecule DR1. It has been proposed that the finding that SEB can form complexes with TcR in both the absence and presence of MHC class

II provides a mechanism for the ability of SEB to induce anergy in some cases and activation in others (11).

SEB is excreted by *S. aureus* strains from diverse clonal complexes. Most, if not all, staphylococcal strains designated as part of the CDC USA400 clonal group (by pulsed-field gel electrophoresis) produce large amounts of SEB or SEC. One study with isolates derived from New York identified SEB in four clonal complexes, with CC8 being the most common, followed by CC59, CC20, and one unassigned strain (12). Sequence analysis of 20 different *S. aureus* strains identified amino acid substitutions when compared to the SEB of strains COL and MNHO. These amino acid mutations involve positions 7 (lysine-asparagine), 14 (serine-alanine), 35 (alanine-serine), 125 (glutamine-histidine), 192 (asparagine-serine), and

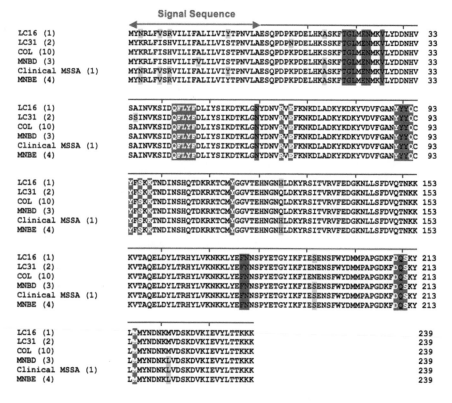

FIGURE 1 Alignment of amino acid sequences of SEB derived from *S. aureus* clinical isolates. Amino acid mutations are highlighted in green. MHC- and TcR-interacting residues are shown in blue and magenta, respectively. doi:10.1128/microbiolspec.AID-0002-2012.f1

222 (methionine-leucine) (13) (Fig. 1). It is noteworthy that these amino acid sequences lie outside the residues that are responsible for binding to MHC class II molecule and the TcR (Fig. 2). Investigations with purified, variant SEBs indicated that they varied in inducing proliferation of rabbit splenocytes in vitro as well as in lethality in a rabbit model of toxic shock syndrome (TSS) (13). Enzyme-linked immunosorbent assay (ELISA)-based quantification of SEB in supernatants of cultures in log phase demonstrates great variability among clinical *S. aureus* isolates, including sequential isolates derived from the same patient (12).

Interaction of Immune Cells with SEB

The primary targets of SEB are the TcR on T cells and the MHC class II molecules on APCs, resulting in a ternary complex between MHC class II molecules and specific Vβ chains of the TcR (6, 8, 9, 10) formed by this cross-linking. SEB binds to the MHC molecule outside the peptide-binding groove without prior processing, stimulating one of the seven Vh subclasses of the TcR (3, 12, 13.2, 14, 15, 17, or 20). Stimulated T cells then release large amounts of cytokines, namely interleukin-2 (IL-2), tumor necrosis factor alpha (TNF-α), and gamma interferon (IFN-γ), and undergo hyperproliferation and ultimately depletion. Cell adhesion molecules such as CD2 and ELAM on endothelial cells can also function as coreceptors for SEB-induced T-cell activation and cytokine production (14). The trimer complex activates intracellular signaling, which elicits phosphotidylinositol production and intracellular Ca^{2+} flux. This is followed by a rapid activation of membrane-associated protein tyrosine kinase and protein kinase C (15). Activation of the CD28-regulated signal transduction pathway is required for SAg stimulation in T cells and subsequent IL-2

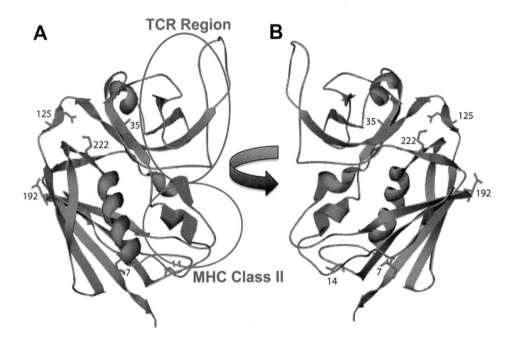

FIGURE 2 (A) Ribbon structure of SEB protein showing amino acid mutations in *S. aureus* isolates. Residues which interact with MHC and TcR are shown in blue and magenta, respectively. **(B)** View after rotating 180 degrees around vertical axis. doi:10.1128/microbiolspec.AID-0002-2012.f2

production. Activation of transcriptional factors NF-κB and AP-1 result in high-level expression of cytokines, including IL-1 and TNF-α from macrophages and TNF-β, IL-2, and IFN-γ from T cells. Excreted cytokines have potent effects and cause fever, hypotension, multiorgan dysfunction, and ultimately, lethal shock. Table 1 summarizes the biological and pathological effects of SEB.

In Vitro Models to Study SAg Activity of SEB

In vitro cellular responses of SEB have been extensively studied in human peripheral blood mononuclear cells (PBMCs) and murine splenocytes. The MHC of murine cells has a lower affinity to SEB than the human HLA complex. Therefore, humans are many times more sensitive to SEB. Human PBMCs are sensitive to picomolar concentrations of SEB, whereas mouse splenocytes require nanomolar concentrations for stimulation. SEB-induced T-cell proliferation can be measured with different methods and usually peaks at 96 h in the employed in vitro systems. Most cytokine stimulation assays focus on quantification of IFN-γ and IL-2, but other cytokines are also induced, including IL-1, IL-6, IL-12, TNF-α, and IL-8. For optimal induction of proliferation, both T cells and monocytes are required. In vitro studies have demonstrated that SEB can also interact directly with TcR in the absence of MHC class II molecules, which results in an anergic T-cell response (11).

TABLE 1 Major biological and pathological activities of SEB

Superantigenicity: proliferation of CD4 T cells following binding with the Vβ motif of TcR and MHC class II molecules on the surface of APCs

Induction and release of several cytokines

Lethality and shock in experimental animals, including mice, rabbits, piglets, and monkeys

Emetic activity

Direct or indirect involvement in pathogenesis of severe diseases, including TSS, nonmenstrual TSS, atopic dermatitis, asthma, and chronic rhinitis

ANIMAL MODELS TO STUDY THE PATHOGENESIS OF SEB IN VIVO

Murine Models

Clearance of SEB has been investigated in mice after intravenous (i.v.) injection. SEB becomes systemically distributed within 5 to 30 min in blood and in lymph nodes (16). Clearance occurs within 10 to 24 h via glomerular filtration in the kidney. Small amounts of SEB are detectable also in the spleen. Manifestation of functional outcomes such as anergy, clonal expansion, and clonal deletion begins after 24 h.

Murine Models with Potentiating Agents

Standard mice are not very sensitive to SEB due to low-affinity binding of SEB to murine MHC class II. Therefore, a potentiating agent is required to amplify the toxic effect of SEB. The list of potentiating agents includes lipopolysaccharide (LPS), D-galactosamine, and actinomycin D (10, 17). The hepatotoxin D-galactosamine induces TNF-α and produces fulminant liver failure and shock when given in combination with SEB, and higher levels of TNF-α are measured when compared to SEB alone. IL-2-deficient mice are more resistant to SEB-induced lethal shock (SEBILS), supporting the importance of IL-2 in the pathogenesis of SEBILS (18). The lethal shock in this model is associated with high concentrations of IL-1, IL-2, TNF-α, and INF-γ in the serum, which results in shock in mice. Studies that analyzed the cytokine level in the serum of mice treated with SEB or LPS alone or in combination (19) demonstrated higher TNF-α, IL-6, macrophage inflammatory protein 2, and monocyte chemoattractant protein 1 (MCP-1) levels in mice treated with both toxins than in those treated with either alone. Significantly higher levels of IFN-γ and IL-2 were observed at the later time point. However, it remains difficult to discern which cytokine induction is specifically caused by SEB in this model.

Murine Models Without Potentiating Agents

A dual-dose SEB model has been described for C3H/HeJ, a Toll-like receptor 4-defective mouse, and involves giving one dose of SEB (5 μg) administered intranasally followed by another dose of SEB (2 μg) intraperitoneally (i.p.) 2 h later, which results in high serum concentrations of IL-2, IL-6, and MCP-1 as well as elevated MCP-1 levels in the lung (20). The increased concentration of MCP-1, a potent activator and chemotactic factor for T cells and monocytes, may contribute to leukocyte recruitment into the lungs. Lethality and clinical signs of intoxication, such as ruffled fur and hypothermia, are similar to those observed in transgenic mice and nonhuman primates.

Another dual-dosing model for SEBILS is the HLA transgenic mouse model. These MHC class II knockout mice express the human MHC class II determinant DR3 in *trans* and are thus more sensitive to SEBILS. Two doses of SEB (50 μg) given 48 h apart i.p. induce toxic shock and 100% mortality (21). These mice also exhibit high levels of IFN-γ, IL-2, and IL-6 when SEB is administered by aerosol (22).

Rat Model

Rats have been used to study the effect of SEB in the central nervous system and to specifically clarify the role of the vagus nerve in sensation and transmission of abdominal SEB stimulation. In this model, i.p. administration of SEB (1 mg/kg of body weight) induced a robust Fos expression and induced activation of neurons in widespread brain areas, transmitting the signal of abdominal immune stimulation to the brain (23).

Rabbit Model

Rabbits are more sensitive to many staphylococcal toxins and develop pyrogenic symptoms similar to those of humans when SAgs are given by continuous perfusion (24). They also show a toxicity to SEB similar to those observed in staphylococcal food-borne illness, namely emesis when ingested orally, although this is not observed with the streptococcal SAgs or TSST-1. The role of SAgs (TSST-1, SEB, and SEC) in the setting of staphylococcal sepsis has been successfully investigated in a rabbit model of lethal pulmonary infection (25).

Piglet Model

A piglet model has also been used in assessing and understanding pathology and toxicity following native SEB challenge (26). For these models, weaning 7- to 14-day-old Yorkshire piglets are injected with SEB i.v. The clinical signs are biphasic, with pyrexia, vomiting, and diarrhea within 4 h, followed by terminal hypotension and shock by 96 h. Mild lymphoid lesions are identified as early as 24 h, with severe lymphadenopathy, splenomegaly, and prominent Peyer's patches by 72 h. Widespread edema—most prominent in the mesentery, between loops of spiral colon, and in retroperitoneal connective tissue—is found at 72 h. Additional histologic changes included perivascular aggregates of large lymphocytes variably present in the lung and brain, circulating lymphoblasts, and lymphocytic portal hepatitis. The piglet model has also been successfully used in oral vaccine studies. Like human cells, pig leukocytes readily respond to native SEB. Therefore, the piglet model is superior to mouse models which require potentiation of SEB toxicity (27) and the DR3 transgenic mouse model in mirroring the biphasic clinical response and overall pathology observed in humans. It is considerably cheaper than the rhesus macaque model.

Nonhuman Primate Model

In the late 1960s, rhesus monkeys (*Macaca mulatta*) were used to study SEB pathogenesis because they exhibit disease progression similar to that observed in humans (28). They manifest multiorgan failure and shock when injected i.v. Specifically, they exhibit acute renal failure, terminal depression of electro-encephalographic patterns, fever, and emesis. A SEB-induced immediate-type skin reaction was also investigated in unsensitized monkeys. Substance P plays a predominant role in mediating intradermal SEB challenge and exerts its effect on cutaneous mast cells via stimulation of primary sensory neurons that contain substance P (29). The prohibitively high expenses and the limited number of monkeys that can be used per group limit the use of this model.

In summary, several animal models are available to test neutralization of SEB in vivo. It should be pointed out that SEB quantities differ between the models, as do the inherent sensitivities of the animals. This has to be taken into consideration when the efficacies of Abs are compared.

CLINICAL MANIFESTATION AND EPIDEMIOLOGY

SEB can cause several clinical symptoms in exposed humans. Manifestations of intoxication depend on the dose as well as the route of exposure.

Food Poisoning

SEB is one of the most common toxins implicated in toxin-mediated food-borne disease. Typically, heavily colonized food handlers contaminate food products with *S. aureus* via manual contact, coughing, or sneezing. *S. aureus* grows rapidly and excretes enterotoxins, especially in food products such as cream, mayonnaise, unrefrigerated meats, dairy, and bakery products. Heating the contaminated food only kills the bacteria but does not destroy the heat-stable, preformed SEB toxin. After ingestion of the toxin, the incubation period before patients become symptomatic is only approximately 4 to 6 h. This is also supported by data on occupational exposures in three laboratory workers at the U.S. Army Medical Research Institute who developed conjunctivitis with localized cutaneous swelling within 1 to 6 h, followed by gastrointestinal symptoms in two of the three workers after accidental cutaneous or ocular exposure to SEB (30).

Toxic Shock Syndrome (TSS)

TSS is characterized by the occurrence of fever, hypotension, multiple organ system dysfunction, rash, and desquamation, and it is classified as nonmenstrual or menstrual. The latter was first characterized in 1978 (31) in women that used tampons and is associated with TSST-1. The incidence has decreased significantly in past years (32), and nonmenstrual cases account for 55% of all cases (33). Those latter syndromes are commonly associated with SEB. TSS has been reported to occur in association with use of barrier contraceptives and after vaginal and cesarean delivery. It has also been reported in the setting of soft tissue infection, endovascular infection, and visceral abscesses as well as upper and lower respiratory tract infection (34). Up to one-third of patients who have TSS develop recurrent disease. This requires persistent colonization with a toxigenic strain of *S. aureus* and only develops in patients who do not mount a humoral immune response to the implicated staphylococcal toxin (35). It is noteworthy that several case reports of staphylococcal TSS without rash have been described, which can make the diagnosis very difficult. It has been suggested that rash and desquamation result from delayed hypersensitivity, which is amplified by SAgs (36).

Atopic Dermatitis (AD)

AD is a common skin disorder that affects children during early childhood as well as adults. Patients with AD are frequently colonized with *S. aureus* strains. Comparison of colonizing *S. aureus* strains derived from patients with uncomplicated AD versus those derived from patients with chronic steroid-resistant AD indicate that the latter more commonly excrete SAg SEB. SAgs induce immunoglobulin E (IgE) Abs that are thought to exacerbate the skin and allergic inflammation in AD. Approximately 50 to 80% of patients with chronic AD have IgE Abs specific to SEA and SEB (37, 38). This hypothesis is further supported by data derived from a murine model of atopic dermatitis, where topical SAg exposure induces epidermal accumulation of $CD8^+$ T cells, a mixed Th1/Th2 type dermatitis, and production of IgE Abs (39). A recent study observed predominance of SEB and SED in *S. aureus* isolates from AD patients with low IgE titers characterized by the prevalence of $CD8^+$ lymphocytes and a dominant Th1 profile induced by SAgs and elevated IFN-γ expression (40).

Respiratory Diseases, Including Asthma and Nasal Polyps

Several studies suggest an association of colonization with SEB-excreting *S. aureus* and chronic rhinitis. A small clinical study comprised of 32 patients indicated a possible association between chronic rhinosinusitis and ulcerative colitis (UC). After functional endoscopic sinus surgery, the clinical symptom scores of chronic rhinosinusitis and UC severe scores were significantly reduced in these patients. Interestingly, the number of cultured *S. aureus* colonies from the surgically removed sinus mucosa significantly correlated with the decrease in UC severe scores, and high levels of SEB were detected in the sinus wash fluids of these patients.

In summary, SEB-mediated disease is diverse and extends beyond TSS. Recent studies strongly suggest that SEB excretion by colonizing strains may worsen inflammatory responses of allergic diseases.

DIAGNOSIS

SEB-mediated intoxication is usually diagnosed based on clinical suspicion and symptoms. The clinical signs of SEB intoxication are fever, vomiting, myalgia, diarrhea, headache, and in severe cases, lethal shock. Laboratory findings are not specific for the diagnosis of SEB intoxication, as nonspecific neutrophilic leukocytosis and an elevated erythrocyte sedimentation rate are present in many illnesses. A rising Ab titer response to SEB can be helpful to validate the diagnosis retrospectively. Several methods to directly detect and quantify SEB have been developed in recent years. They include immunological assays such as immunodiffusion assays, radioimmunoassay, and ELISA, which have been applied for detection of SEB. Radioimmunoassay can detect up to 1 ng of SEB/ml in food extract; and ELISAs can detect less than 0.1 ng of SEB/ml in urine, blood, or food extract. Development of better instruments for mass spectrometry (MS) techniques has enhanced possibilities of more-precise structure identification and confirmation of proteins. Using this technique in combination with the Abs surface plasmon resonance chip has further enhanced the sensitivity and feasibility of these techniques. Currently, matrix-assisted laser desorption ionization–time of flight and electrospray ionization (ESI)-time of flight MS-based analysis can be completed within 1 h and have a very low detection limit of 3 pmol/ml of water (41). The combination of liquid chromatography-ESI MS/MS allows accurate determination by molecular mass and also by amino acid sequencing after enzymatic digestion. A sensitive laser nephelometric assay was developed to detect SEB in plasma of healthy volunteers as well as patients (42). Despite novel diagnostic approaches, evidence that SEB has actually been detected in human body fluids of either infected or intoxicated patients is scarce (43).

TREATMENT

There is no treatment available for SEB-mediated shock other than symptomatic support. The disease in the setting of food intoxication is usually self-limiting, and patients recover with active hydration and supportive measures. Steroids and antibiotics have not been shown to be effective for SEB intoxication (44). Many approaches to prophylaxis and therapy of SEB-mediated diseases have been explored and are outlined below. They include active immunization with inactivated recombinant SEB vaccines, synthetic peptides, and proteasome-SEB toxoid. Furthermore, Ab-based passive immunoprophylaxis/immunotherapy, as well as synthetic peptide antagonists and receptor mimics, such as chimeric mimics of MHC class II-TcR and of the TcR-Vβ, have been investigated. To date, the FDA has licensed no vaccine and antitoxin. However, numerous studies on various animal models for SEBILS have shown a favorable outcome with these diverse ranges of reagents that inhibit the proliferation of T cells and downregulate the expression of cytokine.

Peptide Antagonists

SEBILS can be successfully blocked with small overlapping antagonist peptides that inhibit the initial step of toxin-receptor interactions. Peptides directed to SEB amino acids 150 to 161 showed antagonist activity and protect mice from lethal shock against SEA, SEB, and TSST-1 when given i.v. 30 min after a lethal toxin dose (45). This conserved domain of SEB is not directly involved in MHC class II or TcR binding; however, it may be involved in interactions with coligands or cytotoxic T-lymphocyte antigen, which are necessary for superantigenic activity. A subsequent study also showed that peptides interfering with SEB domain residues 140 to 151 can block the proliferative effects against all staphylococcal and streptococcal SAgs and antipeptide Ab can protect passively against toxic shock in a rabbit model (46). However, a subsequent study indicated that these peptides were not effective in blocking T-cell activation, cytokine production, and SEB-induced toxic shock in HLA class II transgenic mice as well as human T lymphocytes in vitro (47). Recently, another study demonstrated inhibition using dodecapeptide P72, which does not bind to MHC class II (48).

Vβ Domains

Another method to neutralize SEB action is by employing soluble forms of genetically engineered Vβ domains. These are high-affinity toxin-binding agents. A soluble G5-8 mouse Vβ (Vβ8.2) mutant was generated and shown to be a promising therapeutic agent. Both administration of Vβ-TcR G5-8 as well as prior hyperimmunization to raise neutralizing Abs to SEB dramatically increase survival in a lethal pulmonary disease model in rabbits (49). Only equimolar amounts of these molecules are required to neutralize SEB, which indicates that they could have beneficial pharmacodynamic qualities.

Cytokine Inhibitors

Several drugs can interfere with cytokine induction and T-cell proliferation. They include the antibiotic doxycycline, which downregulates the SEB-induced proinflammatory cytokine and chemokine response as well as SEB-induced T-cell proliferation in human PBMCs (50). Furthermore, pentoxifylline, a methylxanthine derivative, and dexamethasone also inhibit SEB-induced activation of human PBMCs in vitro and also SEBILS in mice (51, 52). Recently, rapamycin, an immunosuppressant, has also been shown to inhibit cytokine release in vitro and toxin-mediated shock in mice (53). All of these therapeutic agents indirectly inhibit SEB-induced effects by downregulating the cytokine responses.

Immunotherapy

Von Behring and Kitasato first established immunotherapy by demonstrating that passive transfer of Abs from immunized animals could protect nonimmune animals against diphtheria. Before the discovery of sulfonamide in the 1930s, serum therapy was a common option to treat infectious diseases (54). Serum therapy remains the only prophylactic and therapeutic option against many toxin-mediated and viral diseases. Toxins are usually structurally distinct from the self-antigens expressed by the host cells and therefore safe targets for Ab therapy. One problem is that most investigators only screened monoclonal Abs (MAbs) alone and characterized them as protective, indifferent, and disease enhancing. This approach neglects the fact that naturally occurring Ab responses are complex polyclonal mixtures of Abs. However, in part, this simplified approach is chosen because the interaction between multiple Abs and toxins is complex and not easily predictable, let alone reproducible. Thus, FDA approval would be more difficult to obtain for mixtures of Abs. Currently, 39 MAbs are licensed by the FDA for human use for diverse indications, in addition to several polyclonal sera from diverse sources. Based on decades of successful use, Abs are considered valuable candidates for novel drug development because of their unique pharmacological qualities and safety profiles.

Epidemiological and Clinical Evidence

Since 11 September 2001, the development of Abs to neutralize toxins that could potentially be used in biological warfare has substantially increased, specifically for toxins like ricin, anthrax, Shiga toxin, pertussis, and SEB (55). For SEB, this research is highly justified because both clinical and experimental data strongly support the concept that immunoglobulins can be used to treat SEB-mediated disease. SEBILS in animals and humans involve induction of several proinflammatory cytokines, including, e.g., TNF-α. Passive immunization with neutralizing anti-TNF-α MAb can prevent SEB-induced lethality. Although this establishes for TNF-α a pivotal role in SEB-mediated disease (10), this MAb does not neutralize SEB but only the effects of SEB induction. Similarly, Abs to costimulatory molecules, like anti-B7.2 MAbs, significantly inhibited T-cell activation by lowering systemic IL-2 release, blastogenesis, and IL-2 receptor expression and thus improved SEBILS survival in mice (56). Specific therapy, how-ever, would be preferable, as it prevents rather than disrupts the cytokine induction.

Epidemiological data is consistent with the notion that Abs matter because older patients and healthy blood donors are more likely to exhibit Abs against SEB- and TSST-1-induced shock and recurrence is more common in younger patients who do not have Abs (34). Titers in patients vary and predict susceptibility to presumed toxin-mediated disease. In addition, investigations with serum from healthy blood donors demonstrated that immunoglobulin counteracted SEB stimulation in T-cell assays (57).

Vaccine Data

Several SEB vaccines have been tested in the past. The U.S. Army Medical Research Institute first started but ultimately abandoned the development of a vaccine to SEB using formalin-inactivated SEB toxin. SEB toxoid can be generated by prolonged incubation of SEB in formalin at pH 7.5. Despite retained immunogenicity and its ability to induce protective Abs in monkeys and rabbits, repeated oral doses of SEB toxoid proved to be poor mucosal immunogens and were thus not efficacious against the enteric ill effects of orally given SEB. Later, SEB toxoids containing a nontoxic biodegradable adjuvant, poly (DL-lactide-co-glycolide) microspheres or proteasomes were shown to be capable of inducing long-lasting, high-titered Abs. This toxoid-elicited immunity promotes neutralization of toxin in vivo and aborts lethality in mice and rhesus monkeys (58, 59). Mucosal vaccination with attenuated recombinant SEB vaccine in conjunction with cholera toxin was explored in mice and nonhuman primate models and shown to be effective after challenge with wild-type SEB toxin (27, 60, 61). Mice immunized intranasally were fully protected against a lethal dose of wild-type SEB, whereas partial (75%) protection was seen when mice were immunized intragastrically. Site-directed mutagenesis of conserved receptor-binding surfaces of SEA and SEB has been employed to generate toxoids for vaccination. Key amino acid residues involved in binding to the TcR Vβ chain (N23) and MHC class II (F44) were substituted. Amino acid substitutions result in toxins with reduced SAg activity (61). A SEB triple mutant with three critical amino acid substitutions in the MHC class II binding portion (L45, Y89) and TcR Vβ chain-binding portion (Y94) also manifests reduced T-cell activation without altering the structure of the Ag (62). This toxoid was also explored as a vaccine candidate in piglets where it induced an adequate Ab response even without the addition of the cholera toxin adjuvant. In summary, results of vaccine studies underscore the importance of the humoral immune response and encourage efforts to generate Abs for passive immunotherapy (62).

Passive Immunotherapy

Murine MAb

Several SEB-specific murine MAbs have been described in the literature. However, the majority of them have not been rigorously tested in animal models, and thus,

their ultimate neutralization capacity is difficult to judge (21, 56, 63, 64). Table 2 summarizes the list of MAbs generated against SEB toxin.

Four murine MAbs, B334 (IgG1), B327 (IgG2b), B87 (IgG1), and 2B33 (IgG1), which exhibit nanomolar range affinity have been described, and they recognized different, non-overlapping epitopes to SEB (64). Of those, B87 and 2B33 inhibited the KS-6.1 (Vβ8.2) T-cell response to SEB. To our knowledge, these MAbs have not been further tested in in vivo models.

A neutralizing murine anti-TSST-1 MAb (MAb5) which cross-reacts with SEB was evaluated for neutralization of SEB-induced superantigenic activities in vitro (63). The Ab was found to partially inhibit SEB-induced T-cell mitogenesis (63%) and TNF secretion (70%) in human PBMCs. Epitope mapping revealed that this Ab bound to TSST-1 residues 47 to 56 ($_{47}$FPSPYYSPAF$_{56}$) and to SEB residues 83 to 92 ($_{83}$DVFGANYYYQ$_{92}$), sequences that are structurally dissimilar. These studies were also not analyzed further in in vivo models.

TABLE 2 List of MAbs generated against SEB toxins

Source	Ab(s)	Affinity unit(s)	In vitro model(s)	In vivo model(s)	Reference
Murine	IFD7, 2DA3 and 2HA10, 2EG5 and 2GD9		BALB/c splenocytes		72
Murine	B334, B327, B87, 2B33	nM	Mouse Vβ8.2 + T cell (KS-6.1)		64
Murine	MAb5 (anti-TSST MAb)		Human PBMCs		63
Chicken	IgY		BALB/c	Rhesus monkeys	66
Murine phage display	Soluble SEB-ScFv	nM			73
Chimeric	Ch82M and Ch63	pM	HLA-DR3 mouse splenocytes		67
Human	10 Fab and 4 full-length MAbs	nM	Human PBMCs	BALB/c	69
Human	Human MAb79G9, human MAb154	pM–nM	Human PBMCs	BALB/c	70
Murine	20B1, 14G8, 6D3, 4C7		Human T cells	BALB/c, HLA-DR3	21
Chimeric + lovastatin	Ch82M and Ch63 with lovastatin		BALB/c mouse splenocytes	HLA-DR3	68
Murine	3F3 (anti-SEA and -SEB)				74
Synthetic human MAb	IgG 075, IgG 079, IgG 079-P, IgG 119, IgG 120, IgG 121	nM	Human PBMCs	BALB/c	71

Recently, four murine MAbs (20B1, 14G8, 6D3, and 4C7) specific to SEB were investigated, and three of four MAbs showed significant inhibition of SEB-induced T-cell proliferation as well as IL-2 and IFN-γ production by human T cells in vitro (21). These MAbs bind to different conformational epitopes that are destroyed by deletion of the distal C terminus of SEB. In spite of inhibition of T-cell proliferation in vitro, these MAbs differed in protective efficacy in a SEBILS mouse model. MAbs 14G8 and 4C7 were not effective in in vivo BALB/c and HLA-DR3 mouse models. MAb 20B1 was 100% protective in both mouse models, whereas 6D3 was partially protective in the BALB/c model but nonprotective in the HLA-DR3 model. In addition, enhanced protection against SEBILS was demonstrated when two nonprotective MAbs, such as 14G8 and 6D3, were combined in vivo even if they were less protective or nonprotective in monotherapy in the HLA-DR3 model. This study was important, as it demonstrated the superiority of combination therapy, possibly because of altered toxin clearance via Fc receptor-mediated uptake.

The SEB-neutralizing MAb-20B1 has also been shown to be an effective treatment in methicillin-resistant *S. aureus* infection in three mouse models. Administration of mAb-20B1 protects mice from lethal sepsis and reduces invasion of skin tissue and deep abscess formation. This study demonstrates further evidence for the role of SEB in *S. aureus* infections and a rationale for anti-SEB IgG as an immunotherapeutic agent for treatment of severe staphylococcal infections (65).

Chicken

SEB-specific Abs generated in chickens (IgY) successfully inhibited SEB-induced T-cell proliferation and cytokine responses in vitro and in passive transfer-protected mice. Rhesus monkeys were also protected from lethal SEB aerosol exposure when treated with the IgY specific for SEB up to 4 h after challenge. The advantage of chicken Abs would be substantial cost savings (66).

Chimeric and Human Abs

In the more recent era of Ab development, construction of chimeric and humanized Abs have been aggressively pursued, as they can be expected to be less immunogenic and can potentially also confer human constant region function. A group of investigators generated chimeric human-mouse SEB-specific Abs (67). Two good candidates were identified and further investigated. At all SEB concentrations, significant neutralization of SEB-induced T-cell proliferation (human and mouse) was achieved with the chimeric Abs Ch82M and Ch63. Interestingly, improved neutralization between the combination of anti-SEBs and either Ab used alone was also noted. These chimeric Abs manifested affinities in the picomolar range. The chimeric Abs have also been tested in HLA-DR3 transgenic mice and achieved partial protection with one and complete protection with a combination of MAbs. In addition, these chimeric Abs were also shown to be effective both in vitro and in vivo when combined with lovastatin (68).

More-recent work has focused on developing human MAbs to SEB. The inhibitory and biophysical properties of 10 human Fabs, derived by panning after vaccination with STEBVax, were examined. These Fabs exhibited binding affinities equal to polyclonal IgG, had low-nanomolar 50% inhibitory concentrations against SEB in cell culture assays, and partially protected mice from SEBILS. This study used an LPS-potentiated model with fairly low doses of SEB (2.5 µg). Fabs also bound to SEC1 and SEC2 as well as streptococcal pyrogenic exotoxin C. Four Fabs against SEB, with the lowest 50% inhibitory concentrations, were converted into native full-length MAbs. Of note is that a 250-fold-greater inhibition of SEB-induced T-cell activation was observed with two MAbs than with their respective Fab fragments, which had equal binding affinities (69). SEB-specific fully human MAbs were also generated using the "human MORPHO-DOMA technology" after isolating B cells from healthy donors whose sera showed preexisting high immune reactivity to SEB. Human MAb 154 showed an inhibitory effect on SEB-induced secretion of proinflammatory cytokines specifically tested for IFN-γ and TNF-α by human PBMCs and protected mice prophylactically from a challenge of up to 100 μg of SEB injected i.p. potentiated by LPS (70).

In addition, using phage display technology, human Ag-binding fragments have been synthesized and converted into fully human IgG Ab. These synthetic human MAbs display affinities in the nanomolar range. They were effective at a dose of 200 μg in the murine SEBILS model using different challenge doses of SEB (71).

FUTURE CHALLENGE

Current data from various studies are encouraging and predict that neutralization of SAgs like SEB is feasible. Future developments should focus on developing high-affinity MAbs that exhibit good pharmacokinetic parameters and will permit treatment with lower doses. Several studies indicate that combination of MAbs may result in more potent neutralization. A major challenge is to define an adequate setting in which these Abs can be tested, as patients with toxic shock are difficult to identify, let alone provide consent for a study. The FDA has recently approved raxibacumab to treat inhalational anthrax. This is the first MAb approved using the animal efficacy rule. So one option would be to test these MAbs only in nonhuman primate models, which is possible under the new FDA animal efficacy rule. Another option would be to better define the SEB-induced allergic syndromes that could constitute human patients to test the effect of neutralizing Abs. Another challenge will be to identify the selective pressures on bacteria expressing SAgs and how the selective pressures influence the interaction between SAg-bearing bacteria and the human immune system. This knowledge may prove invaluable to prevent emerging diseases mediated by SAgs and, most importantly, to improve the management of SAg-associated diseases. In this regard, care will have to be taken to monitor for the emergence of SEB variants that may not be effectively neutralized by all Abs.

ACKNOWLEDGMENTS

We thank Kaushik Dutta for generating the figure.

BCF was supported by NIH grant U54-AI057158 and in part by an award from Pfizer's Centers for Therapeutic Innovation, New York.

Conflicts of interest: We disclose no conflicts.

CITATION

Fries BC, Varshney AK. 2013. Bacterial toxins—staphylococcal enterotoxin B. Microbiol Spectrum 1(2):AID-0002-2012

REFERENCES

1. **Fleischer B.** 1994. Superantigens. *APMIS* **102:**3–12.
2. **Wilson GJ, Seo KS, Cartwright RA, Connelley T, Chuang-Smith ON, Merriman JA, Guinane CM, Park JY, Bohach GA, Schlievert PM, Morrison WI, Fitzgerald JR.** 2011. A novel core genome-encoded superantigen contributes to lethality of community-associated MRSA necrotizing pneumonia. *PLoS Pathog* **7:**e1002271.
3. **Grumann D, Scharf SS, Holtfreter S, Kohler C, Steil L, Engelmann S, Hecker M, Volker U, Broker BM.** 2008. Immune cell activation by enterotoxin gene cluster (egc)-encoded and non-egc superantigens from Staphylococcus aureus. *J Immunol* **181:**5054–5061.
4. **Franz DR, Parrott CD, Takafuji ET.** 1997. The U.S. biological warfare and biological defense programs, p 425–436. *In* Sidell FR, Takafuji E, Franz DR (ed), *Textbook of Military Medicine. Part I. Warfare, Weaponry and the Casualty*, vol 3. U.S. Government. Printing Office, Washington, DC.
5. **Iandolo JJ, Shafer WM.** 1977. Regulation of staphylococcal enterotoxin B. *Infect Immun* **16:**610–616.
6. **Swaminathan S, Furey W, Pletcher J, Sax M.** 1992. Crystal structure of staphylococcal enterotoxin B, a superantigen. *Nature* **359:**801–806.
7. **Papageorgiou AC, Tranter HS, Acharya KR.** 1998. Crystal structure of microbial superantigen

staphylococcal enterotoxin B at 1.5 A resolution: implications for superantigen recognition by MHC class II molecules and T-cell receptors. *J Mol Biol* **277**:61–79.

8. **Kappler JW, Herman A, Clements J, Marrack P.** 1992. Mutations defining functional regions of the superantigen staphylococcal enterotoxin B. *J Exp Med* **175**:387–396.

9. **Faulkner L, Cooper A, Fantino C, Altmann DM, Sriskandan S.** 2005. The mechanism of superantigen-mediated toxic shock: not a simple Th1 cytokine storm. *J Immunol* **175**:6870–6877.

10. **Miethke T, Wahl C, Heeg K, Echtenacher B, Krammer PH, Wagner H.** 1992. T cell-mediated lethal shock triggered in mice by the superantigen staphylococcal enterotoxin B: critical role of tumor necrosis factor. *J Exp Med* **175**:91–98.

11. **Hewitt CR, Lamb JR, Hayball J, Hill M, Owen MJ, O'Hehir RE.** 1992. Major histocompatibility complex independent clonal T cell anergy by direct interaction of Staphylococcus aureus enterotoxin B with the T cell antigen receptor. *J Exp Med* **175**:1493–1499.

12. **Varshney AK, Mediavilla JR, Robiou N, Guh A, Wang X, Gialanella P, Levi MH, Kreiswirth BN, Fries BC.** 2009. Diverse enterotoxin gene profiles among clonal complexes of Staphylococcus aureus isolates from the Bronx, New York. *Appl Environ Microbiol* **75**:6839–6849.

13. **Kohler PL, Greenwood SD, Nookala S, Kotb M, Kranz DM, Schlievert PM.** 2012. Staphylococcus aureus isolates encode variant staphylococcal enterotoxin B proteins that are diverse in superantigenicity and lethality. *PLoS One* **7**:e41157.

14. **Krakauer T.** 1994. Cell adhesion molecules are co-receptors for staphylococcal enterotoxin B-induced T-cell activation and cytokine production. *Immunol Lett* **39**:121–125.

15. **Matsuyama S, Koide Y, Yoshida TO.** 1993. HLA class II molecule-mediated signal transduction mechanism responsible for the expression of interleukin-1 beta and tumor necrosis factor-alpha genes induced by a staphylococcal superantigen. *Eur J Immunol* **23**:3194–3202.

16. **Vabulas R, Bittlingmaier R, Heeg K, Wagner H, Miethke T.** 1996. Rapid clearance of the bacterial superantigen staphylococcal enterotoxin B in vivo. *Infect Immun* **64**:4567–4573.

17. **Stiles BG, Bavari S, Krakauer T, Ulrich RG.** 1993. Toxicity of staphylococcal enterotoxins potentiated by lipopolysaccharide: major histocompatibility complex class II molecule dependency and cytokine release. *Infect Immun* **61**:5333–5338.

18. **Khan AA, Priya S, Saha B.** 2009. IL-2 regulates SEB induced toxic shock syndrome in BALB/c mice. *PLoS One* **4**:e8473.

19. **Krakauer T, Buckley MJ, Fisher D.** 2010. Proinflammatory mediators of toxic shock and their correlation to lethality. *Mediators Inflamm* **2010**:517594.

20. **Huzella LM, Buckley MJ, Alves DA, Stiles BG, Krakauer T.** 2009. Central roles for IL-2 and MCP-1 following intranasal exposure to SEB: a new mouse model. *Res Vet Sci* **86**:241–247.

21. **Varshney AK, Wang X, Cook E, Dutta K, Scharff MD, Goger MJ, Fries BC.** 2011. Generation, characterization, and epitope mapping of neutralizing and protective monoclonal antibodies against staphylococcal enterotoxin B-induced lethal shock. *J Biol Chem* **286**:9737–9747.

22. **Roy CJ, Warfield KL, Welcher BC, Gonzales RF, Larsen T, Hanson J, David CS, Krakauer T, Bavari S.** 2005. Human leukocyte antigen-DQ8 transgenic mice: a model to examine the toxicity of aerosolized staphylococcal enterotoxin B. *Infect Immun* **73**:2452–2460.

23. **Wang X, Wang BR, Zhang XJ, Duan XL, Guo X, Ju G.** 2004. Fos expression in the rat brain after intraperitoneal injection of Staphylococcus enterotoxin B and the effect of vagotomy. *Neurochem Res* **29**:1667–1674.

24. **McCormick JK, Bohach GA, Schlievert PM.** 2003. Pyrogenic, lethal, and emetic properties of superantigens in rabbits and primates. *Methods Mol Biol* **214**:245–253.

25. **Strandberg KL, Rotschafer JH, Vetter SM, Buonpane RA, Kranz DM, Schlievert PM.** 2010. Staphylococcal superantigens cause lethal pulmonary disease in rabbits. *J Infect Dis* **202**:1690–1697.

26. **Bi S, Das R, Zelazowska E, Mani S, Neill R, Coleman GD, Yang DC, Hammamieh R, Shupp JW, Jett M.** 2009. The cellular and molecular immune response of the weanling piglet to staphylococcal enterotoxin B. *Exp Biol Med (Maywood)* **234**:1305–1315.

27. **Boles JW, Pitt ML, LeClaire RD, Gibbs PH, Torres E, Dyas B, Ulrich RG, Bavari S.** 2003. Generation of protective immunity by inactivated recombinant staphylococcal enterotoxin B vaccine in nonhuman primates and identification of correlates of immunity. *Clin Immunol* **108**:51–59.

28. **Hodoval LF, Morris EL, Crawley GJ, Beisel WR.** 1968. Pathogenesis of lethal shock after intravenous staphylococcal enterotoxin B in monkeys. *Appl Microbiol* **16**:187–192.

29. **Alber G, Scheuber PH, Reck B, Sailer-Kramer B, Hartmann A, Hammer DK.** 1989. Role of substance P in immediate-type skin reactions induced by staphylococcal enterotoxin B in unsensitized monkeys. *J Allergy Clin Immunol* **84**:880–885.

30. **Rusnak JM, Kortepeter M, Ulrich R, Poli M, Boudreau E.** 2004. Laboratory exposures to staphylococcal enterotoxin B. *Emerg Infect Dis* **10:**1544–1549.

31. **Todd J, Fishaut M, Kapral F, Welch T.** 1978. Toxic-shock syndrome associated with phage-group-I staphylococci. *Lancet* **ii:**1116–1118.

32. **Hajjeh RA, Reingold A, Weil A, Shutt K, Schuchat A, Perkins BA.** 1999. Toxic shock syndrome in the United States: surveillance update, 1979 1996. *Emerg Infect Dis* **5:**807–810.

33. **Gaventa S, Reingold AL, Hightower AW, Broome CV, Schwartz B, Hoppe C, Harwell J, Lefkowitz LK, Makintubee S, Cundiff DR, et al.** 1989. Active surveillance for toxic shock syndrome in the United States, 1986. *Rev Infect Dis* **11** (Suppl 1):S28–S34.

34. **Andrews MM, Parent EM, Barry M, Parsonnet J.** 2001. Recurrent nonmenstrual toxic shock syndrome: clinical manifestations, diagnosis, and treatment. *Clin Infect Dis* **32:**1470–1479.

35. **Stolz SJ, Davis JP, Vergeront JM, Crass BA, Chesney PJ, Wand PJ, Bergdoll MS.** 1985. Development of serum antibody to toxic shock toxin among individuals with toxic shock syndrome in Wisconsin. *J Infect Dis* **151:**883–889.

36. **John CC, Niermann M, Sharon B, Peterson ML, Kranz DM, Schlievert PM.** 2009. Staphylococcal toxic shock syndrome erythroderma is associated with superantigenicity and hypersensitivity. *Clin Infect Dis* **49:**1893–1896.

37. **Nissen D, Pedersen LJ, Skov PS, Vejlsgaard GL, Poulsen LK, Jarlov JO, Karlsmark T, Nolte H.** 1997. IgE-binding components of staphylococcal enterotoxins in patients with atopic dermatitis. *Ann Allergy Asthma Immunol* **79:**403–408.

38. **Tada J, Toi Y, Akiyama H, Arata J, Kato H.** 1996. Presence of specific IgE antibodies to staphylococcal enterotoxins in patients with atopic dermatitis. *Eur J Dermatol* **6:**552–554.

39. **Savinko T, Lauerma A, Lehtimaki S, Gombert M, Majuri ML, Fyhrquist-Vanni N, Dieu-Nosjean MC, Kemeny L, Wolff H, Homey B, Alenius H.** 2005. Topical superantigen exposure induces epidermal accumulation of CD8+ T cells, a mixed Th1/Th2-type dermatitis and vigorous production of IgE antibodies in the murine model of atopic dermatitis. *J Immunol* **175:**8320–8326.

40. **Bozek A, Fisher A, Filipowska B, Mazur B, Jarzab J.** 2012. Clinical features and immunological markers of atopic dermatitis in elderly patients. *Int Arch Allergy Immunol* **157:**372–378.

41. **Kientz CE, Hulst AG, Wils ER.** 1997. Determination of staphylococcal enterotoxin B by on-line (micro) liquid chromatography-electrospray mass spectrometry. *J Chromatogr A* **757:**51–64.

42. **Hosotsubo KK, Hosotsubo H, Nishijima MK, Nishimura M, Taenaka N, Yoshiya I.** 1989. Rapid screening for Staphylococcus aureus infection by measuring enterotoxin B. *J Clin Microbiol* **27:**2794–2798.

43. **Azuma K, Koike K, Kobayashi T, Mochizuki T, Mashiko K, Yamamoto Y.** 2004. Detection of circulating superantigens in an intensive care unit population. *Int J Infect Dis* **8:**292–298.

44. **Komisar JL, Weng CF, Oyejide A, Hunt RE, Briscoe C, Tseng J.** 2001. Cellular and cytokine responses in the circulation and tissue reactions in the lung of rhesus monkeys (Macaca mulatta) pretreated with cyclosporin A and challenged with staphylococcal enterotoxin B. *Toxicol Pathol* **29:**369–378.

45. **Arad G, Levy R, Hillman D, Kaempfer R.** 2000. Superantigen antagonist protects against lethal shock and defines a new domain for T-cell activation. *Nat Med* **6:**414–421.

46. **Visvanathan K, Charles A, Bannan J, Pugach P, Kashfi K, Zabriskie JB.** 2001. Inhibition of bacterial superantigens by peptides and antibodies. *Infect Immun* **69:**875–884.

47. **Rajagopalan G, Sen MM, David CS.** 2004. In vitro and in vivo evaluation of staphylococcal superantigen peptide antagonists. *Infect Immun* **72:**6733–6737.

48. **Wang S, Li Y, Xiong H, Cao J.** 2008. A broad-spectrum inhibitory peptide against staphylococcal enterotoxin superantigen SEA, SEB and SEC. *Immunol Lett* **121:**167–172.

49. **Buonpane RA, Churchill HR, Moza B, Sundberg EJ, Peterson ML, Schlievert PM, Kranz DM.** 2007. Neutralization of staphylococcal enterotoxin B by soluble, high-affinity receptor antagonists. *Nat Med* **13:**725–729.

50. **Krakauer T, Buckley M.** 2003. Doxycycline is anti-inflammatory and inhibits staphylococcal exotoxin-induced cytokines and chemokines. *Antimicrob Agents Chemother* **47:**3630–3633.

51. **Krakauer T, Stiles BG.** 1999. Pentoxifylline inhibits superantigen-induced toxic shock and cytokine release. *Clin Diagn Lab Immunol* **6:**594–598.

52. **Krakauer T, Buckley M.** 2006. Dexamethasone attenuates staphylococcal enterotoxin B-induced hypothermic response and protects mice from superantigen-induced toxic shock. *Antimicrob Agents Chemother* **50:**391–395.

53. **Krakauer T, Buckley M, Issaq HJ, Fox SD.** 2010. Rapamycin protects mice from staphylococcal enterotoxin B-induced toxic shock and blocks cytokine release in vitro and in vivo. *Antimicrob Agents Chemother* **54:**1125–1131.

54. **Casadevall A.** 2006. The third age of antimicrobial therapy. *Clin Infect Dis* **42:**1414–1416.

55. **Chow SK, Casadevall A.** 2012. Monoclonal antibodies and toxins-a perspective on function and isotype. *Toxins (Basel)* **4:**430–454.

56. **Muraille E, De Smedt T, Urbain J, Moser M, Leo O.** 1995. B7.2 provides co-stimulatory functions in vivo in response to staphylococcal enterotoxin B. *Eur J Immunol* **25:**2111–2114.

57. **LeClaire RD, Bavari S.** 2001. Human antibodies to bacterial superantigens and their ability to inhibit T-cell activation and lethality. *Antimicrob Agents Chemother* **45:**460–463.

58. **Tseng J, Komisar JL, Trout RN, Hunt RE, Chen JY, Johnson AJ, Pitt L, Ruble DL.** 1995. Humoral immunity to aerosolized staphylococcal enterotoxin B (SEB), a superantigen, in monkeys vaccinated with SEB toxoid-containing microspheres. *Infect Immun* **63:**2880–2885.

59. **Lowell GH, Kaminski RW, Grate S, Hunt RE, Charney C, Zimmer S, Colleton C.** 1996. Intranasal and intramuscular proteosome-staphylococcal enterotoxin B (SEB) toxoid vaccines: immunogenicity and efficacy against lethal SEB intoxication in mice. *Infect Immun* **64:**1706–1713.

60. **Stiles BG, Garza AR, Ulrich RG, Boles JW.** 2001. Mucosal vaccination with recombinantly attenuated staphylococcal enterotoxin B and protection in a murine model. *Infect Immun* **69:**2031–2036.

61. **Woody MA, Krakauer T, Stiles BG.** 1997. Staphylococcal enterotoxin B mutants (N23K and F44S): biological effects and vaccine potential in a mouse model. *Vaccine* **15:**133–139.

62. **Ulrich RG, Olson MA, Bavari S.** 1998. Development of engineered vaccines effective against structurally related bacterial superantigens. *Vaccine* **16:**1857–1864.

63. **Pang LT, Kum WW, Chow AW.** 2000. Inhibition of staphylococcal enterotoxin B-induced lymphocyte proliferation and tumor necrosis factor alpha secretion by MAb5, an anti-toxic shock syndrome toxin 1 monoclonal antibody. *Infect Immun* **68:**3261–3268.

64. **Hamad AR, Herman A, Marrack P, Kappler JW.** 1994. Monoclonal antibodies defining functional sites on the toxin superantigen staphylococcal enterotoxin B. *J Exp Med* **180:**615–621.

65. **Varshney AK, Wang X, Scharff MD, Macintyre J, Zollner RS, Kovalenko OV, Martinez LR, Byrne FR, Fries BC.** 2013. Staphylococcal enterotoxin B specific monoclonal antibody 20B1 successfully treats diverse *Staphylococcus aureus* infections. *J Infect Dis* Aug 6. [Epub ahead of print]. doi:10.1093/infdis/jit421

66. **LeClaire RD, Hunt RE, Bavari S.** 2002. Protection against bacterial superantigen staphylococcal enterotoxin B by passive vaccination. *Infect Immun* **70:**2278–2281.

67. **Tilahun ME, Rajagopalan G, Shah-Mahoney N, Lawlor RG, Tilahun AY, Xie C, Natarajan K, Margulies DH, Ratner DI, Osborne BA, Goldsby RA.** 2010. Potent neutralization of staphylococcal enterotoxin B by synergistic action of chimeric antibodies. *Infect Immun* **78:**2801–2811.

68. **Tilahun ME, Kwan A, Natarajan K, Quinn M, Tilahun AY, Xie C, Margulies DH, Osborne BA, Goldsby RA, Rajagopalan G.** 2011. Chimeric anti-staphylococcal enterotoxin B antibodies and lovastatin act synergistically to provide in vivo protection against lethal doses of SEB. *PLoS One* **6:**e27203.

69. **Larkin EA, Stiles BG, Ulrich RG.** 2010. Inhibition of toxic shock by human monoclonal antibodies against staphylococcal enterotoxin B. *PLoS One* **5:**e13253.

70. **Drozdowski B, Zhou Y, Kline B, Spidel J, Chan YY, Albone E, Turchin H, Chao Q, Henry M, Balogach J, Routhier E, Bavari S, Nicolaides NC, Sass PM, Grasso L.** 2010. Generation and characterization of high affinity human monoclonal antibodies that neutralize staphylococcal enterotoxin B. *J Immune Based Ther Vaccines* **8:**9.

71. **Karauzum H, Chen G, Abaandou L, Mahmoudieh M, Boroun AR, Shulenin S, Devi VS, Stavale E, Warfield KL, Zeitlin L, Roy CJ, Sidhu SS, Aman MJ.** 2012. Synthetic human monoclonal antibodies toward staphylococcal enterotoxin B (SEB) protective against toxic shock syndrome. *J Biol Chem* **287:**25203–25215.

72. **Lin YS, Largen MT, Newcomb JR, Rogers TJ.** 1988. Production and characterisation of monoclonal antibodies specific for staphylococcal enterotoxin B. *J Med Microbiol* **27:**263–270.

73. **Singh PK, Agrawal R, Kamboj DV, Gupta G, Boopathi M, Goel AK, Singh L.** 2010. Construction of a single-chain variable-fragment antibody against the superantigen staphylococcal enterotoxin B. *Appl Environ Microbiol* **76:**8184–8191.

74. **Liang B, Zhang Y, Liu A, Zhou Y, Chen F, Wang X.** 2011. Production of a monoclonal antibody by simultaneous immunization of staphylococcal enterotoxin A and B. *Appl Biochem Biotechnol* **164:**831–840.

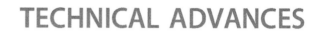

TECHNICAL ADVANCES

Antibody Engineering

19

KIN-MING LO,[1] OLIVIER LEGER,[2] and BJÖRN HOCK[3]

Monoclonal antibodies are enjoying outstanding commercial success, with 4 of the top 10 best-selling drugs. Although most of the preclinical and clinical experiences with therapeutic antibodies have been gained from the treatment of cancer and inflammatory diseases, effective therapy is not limited to these indications. For example, palivizumab (Synagis) has been approved for the prophylactic treatment for respiratory syncytial virus (RSV) infections and remains the only therapeutic antibody for the treatment of infectious diseases to date.

In this article, we review the latest advances in antibody-engineering technologies to make an antibody clinically and commercially successful. We discuss the rationale behind the choice of immunoglobulin isotype and the protein engineering of the constant regions. This is followed by a review of the humanization strategy to minimize immunogenicity and the recent approaches to affinity mature the antigen binding of the antibody. Finally, we have an overview of the next-generation antibodies, such as antibody-drug conjugates, bispecific antibodies, and immunocytokines, which are being developed to meet future challenges.

[1]Department of Protein Engineering and Antibody Technologies, EMD Serono Research Institute, Billerica, MA 01821; [2]Department of Protein Engineering and Antibody Technologies, Merck Serono S.A.—Geneva, 1202 Geneva, Switzerland; [3]Department of Protein Engineering and Antibody Technologies, Merck Serono, Merck KGaA, D-64293 Darmstadt, Germany.

Antibodies for Infectious Diseases
Edited by James E. Crowe, Jr., Diana Boraschi, and Rino Rappuoli
© 2015 American Society for Microbiology, Washington, DC
doi:10.1128/microbiolspec.AID-0007-2012

THE CONSTANT REGIONS: PROTEIN AND GLYCOENGINEERING OF THE Fc

The Fc portion of the antibody, which determines its effector functions and is responsible for its pharmacokinetic properties, has to be carefully chosen to suit its therapeutic applications. To date, all of the approved therapeutic antibodies are of the immunoglobulin G (IgG) isotype, because IgGs are the predominant serum immunoglobulins and are readily manufacturable as biotherapeutics. Furthermore, IgG binds the Fcγ receptors (FcγRs) on immune cells to elicit various effector functions and is the only isotype that binds the protective neonatal Fc receptor FcRn, which gives typical IgGs (IgG1, -2, and -4) their long serum half-lives of about 21 days in humans.

Most of the knowledge gained on antibody therapy is from the treatment of cancer and autoimmune disorders using IgG1, the preferred IgG subclass because its potent effector functions are expected to contribute to the mechanism of action of the antibody. For infectious diseases, the only therapeutic antibody approved to date is palivizumab, also an IgG1, for the prophylactic treatment for RSV. The potent antibody-dependent cellular cytotoxicity (ADCC) and complement-dependent cytotoxicity (CDC) of IgG1 that are desirable for eradicating cancer or autoimmune disease-causing cells, however, may not be ideal for the treatment of certain infectious diseases. In cancer therapy, the major cell types mediating ADCC are NK cells and macrophages, which also eradicate tumor cells by antibody-dependent cellular phagocytosis (ADCP). To maximize cellular cytotoxicity, optimal engagement of the activating receptor FcγRIII on NK cells and macrophage is important. On the other hand, polymorphonuclear (PMN) cells, which are about 10 times more abundant than monocytes and NK cells, constitute the first line of defense against bacteria, and FcγRIIA, the most widely expressed FcγR, is the central initiator of IgG-mediated phagocytosis by human PMN (1).

Therefore, a different strategy for engineering antibodies against infectious agents may be needed. Such a strategy should consider the choice of Ig isotypes and subclasses best suited for the disease, the glycosylation pattern to facilitate the desired mode of action, and the optimal pharmacokinetic and pharmacodynamic properties. These considerations will in turn determine the expression system, host cell lines, and production method.

Choice of Ig Isotypes and Subclasses

IgA as a Potential Isotype for Therapeutic Antibodies Against Infectious Diseases

The majority of the antibodies approved for the treatment of cancer and autoimmune disorders are of the IgG1 subclass. Although isotypes other than IgG have not been successfully developed, IgA presents itself as a logical candidate against infectious diseases because IgAs in nature provide the principal defense against pathogens, in the first line, as IgA dimers against invasion by preventing the attachment of microbes or toxins to the mucosal lining, and, in the second line, as IgA monomers in circulation to neutralize pathogens that have breached the mucosal barrier. Furthermore, IgA represents the most abundantly produced antibody and is the second most prevalent isotype in the blood behind IgG.

IgA has two subclasses, IgA1 and IgA2. IgA1 with an extended hinge region may offer higher avidity antigen binding with distantly spaced antigens, but it is more vulnerable to proteolysis by enzymes from pathogenic bacteria (2). IgA, especially the IgA2 isoform, has been shown to be superior to IgG1 in recruiting human PMN as effector cells to mediate ADCC (3). In addition, ADCP by human peripheral blood neutrophils is more effectively mediated by IgA than by IgG (4).

The IgA dimer format may be preferable in certain disease settings. However, the development of an IgA dimer is more challenging than that of a monomer. Toward that end, a recombinant dimeric IgA against epidermal growth factor receptor (EGFR) was produced and shown to mediate effective tumor cell killing. Importantly, the dimeric IgA, but not the monomeric IgA or IgG, was directionally transported by the polymeric Ig receptor through an epithelial cell monolayer in vitro (5). This has important implications for the IgA dimer as a potential anti-infectious agent at the mucosa.

IgG and its Subclasses

IgG1

The human IgG1 subclass was chosen almost a priori for therapeutic antibodies. Besides being the one that is most abundant in circulation, it has potent ADCC and CDC activities, and also the most desirable chemical, manufacturing, and control (CMC) properties as a biotherapeutic, e.g., it does not have the problems that IgG2 and IgG4 have (see below). Most of the experience with therapeutic IgG1 antibodies has been for the treatment of cancer, where the importance of CDC to the mechanism of action is controversial. Based on studies in complement-deficient mice, it has been shown that the contribution of the complement pathway to proinflammatory responses initiated by IgG is minor (6). However, complement plays an important role in the phagocytosis of opsonized bacteria mediated by the complement receptors (7). Therefore, we need to take a critical look to engineer the most effective human isotype to provide protection against infectious agents because of the different biology involved.

IgG1 binds all three classes of FcγR. Normally, FcγRI is saturated with serum IgG, which explains why this high-affinity FcγR may play only a minor role in IgG-mediated cellular responses such as ADCC and ADCP (6). The binding of IgG1 to the inhibitory FcγRIIB and the glycosylphosphatidylinositol-anchored FcγRIIIB, which does not signal, may render IgG1 suboptimal in triggering effector functions by PMN (4). Surprisingly, in a mouse study designed to compare the efficacies of human IgG subclasses with identical V regions against

a yeast infection (*Cryptococcus neoformans*, which causes meningitis in AIDS patients), IgG2 and IgG4, which have few ADCC/ADCP and CDC activities, respectively, protected the mice, whereas for the effector functions competent counterparts, IgG3 had no effect and IgG1 actually potentiated the infection (8). This unexpected result was explained by the observation that phagocytosed yeast was not killed to a significant extent, and the macrophages can possibly act as a Trojan horse for its survival and dissemination (9). Interestingly, studies in complement-deficient mice suggested that complement may also play a role in the antibody-mediated enhancement of cryptococcal infection (10).

IgG2

Although IgG2 is often considered as the effector-silent isotype in cancer treatment, it should be noted that the principal effector cells in the human peripheral blood mononuclear cell used in the classical in vitro ADCC assay are NK cells, which express only FcγRIII. In this assay, IgG1 and IgG3 are the most potent, while IgG2 and IgG4 have no detectable activity.

However, it has been reported that IgG2 can trigger ADCC by neutrophils mediated by FcγRIIA (11). This finding may explain the discrepancy between the lack of in vitro ADCC using NK cells, and yet readily detectable cytolytic activities of anti-CD8 IgG2 and IgG4 in mice (12), and, more importantly, the cytolytic activity of alemtuzumab (Campath) IgG4 in humans (13, 14). In addition, although complement plays a role in the phagocytosis of opsonized bacteria mediated by the complement receptors, IgG2 engagement of FcRIIA alone on phagocytic cells can lead to phagocytosis of opsonized bacteria (7).

IgG2 exhibits disulfide structural heterogeneity, resulting in at least three isoforms which differ by the disulfide connectivity at the hinge region (15). This can be more than a CMC issue on the homogeneity of the product, since some of the isoforms have been shown to affect binding affinity (16). IgG2 hinge region homogeneity with uniform disulfide bonds can be readily achieved by the use of a modified IgG1 hinge (17).

IgG3

IgG3 has an extended hinge region that imparts greater segmental flexibility and motion, resulting in a larger angle and longer distance between the two binding sites, to attain bivalent binding (18). It is for this reason that the IgG3 subclass was chosen for the development of a class of antibody cytokine fusion proteins (19). This extra spacing and flexibility provided by the IgG3 hinge may be particularly relevant for antiviral antibodies, because viruses such as the human immunodeficiency virus (HIV) have envelope spikes that are few and far between (20). Such spacing between epitopes is a strategy HIV has evolved to avoid bivalent binding to thwart neutralization by antibodies. For development as a biotherapeutic, IgG3 suffers from the fact that it has a relatively short serum half-life of about 7 days in humans.

IgG4

The IgG4 subclass is usually chosen for its complete lack of CDC, low ADCC (despite its high binding affinity for FcγRI [21]), and anti-inflammatory activity (22). The hinge region of the IgG4 H chain has two cysteine residues that can form either an intrachain disulfide bond or two interchain disulfide bonds with its partner H chain, and this accounts for the presence of about 50% of half-molecules (HL, a light chain bound to one heavy chain) when IgG4 is analyzed by sodium dodecyl sulfate-gel electrophoresis under non-reducing conditions. This heterogeneity is more than a CMC issue because recently it has been shown that therapeutic IgG4 antibodies can engage in Fab-arm exchange with endogenous human IgG4 in vivo (23), resulting in the functional monovalency of IgG4, with the loss of binding avidity and cross-linking effects. It is noteworthy that of the two approved therapeutic IgG4 antibodies, only gemtuzumab contains a hinge modification, whereas natalizumab does not

(24). Indeed, natalizumab showed significant levels of Fab-arm exchange in 15 of 16 patients, as early as 1 h after infusion (23). Therefore, therapeutic IgG4 antibodies should be designed to prevent the Fab-arm exchange by introducing the S228P mutation to stabilize the hinge region, and, more importantly, the R409 K mutation to stabilize the CH3 region (25). On the other hand, this Fab-arm exchange property of IgG4 can be exploited to generate recombinant bispecific therapeutic antibody, such as the Duobody of Genmab (Utrecht, The Netherlands).

Fc Glycosylation and Effector Functions

The N-glycan in the Fc is essential for the engagement of the FcγRs (but not FcRn) and hence important for effector functions. Therefore, antibodies whose effector functions are important for their mechanisms of action have to be produced in mammalian cells, or, more recently, in glycoengineered yeast (26). Importantly, the nature of the N-glycan chain, such as the presence of the bisecting N-acetylglucosamine (GlcNAc), fucose, and terminal sialic acids, modulates the activation of the FcγRs and immune cells.

Bisecting GlcNAc and Fucosylation Impact ADCC

It was recognized early on that the glycosylation pattern and biological activity of alemtuzumab expressed in different cell lines varied. The alemtuzumab produced from rat myeloma cells had a bisecting GlcNAc and a low extent of fucosylation, and it showed the highest ADCC (27). Although antibodies produced in β(1,4)-N-acetylglucosaminyltransferase III (GnTIII) transfected Chinese hamster ovary (CHO) cells had improved ADCC because of the addition of the bisecting GlcNAc (28), it was recognized later that the absence of fucose was dominant over bisecting GlcNAc in enhancing the ADCC. Indeed, the enhancement effect of bisecting GlcNAc was only observed in highly fucosylated IgG1, which has low ADCC activity (29).

Since ADCC was considered as an important mechanism of action for a number of therapeutic antibodies, and NK cells, the effector cells used in standard ADCC assays in vitro, express only FcγRIIIA, technology to improve FcγRIIIA binding of antibodies received a lot of attention. Furthermore, increased FcγRIIIA binding may also enhance antigen uptake by FcγRIIIA-expressing dendritic cells and macrophages, thus potentiating the adaptive immune surveillance.

The importance of ADCC to antitumor activity was supported by clinical data, which showed that response to antibody therapy was positively correlated to the binding affinity of FcγRIIIA to IgG1. For rituximab (Rituxan) in the treatment of non-Hodgkin's lymphoma, Waldenströms macroglobulinemia, and follicular lymphoma, FcγRIIIA polymorphism was found to be a good predictor of clinical outcome, with patients expressing the 158V variant, which has a higher binding affinity for IgG1, responding better than patients expressing the 158F variant (30, 31). Similar positive correlation was also reported for trastuzumab (Herceptin) in the treatment of metastatic breast cancer (32), and for Erbitux in the treatment of metastatic colorectal cancer (33). There is also direct evidence that increasing the binding affinity of an antibody for FcγRIIIA translates to improved efficacy in the clinic. Anti-RhD monoclonal antibodies (mAbs) produced in YB2/0 cells, which have low fucose levels, demonstrated superior clearance of RhD-positive red blood cells, relative to monoclonal antibodies produced in other producer lines (34).

It should be noted that, while antibodies with low fucose levels have enhanced ADCC mediated by NK cells, they were found to be less potent in inducing ADCC mediated by activated PMN, in comparison with antibodies with high fucose levels. PMN express FcγRIIA, and, instead of FcγRIIIA, the glycosylphosphatidylinositol anchored FcγRIIIB, which does not have the signaling ability to trigger effector functions by PMN. Since fucosylation levels on antibodies are not known to affect binding to FcγRIIA, it is possible that the higher-affinity binding of antibodies with low fucose levels to FcγRIIIB acts as a decoy mechanism, resulting in less binding to FcγRIIA, the receptor responsible for activating the PMN-mediated ADCC (35). This shows that the impact of Fc glycosylation on ADCC is critically dependent on the recruited effector cell type, an important point to consider when designing antibodies for the treatment of infectious diseases.

Manipulating Effector Functions and Pharmacokinetic Properties

In addition to the aforementioned GnTIII-transfected CHO cells by Roche Glycart (Schlieren, Switzerland) to produce antibodies with bisecting GlcNAc, an α-1,6-fucosyltransferase (FUT8) knockout CHO cell line was developed by Kyowa Hakko Kogyo (Tokyo, Japan) to produce nonfucosylated antibodies (36). Furthermore, glyco-optimized and fully human glycosylated antibodies can be produced from glycoengineered mammalian cells (Glycotope, Berlin, Germany) or yeast (GlycoFi Merck, Lebanon, New Hampshire) (25).

Instead of glycoengineering, Fc mutations can be introduced to optimize binding to specific FcγRs, such as increased binding to activating FcγRs and decreased binding to the inhibitory FcγRIIB, thereby improving the so-called A/I ratio, to enhance ADCC and ADCP (37, 38, 39). On the other hand, for therapeutic applications where effector functions are undesirable, mutations to abrogate ADCC and CDC are well described in the literature. One common strategy is to incorporate natural motifs from IgG2 and IgG4 to decrease binding to FcγRs and complement, respectively, while keeping potential immunogenicity of the changes to a minimum. For example, Armour et al. (40) replaced residues 233 to 236 in the lower hinge region of IgG1 responsible for FcγR binding with the corresponding residues from IgG2, and introduced IgG4 residues at position 327, 330, and 331 to abolish binding to C1q. Similarly, the "effector silent" IgG2/G4 composite antibody of Mueller et al (41) and the IgG2m4 of An et al. (42) were all based on incorporating the nonbinding motifs of IgG2 and IgG4. However, as mentioned earlier, incorporating natural motifs from IgG2 and IgG4 does not necessarily mean complete elimination of binding. In fact, it was recognized that IgG2 and IgG4 can lead to unwanted side effects, presumably caused by residual interactions with FcγRIIA (H131) and FcγRI (43). It should be pointed out that complete removal of N-glycan greatly impaired binding to cellular FcγRs and C1q (44), without affecting the interaction with FcRn (37, 45). Therefore, an aglycosylated form of IgG2 may offer the best approach to "effector silent" antibodies (46). This is supported by the alemtuzumab study, which showed that the IgG4 subclass, despite the lack of ADCC in vitro, had cytolytic activities in humans, whereas the aglycosylated form had neither in vitro nor in vivo cytolytic activities (13, 14).

In addition to optimizing the binding to FcγRs selectively, Fc mutations were also introduced to increase binding to FcRn at acidic pH, but not at neutral pH, thereby enhancing the recycling of IgG from the endosomes back to the circulation. The affinities of therapeutic IgGs and Fc-containing proteins for FcRn at pH 6.0 were shown to be closely correlated with their serum half-lives from clinical studies (47). One well-characterized Fc mutant with enhanced binding to FcRn has the triple mutations YTE (M252Y/S254T/T256E) introduced into the Fc portion of an anti-RSV monoclonal antibody, resulting in 10-fold increase in binding to human and monkey FcRn at pH 6.0 but not pH 7.4. This translates to a fourfold improvement in serum half-life in monkeys (48). With human FcRn knock-in mice being commercially available now, serum half-life of therapeutic antibody candidates can be compared conveniently in this surrogate host (49).

It should be noted that FcRn, while primarily known as a neonatal receptor and a protective receptor for IgG, can also be exploited to mediate immune functions against infections. Its expression is not restricted to endothelial and epithelial cells, but also found in human monocytes and dendritic cells. FcRn on these immune cells can translocate to nascent phagosomes, thereby facilitating IgG-mediated bacterial phagocytosis (50).

Fc Sialylation

High levels of sialylation of the Fc glycans in IgGs are associated with reduced binding to FcγRIIIA on NK cells, resulting in lower ADCC both in vitro (51) and in an in vivo model of immune thrombocytopenia (52). However, it is not clear whether this is entirely due to lower-affinity binding to FcγRIIIA specifically, or also partly due to lower binding to cell surface antigens in general, because many cell surface antigens and receptors have terminal sialic acids (51). What is certain is that the effect of sialylation on FcγR binding was independent of the 2,3- and 2,6-linkage of the sialic acid to the penultimate galactose on the complex biantennary N-linked glycan (52).

The 2,6-linkage, however, is definitely responsible for the anti-inflammatory activity of intravenous immunoglobulin treatment, which has been widely used to treat autoimmune diseases such as immune thrombocytopenia, rheumatoid arthritis, and systemic lupus erythematosus. Interestingly, the receptor responsible for the binding of 2,6-sialylated IgG is not one of the canonical FcγRs, but a C-type lectin receptor DC-SIGN on dendritic cells, resulting in the secretion of soluble anti-inflammatory mediators that increase surface expression of FcγRIIB on macrophages found at the site of inflammation (53). Subsequent cross-linking of FcγRIIB and activating FcγRs on the macrophage by the autoantibody in the immunocomplex results in inhibition of macrophage activation, which accounts for the anti-inflammatory activity of intravenous immunoglobulin. Therefore, enhancing the 2,6-linkage sialylation of IgG may be an effective way of increasing anti-inflammatory activity of therapeutic antibodies, e.g., in the treatment of infectious diseases where controlling inflammation is of paramount importance. It is interesting to note that, despite that only 5%

of the total serum IgG is fully sialylated, innate IgGs are generally anti-inflammatory in the steady state; the extent of sialylation is reduced in the course of an antigen-specific immune response so that the IgGs become more proinflammatory (54).

Aglycosylated Fc

Production of full-length antibodies has been done exclusively in eukaryotic cells because of their complex tetrameric structure and the posttranslational glycosylation critical for effector functions. The demonstration that heavy and light chains can be efficiently secreted and assembled in the *Escherichia coli* periplasm paved the way to an inexpensive method for the manufacture of therapeutic antibodies, especially for treatment in which effector functions are not desirable (55).

Aglycosylated antibodies retain binding to FcRn (37) and have been shown to have normal pharmacokinetic profiles in the clinic (56). If effector functions are desirable, point mutations can be readily introduced to restore FcγR and complement binding, and, better still, selectively engage certain FcγRs to achieve a more favorable A/I ratio (56, 57, 58), especially for the treatment of certain infectious diseases in which enhancing phagocytosis is important.

HUMANIZATION

The key factor to reducing the inherent immunogenicity of a product candidate is to make the therapeutic monoclonal antibody as similar as possible to naturally occurring human immunoglobulin sequences without losing the changes that result in the desired functional properties.

Humanized antibodies are antibodies from non-human species whose amino acid sequences have been changed to improve their similarity to antibody variants produced naturally in humans. Before rodent antibodies can be used in clinical application, it is essential to humanize them to decrease their immunoge-

nicity and increase their activity in the human immune system.

Antibody humanization comprises proven strategies for lessening the immunogenicity of well-characterized mAbs from animal sources (commonly mice) and for ameliorating their activation of the effector functions of the human immune system, thus producing clinical diagnostics and therapeutics. To overcome the immunogenicity triggered by non-human biologics, approaches such as the development of hybridomas and B-cell cloning from antibody-secreting cells from human peripheral blood and the production of human antibody repertoires in transgenic mice or on the surface of different display systems have emerged as platforms for engineering fully human therapeutic antibodies. However, because there are neither royalties nor license fees attached to the use of the hybridoma technology, the development of animal (mainly mouse) monoclonal antibodies as therapeutics remains a very attractive alternative providing that they are humanized to translate high-quality non-human antibodies to the clinic.

CDR Grafting: Standard Technology

In the past 25 years, multiple strategies for the humanization of mAbs have been reported in the literature. However, complementarity determining region (CDR) grafting onto a homologous (high-sequence homology) human antibody framework (acceptor) remains the most utilized technique for mAb humanization (59). Strict CDR grafting usually results in significant to complete loss of antigen recognition by the acceptor antibody. This problem can be resolved by backmutating critical framework sites on the acceptor to the corresponding amino acid residues in the donor sequence. These critical framework residues for back-mutation are selected from the wealth of published structural data on antibodies and/ or from the homology-modeled structure of the mouse Fv sequence that reveals the framework positions important for maintaining the integrity of the Ig fold or for supporting the conformation of the CDR (canonical residues). Figure 1 describes the main decision-making points during the CDR-grafting process and their evolution over the years. CDR grafting guided by molecular modeling is a well-validated approach that has been instrumental for the development of several FDA-approved antibodies, such as Tysabri (60) and Actemra (61). For a detailed description of the standard technology, see review by Leger and Saldanha (62).

Alternative Approaches

Veneering or Resurfacing
It was proposed by Padlan (63) that murine variable domains could be veneered to reduce their antigenicity. Veneering, also known as resurfacing, is a technique whereby the exposed framework residues are replaced by amino acids found at corresponding positions in human antibody sequences. Although many antibodies have been humanized by variable domain resurfacing, to our knowledge, no clinical studies with these antibodies have been published until now.

Grafting of Abbreviated CDRs Containing SDRs
CDR-grafted humanized antibodies carry xenogeneic CDRs which may evoke antivariable region, including anti-idiotypic, responses. Not all the CDR residues of a murine antibody are essential for antigen binding; this rationale comes from a comprehensive analysis of the three-dimensional structures of the antibody

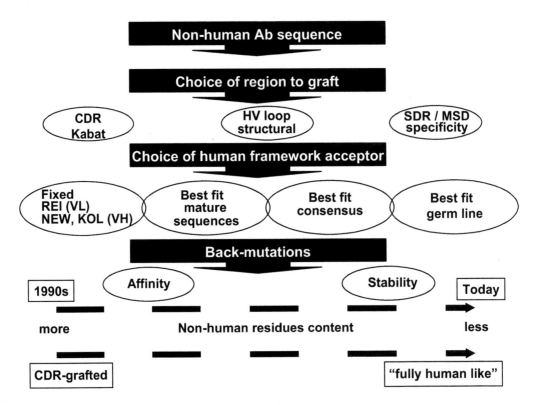

FIGURE 1 Flow chart describing the main decision-making points and their evolution over the years, in a typical CDR-grafting protocol. CDR, complementarity-determining region; HV, hypervariable loops; SDR, specificity-determining regions; MSD, minimum specificity determinant. REI, NEW, and KOL are light or heavy variable region sequences derived from human myeloma cell lines. doi:10.1128/microbiolspec.AID-0007-2012.f1

combining site where it was suggested that only 20 to 33% of the CDR residues are critical in the antigen-antibody interaction (64). These residues, located in the regions of high variability and most likely unique to each antibody, are designated as specificity-determining residues (SDRs). A new approach to the humanization of antibodies, therefore, was based on grafting only the SDRs of a xenogeneic antibody into the human antibody frameworks. The immunogenicity of an antibody therefore could be reduced by transplanting only those parts of the CDRs that contain the SDRs. The "abbreviated" CDRs have been defined (65) as the boundaries of the potential SDRs in various antigen combining sites.

Superhumanization

This humanization strategy is based on structural homologies between mouse and human CDRs and essentially ignores the frameworks. The first step of this CDR-grafting method is to identify human germ line V genes that in combination have the same canonical structure class as the mouse antibody to be humanized. Within that matching subset, typically a half-dozen genes from 44 functional VH or 41 functional VL genes in the human genome, H and L chain gene segments are picked whose CDRs have the best residue-to-residue homology to the mouse antibody. In the selected sequences, the remaining nonhomologous CDR residues are simply converted to the mouse antibody sequence. mAbs constructed by this strategy retain the ability to bind antigen, and, because they are CDR grafted in a way that minimizes deviation from human sequences, such Abs are called "superhumanized" (66).

Because the choice of the human frameworks is driven by the sequence and structure of the CDRs, this strategy has the potential to generate humanized antibodies that retain good binding to their cognate antigen. However, the general applicability of such a framework-ignoring strategy is uncertain since (i) favorable conformation(s) of a given CDR can be uniquely dependent on some specific source framework residues (canonical residues), and (ii) particular source framework residues may, in some cases, actively participate in direct interactions with the antigen as has been observed in certain antigen/antibody complexes.

Human String Content Optimization

Recently, Lazar et al. (67) have introduced a new method of humanization based on a novel and immunologically relevant metric of antibody humanness, termed human string content, that quantifies a sequence at the level of potential major histocompatibility complex/T-cell epitopes. Human identity is defined as the number of total "human 9-mers," which is an exact count of 9-mer stretches in the Fv that perfectly match any one of the corresponding stretches of nine amino acids in their set of functional human germ line sequences. Human 9-mer content is used as a measure of T-cell tolerance (i.e., if a stretch of nine consecutive amino acids matches one of the human germ line segments, it is more likely that T cells will not recognize it because of developmental tolerance for the original human 9-mer). This approach utilizes the homology present in human germ line sequences to make murine-to-human substitutions that increase the human sequence content of the Fv.

Framework Shuffling and Human Framework Adaptation

Dall'Acqua et al. (68) describes a new humanization approach called "framework shuffling" that does not require any rational design or structural information and for which there is no need to design backmutations. In this method, a given non-human monoclonal antibody is humanized by synthesizing a combinatorial library comprising its six CDRs fused in frame to a pool of mixed and matched human germ line frameworks. These human frameworks encompassed all known heavy- and light-chain human germ line genes. Libraries were cloned into an M13-based phage expression vector. The primary screen consists of a single-point enzyme-linked immunosorbent assay using periplasmic extracts prepared from individual recombinant M13 clones.

Recently, an alternative to the FR shuffling, human framework selection, was described by Fransson et al. (69) as the first step of a new humanization method called human framework adaptation. In this method, the human germ line genes are selected based on sequence and structural considerations. This is followed by a second step of SDR optimization.

Combinatorial Library Approaches

Guided selection

An alternative method, guided selection, has been developed to convert murine antibodies into completely human antibodies with similar binding characteristics. This methodology was originally developed by Jespers et al. (70). In this method, mouse VH and VL domains are sequentially or in parallel replaced by human VH and VL domains, respectively, using phage selection to derive human antibodies with best affinity. A potential disadvantage of the guided selection approach is that shuffling one or both antibody chains can result in epitope drift (71). This can however be seen as an advantage for introducing minor but essential changes in specificity such as removing cross-reactivities to unwanted antigens (72). To maintain the epitope recognized by the source non-human antibody, CDRs can be conserved. In this alternative method, one or both non-human CDR3s are commonly retained since they usually play a critical role in the recognition of the antigen.

Combinatorial Library Strategy

Rosok et al. (73), using a combinatorial approach and colony lift as selection method, have described a general antibody-engineering strategy that combines elements of structure-based approaches with in vitro evolution strategies to address the difficulty of maintaining antibody binding activity following humanization. More recently, also using the combinatorial approach but phage display as selection method, Rader et al. (74) and

Nishibori et al. (75) humanized a rabbit and chicken antibody, respectively.

Concluding Remarks on Humanization

There is no simple correlation between sequence humanness and immune response, as illustrated by the virtual absence of immunogenicity for the CDR-grafted humanized antibody trastuzumab and the 5 to 89% neutralizing response rate in a subset of patients, which varies depending on the disease and the therapy, to the fully human mAb adalimumab (Humira) (76). Many factors in addition to protein sequence can affect immunogenicity, such as dose and administration parameters (route, duration, and frequencies, as well as target-specific effects), but one of the most critical factors is the biophysical properties of the final molecule (77). These properties should be carefully monitored during the humanization process.

To conclude, we propose that a mixing and matching of techniques could be used in future protocols to take into consideration all the different aspects of humanization that we considered above with the ultimate goal of engineering fully human monoclonal antibodies. Such an attempt has recently been reported by Bernett et al. (78). Starting from the source murine variable regions of three currently marketed mAbs targeting CD25 (daclizumab), vascular endothelial growth factor (bevacizumab), and tumor necrosis factor alpha (infliximab), they generated "fully human" antibodies. All three engineered mAbs had levels of sequence humanness comparable to other fully human mAbs and yet maintained antigen binding and in vitro activity comparable to the three marketed drugs.

AFFINITY MATURATION

The antibody leads resulting from the discovery efforts meet established criteria regarding affinity and specificity. Affinity to the target molecule defines the future monoclonal antibody drug's efficacy and influences the drug dose required to obtain the desired effectiveness. A key requirement during antibody development is therefore to engineer a molecule with sufficiently high affinity to guarantee effective occupancy over prolonged periods. On one hand, for neutralization of soluble antigens, like cytokines, or viruses, the neutralization efficiency seems to be well correlated with the binding affinity. On the other hand, the assessment of affinity goals for antibodies against membrane receptors is often challenging.

In Vivo Affinity Maturation

The affinities of antibodies obtained in vivo tend to fall within characteristic ranges constrained by biological requirements imposed during the ontogeny of B cells. Specific antigen recognition by a surface antibody on a B cell, followed by endocytosis, leads to efficient antigen presentation (79), initiating cytokine release, B- and T-cell proliferation and differentiation, somatic hypermutation, and so on. Foote and Eisen (80, 81) argued that the residence time of an antigen complexed to a B-cell surface antibody would constrain the dissociation rate constant (k_{off}) selectable in vivo. The essence of their proposal was that antibody-antigen complexes with lifetimes much longer than the time necessary for uptake would all be processed equally well, hence, could not be distinguished. This idea of an intrinsic affinity ceiling for the selection of antibodies generated in vivo was supported by the result of a study by Batista and Neuberger (82). To study how signaling and antigen presentation through B-cell receptors depend on antigen/B-cell receptor affinity, lysozyme-specific B-cell transfectants were challenged with mutated lysozymes differing in their binding kinetics. The results of their study confirmed the predicted ceiling value for K_a in the order of 10^{10} M^{-1} (K_d of 100 pM) proposed by Foote and Eisen. This, of course, does not imply that antibodies with affinities greater than 100 pM cannot be obtained; rather, there is unlikely to be actual selection in favor of mutations that take affinities beyond this value. This prediction of an in vivo affinity ceiling has been frequently challenged. Indeed, with the use of transgenic mice producing fully human antibodies, the generation of antibodies with subnanomolar affinities (less than 10 pM) has frequently been reported (83). The existence of an in vivo generated antibody to interleukin-8 with a subpicomolar affinity (610 fM) has also been reported (84). This confirms that, by using efficient antibody generation procedures to screen a larger proportion of the available immune repertoire in hyperimmune animals, it is possible to isolate antibodies with exceptionally high affinities well beyond the proposed affinity ceiling.

Generation of high-affinity antibody against T cell-dependent antigen has also been described in germinal center-associated DNA primase gene-transgenic C57BL/6 mice (Ganp^{Tg}). Recent data suggest that germinal center-associated DNA primase may serve as an essential link required to transport activation-induced cytidine deaminase (AID), whose action during transcription is necessary for somatic hypermutation (SHM) (85), to actively transcribed immunoglobulin variable regions (86). These Ganp^{Tg} mice generate exceptionally high-affinity monoclonal antibodies against nitrophenyl-hapten, HIV-1 (V3 peptide)-epitope (87) and SARS-CoV-epitope ($K_d > 10^{-11}$ M) (86). These mice develop Hodgkin-like lymphomas of non-T and non-B surface phenotype with multiple mutations at immunoglobulin variable heavy chain region genes (88). Custom production of antibodies using these mice is offered by Trans Genic Inc.

In Vitro Mutagenesis, Display, and Selection

In vitro mutagenesis remains one of the most commonly used and widely accepted strategies for affinity maturating antibodies to the nanomolar (89), picomolar (90), or even femtomolar (91) range. In vitro antibody display technologies, such as phage, yeast, and ribosome display, have been widely utilized to increase antibody affinity. There are many options for diversifying V genes for affinity maturation, including the random introduction of mutations, for example, by error-prone PCR, CDR mutagenesis using spiked oligonucleotides and chain shuffling. These different strategies have been reviewed extensively (92, 93). Here we are going to describe some alternative and new developments for in vitro affinity maturation of antibodies.

In Vitro Affinity Maturation by Somatic Hypermutation

The genetic diversity created by the immune system is so large that, for nearly every foreign antigen, an antibody can be generated to bind it. After combinatorial rearrangement of gene segments, the antibody variable region is mutated at a rate orders of magnitude greater than the spontaneous mutation rate. This occurs when activated B cells encounter antigen and is termed immunoglobulin (Ig) SHM. AID is essential for the initiation of SHM in B cells by the deamination of cytidine residues directly in Ig genes (94). To achieve this, AID is targeted to V-region DNA sequences, termed hotspots (e.g., WRCH) that result in mutations and amino acid substitutions, which are frequently in positions biased to modulate antigen binding (95). Expression of AID alone has been shown to be sufficient to reproduce the salient features of SHM in both B cells (96, 97) and other mammalian cells (98). However, these cell lines are difficult to transfect at efficiencies suitable for use with diverse libraries. Nevertheless, the potential of using SHM in vitro has been apparent since Cumbers et al. (99) were able to evolve the endogenous IgM in Ramos cells to recognize streptavidin with an apparent affinity of 11 nM after 19 rounds of fluorescence-activated cell sorting; demonstrating that hypermutating cell lines can be used for iterative maturation of antibodies in vitro (99). More recently, Bowers et al. (100) have developed a novel approach where, by coupling in vitro SHM with mammalian display, they were

able to affinity mature an antibody to human β-nerve growth factor, as full-length, glycosylated IgGs, to low pM K_d.

Affinity Maturation of Antibody by Mammalian display

Problems with protein folding, posttranslational modification, and codon usage still limit the number of improved antibodies that can be obtained by display of antibodies on the surface of microorganisms (phage, bacteria, and yeast). An ideal system would select and improve antibodies in a mammalian cell environment where they are naturally made. Ho et al. have described a system to display single-chain anti-CD22 Fv fragments on human embryonic kidney 293T cells (101). In a proof-of-concept experiment, cells expressing a rare mutant antibody with higher affinity were enriched 240-fold by a single-pass cell sorting from a large excess of cells expressing wild-type antibody with a slightly lower affinity. Furthermore, they successfully obtained a highly enriched mutant with increased binding affinity for CD22 after a single selection of a combinatory library randomizing an intrinsic antibody hotspot. Standard transfection or electroporation methods, however, will typically introduce multiple copies of vectors into each cell. It is difficult to control the number of vectors introduced into each cell and, more importantly, the location of the integration into the host cell genome. Multiple copies of vectors and multiple integration sites in the host cell create a time-consuming process for screening and characterization. It also becomes extremely difficult to compare precisely the affinity and expression on the mammalian cell surface and isolate the desired cell clones efficiently. Zhou et al. described a novel mammalian full-length IgG display system successful in solving the critical issues of single specificity and relatively equal expression through the recombinase Flp-mediated single-copy integration. They demonstrated the application of their system in affinity maturation, identifying anti-OX40 ligand mutants of parental mAb40-L11 antibody with significantly improved neutralizing activity from a randomly mutagenized library (102). More recently, two other mammalian cell-displayed full-length antibody display systems that could be used for affinity maturation have been described (103, 104).

Affinity Maturation by Somatic Mutations and Computational Design

Recent advances in computational technologies combined with dramatic advances in high-throughput technology have the potential to make important contributions to the development of biological therapeutic antibodies (105). In the ideal case where high-resolution antibody structures or, preferably, antibody-antigen complex structures are available, determination of contact residues is straightforward, and this information can be applied to guide the maturation process (106). If experimentally determined structures are not available, but the paratope has been reliably mapped, a three-dimensional model of the variable domains can be constructed (107) and the residues affecting affinity can be projected onto it (108), thereby facilitating the selection of candidate positions for maturation. For review of recent progress in the field of computer-aided antibody development mainly focusing on antibody modeling, see Kuroda et al. (109). Improvements are still needed in all of the computational approaches; for example, understanding loop flexibility is particularly important in antibody design because large conformational changes can occur upon antigen binding, and affinity maturation can modulate both the conformation and dynamics of the CDR loops.

In terms of improvements of the properties in antibodies, such as immunogenicity and solubility, sequence-based methods have shown promise in antibody engineering (110, 111).

In Vitro Affinity Maturation without Display

The widespread use of phage and yeast display can be attributed largely to the fact that, when well implemented, very complex libraries can be screened relatively easily by panning or cell sorting, respectively. However, the "single-pot" phage display panning approach of large libraries has well-documented drawbacks with respect to selection bias toward variants that are better displayed or that allow faster growth of the expressing host cell (112, 113). The effects are magnified over the multiple rounds of selection and amplification, so that useful candidates may be lost, if they do not also compete well in these therapeutically irrelevant selection criteria. In addition, it is impractical to generate and screen by display methods many dozens of mutagenic libraries simultaneously but individually, an approach that proved important in the present work. Finally, display methods generally have an insufficient dynamic range to allow reliable isolation of the tightest protein target binders when starting with an already tightly binding antibody. As an alternative to display methods, antibody variants can be tested in a clonal, well-based, high-throughput screening process with quantitative determination of properties to ensure selection of candidates with the best mix of desired characteristics.

Votsmeier et al. (91) describe an elegant and generic method to improve antibody affinities without phage or cell surface display. In their approach, they used clonal, quantitative, well-based high-throughput screening for selection of soluble Fab (fragment antigen binding) expression of the library variants and limited library diversification to CDRs only. In each library, two neighboring residues were fully diversified. The mutation pairs in each screening hit were deconvoluted to identify contributions from each individual residue change. In total, 33 double-NNK libraries were generated, encompassing all 62 CDR positions of adalimumab (114). Their multistep optimization approach includes a first "mutation gathering" round of library generation and screening, followed by rounds in which the gathered mutations are recombined. They applied their approach to the affinity maturation of antitumor necrosis factor (TNF) antibody adalimumab, which binds TNF with ~100 pM affinity, and achieved ~500-fold affinity improvement, resulting in femtomolar binding. With similar reasoning, adalimumab was previously subjected to affinity maturation by using a single-chain variable fragment (scFv) yeast display approach including diversity generation at every CDR residue position and recombination of the beneficial mutations (115). In comparison with Rajpal et al., the Votsmeier et al. process resulted in fewer mutations for a given affinity increase. Given the large flexibility in assay design of well-based screening, the approach described by Votsmeier et al. has clear applications to other antibody properties, such as stability, solubility, selectivity, species cross-reactivity, expression yield, receptor modulation, or cellular responses.

THE NEXT-GENERATION ANTIBODIES TO MEET FUTURE CHALLENGES

Despite mAbs having outstanding commercial success with 4 of the top 10 best-selling drugs in 2009 (116), they suffer from several shortcomings. First, the addressable target space appears to be limited, causing fierce competition. In oncology, for example, nine marketed products correspond to only six different targets (vascular endothelial growth factor, EGFR, Her2, CD20, CD33, and CD52). For autoimmune and inflammatory diseases, four TNFα-neutralizing mAbs have been marketed (infliximab, adalimumab, golimumab, and certolizumab PEGol) (117). The number of mAb launches validating new targets is limited to only a few per year, demonstrating that new therapeutic target discovery is an elusive and costly business. Another major drawback is that mAbs have relatively low clinical efficacy and are usually not effective as monotherapy in cancer. As a consequence of their large molecular weight and complex structure, mAbs do not penetrate tissues very well and need to be administered parenterally. In addition, manufacturing of mAbs is complex and costly.

Several "Next-Generation Antibody" technologies have been developed to overcome one or more of the liabilities mentioned above. The smaller size and less complex structure of antibody fragments and alternative scaffold binders are cheaper to produce and may have better tumor penetration (118). Antibody drug conjugates (ADCs), bispecific antibodies, and the glycoengineering of the Fc glycan mentioned above may result in antibodies with improved efficacy (119). However, all these technologies have one thing in common: they are still nascent and it remains to be shown that the innovation translates into clinical and commercial success.

Antibody Drug Conjugates

One approach to increase the efficacy of mAbs in the treatment of cancer and virally infected cells is the antibody drug conjugates (ADC) concept (120, 121). Because small-molecule cancer drugs often have issues with dose-limiting systemic toxicities, the concept of ADC is to use mAbs to target those compounds directly to the tumor. To this end, conjugated agents may include small-molecule drugs, toxins, radionuclides, proteins, peptides, and other classes (122). Although two radionuclide conjugates, Zevalin and Bexxar (123), have been marketed, neither of those molecules is a particular commercial success, and it appears that industry nowadays has regained interest for conjugation of small-molecule drugs to antibodies (124). The idea of using an antibody chemically linked to a cytotoxic small molecule to target a tumor is more than 25 years old, but the therapeutic index appeared to be an issue. Gemtuzumab ozogamicin (125), a conjugate of calicheamicin to a humanized anti-CD33 mAb, was released in 2000 but subsequently withdrawn because of production and safety concerns (126). Only recently, another ADC was launched, and some 20 are in the clinical pipeline (124). Brentuximab vedotin, a conjugate of an auristatin derivative to an anti-CD30 antibody (127), was developed by Seattle Genetics in collaboration with Millenium, and approved for the treatment of relapsed and refractory Hodgkin's lymphoma. Another advanced clinical candidate, T-DM1, which is a maytansinoid fusion with Roche Genentech's Trastuzumab, is currently in Phase 3 for Her2+ metastatic breast cancer (128). T-DM1 exploits the ADC technology developed by Immunogen, Seattle Genetics' major competitor. Both types of payloads, Seattle Genetics' auristatins and Immunogen's maytansinoids, are highly potent antimitotic agents that show intrinsic activity in proliferating cells.

To achieve an optimal ADC, several parameters need to be considered. In general, it is important to utilize a highly selective antibody directed against a cell surface receptor that is overexpressed on tumor cells relative to normal tissues to avoid unwanted side effects. If the toxin is active inside the cell, such as the tubulin blockers or DNA-methylating agents, the ADC needs to be internalized by the target cell after ligand binding and the toxin released to initiate the cytotoxic activity. The chemical linker connecting the small-molecule toxin and the antibody plays a critical role for every ADC concept, and cleavable and noncleavable linkers have been described. While noncleavable linkers release the toxin by degradation of the antibody in the lysosomal pathway, release of the payload from cleavable linkers is either driven by enzymatic activity or by acidic pH in the hypoxic environment inside a tumor (129).

On the CMC side, ADC appears to be particularly challenging (130). Chemical conjugation of drug-linker complexes to mAbs needs to be carefully controlled to guarantee product homogeneity. Depending on the chemistry utilized, several conjugations can take place at multiple sites of a single mAb molecule, and the number of toxins added needs to be optimized and controlled. In addition, conjugation of a drug-linker complex may change the CMC properties of the ADC relative to the parental antibody requiring more complex production processes and analytics. In summary, developing an ADC is challenging, and, thus, it is no surprise that

these medicines come along with a steep price tag. In 2011, Seattle Genetics announced that the treatment with brentuximab vedotin will cost $13,500 per dose with seven to nine doses per trial treatment (124).

Immunocytokine (ICK) can be considered another form of ADC with cytokine as a payload (131). As a recombinant antibody-cytokine fusion protein instead of a chemical conjugate, ICK does not have the production issues of a typical ADC. Also, its cytokine is not packaged in the ICK as an inactive "pro-drug," and hence it exerts its biological activity once in circulation. Therefore, the concept of ICK relies on the specific targeting by the antibody moiety to bring the potent cytokine moiety to the tumor site to activate the tumor-infiltrating immune cells, resulting in the induction of a long-term protective immune response. Similar to ADC, the specificity of the antibody is of utmost importance to minimize its side effects. For treatment of infectious diseases, the cytokine can be chosen for its proinflammatory/anti-inflammatory profile to suit the application. Furthermore, the cytokine can be further engineered to decrease systemic toxicity and increase the therapeutic index, as demonstrated by a low-toxicity IL-2 ICK (132).

Bispecific Antibodies

Combining mAbs with different mechanisms of action (MOAs) is another approach for improving the efficacy of mAbs, and is currently being explored in a number of clinical and preclinical programs. For example, different targets such as EGFR and insulin growth factor receptor can be combined to explore synergistic MOAs (133) or to suppress resistance mechanisms as described for EGFR and cMET (134).

Monoclonal antibody combinations are challenging from a development and marketing perspective, since each single antibody as well as the combination will likely require regulatory testing and approval from authorities such as the FDA and European Medicines Evaluation Agency, leading to delays and a significant increase in development costs. In addition, the interdependency of efficacy and pharmacokinetics needs to be carefully studied. Bispecific antibody (bsAb) technologies appear to be an attractive alternative, because they offer a solution to combine synergistic MOAs in a single entity. In addition, bsAbs open new MOAs as demonstrated by Micromet's BiTE (135), which physically links the effector cell to the target cell through a bridging mechanism that cannot be achieved by a combination of the two separate antibodies.

Although the bsAb concept provides a striking solution for the combination of different MOAs, production of these molecules turned out to be very challenging. Shortly after the invention of the mAb technology, Milstein and Cuello (136, 137) described the Quadroma technology for the production of bsAb which was essentially a hybrid of two hybridomas. Although scientifically very elegant, it became apparent that production in industrial scale was not feasible because of the complexity of the molecular species produced (138). Other early approaches included chemical cross-linking (139, 140), tandem fusions of ScFv or V domains (141, 142), or their fusion to the C terminus of heavy chains. Up to now, only one bsAb, the anti-EpCAM x anti-CD3 catumaxomab (143), has been approved in Europe for the treatment of malignant ascites. Catumaxomab is a rat/mouse chimeric IgG2a that is very immunogenic. Other bsAbs in advanced clinical development, such as the anti-CD19 x anti-CD3 blinatumomab (Micromet), are based on tandem fusions of scFvs and therefore do not display mAb effector functions or favorable pharmacokinetic properties such as a long serum half-life in humans.

A heterodimeric human Fc fusion retaining a long serum half-life and mAb-like effector functions is the ideal vehicle for engineering therapeutic bsAbs. Genentech's "knobs-into-holes" technology (144) offered a first technical solution by introducing different complementary mutations in the two CH3 domains that favor heterodimerization. Instead of designs based on steric considerations, heterodimerization could also be achieved by electrostatic steering (145). Recently, Davis et al. (146) designed strand-exchange engineered domains (SEED), a novel bsAb platform based on the engineering of the CH3 domain. SEED is based on a rational design strategy that combines structurally related and conserved sequences of human IgG and IgA CH3 domains. By alternating sequences derived from both CH3 domains, two distinct SEED protein chains (designated AG and GA) were generated, creating asymmetric interfaces with modified β-sheet structures that preferentially heterodimerize. Because CH3 domains drive the heterodimerization of immunoglobulin heavy chains, AG and GA chains expressed in the context of antibody heavy chains can be utilized to produce monovalent and monospecific or bivalent and bispecific antibody-like molecules.

Since light chain pairing to the heavy chain is random during the assembly of a bispecific antibody, there is a need for a technology that can direct the specific pairing of the free light chain to its cognate heavy chain. The Crossmab approach uses immunoglobulin domain crossover (147) to get around this, while some technologies screen for a common light chain for the two different Fabs (148), or use single variable domains to avoid the use of the light chain altogether (149). One approach succeeded to provide a completely natural antibody with bispecific targeting by screening for a single Fv that can bind two different antigens. This "two-in-one" antibody uses an Fv variant of the antibody trastuzumab that interacts with both Her2 and vascular endothelial growth factor (150). On the other hand, the dual variable domains-Ig approach covalently links the two VLs of different specificities, which then pair up with the two cognate VHs also similarly linked, thus creating the two variable domains of different specificities in tandem (151).

In the development and design of the heterodimeric molecules, special care has to be taken so that the resulting bispecific molecule bears the same biological properties as the parental IgG molecule. This includes long serum half-life, ADCC and CDC, as well as excellent biophysical properties such as high protein homogeneity, protein A binding, and thermal stability. In addition, it is important to evaluate the manufacturability of this new molecule, including expression levels, ease of purification, thermal stability, and long-term storage potential. Only a molecule that has passed all of these tests would be ready for incorporation into the therapeutic pipeline.

ACKNOWLEDGMENT

Conflicts of interest: We disclose no conflicts.

CITATION

Lo K-M, Leger O, Hock B. 2014. Antibody engineering. Microbiol Spectrum 2(1):AID-0007-2012

REFERENCES

1. **Rodriguez ME, van der Pol WL, Sanders LA, van de Winkel JG.** 1999. Crucial role of FcgammaRIIa (CD32) in assessment of functional anti-*Streptococcus pneumoniae* antibody activity in human sera. *J Infect Dis* **179:**423–433.
2. **Woof JM, Kerr MA.** 2004. IgA function—variations on a theme. *Immunology* **113:**175–177.
3. **Dechant M, Beyer T, Schneider-Merck T, Weisner W, Peipp M, van de Winkel JG, Valerius T.** 2007. Effector mechanisms of recombinant IgA antibodies against epidermal growth factor receptor. *J Immunol* **179:**2936–2943.
4. **Weisbart RH, Kacena A, Schuh A, Golde DW.** 1988. GM-CSF induces human neutrophil IgA-mediated phagocytosis by an IgA Fc receptor activation mechanism. *Nature* **332:**647–648.
5. **Lohse S, Derer S, Beyer T, Klausz K, Peipp M, Leusen JH, van de Winkel JG, Dechant M, Valerius T.** 2011. Recombinant dimeric IgA antibodies against the epidermal growth factor receptor mediate effective tumor cell killing. *J Immunol* **186:**3770–3778.
6. **Nimmerjahn F, Ravetch JV.** 2010. Antibody-mediated modulation of immune responses. *Immunol Rev* **236:**265–275.
7. **Noya FJ, Baker CJ, Edwards MS.** 1993. Neutrophil Fc receptor participation in phagocytosis of type III group B streptococci. *Infect Immun* **61:**1415–1420.
8. **Beenhouwer DO, Yoo EM, Lai CW, Rocha MA, Morrison SL.** 2007. Human immunoglobulin G2 (IgG2) and IgG4, but not IgG1 or IgG3, protect mice against Cryptococcus *neoformans infection.* *Infect Immun* **75:**1424–1435.
9. **Tucker SC, Casadevall A.** 2002. Replication of *Cryptococcus neoformans* in macrophages is accompanied by phagosomal permeabilization and accumulation of vesicles containing polysaccharide in the cytoplasm. *Proc Natl Acad Sci USA* **99:**3165–3170.
10. **Zebedee SL, Koduri RK, Mukherjee J, Mukherjee S, Lee S, Sauer DF, Scharff MD, Casadevall A.** 1994. Mouse-human immunoglobulin G1 chimeric antibodies with activities against *Cryptococcus neoformans.* *Antimicrob Agents Chemother* **38:**1507–1514.
11. **Schneider-Merck T, Lammerts van Bueren JJ, Berger S, Rossen K, van Berkel PH, Derer S, Beyer T, Lohse S, Bleeker WK, Peipp M, Parren PW, van de Winkel JG, Valerius T, Dechant M.** 2010. Human IgG2 antibodies against epidermal growth factor receptor effectively trigger antibody-dependent cellular cytotoxicity but, in contrast to IgG1, only by cells of myeloid lineage. *J Immunol* **184:**512–520.
12. **Isaacs JD, Clark MR, Greenwood J, Waldmann H.** 1992. Therapy with monoclonal antibodies. An in vivo model for the assessment of therapeutic potential. *J Immunol* **148:**3062–3071.
13. **Isaacs JD, Wing MG, Greenwood JD, Hazleman BL, Hale G, Waldmann H.** 1996. A therapeutic human IgG4 monoclonal antibody that depletes target cells in humans. *Clin ExpImmunol* **106:**427–433.
14. **Isaacs JD.** 2001. From bench to bedside: discovering rules for antibody design, and improving serotherapy with monoclonal antibodies. *Rheumatology* **40:**724–738.
15. **Wypych J, Li M, Guo A, Zhang Z, Martinez T, Allen MJ, Fodor S, Kelner DN, Flynn GC, Liu YD, Bondarenko PV, Ricci MS, Dillon TM, Balland A.** 2008. Human IgG2 antibodies display disulfide-mediated structural isoforms. *J Biol Chem* **283:**16194–16205.
16. **Dillon TM, Ricci MS, Vezina C, Flynn GC, Liu YD, Rehder DS, Plant M, Henkle B, Li Y, Deechongkit S, Varnum B, Wypych J, Balland A, Bondarenko PV.** 2008. Structural and functional characterization of disulfide isoforms of the human IgG2 subclass. *J Biol Chem* **283:**16206–16215.
17. **Lo KM, Zhang J, Sun Y, Morelli B, Lan Y, Lauder S, Brunkhorst B, Webster G, Hallakou-Bozec S, Doaré L, Gillies SD.** 2005. Engineering a pharmacologically superior form of leptin for the treatment of obesity. *Protein Eng Des Sel* **18:**1–10.

18. **Tan LK, Shopes RJ, Oi VT, Morrison SL.** 1990. Influence of the hinge region on complement activation, C1q binding, and segmental flexibility in chimeric human immunoglobulins. *Proc Natl Acad Sci USA* **87:**162–166.

19. **Dela Cruz JS, Huang TH, Penichet ML, Morrison SL.** 2004. Antibody-cytokine fusion proteins: innovative weapons in the war against cancer. *Clin Exp Med* **4:**57–64.

20. **Klein JS, Bjorkman PJ.** 2010. Few and far between. How HIV may be evading antibody avidity. *PLoS Pathogens* **6:**1–6.

21. **Bruhns P.** 2012. Properties of mouse and human IgG receptors and their contribution to disease models. *Blood* **119:**5640–5649.

22. **van der Neut Kolfschoten M, Schuurman J, Losen M, Bleeker WK, Martínez-Martínez P, Vermeulen E, den Bleker TH, Wiegman L, Vink T, Aarden LA, De Baets MH, van de Winkel JG, Aalberse RC, Parren PW.** 2007. Anti-inflammatory activity of human IgG4 antibodies by dynamic Fab arm exchange. *Science* **317:**1554–1557.

23. **Labrijn AF, Buijsse AO, van den Bremer ET, Verwilligen AY, Bleeker WK, Thorpe SJ, Killestein J, Polman CH, Aalberse RC, Schuurman J, van de Winkel JG, Parren PW.** 2009. Therapeutic IgG4 antibodies engage in Fab-arm exchange with endogenous human IgG4 in vivo. *Nat Biotechnol* **27:**767–771.

24. **Shapiro RI, Plavina T, Schlain BR, Pepinsky RB, Garber EA, Jarpe M, Hochman PS, Wehner NG, Bard F, Motter R, Yednock TA, Taylor FR.** 2011. Development and validation of immunoassays to quantify the half-antibody exchange of an IgG4 antibody, natalizumab (Tysabri®) with endogenous IgG4. *J Pharm Biomed Anal* **55:**168–175.

25. **Rispens T, Meesters J, den Bleker TH, Ooijevaar-De Heer P, Schuurman J, Parren PW, Labrijn A, Aalberse RC.** 2013. Fc-Fc interactions of human IgG4 require dissociation of heavy chains and are formed predominantly by the intra-chain hinge isomer. *Mol Immunol* **53:**35–42.

26. **Li H, Sethuraman N, Stadheim TA, Zha D, Prinz B, Ballew N, Bobrowicz P, Choi BK, Cook WJ, Cukan M, Houston-Cummings NR, Davidson R, Gong B, Hamilton SR, Hoopes JP, Jiang Y, Kim N, Mansfield R, Nett JH, Rios S, Strawbridge R, Wildt S, Gerngross TU.** 2006. Optimization of humanized IgGs in glycoengineered *Pichia pastoris. Nat Biotechnol* **24:**210–215.

27. **Lifely MR, Hale C, Boyce S, Keen MJ, Phillips J.** 1995. Glycosylation and biological activity of CAMPATH-1H expressed in different cell lines and grown under different culture conditions. *Glycobiology* **5:**813–822.

28. **Umaña P, Jean-Mairet J, Moudry R, Amstutz H, Bailey JE.** 1999. Engineered glycoforms of an antineuroblastoma IgG1 with optimized antibody-dependent cellular cytotoxic activity. *Nat Biotechnol* **17:**176–180.

29. **Shinkawa T, Nakamura K, Yamane N, Shoji-Hosaka E, Kanda Y, Sakurada M, Uchida K, Anazawa H, Satoh M, Yamasaki M, Hanai N, Shitara K.** 2003. The absence of fucose but not the presence of galactose or bisecting N-acetylglucosamine of human IgG1 complex-type oligosaccharides shows the critical role of enhancing antibody-dependent cellular cytotoxicity. *J Biol Chem* **278:**3466–3473.

30. **Cartron G, Dacheux L, Salles G, Solal-Celigny P, Bardos P, Colombat P, Watier H.** 2002. Therapeutic activity of humanized anti-CD20 monoclonal antibody and polymorphism in IgG Fc receptor FcγRIIIa gene. *Blood* **99:**754–758.

31. **Treon SP, Hansen M, Branagan AR, Verselis S, Emmanouilides C, Kimby E, Frankel SR, Touroutoglou N, Turnbull B, Anderson KC, Maloney DG, Fox EA.** 2005. Polymorphisms in FcγRIIIA (CD16) receptor expression are associated with clinical response to rituximab in Waldenström's macroglobulinemia. *J Clin Oncol* **23:**474–481.

32. **Musolino A, Naldi N, Bortesi B, Pezzuolo D, Capelletti M, Missale G, Laccabue D, Zerbini A, Camisa R, Bisagni G, Neri TM, Ardizzoni A.** 2008. Immunoglobulin G fragment C receptor polymorphisms and clinical efficacy of trastuzumab-based therapy in patients with HER-2/neu-positive metastatic breast cancer. *J Clin Oncol* **26:**1789–1796.

33. **Bibeau F, Lopez-Crapez E, Di Fiore F, Thezenas S, Ychou M, Blanchard F, Lamy A, Penault-Llorca F, Frébourg T, Michel P, Sabourin JC, Boissière-Michot F.** 2009. Impact of FcγRIIa-FcγRIIIa polymorphisms and *KRAS* mutations on the clinical outcome of patients with metastatic colorectal cancer treated with cetuximab plus irinotecan. *J Clin Oncol* **27:**1122–1129.

34. **Kumpel BM.** 2007. Efficacy of RhD monoclonal antibodies in clinical trials as replacement therapy for prophylactic anti-D immunoglobulin: more questions than answers. *Vox Sang* **93:**99–111.

35. **Peipp M, Lammerts van Bueren JJ, Schneider-Merck T, Bleeker WW, Dechant M, Beyer T, Repp R, van Berkel PH, Vink T, van de Winkel JG, Parren PW, Valerius T.** 2008. Antibody fucosylation differentially impacts cytotoxicity mediated by NK and PMN effector cells. *Blood* **112:**2390–2399.

36. **Mori K, Iida S, Yamane-Ohnuki N, Kanda Y, Kuni-Kamochi R, Nakano R, Imai-Nishiya H, Okazaki A, Shinkawa T, Natsume A, Niwa R, Shitara K, Satoh M.** 2007. Non-fucosylated

therapeutic antibodies: the next generation of therapeutic antibodies. *Cytotechnology* **55**:109–114.

37. **Shields RL, Namenuk AK, Hong K, Meng YG, Rae J, Briggs J, Xie D, Lai J, Stadlen A, Li B, Fox JA, Presta LG.** 2001. High resolution mapping of the binding site on human IgG1 for FcγRI, FcγRII, FcγRIII, and FcRn and design of IgG1 variants with improved binding to the FcγR. *J Biol Chem* **276**:6591–6604.

38. **Nimmerjahn F, Ravetch JV.** 2005. Divergent immunoglobulin G subclass activity through selective Fc receptor binding. *Science* **310**:1510–1512.

39. **Lazar GA, Dang W, Karki S, Vafa O, Peng JS, Hyun L, Chan C, Chung HS, Eivazi A, Yoder SC, Vielmetter J, Carmichael DF, Hayes RJ, Dahiyat BI.** 2006. Engineered antibody Fc variants with enhanced effector function. *Proc Natl Acad Sci USA* **103**:4005–4010.

40. **Armour KL, Clark MR, Hadley AG, Williamson LM.** 1999. Recombinant human IgG molecules lacking Fcγ receptor I binding and monocyte triggering activities. *Eur J Immunol* **29**:2613–2624.

41. **Mueller JP, Giannoni MA, Hartman SL, Elliott EA, Squinto SP, Mathis LA, Evans MJ.** 1997. Humanized porcine VCAM-specific monoclonal antibodies with chimeric IgG2/G4 constant regions block human leukocyte binding to porcine endothelial cells. *Mol Immunol* **34**:441–452.

42. **An Z, Forrest G, Moore R, Cukan M, Haytko P, Huang L, Vitelli S, Zhao JZ, Lu P, Hua J, Gibson CR, Harvey BR, Montgomery D, Zaller D, Wang F, Strohl W.** 2009. IgG2m4, an engineered antibody isotype with reduced Fc function. *MAbs* **1**:572–579.

43. **Labrijn AF, Aalberse RC, Schuurman J.** 2008. When binding is enough: nonactivating antibody formats. *Curr Opin Immunol* **20**:479–485.

44. **Tao MH, Morrison SL.** 1989. Studies of aglycosylated chimeric mouse-human IgG. Role of carbohydrate in the structure and effector functions mediated by the human IgG constant region. *J Immunol* **143**:2595–2601.

45. **Nimmerjahn F, Ravetch JV.** 2008. Fcγ receptors as regulators of immune responses. *Nat Rev Immunol* **8**:34–47.

46. **Jefferis R.** 2007. Antibody therapeutics: isotype and glycoform selection. *Expert Opin Biol Ther* **7**:1401–1413.

47. **Suzuki T, Ishii-Watabe A, Tada M, Kobayashi T, Kanayasu-Toyoda T, Kawanishi T, Yamaguchi T.** 2010. Importance of neonatal FcR in regulating the serum half-life of therapeutic proteins containing the Fc domain of human IgG1: a comparative study of the affinity of monoclonal antibodies and Fc-fusion proteins to human neonatal FcR. *J Immunol* **184**:1968–1976.

48. **Dall'Acqua WF, Kiener PA, Wu H.** 2006. Properties of human IgG1s engineered for enhanced binding to the neonatal Fc receptor (FcRn). *J Biol Chem* **281**:23514–23524.

49. **Petkova SB, Akilesh S, Sproule TJ, Christianson GJ, Al Khabbaz H, Brown AC, Presta LG, Meng YG, Roopenian DC.** 2006. Enhanced half-life of genetically engineered human IgG1 antibodies in a humanized FcRn mouse model: potential application in humorally mediated autoimmune disease. *Int Immunol* **18**:1759–1769.

50. **Vidarsson G, Stemerding AM, Stapleton NM, Spliethoff SE, Janssen H, Rebers FE, de Haas M, van de Winkel JG.** 2006. FcRn: an IgG receptor on phagocytes with a novel role in phagocytosis. *Blood* **108**:3573–3579.

51. **Scallon BJ, Tam SH, McCarthy SG, Cai AN, Raju TS.** 2007. Higher levels of sialylated Fc glycans in immunoglobulin G molecules can adversely impact functionality. *Mol Immunol* **44**:1524–1534.

52. **Anthony RM, Nimmerjahn F, Ashline DJ, Reinhold VN, Paulson JC, Ravetch JV.** 2008. Recapitulation of IVIG anti-inflammatory activity with a recombinant IgG Fc. *Science* **320**:373–376.

53. **Anthony RM, Wermeling F, Karlsson MC, Ravetch JV.** 2008. Identification of a receptor required for the anti-inflammatory activity of IVIG. *Proc Natl Acad Sci USA* **105**:19571–19578.

54. **Kaneko Y, Nimmerjahn F, Ravetch JV.** 2006. Anti-inflammatory activity of immunoglobulin G resulting from Fc sialylation. *Science* **313**:670–673.

55. **Simmons LC, Reilly D, Klimowski L, Raju TS, Meng G, Sims P, Hong K, Shields RL, Damico LA, Rancatore P, Yansura DG.** 2002. Expression of full-length immunoglobulins in *Escherichia coli*: rapid and efficient production of aglycosylated antibodies. *J Immunol Methods* **263**:133–147.

56. **Jung ST, Kang TH, Kelton W, Georgiou G.** 2011. Bypassing glycosylation: engineering aglycosylated full-length IgG antibodies for human therapy. *Curr Opin Biotechnol* **22**:858–867.

57. **Sazinsky SL, Ott RG, Silver NW, Tidor B, Ravetch JV, Wittrup KD.** 2008. Aglycosylated immunoglobulin G1 variants productively engage activating Fc receptors. *Proc Natl Acad Sci USA* **105**:20167–20172.

58. **Jung ST, Reddy ST, Kang TH, Borrok MJ, Sandlie I, Tucker PW, Georgiou G.** 2010. Aglycosylated IgG variants expressed in bacteria that selectively bind FcγRI potentiate tumor cell killing by monocyte-dendritic cells. *Proc Natl Acad Sci USA* **107**:604–609.

59. **Jones TP, Dear PH, Foote J, Neuberger MS, Winter G.** 1986. Replacing the complementarity-determining regions in a human antibody with those from a mouse. *Nature* **321**:522–525.

60. **Léger OJ, Yednock TA, Tanner L, Horner HC, Hines DK, Keen S, Saldanha J, Jones ST, Fritz LC, Bendig MM.** 1997. Humanization of a mouse antibody against human alpha-4 integrin: a potential therapeutic for the treatment of multiple sclerosis. *Hum Antibodies* **8:**3–16.

61. **Sato K, Tsuchiya M, Saldanha J, Koishihara Y, Ohsugi Y, Kishimoto T, Bendig MM.** 1994. Humanization of a mouse anti-human interleukin-6 receptor antibody comparing two methods for selecting human framework regions. *Mol Immunol* **31:**371–381.

62. **Leger O, Saldanha WJ.** 2012. Humanization of antibodies, p 1–23. *In* Wood CR (ed), Molecular Medicine and Medicinal Chemistry, vol **4**. *Antibody Drug Discovery*. Imperial College Press, London, United Kingdom.

63. **Padlan EA.** 1991. A possible procedure for reducing the immunogenicity of antibody variable domains while preserving their ligand-binding properties. *Mol Immunol* **28:**489–498.

64. **Padlan EA.** 1994. Anatomy of the antibody molecule. *Mol Immunol* **31:**169–217.

65. **Padlan EA, Abergel C, Tipper JP.** 1995. Identification of specificity-determining residues in antibodies. *FASEB J* **9:**133–139.

66. **Tan P, Mitchell DA, Buss TN, Holmes MA, Anasetti C, Foote J.** 2002. "Superhumanized" antibodies: reduction of immunogenic potential by complementarity-determining region grafting with human germline sequences: application to an anti-CD28. *J Immunol* **169:**1119–1125.

67. **Lazar GA, Desjarlais JR, Jacinto J, Karki S, Hammond PW.** 2007. A molecular immunology approach to antibody humanization and functional optimization. *Mol Immunol* **44:**1986–1998.

68. **Dall'Acqua WF, Damschroder MM, Zhang J, Woods RM, Widjaja L, Yu J, Wu H.** 2005. Antibody humanization by framework shuffling. *Methods* **36:**43–60.

69. **Fransson J, Teplyakov A, Raghunathan G, Chi E, Cordier W, Dinh T, Feng Y, Giles-Komar J, Gilliland G, Lollo B, Malia TJ, Nishioka W, Obmolova G, Zhao S, Zhao Y, Swanson RV, Almagro JC.** 2010. Human framework adaptation of a mouse anti-human IL-13 antibody. *J Mol Biol* **398:**214–231.

70. **Jespers LS, Roberts A, Mahler SM, Winter G, Hoogenboom HR.** 1994. Guiding the selection of human antibodies from phage display repertoires to a single epitope of an antigen. *Biotechnology (NY)* **12:**899–903.

71. **Kang AS, Jones TM, Burton DR.** 1991. Antibody redesign by chain shuffling from random combinatorial immunoglobulin libraries. *Proc Natl Acad Sci USA* **88:**11120–11123.

72. **Christensen PA, Danielczyk A, Ravn P, Larsen M, Stahn R, Karsten U, Goletz S.** 2009. Modifying antibody specificity by chain shuffling of V/V between antibodies with related specificities. *Scand J Immunol* **69:**1–10.

73. **Rosok MJ, Yelton DE, Harris LJ, Bajorath J, Hellström KE, Hellström I, Cruz GA, Kristensson K, Lin H, Huse WD, Glaser SM.** 1996. A combinatorial library strategy for the rapid humanization of anticarcinoma BR96 Fab. *J Biol Chem* **271:**22611–22618.

74. **Rader C, Ritter G, Nathan S, Elia M, Gout I, Jungbluth AA, Choen LS, Welt S, Old LJ, Barbas CF 3rd.** 2000. The rabbit antibody repertoire as a novel source for the generation of therapeutic human antibodies. *J Biol Chem* **275:**13668–13676.

75. **Nishibori N, Horiuchi H, Furusawa S, Matsuda H.** 2006. Humanization of chicken monoclonal antibody using phage-display system. *Mol Immunol* **43:**634–642.

76. **Radstake TR, Svenson M, Eijsbouts AM, van den Hoogen FH, Enevold C, van Riel PL, Bendtzen K.** 2009. Formation of antibodies against infliximab and adalimumab strongly correlates with functional drug levels and clinical responses in rheumatoid arthritis. *Ann Rheum Dis* **68:**1739–1745.

77. **De Groot AS, Scott DW.** 2007. Immunogenicity of protein therapeutics. *Trends Immunol* **28:**482–490.

78. **Bernett MJ, Karki S, Moore GL, Leung IW, Chen H, Pong E, Nguyen DH, Jacinto J, Zalevsky J, Muchhal US, Desjarlais JR, Lazar GA.** 2010. Engineering fully human monoclonal antibodies from murine variable regions. *J Mol Biol* **396:**1474–1490.

79. **Lanzavecchia A.** 1985. Antigen-specific interaction between T and B cells. *Nature* **314:**537–539.

80. **Foote J, Eisen HN.** 1995. Kinetic and affinity limits on antibodies produced during immune responses. *Proc Natl Acad Sci USA* **92:**1054–1056.

81. **Foote J, Eisen HN.** 2000. Breaking the affinity ceiling for antibodies and T cell receptors. *Proc Natl Acad Sci USA* **97:**10679–10681.

82. **Batista FD, Neuberger MS.** 1998. Affinity dependence of the B cell response to antigen: a threshold, a ceiling, and the importance of off-rate. *Immunity* **8:**751–759.

83. **Drake AW, Myszka DG, Klakamp SL.** 2004. Characterizing high-affinity antigen/antibody complexes by kinetic- and equilibrium-based methods. *Anal Biochem* **328:**35–43.

84. **Rathanaswami P, Roalstad S, Roskos L, Su QJ, Lackie S, Babcook J.** 2005. Demonstration of an in vivo generated sub-picomolar affinity fully

human monoclonal antibody to interleukin-8. *Biochem Biophys Res Commun* **334**:1004–1013.

85. Liu M, Duke JL, Richter DJ, Vinuesa CG, Goodnow CC, Kleinstein SH, Schatz DG. 2008. Two levels of protection for the B cell genome during somatic hypermutation. *Nature* **451**:841–845.

86. Maeda K, Singh SK, Eda K, Kitabatake M, Pham P, Goodman MF, Sakaguchi N. 2010. GANP-mediated recruitment of activation-induced cytidine deaminase to cell nuclei and to immunoglobulin variable region DNA. *J Biol Chem* **285**:23945–23953.

87. Sakaguchi N, Kimura T, Matsushita S, Fujimura S, Shibata J, Araki M, Sakamoto T, Minoda C, Kuwahara K. 2005. Generation of high-affinity antibody against T cell-dependent antigen in the Ganp gene-transgenic mouse. *J Immunol* **174**:4485–4494.

88. Fujimura S, Xing Y, Takeya M, Yamashita Y, Ohshima K, Kuwahara K, Sakaguchi N. 2005. Increased expression of germinal center-associated nuclear protein RNA-primase is associated with lymphomagenesis. *Cancer Res* **65**:5925–5934.

89. de Haard HJ, van Neer N, Reurs A, Hufton SE, Roovers RC, Henderikx P, de Bruïne AP, Arends JW, Hoogenboom HR. 1999. A large non-immunized human Fab fragment phage library that permits rapid isolation and kinetic analysis of high affinity antibodies. *J Biol Chem* **274**:18218–18230.

90. Schier R, McCall A, Adams GP, Marshall KW, Merritt H, Yim M, Crawford RS, Weiner LM, Marks C, Marks JD. 1996. Isolation of picomolar affinity anti-c-erbB-2 single-chain Fv by molecular evolution of the complementarity determining regions in the center of the antibody binding site. *J Mol Biol* **263**:551–567.

91. Votsmeier C, Plittersdorf H, Hesse O, Scheidig A, Strerath M, Gritzan U, Pellengahr K, Scholz P, Eicker A, Myszka D, Coco WM, Haupts U. 2012. Femtomolar Fab binding affinities to a protein target by alternative CDR residue co-optimization strategies without phage or cell surface display. *MAbs* **4**:341–348.

92. Wark KL, Hudson PJ. 2006. Latest technologies for the enhancement of antibody affinity. *Adv Drug Deliv Rev* **58**:657–670.

93. Lowe D, Wilkinson T, Vaughan TJ. 2012. Affinity maturation approaches for antibody lead optimization, p 85–119. *In* Wood CR (ed), Molecular Medicine and Medicinal Chemistry, vol 4. *Antibody Drug Discovery*. Imperial College Press, London, United Kingdom.

94. Maul RW, Gearhart PJ. 2010. AID and somatic hypermutation. *Adv Immunol* **105**:159–191.

95. Goodman MF, Scharff MD, Romesberg FE. 2007. AID-initiated purposeful mutations in immunoglobulin genes. *Adv Immunol* **94**:127–155.

96. Delker RK, Fugmann SD, Papavasiliou FN. 2009. A coming-of-age story: activation-induced cytidine deaminase turns 10. *Nat Immunol* **10**:1147–1153.

97. Kajita M, Okazawa T, Ikeda M, Todo K, Magari M, Kanayama N, Ohmori H. 2010. Efficient affinity maturation of antibodies in an engineered chicken B cell line DT40-SW by increasing point mutation. *J Biosci Bioeng* **110**:351–358.

98. Martin A, Scharff MD. 2002. Somatic hypermutation of the AID transgene in B and non-B cells. *Proc Natl Acad Sci USA* **99**:12304–12308.

99. Cumbers SJ, Williams GT, Davies SL, Grenfell RL, Takeda S, Batista FD, Sale JE, Neuberger MS. 2002. Generation and iterative affinity maturation of antibodies in vitro using hypermutating B-cell lines. *Nat Biotechnol* **20**:1129–1134.

100. Bowers PM, Horlick RA, Neben TY, Toobian RM, Tomlinson GL, Dalton JL, Jones HA, Chen A, Altobell L 3rd, Zhang X, Macomber JL, Krapf IP, Wu BF, McConnell A, Chau B, Holland T, Berkebile AD, Neben SS, Boyle WJ, King DJ. 2011. Coupling mammalian cell surface display with somatic hypermutation for the discovery and maturation of human antibodies. *Proc Natl Acad Sci USA* **108**:20455–20460.

101. Ho M, Nagata S, Pastan I. 2006. Isolation of anti-CD22 Fv with high affinity by Fv display on human cells. *Proc Natl Acad Sci USA* **103**:9637–9642.

102. Zhou C, Jacobsen FW, Cai L, Chen Q, Shen WD. 2010. Development of a novel mammalian cell surface antibody display platform. *MAbs* **2**:508–518.

103. Li CZ, Liang ZK, Chen ZR, Lou HB, Zhou Y, Zhang ZH, Yu F, Liu S, Zhou Y, Wu S, Zheng W, Tan W, Jiang S, Zhou C. 2012. Identification of HBsAg-specific antibodies from a mammalian cell displayed full-length human antibody library of healthy immunized donor. *Cell Mol Immunol* **9**:184–190.

104. Li F, Liu YH, Li YW, Ju Q, Chen L, Xie PL, Li YH, Li GC. 2012. Human anti-EGFL7 recombinant full-length antibodies selected from a mammalian cell-based antibody display library. *Mol Cell Biochem* **365**:77–84.

105. Reddy ST, Georgiou G. 2011. Systems analysis of adaptive immunity by utilization of high-throughput technologies. *Curr Opin Biotechnol* **22**:584–589.

106. Clark LA, Boriack-Sjodin PA, Eldredge J, Fitch C, Friedman B, Hanf KJ, Jarpe M, Liparoto SF, Li Y, Lugovskoy A, Miller S, Rushe M, Sherman

W, Simon K, Van Vlijmen H. 2006. Affinity enhancement of an in vivo matured therapeutic antibody using structure-based computational design. *Protein Sci* 15:949–960.

107. **Fontayne A, De Maeyer B, De Maeyer M, Yamashita M, Matsushita T, Deckmyn H.** 2007. Paratope and epitope mapping of the antithrombotic antibody 6B4 in complex with platelet glycoprotein Ibα. *J Biol Chem* 282:23517–23524.

108. **Fontayne A, Vanhoorelbeke K, Pareyn I, Van Rompaey I, Meiring M, Lamprecht S, Roodt J, Desmet J, Deckmyn H.** 2006. Rational humanization of the powerful antithrombotic anti-GPIbα antibody: 6B4. *Thromb Haemost* 96:671–684.

109. **Kuroda D, Shirai H, Jacobson MP, Nakamura H.** 2012. Computer-aided antibody design. *Protein Eng Des Sel* 25:507–522.

110. **Abhinandan KR, Martin AC.** 2007. Analyzing the "degree of humanness" of antibody sequences. *J Mol Biol* 369:852–862.

111. **David MP, Concepcion GP, Padlan EA.** 2010. Using simple artificial intelligence methods for predicting amyloidogenesis in antibodies. *BMC Bioinformatics* 11:79.

112. **Clackson T, Wells JA.** 1994. In vitro selection from protein and peptide libraries. *Trends Biotechnol* 12:173–184.

113. **Derda R, Tang SK, Li SC, Ng S, Matochko W, Jafari MR.** 2011. Diversity of phage-displayed libraries of peptides during panning and amplification. *Molecules* 16:1776–1803.

114. **Salfeld JG, Allen DJ, Hoogenboom HR, Kaymakcalan Z, Labkovsky B, Mankovich JA, McGuinness BT, Roberts AJ, Sakorafas P, Schoenhaut D, Vaughan TJ, White M, Wilton AJ.** 2003. *Human antibodies that bind human TNFα.* US Patent 6090382.

115. **Rajpal A, Beyaz N, Haber L, Cappuccilli G, Yee H, Bhatt RR, Takeuchi T, Lerner RA, Crea R.** 2005. A general method for greatly improving the affinity of antibodies by using combinatorial libraries. *Proc Natl Acad Sci USA* 102:8466–8471.

116. **Via MC.** 2009. *Monoclonal Antibodies: Pipeline Analysis and Competitive Assessment.* Cambridge Healthtech Institute, Needham, MA.

117. **Licastro F, Chiappelli M, Ianni M, Porcellini E.** 2009. Tumor necrosis factor-alpha antagonists: differential clinical effects by different biotechnological molecules. *Int J Immunopathol Pharmacol* 22:567–572.

118. **Gebauer M, Skerra A.** 2009. Engineered therapeutic scaffolds as next generation antibody therapeutics. *Curr Opin Chem Biol* 13:245–255.

119. **Beck A, Wurch T, Bailly C, Corvaia N.** 2010. Strategies and challenges for the next generation of theraputic antibodies. *Nat Rev Immunol* 10:345–352.

120. **Teicher BVA, Chati RVJ.** 2011. Antibody conjugate therapeutics: challenges and potential. *Clin Cancer Res* 17:6389–6397.

121. **Mayes S, Brown N, Illidge TM.** 2011. New antibody drug treatments for lymphoma. *Expert Opin Biol Ther* 11:623–640.

122. **Visiongain.** 2012. Next generation antibody therapies: pipeline and market 2011–2012. Visiongain Ltd., London, United Kingdom.

123. **Stasi R.** 2008. Gemtuzuman Ozogamicin: An anti-CD33 immunoconjugate for the treatment of acute myeloid leukemia. *Expert Opin Biol Ther* 8:527–540.

124. **Gualberto A.** 2012. Brentuximab Vedotin (SGN-35), an antibody-drug conjugate for the treatment of CD30-positive malignancies. *Expert Opin Investig Drugs* 21:205–216.

125. **Burris HA 3rd, Tibbitts J, Holden SN, Sliwkowski MX, Lewis Phillips GD.** 2011. Trastuzumab emtansine (T-DM1): a novel agent for targeting HER2+ breast cancer. *Clin Breast Cancer* 11:275–282.

126. **Alley SC, Okeley NM, Senter PD.** 2010. Antibody-drug conjugates: targeted drug delivery for cancer. *Curr Opin Chem Biol* 14:529–537.

127. **Hughes B.** 2010. Antibody-drug conjugates for cancer: poised to deliver? *Nat Rev Drug Discov* 9:665–667.

128. **Löwenberg B, Beck J, Graux C, van Putten W, Schouten HC, Verdonck LF, Ferrant A, Sonneveld P, Jongen-Lavrencic M, von Lilienfeld-Toal M, Biemond BJ, Vellenga E, Breems D, de Muijnck H, Schaafsma R, Verhoef G, Döhner H, Gratwohl A, Pabst T, Ossenkoppele GJ, Maertens J; Dutch-Belgian Hemato-Oncology Cooperative Group (HOVON); German Austrian AML Study Group (AMLSG); Swiss Group for Clinical Cancer Research Collaborative Group (SAKK).** 2010. Gemtuzumab ozogamicin as postremission treatment in AML at 60 years of age or more: results of a multicenter phase 3 study. *Blood* 115:2586–2591.

129. **Ducry L, Stump B.** 2010. Antibody-drug conjugates: linking cytotoxic payloads to monoclonal antibodies. *Bioconjugate Chem* 21:5–13.

130. **Lin K, Tibbitts J.** 2012. Pharmacokinetic considerations for antibody drug conjugates. *Pharm Res* 29:2354–2366.

131. **Gillies SD, Lan Y, Wesolowski JS, Qian X, Reisfeld RA, Holden S, Super M, Lo K-M.** 1998. Antibody-IL-12 fusion proteins are effective in SCID mouse models of prostate and colon carcinoma metastases. *J Immunol* 160:6195–6203.

132. **Gillies SD, Lan Y, Hettmann T, Brunkhorst B, Sun Y, Mueller SO, Lo K-M.** 2011. A low-toxicity

IL-2 based immunocytokine retains anti-tumor activity despite its high degree of IL-2 receptor selectivity. *Clin Cancer Res* **17:**3673–3685.

133. Lu D, Zhang H, Ludwig D, Persaud A, Jimenez X, Burtrum D, Balderes P, Liu M, Bohlen P, Witte L, Zhu Z. 2004. Simultaneous blockade of both the epidermal growth factor receptor and the insulin-like growth factor receptor signaling pathways in cancer cells with a fully human recombinant bispecific antibody. *J Biol Chem* **279:**2856–2865.

134. Stommel JM, Kimmelman AC, Ying H, Nabioullin R, Ponugoti AH, Wiedemeyer R, Stegh AH, Bradner JE, Ligon KL, Brennan C, Chin L, DePinho RA. 2007. Coactivation of receptor tyrosine kinases affects the response of tumor cells to targeted therapies. *Science* **318:**287–290.

135. Baeuerle PA, Reinhardt C. 2009. Bispecific T-cell engaging antibodies for cancer therapy. *Cancer Res* **69:**4941–4944.

136. Milstein C, Cuello AC. 1983. Hybrid hybridomas and their use in immunohistochemistry. *Nature* **305:**537–540.

137. Milstein C, Cuello AC. 1984. Hybrid hybridomas and the production of bi-specific monoclonal antibodies. *Immunology Today* **5:**299–304.

138. Carter P. 2001. Bispecific human IgG by design. *J Immunol Methods* **248:**7–15.

139. Brennan M, Davison PF, Paulus H. 1985. Preparation of bispecific antibodies by chemical recombination of monoclonal immunoglobulin G1 fragments. *Science* **229:**81–83.

140. Glennie MJ, McBride HM, Worth AT, Stevenson GT. 1987. Preparation and performance of bispecific F(ab' gamma)2 antibody containing thioether-linked Fab' gamma fragments. *J Immunol* **139:**2367–2375.

141. Atwell JL, Pearce LA, Lah M, Gruen LC, Kortt AA, Hudson PJ. 1996. Design and expression of a stable bispecific scFv dimer with affinity for both glycophorin and N9 neuraminidase. *Mol Immunol* **33:**1301–1312.

142. Huston JS, George AJ. 2001. Engineered antibodies take center stage. *Hum Antibodies* **10:**127–142.

143. Seimetz D, Lindhofer H, Bokemeyer C. 2010. Development and approval of the trifunctional antibody catumaxomab (anti-EpCAM x anti-CD3) as a targeted cancer immunotherapy. *Cancer Treat Rev* **36:**458–467.

144. Ridgway JB, Presta LG, Carter P. 1996. 'Knobs-into-holes' engineering of antibody CH3 domains for heavy chain heterodimerization. *Protein Eng* **9:**617–621.

145. Gunasekaran K, Pentony M, Shen M, Garrett L, Forte C, Woodward A, Ng SB, Born T, Retter M, Manchulenko K, Sweet H, Foltz IN, Wittekind M, Yan W. 2010. Enhancing antibody Fc heterodimer formation through electrostatic steering effects: applications to bispecific molecules and monovalent IgG. *J Biol Chem* **285:**19637–19646.

146. Davis JH, Aperlo C, Li Y, Kurosawa E, Lan Y, Lo K-M, Huston JS. 2010. SEEDbodies: fusion proteins based on strand-exchange engineered domain (SEED) CH3 heterodimers in an Fc analogue platform for asymmetric binders or immunofusions and bispecific antibodies. *Protein Eng Des Sel* **23:**195–202.

147. Schaefer W, Regula JT, Bähner M, Schanzer J, Croasdale R, Dürr H, Gassner C, Georges G, Kettenberger H, Imhof-Jung S, Schwaiger M, Stubenrauch KG, Sustmann C, Thomas M, Scheuer W, Klein C. 2011. Immunoglobulin domain crossover as a generic approach for the production of bispecific IgG antibodies. *Proc Natl Acad Sci USA* **108:**11187–11192.

148. Merchant AM, Zhu Z, Yuan JQ, Goddard A, Adams CW, Presta LG, Carter P. 1998. An efficient route to human bispecific IgG. *Nat Biotechnol* **16:**677–681.

149. Shen J, Vil MD, Jimenez X, Zhang H, Iacolina M, Mangalampalli V, Balderes P, Ludwig DL, Zhu Z. 2007. Single variable domain antibody as a versatile building block for the construction of IgG-like bispecific antibodies. *J Immunol Methods* **318:**65–74.

150. Bostrom J, Yu SF, Kan D, Appleton BA, Lee CV, Billeci K, Man W, Peale F, Ross S, Wiesmann C, Fuh G. 2009. Variants of the antibody herceptin that interact with HER2 and VEGF at the antigen binding site. *Science* **323:**1610–1614.

151. Wu C, Ying H, Grinnell C, Bryant S, Miller R, Clabbers A, Bose S, McCarthy D, Zhu RR, Santora L, Davis-Taber R, Kunes Y, Fung E, Schwartz A, Sakorafas P, Gu J, Tarcsa E, Murtaza A, Ghayur T. 2007. Simultaneous targeting of multiple disease mediators by a dual-variable-domain immunoglobulin. *Nat Biotechnol* **25:**1290–1297.

High-Throughput DNA Sequencing Analysis of Antibody Repertoires

20

SCOTT D. BOYD[1] and SHILPA A. JOSHI[1]

INTRODUCTION

New high-throughput DNA sequencing (HTS) technologies developed in the past decade have rapidly increased the scale of data collection for all aspects of human genetics (1, 2). The complex somatic gene rearrangements of immunoglobulin (Ig) and T-cell antigen receptors (TCRs) in the adaptive immune system are particularly appropriate targets for investigation using these new technologies. The antigen specificity of adaptive human immune responses and the storage of specific immunological memory depend on the sequences of the Ig and TCR gene rearrangements expressed by B cells and T cells. Until recently, the difficulty and cost of obtaining sequence data limited the kinds of immunological research questions that could be studied. Pioneering work examining dozens to hundreds of Ig rearrangements with Sanger sequencing has revealed some overall features of the repertoires of these receptors, while physical selection and sorting of B-cell populations of interest has led to the identification of antibodies specific for a variety of infectious agents and vaccine components. However, given that a single human body contains an estimated 10^{11} B cells representing, at a minimum, millions of distinct clonal populations, experiments using Sanger sequencing were underpowered to evaluate the full scale of antibody repertoires.

[1]Department of Pathology, Stanford University, Stanford, CA 94305.
Antibodies for Infectious Diseases
Edited by James E. Crowe, Jr., Diana Boraschi, and Rino Rappuoli
© 2015 American Society for Microbiology, Washington, DC
doi:10.1128/microbiolspec.AID-0017-2014

This chapter first reviews genetic features of Ig loci and the HTS technologies that have been applied to human repertoire studies, then discusses experimental design, data analysis choices in these experiments, and insights gained in immunological and infectious disease studies using these approaches.

ANTIBODY GENE REARRANGEMENTS

Antibodies in humans are protein complexes whose basic unit is a disulfide-linked pair of heavy chain proteins, each with an associated light chain (Fig. 1). The N-terminal regions of heavy and light chains arc highly variable in their sequences, and are the antigen-binding portions of the antibody. The C-terminal regions of the proteins are termed the constant regions. Light chains are of two types, kappa (IgK) or lambda (IgL), while heavy chains (IgH) are of five major isotypes (IgM, IgD, IgG, IgA, and IgE), with four subtypes of IgG and two subtypes of IgA. Developing B cells assemble the genes encoding the antigen-binding regions of their immunoglobulin heavy chains from germ line arrays of variable (V), diversity (D), and joining (J) gene segments, by first joining a D and J segment together, and then selecting a V segment to join to the newly generated D-J product. During joining, the ends of the gene segments are subject to exonuclease digestion, and nontemplated randomized bases (N bases) are added at the segment junctions. In the developing B cell, an initial attempt to rearrange the immunoglobulin heavy chain locus on one copy of chromosome 14 can potentially give rise to an out-of-frame product; if this happens, then the B cell attempts to rearrange the other copy of the locus. After a productive IgH is expressed, an analogous rearrangement of V and J segments at the kappa or lambda immunoglobulin light chain locus takes place. The mechanistic details and regulation of these events have been reviewed

elsewhere (3). The region of the antibody heavy or light chain structure encoded by the fusion of V, (D), and J segments forms a loop that is the most diverse region of the antibody and is termed the complementarity-determining region 3 (CDR3). CDR3 is often the most important portion of the antibody for binding to antigen, but two other loops (CDR1 and CDR2) encoded by the variable gene segment can also contribute significantly to antigen specificity.

The genetic complexity of the antibody repertoire in an individual's B cells prior to exposure to antigen derives from the combinatorial assembly of V, (D), and J segments, the diversification at the segment junctions encoding the CDR3 loops of the antibody heavy or light chain, and the pairwise combination of heavy and light chains. Earlier rough estimates of the potential number of different antibodies that can be generated by these mechanisms were greater than 10^{11} (4). Such figures are undoubtedly underestimates, because the theoretical number of unique heavy or light chains is limited only by the maximal length of the nontemplated junctional base sequences considered in the calculation. Antigen-stimulated B cells activate an additional program of antibody sequence diversification called somatic hypermutation that generates new point mutations throughout the rearranged V(D)J sequence, creating clonal offspring whose antibodies may possess increased binding affinity for the antigen. Rarer processes such as receptor editing contribute further mechanisms for antibody repertoire generation by enabling secondary rearrangements and replacement of V gene segments. At the level of human populations, additional genetic diversity of antibody repertoires results from allelic variants for immunoglobulin gene segments and structural variants within the immunoglobulin loci that delete or increase the copy number of particular gene segments.

Current understanding of the human germ line DNA sequence for the immunoglobulin

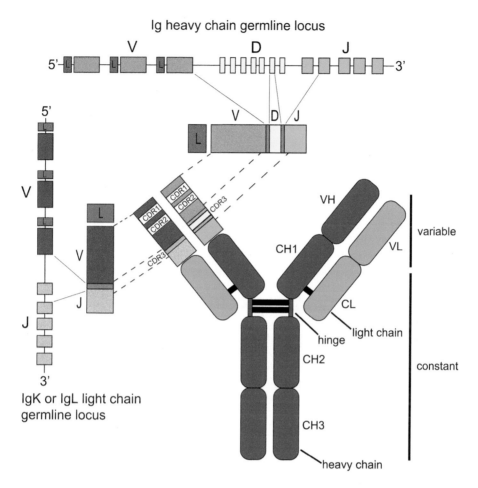

FIGURE 1 Antibody structure and genetic encoding. The germ line (unrearranged) genomic DNA configuration of the immunoglobulin heavy chain locus is depicted at the top of the figure, showing the tandem arrays of V, D, and J gene segments (not to scale). A germ line kappa or lambda light chain locus is depicted on the left-hand side, with unrearranged V and J segments. Stepwise rearrangement of the germ line DNA results in the joining of a heavy chain D and J gene segment, followed by joining of a V segment to the D-J product, to generate the DNA encoding the heavy chain variable region. In the process of rearrangement, the ends of the gene segments are subject to variable amounts of exonuclease digestion, and randomized nontemplated bases are added at the segment ends, to produce additional sequence diversity at the VDJ junctional region that encodes the complementarity-determining region 3 (CDR3) loop, which is often the region of the antibody heavy chain that has the greatest impact on antigen specificity. A similar process of V and J gene rearrangement with diversification of the VJ junction occurs in the light chain locus, to produce the rearranged light chain gene. The constant regions of the heavy and light chains (domains CH1, CH2, and CH3 for the heavy chain, and CL for the light chain) are encoded by downstream exons that are joined to the rearranged V (D)J gene by mRNA splicing. Disulfide bridges joining protein chains in the full antibody structure are shown with black line segments. doi:10.1128/microbiolspec.AID-0017-2014.f1

heavy chain locus, and the number of V, D, and J segments it contains, remains heavily indebted to the initial sequence generated by Matsuda et al. in 1998 (5). Recent human genome-

sequencing efforts have often been less helpful for evaluating immunoglobulin loci, in part, because of the widespread use of oligoclonal Epstein-Barr virus (EBV)-transformed B-cell lines with rearranged Ig genes as the source of DNA for sequencing, resulting in the loss of information about gene segments deleted during rearrangement, as well as the relatively shallow depth of sequencing performed in population-level studies (6). In contrast, HTS has very recently been used to study the germ line locus in particularly tractable human samples, such as cells from a haploid hydatidiform mole, and to survey the haplotypes in this locus in different human population groups (7). The curated sequences in the IMGT database (www.imgt.org) for the human IGH locus at 14q32 indicate that most humans, depending on their haplotypes, have 123 to 129 *IGHV* gene segments, of which 43 to 46 are able to form functional rearrangements; 27 *IGHD* gene segments (23 functional); and 9 *IGHJ* segments (6 functional) (8, 9). The IGK locus at 2p11 encodes 76 *IGKV* in most individuals (31 to 36 functional), and 5 *IGKJ* gene segments (5 functional), while the IGL locus at 22q11 contains 73 to 74 *IGLV* segments (29 to 33 functional) and 7 to 11 *IGLJ* segments (4 to 5 functional) (8, 9). Allelic and copy number variation in Ig loci in different human populations were identified in earlier literature, but the pace of identification of new variants has now accelerated, making it clear that the currently curated variants represent only a small sampling of the total variation that is likely to be present across all human groups (7, 10, 11, 12).

The genetic structure of V gene segments includes a small upstream exon encoding most of a leader peptide, followed by a short intron and a second exon encoding the rest of the leader peptide and the V segment itself. In the unrearranged human germ line loci, the V, D, and J regions are separated from each other by kilobases of sequence, and the constant regions, encoded by single exons (for kappa or lambda) or several exons (for the heavy chain isotypes) are located kilobases downstream of the J segments, with the exception of the lambda locus, where a few J segments are interspersed among the most upstream constant regions. The process of rearranging the genomic DNA at heavy and light chain loci to generate in-frame heavy and light chains results in a compact V(D)J gene that is approximately 400 bases in length.

Somatic hypermutation of human antibodies occurs primarily in the specialized microenvironments of secondary lymphoid tissues, where B cells have access to antigen, specialized dendritic and stromal cells, and T cells that stimulate B cells via soluble mediators and cell-cell contact (13). Human plasmablasts observed after acute antigenic stimulation such as influenza vaccination usually show mutation levels in the range of 5 to 15% in the *IGHV* segment, while memory B cells show somewhat lower mutation levels (14). In unusual circumstances such as chronic exposure to viral antigens in the perturbed immune systems of HIV-infected individuals, much higher mutation levels (over 30%) can be observed in some antibody lineages (15). Mutational events are targeted relatively precisely in a region extending from upstream of, or within, the leader sequence through the V(D)J rearrangement, and taper off in the intron separating the J segments from the constant regions (16, 17). Notably, leader sequences in some loci may be less mutated than the rest of the Ig gene rearrangement, as best documented in mouse kappa light chains (17).

HIGH-THROUGHPUT DNA SEQUENCING INSTRUMENTS

Soon after the completion of the first human genome draft sequence in 2001, a technological race between several different companies and academic laboratories led to the development of a handful of competing platforms for determining DNA sequences in a more highly parallel, miniaturized, and efficient manner than was possible with Sanger sequencing. Common features among these methods were the use of miniaturized microwell plates or flow cells that could capture DNA molecules at particular spatial positions, methods of generating locally amplified template from single DNA molecules for sequencing, and a method of detection of nucleotide sequence that could occur in parallel for thousands to millions of distinct templates at the same time. The platforms that have been most widely used for Ig sequencing in the published literature have been those from Roche/454, Illumina, and Ion Torrent. A brief overview of the features of these instruments is given below. Other promising technologies, including true single-molecule sequencing approaches, have been less widely used so far.

In brief, the Roche/454 and Ion Torrent methods spatially separate and amplify single-template molecules by limiting dilution of the template in aqueous solution followed by production of an aqueous-in-oil emulsion. The template is diluted so that less than one template molecule is present on average per aqueous droplet. The aqueous phase contains the enzymes, primers, nucleotides, and buffers for PCR, as well as capture beads to which the amplified template becomes attached. After PCR, the emulsion is broken and the beads are positioned in microfabricated wells of a plate. Both the Roche/454 and Ion Torrent platforms use a sequencing-by-synthesis approach in which reaction mixtures containing only one of the deoxyribonucleotide triphosphates (dATP, dCTP, dGTP, or dTTP) are sequentially used in cycles of extension of a DNA strand complementary to the template. In 454 sequencing, incorporation of one or more nucleotides during an extension step is detected by a coupled enzymatic reaction in the sequencing plate well, in which pyrophosphate liberated from the nucleotide triphosphate added to the growing DNA strand drives the generation of photons of light by luciferase enzyme (18). The Ion Torrent platform detects nucleotide incorporation during DNA synthesis via miniaturized ion sensors in the sequencing plate that detect the release of protons occurring upon nucleotide addition (19). In both the Roche/454 and Ion Torrent protocols, homo-

polymer tracts of a particular nucleotide are sequenced with decreased accuracy, because it is more difficult to distinguish between the levels of signal produced by, for example, 14 incorporation events compared with 15 incorporation events in a sequencing step. Error rates are discussed in greater detail below. Current versions of these instruments give approximately one million sequences with read lengths of over 500 bases in the case of Roche/454, and 10 million sequences of 100 bases for the Ion Torrent PGM. The majority of the published literature on HTS of immunoglobulin genes has used the Roche/454 methodology, but Roche has indicated that it is no longer developing the 454 platform and will not support it in the future.

In contrast, the Illumina platform, which has now become the dominant HTS method for most applications, performs template separation and amplification of diluted template DNA on the surface of a flow cell (20). The flow cell is functionalized with oligonucleotides that capture the template and prime "bridging PCR" amplifications that use linker sequences introduced at the ends of the template during library construction. The bridging PCR yields focal clusters of amplified template molecules that are covalently attached to the flow cell. The amplified clusters are then sequenced with cycles of single-base extension sequencing-by-synthesis. In this strategy, each nucleotide is labeled with a fluorophore that identifies the incorporated nucleotide and blocks further extension of the template once the nucleotide is added to the growing DNA strand. A mixture of all four nucleotide triphosphates is used in each cycle of synthesis. Nucleotide incorporation into each template cluster during each sequencing cycle can be detected by imaging the flow cell and detecting what fluorophore is present. Once the flow cell is imaged, the fluorescent labels are cleaved off and the next cycle of extension and imaging begins. Until recently, a disadvantage of the Illumina instruments was their relatively short read lengths (initially 35 bases), but continual improvements in the methodology have led to current instruments and kits that give total read lengths of sequence that are comparable to the those of the 454 platform. The Illumina MiSeq instrument can sequence approximately 15 million templates per run, yielding up to 300 bases of sequence from each end of the template molecules, while the HiSeq 2500 model can sequence 2 billion templates, reading 125 bases from each end of the template.

EXPERIMENTAL STRATEGIES FOR SEQUENCING Ig REPERTOIRES

Sequencing Ig V(D)J rearrangements in human samples is conceptually straightforward. As a result of the close juxtaposition of V, (D), and J gene segments following genomic rearrangement, short V(D)J PCR amplicons (<500 bp, excluding the lengths of sequencing instrument linkers and barcodes) can be amplified efficiently from genomic DNA or complementary DNA from samples containing B cells. The kilobases of sequence that separate the gene segments in the unrearranged genomic DNA prevent significant amplification from non-B-cell templates in the sample. The incorporation of oligomer nucleotide "barcodes" in the primers or linkers used in library preparation can be used for sample multiplexing in a single sequencing run with any of the HTS instruments, permitting samples to be sequenced together but allowing the sequencing data to be assigned back to the samples by sorting based on the unique sample barcodes. Beyond these similarities, a number of important experimental design choices influence the kinds of interpretation that can be reliably made from sequencing libraries generated by using different approaches, as detailed below.

Cell Populations

High-quality DNA sequencing libraries of V(D)J rearrangements can be produced from templates isolated from total leukocytes, peripheral blood mononuclear cells (PBMCs),

or any tissue containing B cells. In order to identify sequences that are derived from B cells that have undergone somatic mutation, the sequences in such libraries can be evaluated for the presence of mutated nucleotide positions in V, D, or J gene segments (21). However, a number of specialized B-cell subsets in humans, such as memory B cells, plasmablasts, transitional B cells, and suppressor B cells, among others, have been defined on the basis of cell surface receptors, intracellular protein expression, or other phenotypic features, and there can be additional experimental value added by using flow cytometry or other methods to sort out particular B-cell or plasma cell subsets of interest prior to generating libraries (14, 22, 23, 24). It is clear, however, that the cell subset definitions and the functions ascribed to them are subject to progressive refinement and revision over time in the immunological literature, meaning that comparisons of Ig repertoire data based on cell subsets should be made with caution unless identical protocols and definitions are used (22). As a practical matter, sorting of small cell subsets can also make it more difficult to isolate nucleic acids for sequencing with the use of standard methods and can require additional rounds of PCR to generate enough amplified material for accurate quantitation prior to sequencing. Another consideration in human studies is that sometimes samples that are precious because of the rarity of the clinical phenotype, pathogen exposure, or other immunological stimulus may only be available in the form of frozen nonviable cells or leukocyte- or PBMC-derived RNA or DNA, owing to the sample collection and storage protocols or resource limitations in clinical studies. In such cases, valuable data can still be obtained from total Ig repertoires without cell surface phenotype information, and antibody isotype expression and mutation status can be interpreted.

Targeted PCR versus 5′ RACE

The 5′ rapid amplification of cDNA ends (5′ RACE) for library preparation requires only a single primer to hybridize to a known region of the target mRNA. cDNA synthesis proceeds until the 5′ end of the target mRNA is reached, and then one of several approaches can be used to add a known, unrelated primer sequence to the 3′ end of the cDNA strand, permitting subsequent PCR amplification (25). This method has begun to be applied to generate Ig HTS libraries, and may be less subject to primer bias and multiplexed PCR artifacts that can result from using primers within the V, J, or constant regions, while also being better at amplifying heavily mutated Ig sequences where primer binding sites may be altered (26, 27). Limitations of 5′ RACE methods are the requirement for RNA as the starting material, precluding analysis of genomic DNA rearrangements, and more variable performance with RNA of suboptimal quality or limiting quantity. The alternative approach of using multiplexed primer mixtures targeting the V, D, J, or constant regions, and performing PCR from either cDNA or genomic DNA template, has been the predominant method used in the literature to date (Fig. 2). This method is subject to a few potential problems, including PCR amplification bias, as a result of different primer annealing efficiencies to particular gene segments; the need to select primers that can be multiplexed without producing off-target primer dimers or other artifacts; and potential loss of highly mutated sequences from sequencing libraries as a result of the somatic mutation preventing primer annealing. Selection of primers for human Ig rearrangements has focused on the framework (FR) regions FR1, FR2, and FR3, which are relatively less mutated than the CDR sequences in B cells that survive to be observed in human samples, likely because mutated framework regions that destabilize the antibody structure are not compatible with the persistence of the B cell in the body (28, 29, 30). Primers targeting the leader sequences have also been used in a number of publications, particularly those studying highly

mutated antibody lineages such as broadly neutralizing anti-HIV antibodies (31, 32).

Choice of Template

Ig sequencing libraries can be generated from genomic DNA template, typically with V-and J-segment primers, or from cDNA template using V-leader primers, internal V primers, J primers, or constant region primers (Fig. 2). In addition to the considerations related to potential effects of somatic mutation on primer binding, as outlined above, there are several other reasons to select either genomic DNA template, cDNA template, or both, depending on the goals of a particular experiment. One advantage of genomic DNA template is that it permits analysis of both productively rearranged Ig sequences that yield a protein product, as well as unproductively rearranged loci where a stop codon or reading frame incompatibility between the V segment and the downstream gene segments has been introduced during V(D)J rearrangement. While not giving rise to functional protein, the unproductive rearrangements provide a record of the features of the Ig locus rearrangement, such as gene-segment rearrangement frequencies, segment chewback by exonucleases, and nontemplated base addition levels prior to selection of the B cell based on expressed Ig protein. This can be useful in evaluating immunological phenotypes related to receptor gene rearrangements or B-cell selection, such as in immunodeficiency disorders (K. Roskin, submitted for publication). In addition, the fact that there is only one productively rearranged IGH, IGK, or IGL locus per cell can be used to evaluate the sizes of B-cell clones in the cell populations studied, because multiple replicate libraries for sequencing can be generated from independent aliquots of genomic DNA template, and V(D)J rearrangements from different members of the same clone of B cells can later be identified in data analysis (21, 33). In contrast, the many copies of Ig mRNA produced within a single B cell, and the differing

IgH library generation from gDNA template:

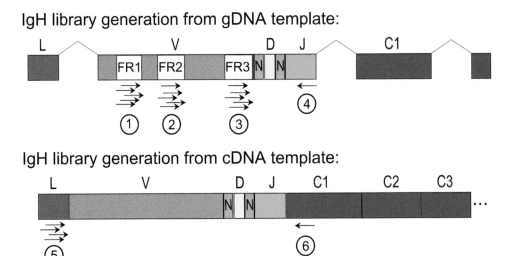

FIGURE 2 **IgH library production from genomic DNA (gDNA) or complementary DNA (cDNA). The top diagram shows the rearranged gDNA encoding an antibody heavy chain. Primer sets designed to hybridize in the framework 1, 2, or 3 (FR1, FR2, FR3) regions (labeled with circled numbers 1, 2, and 3), together with a primer complementary to the J gene segments (labeled 4), can be used for PCR to amplify the VDJ gene rearrangement. Multiple primers are shown for the framework primer sets, indicating the different primers required for amplification of V segments belonging to different families. The leader peptide exon is separated from the V segment by a short intron in the genomic DNA. The lower diagram shows cDNA generated from spliced mRNA encoding a heavy chain. Primers hybridizing to the constant region (labeled 6) can be used as the initial gene-specific primer for 5' RACE protocols (see main text), or else can be used in PCR with primers in the leader sequences (labeled 5), or framework primers, to amplify the VDJ gene rearrangements. The constant region isotype associated with the VDJ gene rearrangement can be identified in such libraries. doi:10.1128/microbiolspec.AID-0017-2014.f2**

levels of mRNA expression for Ig genes in different subsets of B cells, such as relatively low expression in naïve cells and high expression in plasmablasts, mean that it is not possible to reliably distinguish between the presence of cells with high Ig mRNA expression versus the presence of a clone containing many cells with lower Ig mRNA expression, if only a single RNA sample is available for analysis. However, using RNA as the starting material for repertoire sequencing experiments has other important advantages, chiefly that it enables identification of the heavy chain isotype associated with a particular V(D)J rearrangement. Another potential advantage of RNA template is that it should preserve a more complete representation of the B-cell clones present in the cell sample, because each B cell can contribute multiple mRNA copies of its Ig rearrangements, so that, if some template

is lost during purification owing to less than 100% yield, there will not be a linear reduction in the number of B-cell clones represented in the sample, as is the case with genomic DNA. Finally, cDNA contains more amplifiable Ig templates per nanogram of template amplified, compared with genomic DNA where the rearranged Ig loci are a tiny fraction of the total DNA quantity. Because there is a limit to the amount of DNA template that can be added to a PCR reaction, more complex libraries of Ig rearrangements therefore can be generated with fewer PCR reactions by the use of the cDNA template compared with the genomic DNA template.

Multiplexing and Chimeric Sequences

Another kind of artifact that can arise in library preparation is the chimeric sequence, usually generated when a DNA strand is incompletely extended in one PCR cycle, and can then hybridize to an unrelated template and be extended further in a subsequent cycle. If PCR amplifications are performed with several different heavy chain isotype primers in the same reaction, such chimeras may lead to errors of assignment of particular VDJ rearrangements to particular isotypes. Otherwise, they can yield apparent regions of highly increased somatic mutation in the V(D)J rearrangement, and other artifactual results. Bioinformatic filtering to remove sequences with such unusual features is one way of attempting to minimize such effects, but other approaches such as performing PCR with templates at limiting dilution in aqueous-in-oil emulsions or microtiter plates have been proposed and used as alternatives, although these dilution methods raise other challenges of sample throughput (34, 35).

Replicate Library Preparation

As noted above, the preparation of multiple libraries from a sample by using independent template aliquots (either by using a genomic DNA template, or by separating cells into separate aliquots prior to isolating RNA template) permits reliable detection of expanded clonal B-cell populations and distinction between an expanded clone of cells versus a single cell expressing high levels of Ig mRNA (21, 33). As with any experimental methodology, conducting experiments with replicate sampling and library generation helps to distinguish between real signals compared with statistical noise in the dataset and also gives a basis for assessing the robustness of any other secondary results derived from the data.

Error Correction Strategies

The combined frequency of PCR errors and sequencing errors for Ig amplicon libraries sequenced with current HTS platforms are usually less than 0.5% per base, with the exception of polynucleotide tract regions in data gathered with 454/Roche or Ion Torrent instruments. A recent comparison of error rates of benchtop HTS instruments sequencing *Escherichia coli* genomic DNA found that the insertion and deletion (indel) rate was 0.38% per base for the 454 GS Junior, 1.5% per base for the Ion Torrent PGM, and <0.001% per base for the Illumina MiSeq (36). In this comparison, the substitution error rate of the MiSeq instrument was the lowest measured, at 0.1 per 100 bases. The quality of the sequence data with all of these instruments decreases toward the distal ends of the reads. When applied to Ig templates, reported error rates for the combination of PCR and sequencing error, excluding indels, have been reported in the literature and seen in our own experiments, to be approximately 0.1 to 0.3% per base for the 454 platform and 0.1 to 0.2% for Illumina sequencing (21, 29, 36, 37, 38). One approach to detecting potential PCR or sequencing errors, and distinguishing these from true somatic mutation positions or allelic variants of gene segments, is to obtain manyfold more sequencing reads than the number of template molecules in the original sample. Errors occurring early in PCR cannot be corrected with this approach, but, together with the evaluation of sequences derived from known templates (such as sequences cloned into plasmids), this approach can be used to correct many sequencing-derived errors, and give an upper bound of remaining PCR and sequencing errors in the data. An alternative method of detecting errors from amplification or sequencing has been adapted for Ig sequencing from earlier approaches of adding highly diverse sequence tags to nucleic acid templates prior to amplification of libraries from the templates (39, 40, 41, 42). Incorporation of a randomized sequence tag in the primer used for reverse transcription of Ig mRNA enables later comparison of the data from reads sharing the same sequence of randomized tag, and helps the inference of which variant bases are likely to be errors in such sequences (38).

Paired Heavy and Light Chain Sequencing

A long-awaited experimental breakthrough in Ig repertoire studies has been the efficient high-throughput sequencing of native pairs of heavy and light chain (H+L) sequences from large numbers of individual B cells. In 2013, the proof of concept of a method of generating paired H+L sequence libraries from tens of thousands of individual B cells was described, making use of high-density microtiter plates with 125-pl well volumes to separate the cells and enable capture of mRNA from each cell on an oligo-dT functionalized polymer bead, followed by reverse transcription and joining PCR to covalently link the heavy and light chain sequences (43). While the data sets from these initial experiments contained thousands of natively paired sequences, it is likely that the protocols will improve their throughput with the use of emulsion strategies or potentially even the use of microfluidic devices (44).

DATA ANALYSIS APPROACHES

A variety of data analysis methods have been applied to Ig sequence data sets, with many laboratories developing their own pipelines of publicly available software, customized scripts and programs, and databases to manage the data. Owing to the numerous experimental strategies for library preparation being explored in the literature, and the idiosyncrasies of each group's data analysis approaches, direct comparison of reported results is challenging. This is not an insurmountable problem, so long as the experimental protocols are described in sufficient detail, and the raw sequence data are made available to other investigators who wish to evaluate the results by using their own analysis pipeline. It is not realistic to expect that all research laboratories will converge on a single experimental and data analysis approach, but full transparency about library preparation methods and software, including sharing of the scripts used for analysis, should enable appropriate verification of reported results. One overall limitation of many published articles to date has been the relatively low number of samples analyzed and the rare to absent consideration of statistical correction for multiple hypothesis testing in data sets that have many different features that can be compared between samples.

Sequence Barcode Analysis, Filtering, Primer Trimming, and Quality Score Use

As with other amplicon-sequencing experiments, data analysis of Ig libraries typically includes early steps of identifying the sequence barcodes that identify the sample of origin of a sequence. Many groups have designed barcodes that are relatively resistant to sequencing error, in that they are different from each other at two or more positions (i.e., are separated by a Hamming distance of two or more). If gene-specific primers are used in the amplification strategy and a primer is not a perfect match to the gene segment it amplified, trimming of primers is necessary to avoid spurious introduction or loss of point mutations. Quality scores for each nucleotide position are a feature calculated by all of the HTS platforms and agree fairly well with actual error rates in experiments performed with known template sequences (36). Quality scores can be used to exclude sequences of excessively poor quality from further analysis; as an alternative approach, such reads can be carried forward in the analysis and removed from consideration later if they do not align well enough to gene segments of the locus of interest.

Alignment and Parsing Programs

In the place of traditional mapping of reads to a reference scaffold, as is performed for genome or exome sequence analysis, the next step in Ig sequence analysis is determining which regions of the rearranged Ig align with germ line V, D, and J gene segments and constant region sequences in the locus that was amplified, parsing the nontemplated regions at the segment junctions and determining the positions of somatic mutation in the sequence. A number of programs have been devised for this purpose, including IgBlast, V-QUEST, and the hidden Markov model-based programs iHMMune-align and SoDA2 (45, 46, 47, 48). In response to the increasing demand for higher-throughput analysis of large sequence data sets, the IMGT website (www.imgt.org) has introduced a new next-generation sequencing data set portal for sequence alignment and analysis, HighV-QUEST (49). Many of these published analysis programs claim superiority for their approach to sequence analysis, but, in our laboratory, evaluation of the alignments generated by IgBlast, V-QUEST, and iHMMune-align are identical or very similar for most sequences, and differ most in junctional parsing of sequences where the true answer may be unknowable. For example, IGH sequences in which the D segment is very short owing to exonuclease digestion during rearrangement, so that the true germ line D segment identity cannot be determined would be such a case. An important consideration for any of these utilities is the choice of germ line V, D, and J gene segment repertoires used for alignment, because current curated databases are not complete, so depending on the population group studied, rarer and unreported alleles can appear to carry somatic mutations as a result of misalignment to other gene segments (11, 12).

HTS Ig DATA ANALYSIS: APPLICATIONS IN INFECTIOUS DISEASE RESEARCH

A wide variety of secondary analyses can be performed on Ig repertoire data once the sequences are aligned and parsed, depending on the experimental question being asked. Often, particularly if replicate libraries have been generated from a sample, it can be helpful to collapse identical sequences into a single representative, to minimize PCR amplification biases or stochastic PCR jackpots that cause some sequences to appear in increased copy numbers in the sequencing data. Overall features of Ig repertoires, or the repertoires derived from particular B-cell subsets, can be readily determined from the parsed sequence output of any of the alignment utilities described above. Features that have been reported in many studies include gene segment usage frequencies; length, composition, and amino acid sequences of CDR3 regions; mutation levels and distributions; and heavy chain isotype associated with particular V(D)J rearrangements, among other metrics.

Recent articles have provided more detailed insights into baseline human Ig repertoires than were previously known from lower-throughput data, including the individual specific usage frequencies of V, D, and J gene segments, and the presence of copy number variants and allelic variants within particular haplotypes (11, 29, 50). Glanville et al. observed a strong influence of the germ line genome on V, D, and J gene segment usage (probably combining the effects of receptor rearrangement frequencies, and selection acting on the expressed protein) in repertoires sequenced from two pairs of identical twins (51). HTS has also enabled better measurement of the frequencies of uncommon features in Ig repertoires, such as rearrangements using two D segments in the heavy chain and indels generated as a by-product of somatic hypermutation (52, 53, 54). The distinct features of the repertoires of different B-cell subsets, such as class-switched or IgM-expressing memory cells, compared with naïve B cells, at the level of gene segment usage and junctional features, have been reported by several groups (21, 24, 30, 55). Analysis of somatic mutation patterns in Ig rearrangements, and detection of evidence of selection, has also been enhanced in part by the availability of larger data sets for evaluation, and has prompted the development of new tools and interfaces to facilitate analysis of larger sequence sets (56, 57). The influx of much larger datasets of Ig sequences that often contain many representatives of clonally expanded B-cell lineages has also stimulated new approaches for inferring the relationships of descent and genetic inheritance between individual cells within the clone (58).

Determining whether sequences derived from the same B-cell clone are present in different samples of a longitudinal time course, or different tissue sites, sample types, or B-cell subsets, is often of interest and can be approached in several different ways. For initial analyses, we often use a clone definition for comparing two heavy chain sequences requiring that the V and J segments be the same, or of the same subgroup, and that the CDR3 sequence be the same length and match at 80% of the nucleotides. Depending on the experimental question being asked, different thresholds for clonal similarity may be more appropriate. For example, in searching for members of a clonal lineage that matures from the germ line sequence state to a highly mutated state (as in the case of some broadly neutralizing antibodies against HIV), a more permissive definition of CDR3 similarity could be used, and then the putative clone members could be tested for other inherited features such as somatic hypermutation positions. Ensuring that the conclusions drawn in a study are not overly sensitive to minor differences in clonal definitions is a conservative and prudent approach. A number of groups have made striking progress in recent years by using HTS to track the clonal evolution and mutational and selection histories of B-cell lineages making antibodies specific for particular pathogens or vaccine components. Such analyses have been performed most extensively in studies of HIV, identifying putative germ line ancestral sequences of highly mutated antibody lineages that acquire virus neutralization breadth only after many months to years of chronic infection, and identifying shared sequence features of antibodies that bind to particular epitopes of HIV (31, 32, 58, 59, 60, 61, 62, 63, 64). Similar approaches may offer insights into many other infectious diseases and chronic or recurrent infections.

Quantitation or normalization of the contribution of clonally expanded B-cell populations to an observed repertoire can be performed from multiple-replicate library data, using a modified form of the Gini-Simpson index adapted for HTS data; we have termed this a "clonality score" or "coincidence index," in recent articles. This measure can distinguish between individuals responding to acute Dengue virus infection from those who are convalescent or uninfected (21, 33). The presence of expanded B-cell clones that persist in the circulation of individuals, as measured with a similar clonality score from samples collected a year apart, is significantly associated with EBV infection status in healthy subjects (21). We have also observed that this measure of clonality is closely correlated with the increase in numbers of plasmablasts observed in the blood 7 days after vaccination with inactivated trivalent influenza vaccine, and that the clonality score is correlated with seroconversion following vaccination. Other recent studies of vaccination for influenza or pneumococcus have highlighted sequences that appear at higher copy number in sequencing libraries following vaccination, which may correspond to expanded clones stimulated by the vaccine, or cells producing higher levels of Ig mRNA, or both (37, 38, 65).

Estimation of the size of the B-cell repertoire has been attempted in a number of prior studies, but is subject to high degrees of uncertainty and underbias when extrapolated from peripheral blood samples that typically contain millions of B cells, representing less than 0.1% of the approximately 100 billion B cells in an individual's body (29). Parametric approaches that make assumptions about the distribution of clone sizes in the repertoire may be particularly unreliable, but even nonparametric estimates such as the lower bound of the "Chao 2" metric are likely to underestimate the minimal size of the repertoire (Y. Liu, personal communication, and reference 66). In our view, currently published estimates of naïve B-cell and T-cell receptor diversity are underestimates of the true values; it will await larger data sets collected with multiple independent samples from each human subject to arrive at better estimates in the future.

In light of the enormous size of the potential antibody repertoire, it has been an open question whether different humans raise similar antibodies in response to the same infectious or vaccination challenge. Previous studies using Sanger sequencing identified some circumstances where highly similar "convergent" antibodies could be detected in different people, such as immunization with *Haemophilus influenzae* type b polysaccharide vaccine or pneumococcal vaccine (67, 68). HTS of Ig repertoires has greatly increased the ability to detect such convergent sequences, and pathogen-specific antibody rearrangements have now been detected in patients infected with Dengue virus and HIV (32, 33, 63) as well as in subjects vaccinated with trivalent inactivated influenza (69). It appears that the stimulation of convergent antibodies that are specific for particular pathogens is a widespread phenomenon. Once more data are gathered for a variety of different pathogens and antigens, it may become possible to read an individual's history of pathogen exposure from the Ig sequences in their memory B-cell repertoire.

CONCLUSIONS AND FUTURE DIRECTIONS

The application of HTS methods to the study of B-cell responses and immunoglobulin structure-function relationships is now well started, and most of the cost limitations and technological shortcomings of the earlier generations of HTS instruments have been overcome. Well-designed experimental protocols and data analysis approaches promise to provide unprecedentedly accurate, extensive, and exact tracking of B-cell populations of biological or medical interest in any immunological context. Initial studies in infectious disease topics have provided new knowledge about the numbers and diversity of B-cell clones stimulated by infection or vaccination by a variety of agents, and have been especially useful in documenting the pathways of mutation and selection followed by antibodies responding to HIV. Clear and explicit documentation of the experimental methods used and data analysis approaches applied to Ig HTS data sets, along with sharing of primer sequences, scripts for analysis, and other important experimental features along with raw and processed data, will help to ensure the reproducibility and broader scientific value of studies in this area. As with any other research area generating and analyzing large and complex molecular datasets, Ig sequence analysis will benefit from a greater emphasis on the use of sample sets with larger numbers of individual patients or subjects, collection of longitudinal repeat sampling from individuals when possible, appropriate statistical analysis to correct for multiple hypothesis testing, and validation of results with training and test sets of data. A particularly promising area is the coupling of HTS studies of immune response genetics (Ig and TCR sequencing, as well as analysis of other host genetic features) with equally powerful genetic analysis of the populations of pathogens seeking to infect the host and evade the immune system. The coming years should offer a ringside seat to researchers intent on observing these fascinating battles.

ACKNOWLEDGMENT

Conflicts of interest: We disclose no conflicts.

CITATION

Boyd SD, Joshi SA. 2014. High-throughput DNA sequencing analysis of antibody repertoires. Microbiol Spectrum 2(5):AID-0017-2014

REFERENCES

1. **Gonzaga-Jauregui C, Lupski JR, Gibbs RA.** 2012. Human genome sequencing in health and disease. *Annu RevMed* **63**:35–61.

2. **Boyd SD.** 2013. Diagnostic applications of high-throughput DNA sequencing. *Annu Rev Pathol* **8**:381–410.

3. **Jung D, Giallourakis C, Mostoslavsky R, Alt FW.** 2006. Mechanism and control of V(D)J recombination at the immunoglobulin heavy chain locus. *Annu Rev Immunol* **24**:541–570.

4. **Janeway CAJ, Travers P, Waport M, Shlomchik MJ.** 2001. *Immunobiology: The Immune System in Health and Disease*, 5th ed. Garland Science, New York.

5. **Matsuda F, Ishii K, Bourvagnet P, Kuma K, Hayashida H, Miyata T, Honjo T.** 1998. The complete nucleotide sequence of the human immunoglobulin heavy chain variable region locus. *J Exp Med* **188**:2151–2162.

6. **Abecasis GR, Altshuler D, Auton A, Brooks LD, Durbin RM, Gibbs RA, Hurles ME, McVean GA.** 2010. A map of human genome variation from population-scale sequencing. *Nature* **467**:1061–1073.

7. **Watson CT, Steinberg KM, Huddleston J, Warren RL, Malig M, Schein J, Willsey AJ, Joy JB, Scott JK, Graves TA, Wilson RK, Holt RA, Eichler EE, Breden F.** 2013. Complete haplotype sequence of the human immunoglobulin heavy-chain variable, diversity, and joining genes and characterization of allelic and copy-number variation. *Am J Hum Genet* **92**:530–546.

8. **Lefranc MP.** 2011. IMGT, the International ImMunoGeneTics Information System. *Cold Spring Harb Protoc* **2011**:595–603.

9. **Lefranc MP, Lefranc G.** 2001. *The Immunoglobulin FactsBook*. Academic Press, New York, NY.

10. **Wang Y, Jackson KJ, Gaeta B, Pomat W, Siba P, Sewell WA, Collins AM.** 2011. Genomic screening by 454 pyrosequencing identifies a new human IGHV gene and sixteen other new IGHV allelic variants. *Immunogenetics* **63**:259–265.

11. **Boyd SD, Gaeta BA, Jackson KJ, Fire AZ, Marshall EL, Merker JD, Maniar JM, Zhang LN, Sahaf B, Jones CD, Simen BB, Hanczaruk B, Nguyen KD, Nadeau KC, Egholm M, Miklos DB, Zehnder JL, Collins AM.** 2010. Individual variation in the germline Ig gene repertoire inferred from variable region gene rearrangements. *J Immunol* **184**:6986–6992.

12. **Wang Y, Jackson KJ, Sewell WA, Collins AM.** 2008. Many human immunoglobulin heavy-chain IGHV gene polymorphisms have been reported in error. *Immunol Cell Biol* **86**:111–115.

13. **Klein U, Dalla-Favera R.** 2008. Germinal centres: role in B-cell physiology and malignancy. *Nat Rev Immunol* **8**:22–33.

14. **Wrammert J, Smith K, Miller J, Langley WA, Kokko K, Larsen C, Zheng NY, Mays I, Garman L, Helms C, James J, Air GM, Capra JD, Ahmed R, Wilson PC.** 2008. Rapid cloning of high-affinity human monoclonal antibodies against influenza virus. *Nature* **453**:667–671.

15. **Mascola JR, Haynes BF.** 2013. HIV-1 neutralizing antibodies: understanding nature's pathways. *Immunol Rev* **254**:225–244.

16. **Lebecque SG, Gearhart PJ.** 1990. Boundaries of somatic mutation in rearranged immunoglobulin genes: 5′ boundary is near the promoter, and 3′ boundary is approximately 1 kb from V(D)J gene. *J Exp Med* **172**:1717–1727.

17. **Rada C, Gonzalez-Fernandez A, Jarvis JM, Milstein C.** 1994. The 5′ boundary of somatic hypermutation in a V kappa gene is in the leader intron. *Eur J Immunol* **24**:1453–1457.

18. **Margulies M, Egholm M, Altman WE, Attiya S, Bader JS, Bemben LA, Berka J, Braverman MS, Chen YJ, Chen Z, Dewell SB, Du L, Fierro JM, Gomes XV, Godwin BC, He W, Helgesen S, Ho CH, Irzyk GP, Jando SC, Alenquer ML, Jarvie TP, Jirage KB, Kim JB, Knight JR, Lanza JR, Leamon JH, Lefkowitz SM, Lei M, Li J, Lohman KL, Lu H, Makhijani VB, McDade KE, McKenna MP, Myers EW, Nickerson E, Nobile JR, Plant R, Puc BP, Ronan MT, Roth GT, Sarkis GJ, Simons JF, Simpson JW, Srinivasan M, Tartaro KR, Tomasz A, Vogt KA, Volkmer GA, Wang SH, Wang Y, Weiner MP, Yu P, Begley RF, Rothberg JM.** 2005. Genome sequencing in microfabricated high-density picolitre reactors. *Nature* **437**:376–380.

19. **Rothberg JM, Hinz W, Rearick TM, Schultz J, Mileski W, Davey M, Leamon JH, Johnson K, Milgrew MJ, Edwards M, Hoon J, Simons JF, Marran D, Myers JW, Davidson JF, Branting A, Nobile JR, Puc BP, Light D, Clark TA, Huber M, Branciforte JT, Stoner IB, Cawley SE, Lyons M, Fu Y, Homer N, Sedova M, Miao X, Reed B, Sabina J, Feierstein E, Schorn M, Alanjary M, Dimalanta E, Dressman D, Kasinskas R, Sokolsky T, Fidanza JA, Namsaraev E, McKernan KJ, Williams A, Roth GT, Bustillo J.** 2011. An integrated semiconductor device enabling non-optical genome sequencing. *Nature* **475**:348–352.

20. **Bentley DR, Balasubramanian S, Swerdlow HP, Smith GP, Milton J, Brown CG, Hall KP, Evers DJ, Barnes CL, Bignell HR, Boutell JM, Bryant J, Carter RJ, Keira Cheetham R, Cox AJ, Ellis DJ, Flatbush MR, Gormley NA,**

Humphray SJ, Irving LJ, Karbelashvili MS, Kirk SM, Li H, Liu X, Maisinger KS, Murray LJ, Obradovic B, Ost T, Parkinson ML, Pratt MR, Rasolonjatovo IM, Reed MT, Rigatti R, Rodighiero C, Ross MT, Sabot A, Sankar SV, Scally A, Schroth GP, Smith ME, Smith VP, Spiridou A, Torrance PE, Tzonev SS, Vermaas EH, Walter K, Wu X, Zhang L, Alam MD, Anastasi C, Aniebo IC, Bailey DM, Bancarz IR, Banerjee S, Barbour SG, Baybayan PA, Benoit VA, Benson KF, Bevis C, Black PJ, Boodhun A, Brennan JS, Bridgham JA, Brown RC, Brown AA, Buermann DH, Bundu AA, Burrows JC, Carter NP, Castillo N, Chiara ECM, Chang S, Neil Cooley R, Crake NR, Dada OO, Diakoumakos KD, Dominguez-Fernandez B, Earnshaw DJ, Egbujor UC, Elmore DW, Etchin SS, Ewan MR, Fedurco M, Fraser LJ, Fuentes Fajardo KV, Scott Furey W, George D, Gietzen KJ, Goddard CP, Golda GS, Granieri PA, Green DE, Gustafson DL, Hansen NF, Harnish K, Haudenschild CD, Heyer NI, Hims MM, Ho JT, Horgan AM, Hoschler K, Hurwitz S, Ivanov DV, Johnson MQ, James T, Huw Jones TA, Kang GD, Kerelska TH, Kersey AD, Khrebtukova I, Kindwall AP, Kingsbury Z, Kokko-Gonzales PI, Kumar A, Laurent MA, Lawley CT, Lee SE, Lee X, Liao AK, Loch JA, Lok M, Luo S, Mammen RM, Martin JW, McCauley PG, McNitt P, Mehta P, Moon KW, Mullens JW, Newington T, Ning Z, Ling Ng B, Novo SM, O'Neill MJ, Osborne MA, Osnowski A, Ostadan O, Paraschos LL, Pickering L, Pike AC, Chris Pinkard D, Pliskin DP, Podhasky J, Quijano VJ, Raczy C, Rae VH, Rawlings SR, Chiva Rodriguez A, Roe PM, Rogers J, Rogert Bacigalupo MC, Romanov N, Romieu A, Roth RK, Rourke NJ, Ruediger ST, Rusman E, Sanches-Kuiper RM, Schenker MR, Seoane JM, Shaw RJ, Shiver MK, Short SW, Sizto NL, Sluis JP, Smith MA, Ernest Sohna Sohna J, Spence EJ, Stevens K, Sutton N, Szajkowski L, Tregidgo CL, Turcatti G, Vandevondele S, Verhovsky Y, Virk SM, Wakelin S, Walcott GC, Wang J, Worsley GJ, Yan J, Yau L, Zuerlein M, Mullikin JC, Hurles ME, McCooke NJ, West JS, Oaks FL, Lundberg PL, Klenerman D, Durbin R, Smith AJ. 2008. Accurate whole human genome sequencing using reversible terminator chemistry. *Nature* **456**:53–59.

21. Wang C, Liu Y, Xu LT, Jackson KJ, Roskin KM, Pham TD, Laserson J, Marshall EL, Seo K, Lee JY, Furman D, Koller D, Dekker CL, Davis MM, Fire AZ, Boyd SD. 2014. Effects of aging, cytomegalovirus infection, and EBV infec-

tion on human B cell repertoires. *J Immunol* **192**:603–611.

22. Jackson SM, Wilson PC, James JA, Capra JD. 2008. Human B cell subsets. *Adv Immunol* **98**:151–224.

23. Mauri C, Blair PA. 2010. Regulatory B cells in autoimmunity: developments and controversies. *Nat Rev Rheumatol* **6**:636–643.

24. Mroczek ES, Ippolito GC, Rogosch T, Hoi KH, Hwangpo TA, Brand MG, Zhuang Y, Liu CR, Schneider DA, Zemlin M, Brown EE, Georgiou G, Schroeder HW Jr. 2014. Differences in the composition of the human antibody repertoire by B cell subsets in the blood. *Front Immunol* **5**:96. doi:10.3389/fimmu.2014.00096.

25. Frohman MA, Dush MK, Martin GR. 1988. Rapid production of full-length cDNAs from rare transcripts: amplification using a single gene-specific oligonucleotide primer. *Proc Natl Acad Sci USA* **85**:8998–9002.

26. Aoki-Ota M, Torkamani A, Ota T, Schork N, Nemazee D. 2012. Skewed primary Igkappa repertoire and V-J joining in C57BL/6 mice: implications for recombination accessibility and receptor editing. *J Immunol* **188**:2305–2315.

27. Choi NM, Loguercio S, Verma-Gaur J, Degner SC, Torkamani A, Su AI, Oltz EM, Artyomov M, Feeney AJ. 2013. Deep sequencing of the murine IgH repertoire reveals complex regulation of nonrandom v gene rearrangement frequencies. *J Immunol* **191**:2393–2402.

28. van Dongen JJ, Langerak AW, Bruggemann M, Evans PA, Hummel M, Lavender FL, Delabesse E, Davi F, Schuuring E, Garcia-Sanz R, van Krieken JH, Droese J, Gonzalez D, Bastard C, White HE, Spaargaren M, Gonzalez M, Parreira A, Smith JL, Morgan GJ, Kneba M, Macintyre EA. 2003. Design and standardization of PCR primers and protocols for detection of clonal immunoglobulin and T-cell receptor gene recombinations in suspect lymphoproliferations: report of the BIOMED-2 Concerted Action BMH4-CT98-3936. *Leukemia* **17**:2257–2317.

29. Boyd SD, Marshall EL, Merker JD, Maniar JM, Zhang LN, Sahaf B, Jones CD, Simen BB, Hanczaruk B, Nguyen KD, Nadeau KC, Egholm M, Miklos DB, Zehnder JL, Fire AZ. 2009. Measurement and clinical monitoring of human lymphocyte clonality by massively parallel VDJ pyrosequencing. *Sci Transl Med* **1**:12ra23. doi:10.1126/scitranslmed.3000540.

30. Briney BS, Willis JR, McKinney BA, Crowe JE Jr. 2012. High-throughput antibody sequencing reveals genetic evidence of global regulation of the naive and memory repertoires that extends across individuals. *Genes Immun* **13**:469–473.

31. Wu X, Zhou T, Zhu J, Zhang B, Georgiev I, Wang C, Chen X, Longo NS, Louder M, McKee K, O'Dell S, Perfetto S, Schmidt SD, Shi W, Wu L, Yang Y, Yang ZY, Yang Z, Zhang Z, Bonsignori M, Crump JA, Kapiga SH, Sam NE, Haynes BF, Simek M, Burton DR, Koff WC, Doria-Rose NA, Connors M, Mullikin JC, Nabel GJ, Roederer M, Shapiro L, Kwong PD, Mascola JR. 2011. Focused evolution of HIV-1 neutralizing antibodies revealed by structures and deep sequencing. *Science* **333**:1593–1602.

32. Scheid JF, Mouquet H, Ueberheide B, Diskin R, Klein F, Oliveira TY, Pietzsch J, Fenyo D, Abadir A, Velinzon K, Hurley A, Myung S, Boulad F, Poignard P, Burton DR, Pereyra F, Ho DD, Walker BD, Seaman MS, Bjorkman PJ, Chait BT, Nussenzweig MC. 2011. Sequence and structural convergence of broad and potent HIV antibodies that mimic CD4 binding. *Science* **333**:1633–1637.

33. Parameswaran P, Liu Y, Roskin KM, Jackson KK, Dixit VP, Lee JY, Artiles KL, Zompi S, Vargas MJ, Simen BB, Hanczaruk B, McGowan KR, Tariq MA, Pourmand N, Koller D, Balmaseda A, Boyd SD, Harris E, Fire AZ. 2013. Convergent antibody signatures in human dengue. *Cell Host Microbe* **13**:691–700.

34. Rubelt F, Sievert V, Knaust F, Diener C, Lim TS, Skriner K, Klipp E, Reinhardt R, Lehrach H, Konthur Z. 2012. Onset of immune senescence defined by unbiased pyrosequencing of human immunoglobulin mRNA repertoires. *PloS One* **7**: e49774. doi:10.1371/journal.pone.0049774.

35. Tan YC, Blum LK, Kongpachith S, Ju CH, Cai X, Lindstrom TM, Sokolove J, Robinson WH. 2014. High-throughput sequencing of natively paired antibody chains provides evidence for original antigenic sin shaping the antibody response to influenza vaccination. *Clin Immunol* **151**:55–65.

36. Loman NJ, Misra RV, Dallman TJ, Constantinidou C, Gharbia SE, Wain J, Pallen MJ. 2012. Performance comparison of benchtop high-throughput sequencing platforms. *Nat Biotechnol* **30**:434–439.

37. Jiang N, He J, Weinstein JA, Penland L, Sasaki S, He XS, Dekker CL, Zheng NY, Huang M, Sullivan M, Wilson PC, Greenberg HB, Davis MM, Fisher DS, Quake SR. 2013. Lineage structure of the human antibody repertoire in response to influenza vaccination. *Sci Transl Med* **5**:171ra119. doi:10.1126/scitranslmed.3004794.

38. Vollmers C, Sit RV, Weinstein JA, Dekker CL, Quake SR. 2013. Genetic measurement of memory B-cell recall using antibody reper-

toire sequencing. *Proc Natl Acad Sci USA* **110**:13463–13468.

39. Shiroguchi K, Jia TZ, Sims PA, Xie XS. 2012. Digital RNA sequencing minimizes sequence-dependent bias and amplification noise with optimized single-molecule barcodes. *Proc Natl Acad Sci USA* **109**:1347–1352.

40. Miner BE, Stoger RJ, Burden AF, Laird CD, Hansen RS. 2004. Molecular barcodes detect redundancy and contamination in hairpin-bisulfite PCR. *Nucleic Acids Res* **32**:e135. doi:10.1093/nar/gnh132.

41. McCloskey ML, Stoger R, Hansen RS, Laird CD. 2007. Encoding PCR products with batch-stamps and barcodes. *Biochem Genet* **45**:761–767.

42. Kinde I, Wu J, Papadopoulos N, Kinzler KW, Vogelstein B. 2011. Detection and quantification of rare mutations with massively parallel sequencing. *Proc Natl Acad Sci USA* **108**:9530–9535.

43. DeKosky BJ, Ippolito GC, Deschner RP, Lavinder JJ, Wine Y, Rawlings BM, Varadarajan N, Giesecke C, Dorner T, Andrews SF, Wilson PC, Hunicke-Smith SP, Willson CG, Ellington AD, Georgiou G. 2013. High-throughput sequencing of the paired human immunoglobulin heavy and light chain repertoire. *Nat Biotechnol* **31**:166–169.

44. Georgiou G, Ippolito GC, Beausang J, Busse CE, Wardemann H, Quake SR. 2014. The promise and challenge of high-throughput sequencing of the antibody repertoire. *Nat Biotechnol* **32**:158–168.

45. Munshaw S, Kepler TB. 2010. SoDA2: a Hidden Markov Model approach for identification of immunoglobulin rearrangements. *Bioinformatics* **26**:867–872.

46. Gaeta BA, Malming HR, Jackson KJ, Bain ME, Wilson P, Collins AM. 2007. iHMMune-align: hidden Markov model-based alignment and identification of germline genes in rearranged immunoglobulin gene sequences. *Bioinformatics* **23**:1580–1587.

47. Giudicelli V, Brochet X, Lefranc MP. 2011. IMGT/V-QUEST: IMGT standardized analysis of the immunoglobulin (IG) and T cell receptor (TR) nucleotide sequences. *Cold Spring Harb Protoc* **2011**:695–715.

48. Ye J, Ma N, Madden TL, Ostell JM. 2013. IgBLAST: an immunoglobulin variable domain sequence analysis tool. *Nucleic Acids Res* **41**: W34–W40.

49. Li S, Lefranc MP, Miles JJ, Alamyar E, Giudicelli V, Duroux P, Freeman JD, Corbin VD, Scheerlinck JP, Frohman MA, Cameron PU, Plebanski M, Loveland B, Burrows SR, Papenfuss AT, Gowans EJ. 2013. IMGT/HighV QUEST paradigm for T cell receptor

IMGT clonotype diversity and next generation repertoire immunoprofiling. *Nat Commun* 4:2333. doi:10.1038/ncomms3333.

50. **Kidd MJ, Chen Z, Wang Y, Jackson KJ, Zhang L, Boyd SD, Fire AZ, Tanaka MM, Gaeta BA, Collins AM.** 2012. The inference of phased haplotypes for the immunoglobulin H chain V region gene loci by analysis of VDJ gene rearrangements. *J Immunol* 188:1333–1340.

51. **Glanville J, Kuo TC, von Budingen HC, Guey L, Berka J, Sundar PD, Huerta G, Mehta GR, Oksenberg JR, Hauser SL, Cox DR, Rajpal A, Pons J.** 2011. Naive antibody gene-segment frequencies are heritable and unaltered by chronic lymphocyte ablation. *Proc Natl Acad Sci USA* 108:20066–20071.

52. **Briney BS, Willis JR, Crowe JE Jr.** 2012. Location and length distribution of somatic hypermutation-associated DNA insertions and deletions reveals regions of antibody structural plasticity. *Genes Immun* 13:523–529.

53. **Briney BS, Willis JR, Hicar MD, Thomas JW II, Crowe JE Jr.** 2012. Frequency and genetic characterization of V(DD)J recombinants in the human peripheral blood antibody repertoire. *Immunology* 137:56–64.

54. **Larimore K, McCormick MW, Robins HS, Greenberg PD.** 2012. Shaping of human germline IgH repertoires revealed by deep sequencing. *J Immunol* 189:3221–3230.

55. **Wu YC, Kipling D, Leong HS, Martin V, Ademokun AA, Dunn-Walters DK.** 2010. High-throughput immunoglobulin repertoire analysis distinguishes between human IgM memory and switched memory B-cell populations. *Blood* 116:1070–1078.

56. **Uduman M, Yaari G, Hershberg U, Stern JA, Shlomchik MJ, Kleinstein SH.** 2011. Detecting selection in immunoglobulin sequences. *Nucleic Acids Res* 39:W499–W504.

57. **Yaari G, Uduman M, Kleinstein SH.** 2012. Quantifying selection in high-throughput Immunoglobulin sequencing data sets. *Nucleic Acids Res* 40:e134. doi:10.1093/nar/gks457.

58. **Sok D, Laserson U, Laserson J, Liu Y, Vigneault F, Julien JP, Briney B, Ramos A, Saye KF, Le K, Mahan A, Wang S, Kardar M, Yaari G, Walker LM, Simen BB, St John EP, Chan-Hui PY, Swiderek K, Kleinstein SH, Alter G, Seaman MS, Chakraborty AK, Koller D, Wilson IA, Church GM, Burton DR, Poignard P.** 2013. The effects of somatic hypermutation on neutralization and binding in the PGT121 family of broadly neutralizing HIV antibodies. *PLoS Pathog* 9:e1003754. doi:10.1371/journal.ppat.1003754.

59. **Liao HX, Chen X, Munshaw S, Zhang R, Marshall DJ, Vandergrift N, Whitesides JF,** Lu X, Yu JS, Hwang KK, Gao F, Markowitz M, Heath SL, Bar KJ, Goepfert PA, Montefiori DC, Shaw GC, Alam SM, Margolis DM, Denny TN, Boyd SD, Marshal E, Egholm M, Simen BB, Hanczaruk B, Fire AZ, Voss G, Kelsoe G, Tomaras GD, Moody MA, Kepler TB, Haynes BF. 2011. Initial antibodies binding to HIV-1 gp41 in acutely infected subjects are polyreactive and highly mutated. *J Exp Med* 208:2237–2249.

60. **Kwong PD, Mascola JR.** 2012. Human antibodies that neutralize HIV-1: identification, structures, and B cell ontogenies. *Immunity* 37:412–425.

61. **Liao HX, Lynch R, Zhou T, Gao F, Alam SM, Boyd SD, Fire AZ, Roskin KM, Schramm CA, Zhang Z, Zhu J, Shapiro L, Mullikin JC, Gnanakaran S, Hraber P, Wiehe K, Kelsoe G, Yang G, Xia SM, Montefiori DC, Parks R, Lloyd KE, Scearce RM, Soderberg KA, Cohen M, Kamanga G, Louder MK, Tran LM, Chen Y, Cai F, Chen S, Moquin S, Du X, Joyce MG, Srivatsan S, Zhang B, Zheng A, Shaw GM, Hahn BH, Kepler TB, Korber BT, Kwong PD, Mascola JR, Haynes BF.** 2013. Co-evolution of a broadly neutralizing HIV-1 antibody and founder virus. *Nature* 496:469–476.

62. **Zhou T, Zhu J, Wu X, Moquin S, Zhang B, Acharya P, Georgiev IS, Altae-Tran HR, Chuang GY, Joyce MG, Do Kwon Y, Longo NS, Louder MK, Luongo T, McKee K, Schramm CA, Skinner J, Yang Y, Yang Z, Zhang Z, Zheng A, Bonsignori M, Haynes BF, Scheid JF, Nussenzweig MC, Simek M, Burton DR, Koff WC, Mullikin JC, Connors M, Shapiro L, Nabel GJ, Mascola JR, Kwong PD.** 2013. Multidonor analysis reveals structural elements, genetic determinants, and maturation pathway for HIV-1 neutralization by VRC01-class antibodies. *Immunity* 39:245–258.

63. **Zhu J, Wu X, Zhang B, McKee K, O'Dell S, Soto C, Zhou T, Casazza JP, Mullikin JC, Kwong PD, Mascola JR, Shapiro L.** 2013. De novo identification of VRC01 class HIV-1-neutralizing antibodies by next-generation sequencing of B-cell transcripts. *Proc Natl Acad Sci USA* 110:E4088–E4097.

64. **Doria-Rose NA, Schramm CA, Gorman J, Moore PL, Bhiman JN, Dekosky BJ, Ernandes MJ, Georgiev IS, Kim HJ, Pancera M, Staupe RP, Altae-Tran HR, Bailer RT, Crooks ET, Cupo A, Druz A, Garrett NJ, Hoi KH, Kong R, Louder MK, Longo NS, McKee K, Nonyane M, O'Dell S, Roark RS, Rudicell RS, Schmidt SD, Sheward DJ, Soto C, Wibmer CK, Yang Y, Zhang Z, Nisc Comparative Sequencing Program, Mullikin JC, Binley JM,**

Sanders RW, Wilson IA, Moore JP, Ward AB, Georgiou G, Williamson C, Abdool Karim SS, Morris L, Kwong PD, Shapiro L, Mascola JR. 2014. Developmental pathway for potent V1V2-directed HIV-neutralizing antibodies. *Nature* **509:**55–62.

65. Ademokun A, Wu YC, Martin V, Mitra R, Sack U, Baxendale H, Kipling D, Dunn-Walters DK. 2011. Vaccination-induced changes in human B-cell repertoire and pneumococcal IgM and IgA antibody at different ages. *Aging Cell* **10:**922–930.

66. Chao A. 1987. Estimating the population size for capture-recapture data with unequal catchability. *Biometrics* **43:**783–791.

67. Zhou J, Lottenbach KR, Barenkamp SJ, Lucas AH, Reason DC. 2002. Recurrent variable region gene usage and somatic mutation in the human antibody response to the capsular polysaccharide of Streptococcus pneumoniae type 23F. *Infect Immun* **70:**4083–4091.

68. Lucas AH, McLean GR, Reason DC, O'Connor AP, Felton MC, Moulton KD. 2003. Molecular ontogeny of the human antibody repertoire to the Haemophilus influenzae type B polysaccharide: expression of canonical variable regions and their variants in vaccinated infants. *Clin Immunol* **108:**119–127.

69. Jackson KJL, Liu Y, Roskin KM, Glanville J, Hoh RA, Seo K, Marshall EL, Gurley TC, Moody MA, Haynes BF, Walter EB, Liao H, Albrecht RA, García-Sastre A, Chaparro-Riggers J, Rajpal A, Pons J, Simen BB, Hanczaruk B, Dekker CL, Laserson J, Koller D, Davis MM, Fire AZ, Boyd SD. 2014. Human responses to influenza vaccination show seroconversion signatures and convergent antibody rearrangements. *Cell Host Microbe* doi:10.1016/j.chom.2014.05.013.

Antibody Informatics: IMGT, the International ImMunoGeneTics Information System

21

MARIE-PAULE LEFRANC[1]

INTRODUCTION

The efficiency of the adaptive immune response and its capability of recognizing a large number of different antigens depend on the huge diversity of the antigen receptors, immunoglobulins (IG), or antibodies of the B lymphocytes and T cell receptors (TR) of the T lymphocytes. The genes that code the IG and TR are highly polymorphic and are organized in clusters in several loci (three loci for IG and four for TR in humans) located on different chromosomes (four in humans) in the genome (1, 2). The molecular synthesis of the IG and TR chains is particularly complex and unique. It includes several mechanisms that occur at the DNA level: combinatorial rearrangements of the variable (V), diversity (D), and joining (J) genes that code the IG and TR variable domain, exonuclease trimming at the ends of the V, D, and J genes, and the random addition of nucleotides by the terminal deoxynucleotidyltransferase (TdT) that create the junction N diversity and, for IG, somatic hypermutations (1, 2). The IG and TR repertoires show an extraordinary diversity with a potential of 10^{12} IG and 10^{12} TR per individual, and the only limiting factor is the number of genetically programmed B and T cells for an organism. Therefore, the analysis of the IG and TR genes and of their

[1]IMGT, the international ImMunoGeneTics information system, Laboratoire d'ImmunoGénétique Moléculaire LIGM, Université Montpellier 2, Institut de Génétique Humaine IGH, UPR CNRS 1142, Montpellier, 34396 cedex 5, France.

Antibodies for Infectious Diseases
Edited by James E. Crowe, Jr., Diana Boraschi, and Rino Rappuoli
© 2014 American Society for Microbiology. All rights reserved.
doi:10.1128/microbiolspec.AID-0001-2012

expression represents a crucial challenge for the understanding of the immune response in normal and pathological situations.

IMGT, the international ImMunoGeneTics information system (http://www.imgt.org) (3), was created in 1989 at Montpellier, France (CNRS and Université Montpellier 2) to standardize the immunogenetics data and to manage the huge diversity of the antigen receptors, IG and TR (1, 2). New concepts, databases, and tools were developed by IMGT to explore and to analyze the particular properties of the IG and TR, compared with conventional genes and proteins. They led to the emergence of a new science, immuno-informatics, and, owing to the huge development of therapeutic antibodies, to antibody informatics, the part of immunoinformatics dealing with IG.

THE BASICS FOR ANTIBODY INFORMATICS

IMGT Gene and Allele Nomenclature

The accuracy and the consistency of the IMGT data are based on IMGT-ONTOLOGY, the first and, so far, unique ontology for immuno-genetics and immunoinformatics (4, 5, 6, 7, 8, 9, 10). IMGT-ONTOLOGY defined, for the first time, the concept of 'genes' for the IG and TR, which led to their gene and allele nomencla-ture (e.g., IGHV1-2*01) and allowed their entry in databases and tools (11). The IMGT IG and TR gene nomenclature (1, 2, 12, 13) was approved at the international level by the Human Genome Organisation (HUGO) No-menclature Committee (HGNC) in 1999 (14, 15) and endorsed by the World Health Orga-nization - International Union of Immunolog-ical Societies (WHO-IUIS) Nomenclature Committee (16, 17). The IMGT IG and TR gene names are the official reference for the genome projects and, as such, have been entered in IMGT/GENE-DB (18), in the Genome Database (GDB) (19), in LocusLink at the National Center for Biotechnology

Information (NCBI) (20), in Entrez Gene (NCBI, USA) when this database (now desig-nated as 'Gene') superseded LocusLink (21), in Ensembl at the European Bioinformatics Institute (EBI) (22), and in the Vertebrate Genome Annotation (Vega) Browser (23) at the Wellcome Trust Sanger Institute (UK). HGNC, Gene (NCBI), Ensembl, and Vega have direct links to IMGT/GENE-DB (18), which is the global reference for IG and TR alleles assigned by the WHO-IUIS-IMGT Nomencla-ture Subcommittee and, so far, the only database managing IG and TR alleles. Since 2008, IMGT gene and allele names have been used by the WHO-International Nonpropri-etary Names (WHO-INN) program in the definition of therapeutic monoclonal anti-bodies (mAb, INN suffix -mab), fusion proteins for immune applications (FPIA, INN suffix -cept), and composite proteins for clinical applications (CPCA) with Fc for increased half-life (24, 25), and the corresponding se-quences and data have been entered in IMGT/2Dstructure-DB (26) and in IMGT/mAb-DB (27) (http://www.imgt.org).

IMGT Unique Numbering

A second IMGT-ONTOLOGY revolutionizing concept was the IMGT unique numbering (28, 29, 30, 31, 32, 33), which, with its two-dimensional (2D) representation, the IMGT Collier de Perles (34, 35, 36, 37, 38), bridged for the first time, and definitively, the gap between sequences and structures for the variable (V) and constant (C) domains of the immunoglob-ulin superfamily (IgSF) proteins (28, 29, 30, 31, 32), and for the groove (G) domains of the major histocompatibility (MH) superfamily (MhSF) (32, 33). The V domains include the V-DOMAIN of the IG and TR and the V-LIKE-DOMAIN of the IgSF other than IG and TR; the C domains include the C-DOMAIN of the IG and TR and the C-LIKE-DOMAIN of the IgSF other than IG and TR; whereas the G domains include the G-DOMAIN of the MH and the G-LIKE-DOMAIN of the MhSF other than MH (28, 29, 30, 31, 32, 33, 34, 35, 36, 37, 38).

IMGT Anchors for V and C Domains

One of the IMGT unique numbering major breakthroughs for antibody informatics was to define 'anchors' in the V and C domains, a new and basic concept for *both* sequences and structures, that definitively solved the heterogeneity and complexity of previous numberings, and also is valid for *both* V and C domains (28, 29, 30, 31). A V domain is made of nine antiparallel beta strands on two layers (designated as framework regions (FR) in a V-DOMAIN), forming a barrel structure or 'sandwich' with a hydrophobic inner core, and three loops (designated as complementarity determining regions (CDR) or hypervariable regions in a V-DOMAIN) (28, 29, 30) (Fig. 1A). Compared with a V domain, a C domain has seven antiparallel beta strands instead of nine, two loops instead of three, and a characteristic CD transverse strand (in the absence of a C′ strand, C′C″ loop, and C″ strand) (31) (Fig. 1B).

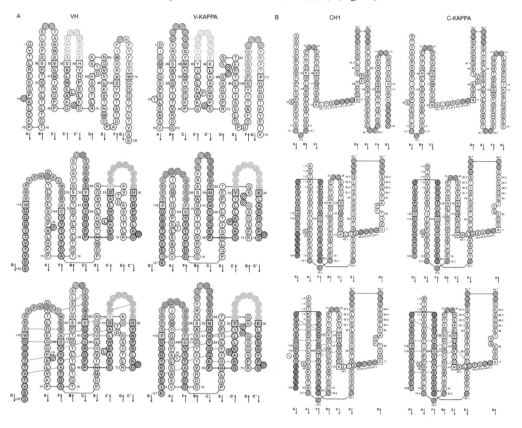

FIGURE 1 IMGT Collier de Perles for V-DOMAIN and C-DOMAIN. A, VH and V-KAPPA. B, CH1 and C-KAPPA. The VH, V-KAPPA, CH1, and C-KAPPA of the motavizumab antibody are shown as examples. IMGT Colliers de Perles are shown on one layer (top), on two layers (middle) (INN, from IMGT/2Dstructure-DB, http://www.imgt.org), and on two layers with hydrogen bonds (bottom) (3ixt_H and 3ixt_L, from IMGT/3Dstructure-DB, http://www.imgt.org) (26, 48). In the V-DOMAIN, anchors (positions 26 and 39, 55 and 66, 104 and 118) support the three CDR (CDR1-IMGT, CDR2-IMGT, and CDR3-IMGT that correspond to the BC, C′C″, and FG loops, respectively) (29, 30, 32). The VH and V-KAPPA CDR-IMGT lengths are [10.7.12] and [5.3.9], respectively. In the C-DOMAIN, anchors (positions 26 and 39, 104 and 118) support the BC and FG loops as in a V-DOMAIN, whereas in the absence of a C′ strand, C′C ″ loops, and C″ strand, anchors 45 and 77 delimit the CD transverse strand (31, 32). A ban symbol indicates an error (K instead of CH1 R120) in the 3D structure PDB file (3ixt), detected by using the IMGT unique numbering and by comparison with the INN sequence. A similar type of error (A instead of CH1 V121) has also been detected by IMGT for the 3D structure of the anti-HIV b12 antibody (1hzh). doi:10.1128/microbiolspec.AID-0001-2012.f1

The IMGT anchors define the positions of the V or C domain strands that support the loops. Anchors are shown in squares in IMGT Colliers de Perles (Fig. 1). In a V domain, these anchors comprise the positions 26 and 39, 55 and 66, 104 and 118 that support the BC, C'C'', and FG loops. In an IG or TR V-DOMAIN, these anchors are the positions of the FR-IMGT that support the CDR-IMGT (28, 29, 30). In a C domain, four anchors are identical to those of a V domain (positions 26 and 39, 104 and 118 that support the BC and FG loops) and two anchors (positions 45 and 77) delimit the CD strand (31).

CDR-IMGT Lengths for Antibody Humanization by Grafting

By allowing a correct delimitation of the FR-IMGT and CDR-IMGT, anchors led to the 'CDR-IMGT lengths' concept. The CDR-IMGT lengths are indicated between brackets and separated by dots, e.g., VH [10.7.12] and V-KAPPA [5.3.9] (see legend to Fig. 1). They are essential information for antibody characterization, used in IMGT databases and tools and in the INN mAb definitions (24) and, experimentally, for antibody humanization. The CDR-IMGT lengths avoid unnecessary extrapolation on canonical structures if the antibody has not yet been crystallized, while, at the same time, they provide the structural delimitations for the V-domain interactions with the antigen (39, 40, 41, 42), as demonstrated by the contact analysis and paratope/epitope details of known 3D structures (40, 41, 42). Moreover, the CDR-IMGT lengths are used whatever the chain type (e.g., heavy, light kappa or lambda for IG) and the species (e.g., human, mouse, rabbit, camel), which is particularly useful for domain comparison in antibody humanization by CDR grafting. For all these reasons, the CDR-IMGT lengths are key criteria for a good grafting in antibody humanization. Grafting CDR-IMGT on a germline-derived human FR-IMGT represents the definitive answer to preserve the specificity and affinity of the original antibody and to obtain, at the same time, a humanized antibody that is the most human as possible (39, 40, 41, 42).

Highly Conserved Amino Acids

In the IMGT unique numbering, amino acids always have the same position number. Highly conserved amino acids of an IG or TR V and C domains are written in red online, in the IMGT Colliers de Perles. They comprise five positions in a V-DOMAIN: cysteine C23 (1st-CYS), tryptophan W41 (CONSERVED-TRP), hydrophobic amino acid 89, cysteine C104 (2nd-CYS), and phenylalanine F118 (J-PHE) or tryptophan W118 (J-TRP) (that belongs to the F/W-G-X-G motif encoded by the J-REGION) (Fig. 1A). In a C domain, there are four highly conserved amino acids: C23 (1st-CYS), W41 (CONSERVED-TRP), hydrophobic 89, and C104 (2nd-CYS), instead of five.

IMGT Standardized and Integrated System

In 2013, IMGT comprised seven databases, seventeen online tools, and more than 15,000 pages of Web resources and is the reference in immunogenetics and immunoinformatics. IMGT-ONTOLOGY concepts (identification, description, classification (11), numerotation (32, 37), and detailed protocols (IMGT/V-QUEST [44], IMGT/JunctionAnalysis [45], IMGT/DomainGapAlign [47], IMGT/3Dstructure-DB [48], IMGT/Collier-de-Perles [38]) have been published in Cold Spring Harbor Protocols ('IMGT booklet' freely downloadable in IMGT references, http://www.imgt.org).

The next sections illustrate the use of IMGT tools for the standardized IG sequences and structures analysis for the IG repertoire analysis in infectious diseases, antibody engineering and humanization, and study of antibody/antigen interactions. Nucleotide sequences from deep sequencing (Next Generation Sequencing [NGS] or High Throughput Sequencing [HTS]) of antibody V domains are analyzed with IMGT/HighV-QUEST (43), the high-throughput version of IMGT/V-QUEST and IMGT/JunctionAnalysis (44, 45, 46). Amino acid sequences of V and C domains are represented with the IMGT/Collier-de-Perles tool (38) and analyzed with IMGT/Domain GapAlign (26, 47). Three-dimensional (3D) structures (including contact analysis and paratope/epitope) are described in IMGT/3Dstructure-DB (26, 48). Based on a friendly interface, IMGT/mAb-DB (27) contains therapeutic monoclonal antibodies (and also FPIA and CPCA with Fc) that can be queried on their specificity, for example, in infectious diseases, on bacterial or viral targets.

ANALYSIS OF ANTIBODY V-DOMAIN NUCLEOTIDE SEQUENCES

IMGT/V-QUEST

Since 1997, IMGT/V-QUEST (44, 46), a highly customized and integrated IMGT online tool, has been the reference for the standardized analysis of IG and TR rearranged V-domain nucleotide sequences. IMGT/V-QUEST identifies the V, D, and J genes and alleles by alignment with the germline IG and TR gene and allele sequences of the IMGT reference directory and, for the IG, the nucleotide (nt) mutations and amino acid (AA) changes resulting from somatic hypermutations. The tool identifies the hot-spot positions in the V-REGION of the closest germline V gene. IMGT/V-QUEST integrates IMGT/JunctionAnalysis (45), for the detailed analysis of the V-J and V-D-J junctions and IMGT/Automat for a complete sequence annotation of the sequences, and also provides IMGT Collier de Perles (37, 38). Customized parameters and results provided by IMGT/V-QUEST and IMGT/JunctionAnalysis have been detailed for antibody informatics (39, 40, 41, 42). The IMGT reference directories against which the tools compare user sequences are regularly updated with new IG and TR data from recently sequenced genomes (rat, rabbit, etc.), annotated in IMGT/LIGM-DB, the IMGT nucleotide sequence database (http://www.imgt.org), and IMGT/GENE-DB, the IMGT gene and allele database (18).

IMGT/HighV-QUEST for Deep Sequencing

Since October 2010, the analysis of IG and TR nucleotide sequences obtained from deep sequencing (NGS or HTS) can be performed with IMGT/HighV-QUEST (43, 46) (http://www.imgt.org) that analyzes 500,000 sequences per run and performs statistical analysis on the results (version July 2012).

The IMGT/HighV-QUEST Search page is very similar to the IMGT/V-QUEST Search page (44, 46). The results are provided in a downloadable main folder with eleven files in CSV format (results equivalent to those of the Excel file of IMGT/V-QUEST online), and one folder with the individual files (up to 500,000) of all the sequences results (results identical for each analyzed sequence to those of IMGT/V-QUEST online in Text, and corresponding to 'Detailed view') (43, 44, 46). Text and CSV formats were chosen to facilitate statistical studies for further interpretation and knowledge extraction. The eleven files of the main folder provide, per analysis, a total of 513 to 576 columns of results (Table 1) and demonstrate that IMGT standards, based on IMGT-ONTOLOGY concepts, fit remarkably well with extensive and detailed NGS data analysis for antibody informatics. The results include the identification of the closest V and J genes and alleles (and D genes for VH), detailed IMGT/JunctionAnalysis results, analysis of the nucleotide (nt) sequence mutations, and analysis of the amino acid (AA) changes in the sequence translations. The AA changes are described for the hydropathy (3 classes), volume (5 classes), and IMGT physicochemical properties (11 classes that comprise aliphatic [A, V, I, L], acid [D, E], basic [H, K, R], amide [N, Q], hydroxyl [S, T], sulfur [C, M], G, P, Y, F, and W) (49) (IMGT Aide-mémoire, in the 'Amino acids' section, http://www.imgt.org). Thus, S40>G (+ + −) means that the two AA involved in the change (S>G) at codon 40 belong to the same hydropathy (+) and volume (+) classes but to different physicochemical properties (−) classes (49). It is the first time

TABLE 1 List of the IMGT/HighV-QUEST[a] results files with number of columns and results content

File number	File name	Number of columns	Results content[b]
1	'Summary'	25–29	• Identity percentage with the closest V, D, and J genes and alleles • FR-IMGT and CDR-IMGT lengths • Amino acid (AA) JUNCTION • Description of insertions and deletions if any
2	'IMGT-gapped-nt-sequences'	18	• Nucleotide (nt) sequences gapped according to the IMGT unique numbering for V-D-J-REGION, V-J-REGION, V-REGION, FR1-IMGT, CDR1-IMGT, FR2-IMGT, CDR2-IMGT, FR3-IMGT • nt sequences of CDR3-IMGT, JUNCTION, J-REGION and FR4-IMGT
3	'Nt-sequences'	63–78	• nt sequences of all labels that can be automatically annotated by IMGT/Automat.
4	'IMGT-gapped-AA-sequences'	18	• AA sequences gapped according to the IMGT unique numbering for the labels V-D-J-REGION, V-J-REGION, V-REGION, FR1-IMGT, CDR1-IMGT, FR2-IMGT, CDR2-IMGT, FR3-IMGT • AA sequences of CDR3-IMGT, JUNCTION, J-REGION and FR4-IMGT
5	'AA-sequences'	18	• Same columns as "IMGT-gapped-AA-sequences" (#4), but sequences of labels are without IMGT gaps.
6	'Junction'	33, 46, 66, or 77	• Results of IMGT/JunctionAnalysis (33 columns for IGL and IGK (also for TRA and TRG) sequences, 46 (if one D), 66 (if two D) or 77 (if 3 D) columns for IGH (also for TRB and TRD) sequences
7	'V-REGION-mutation-and-AA-change table'	11	• List of mutations (nt mutations, AA changes, AA class identity (+) or change (−)) for V-REGION, FR1-IMGT, CDR1-IMGT, FR2-IMGT, CDR2-IMGT, FR3-IMGT, and germline CDR3-IMGT
8	'V-REGION-nt-mutation-statistics'	130	• Number (nb) of nt positions including IMGT gaps, nb of nt, nb of identical nt, total nb of mutations, nb of silent mutations, nb of nonsilent mutations, nb of transitions ($a>g$, $g>a$, $c>t$, $t>c$) and nb of transversions ($a>c$, $c>a$, $a>t$, $t>a$, $g>c$, $c>g$, $g>t$, $t>g$) for V-REGION, FR1-IMGT, CDR1-IMGT, FR2-IMGT, CDR2-IMGT, FR3-IMGT, and germline CDR3-IMGT
9	'V-REGION-AA-change-statistics'	189	• nb of AA positions including IMGT gaps, nb of AA, nb of identical AA, total nb of AA changes, nb of AA changes according to AAclassChangeType (+ + +, + + −, + − −, − − −, ...), and nb of AA class changes according to AAclassSimilarityDegree (nb of Very similar, nb of Similar, nb of Very dissimilar) for V-REGION, FR1-IMGT, CDR1-IMGT, FR2-IMGT, CDR2-IMGT, FR3-IMGT, and germline CDR3-IMGT
10	'V-REGION-mutation-hot spots'	8	• Hot spots motifs ((a/t)a, t(a/t), (a/g)g(c/t)(a/t), (a/t)(a/g)c(c/t) detected in the closest germline V-REGION with positions in FR-IMGT and CDR-IMGT
11	'Parameters'		• Date of the analysis • IMGT/V-QUEST program version, IMGT/V-QUEST reference directory release • Parameters used for the analysis: species, receptor type or locus, IMGT reference directory set, and Advanced parameters.

[a] IMGT/HighV-QUEST (43), freely available for academics on the IMGT Home page (http://www.imgt.org), analyzes up to 500,000 sequences per run. Results in the 11 files are equivalent to those of the Excel file of IMGT/V-QUEST online (46). The statistical analysis (tables and histograms) is performed on the 'Summary' file content and on the CDR3-IMGT results (nt and AA) of results of several runs up to 500,000 sequences and provided as PDF files and PNG figures (detailed in reference 43)

[b] Files 1 to 10 comprise systematically sequence identification (name, functionality, and names of the closest V, D, and J genes and alleles).

that such qualification of AA replacement is provided. This has led us to identify four types of AA changes: very similar (+ + +), similar (++ −, + − +), dissimilar (− − +, − + −, + − −) and very dissimilar (− − −) (44) (file 9 in Table 1).

IMGT/HighV-QUEST performs statistical analysis on the results of several runs up to 500,000 sequences. Detailed statistical analysis tables and histograms (e.g., V, D, and J usage, CDR3-IMGT [nt and AA lengths]), provided as PDF reports and separate graphical elements (figures in PNG format), are described elsewhere (43).

IMGT/HighV-QUEST achieved the same degree of resolution and high-quality results for antibody sequences analysis as IMGT/V-QUEST. Both tools use the same algorithm, and the user can evaluate the quality of his/her sequences before IMGT/HighV-QUEST analysis, by checking the results obtained with IMGT/V-QUEST on a few sequences. The eventual limitations of the IG V domain nucleotide sequence analysis using IMGT/HighV-QUEST are currently *not* on the antibody informatics side, but rather on the experimental and sequencing conditions that need to be improved (sequence length, avoiding PCR or sequencing errors) for a fully reliable and meaningful biological interpretation of the NGS or HTS results. By providing warnings and classification of sequences in categories ('1 copy,' 'More than 1,' 'single allele,' 'several alleles'…), IMGT/HighV-QUEST helps the user in evaluating his/her own data quality and therefore represents the reference tool for antibody-standardized analysis of NGS or HTS data.

ANTIBODY V- AND C-DOMAIN 2D REPRESENTATIONS

IMGT Collier de Perles 2D Representation

IMGT Collier de Perles (34, 35, 36, 37, 38) is a graphical 2D representation of domain, based on the IMGT unique numbering (28, 29, 30, 31, 32, 33). For the IG, the V domains include the V heavy (VH) and V light (VL) domains, the VL being V kappa (V-KAPPA) or V lambda (V-LAMBDA) in higher vertebrates, and V iota (V-IOTA) in fish. The C domains correspond either to a complete C-REGION (C-KAPPA of the IG-Light-Kappa chains or C-LAMBDA of the IG-Light-Lambda chains) or to part of it (e.g., CH1, CH2, and CH3 of the IG-Heavy-Gamma chains) (28, 29, 30, 31,32).

In IMGT Collier de Perles (Fig. 1), amino acids are shown in the one-letter abbreviation. Anchor positions are shown in squares. Hatched circles correspond to missing positions according to the IMGT unique numbering (29, 30, 31, 32). Strand positions at which hydrophobic amino acids (hydropathy index with positive value: I, V, L, F, C, M, A) and tryptophan (W) are found in more than 50% of sequences are shown with a blue background color. Arrows indicate the direction of the beta strands and their designations in 3D structures. The CDR-IMGT of the V-DOMAIN are colored according to the IMGT color menu which indicates the type of rearrangement, V-J or V-D-J (1, 2). Thus, the IMGT color menu for CDR1-IMGT, CDR2-IMGT, and CDR3-IMGT is online red, orange, and purple for VH (encoded by a V-D-J-REGION resulting from a V-D-J rearrangement), and blue, green, and green-blue for V-KAPPA or V-LAMBDA (encoded by a V-J-REGION resulting from a V-J rearrangement) (Fig. 1A).

The IMGT Colliers de Perles of the V and C domains can be displayed on two layers (Fig. 1, middle row) to get a graphical representation closer to the 3D structure, and on two layers with hydrogen bonds (Fig. 1, bottom row) if the mAb has been crystallized and data are in IMGT/3Dstructure-DB (26, 48).

The IMGT/Collier-de-Perles Tool

The IMGT/Collier-de-Perles tool (38) (IMGT Home page, http://www.imgt.org) allows the users to draw IMGT Colliers de Perles, on one or two layers, starting from their own domain amino acid sequences. Sequences have to be gapped according to the IMGT unique numbering (using, for example, IMGT/DomainGapAlign [47]). The IMGT/Collier-de-Perles tool can be customized to display the CDR-IMGT according to the IMGT color menu or the amino acids according to their hydropathy, volume, or the 11 IMGT physicochemical classes (49) (IMGT Aide-Mémoire, in the 'Amino acids' section, http://www.imgt.org).

Importance for Antibody Engineering and Antibody Humanization

The IMGT Colliers de Perles are used in antibody engineering and antibody humanization, and for the evaluation of the immunogenicity of therapeutic monoclonal antibodies (40, 41, 42). The information is particularly useful:

1. to precisely define the CDR1-IMGT, CDR2-IMGT, and CDR3-IMGT to be grafted in antibody humanization design based on CDR grafting. Amino acids of the CDR-IMGT loops are those involved in the interactions with the antigen (40, 41, 42),

2. to compare the physicochemical properties of AA at given positions in the user V-region sequences with those of the IMGT Collier de Perles statistical profiles for the human expressed IGHV, IGKV, and IGLV repertoires (49), and to identify AA that, given their positions, could be potentially immunogenic in chimeric or poorly humanized antibodies. The IMGT statistical profiles comprise 61 positions with conserved properties, among which 13 participate to the inner core, 10 to the inner surface of the ABED and GFCC'C" beta sheet (inside of the 'sandwich'), 21 to the outer surface of the ABED beta sheet and of the F strand, and 10 to turns (exposed to solvent), and seven to the VH-VL interface (detailed in Table 3 of reference 49),

3. to localize unusual amino acid changes, for example, the four AA changes observed between camel IGHV1 genes expressed in conventional IgG1 and those expressed in nonconventional IgG2 and IgG3 (dimer of heavy gamma2 or gamma3 chains with deleted

CH1, without light chain): V42>(F,Y), G49>(E, Q), L50>(C,R) and W52>(F,G,L,W) (IMGT Gene table in IMGT Repertoire, and IMGT Biotechnology page, http://www.imgt.org/IMGTbiotechnology/Camel_IgG.html),

4. to predict important AA interactions, even in the absence of 3D structures, by analyzing the display of conserved hydrogen bonds in crystallized V domains and C domains (Fig. 1) (IMGT Collier de Perles on two layers in IMGT/3Dstructure-DB [26, 48]). Of importance for antibody humanization are the two FR-IMGT positions, 39 and 40, that have hydrogen bonds with a CDR2-IMGT and a CDR3-IMGT position, respectively: anchor 39 with CDR2-IMGT 56 (in VH) or 57 (in VL), and position 40 with CDR3-IMGT 105 (in both VH and VL). These positions eventually need to be kept from the original antibody (26, 48), and

5. to localize the landmarks of the CH domain. These include the conserved N-glycosylation site in the CH2 of the IGHG1, IGHG2, IGHG3, and IGHG4, on the asparagine (Asn) N84.4 at the top of the DE turn. There is also a polymorphic N-glycosylation site N79 in the CH3 strand D of several alleles of the IGHG3 (replaced by a lysine [Lys] K in the other alleles) (Alignment of alleles in IMGT Repertoire, http://www.imgt.org). The positions used for the 'knobs-into-holes' engineering for heavy-chain dimerization and the production of bispecific IgG antibodies involve CH3 positions threonine (Thr) T22 (strand B) and tyrosine (Tyr) Y86 (strand E) with the following AA changes, T22>Y on one CH3 domain and Y86>T on the other one (IMGT Biotechnology page, http://www.imgt.org).

ANALYSIS OF ANTIBODY V- AND C-DOMAIN AMINO ACID SEQUENCES

IMGT/DomainGapAlign

IMGT/DomainGapAlign (26, 47) analyzes the amino acid sequences of the IG and TR variable (V) and constant (C) domains. Several amino acid sequences can be analyzed simultaneously, provided that they belong to the same domain type (V or C). IMGT/DomainGapAlign analyzes the user amino acid domain sequences by comparison with the IMGT reference directory sets (translation of the germline V and J genes and of the C gene domains from IMGT/GENE-DB [18]). These reference amino acid sequences can be displayed by querying IMGT/DomainDisplay (IMGT Home page, http://www.imgt.org).

Antibody V Domain Amino Acid Sequence Analysis

IMGT/DomainGapAlign identifies the closest germline V-REGION and J-REGION alleles. IMGT/DomainGapAlign displays the V region amino acid sequences of the user aligned with the closest V and J regions (Fig. 2A) with IMGT gaps and delimitations of the strands (FR-IMGT) and loops (CDR-IMGT), according to the IMGT unique numbering for V domain (28, 29, 30, 32). For instance, for motavizumab, the V-REGION of the VH domain is identified as having 86.9% identity with the *Homo sapiens* IGHV2-70*01 and the V-REGION of the V-KAPPA as having 83.0% identity with the *H. sapiens* IGKV1-5*01. If several closest alleles are identified, the user can select the display of each corresponding alignment. The amino acid sequence is also displayed online, according to the IMGT color menu, with the delimitations of the V-REGION, J-REGION, and for VH domains, (N-D)-REGION.

The number of amino acid differences in the FR-IMGT and CDR-IMGT is one of the criteria to evaluate the potential immunogenicity (39, 40, 41, 42). The framework of a VH domain comprises 91 positions (25, 17, 38, and 11 positions for FR1-, FR2-, FR3-, and FR4-IMGT, respectively, represented as [25.17.38.11]), whereas the framework of a VL domain comprises 89 positions (26, 17, 36, 10 positions for FR1-, FR2-, FR3-, and FR4-IMGT, respectively, represented as [26.17.36.10]) (26, 47). Thus, for motavizumab, the framework of the VH has 10 AA differences (81/91 identical AA) with the framework

constituted by the closest human germline IGHV2-70*01 and IGHJ6*03, whereas the framework of the V-KAPPA has 5 AA differences (84/89 identical AA) with the framework constituted by the closest human germline IGKV1-5*01 and IGKJ4*01 (Fig. 2A) (in a humanization with a good IMGT grafting, the number of AA differences in the framework is minimal and usually between 0 and 2).

The IMGT/DomainGapAlign results include tables with the characteristics of the AA changes (49) shown in strands and loops, and in FR-IMGT and CDR-IMGT. The IMGT Collier de Perles of the analyzed VH or VL domain (V-D-J region or V-J region, respectively) is also available with highlighted AA differences (in pink circles online) with the closest germline sequence.

Antibody C Domain Amino Acid Sequence Analysis

IMGT/DomainGapAlign displays the C-domain amino acid sequences of the user sequence aligned with the closest C-DOMAIN alleles (Fig. 2B) with IMGT gaps and delimitations of the strands, turns and loops, according to the IMGT unique numbering for C domain (31, 32). The IMGT unique numbering for C-DOMAIN contributes to antibody engineering and humanization by providing a standardized description of the Gm, Am, and Km allotypes, and by establishing, for the first time, the correlation between the G1m, G2m, G3m, A2m, and Km allotypes, and the IGHG1, IGHG2, IGHG3, IGHA2, and IGKC alleles, respectively (50).

For instance, IMGT/DomainGapAlign shows that the C-REGION of motavizumab is 100% identical with the IGHG1*03 allele in its three CH domains and hinge region. The IGHG1*03 allele corresponds to the G1m3 allele (50), characterized by the G1m3 allotype (CH1 arginine [Arg] R120, associated to CH1 isoleucine [Ileu] I103) (Fig. 2B), and to the isoallotypes nG1m17 (CH1 R120) and nG1m1 (CH3 glutamate [Glu] E12 and methionine [Met] M14) (50). The C-KAPPA of

A VH and V-KAPPA

❷ Alignment with the closest gene and allele from the IMGT V domain directory: *Homo sapiens* (human)

```
              FR1-IMGT                CDR1-IMGT      FR2-IMGT      CDR2-IMGT                 FR3-IMGT                          CDR3-IMGT    FR4-IMGT
              (1-26)                  (27-38)        (39-55)       (56-65)                   (66-104)                          (105-117)    (118-128)
          A            B             BC        C       C'    C'C"      C"       D        E         F                  FG          G
        (1-15)        (16-26)        (27-38)  (39-46) (47-55) (56-65) (66-74) (75-84)  (85-96)   (97-104)           (105-117)   (118-128)
        -------->      -------->      ------>  ----->  ----->  ----->  ----->  ----->   ----->    ----->            ------->     ----------
        1     10 15 16   23 26 27      38 3941 46 47   55 56  65 66  74 75   84 85 89  96 97    104 105 11112 117 118      128
        |.........|..| |........|..| |........| |.|..| |.....| |.....| |.....| |.|..| |........| |.|......|      |.....||...| |.......|

8693 H  QVTLRESGP.ALVKP TQTLTLTCTFS GFSLS..TAGMS VGWIRQPP GKALEWLAD IWWD...DKK HYNPSLK.D RLTISKDTSK NQVVLKVTNMDP ADTATYYC ARDMIF.NFYFDV WGQGTTVTVSS
                                                                                                                          ||____||

IGHV2-70*01  QVTLRESGP.ALVKP TQTLTLTCTFS GFSLS..TSGMC VSWIRQPP GKALEWLAL IDWD...DKK YYSTSLK.T RLTISKDTSK NQVVLTMTNMDP VDTATYYC ARI
Homo sapiens                                 A  S  G            D  W     K H NP  D                     KV    A    D        DAFDV WGQGTMVTVSS
                                                                                                                          FY         T

                                                                                                                          IGHJ3*01
                                                                                                                          Homo sapiens
```

❷ Alignment with the closest gene and allele from the IMGT V domain directory: *Homo sapiens* (human)

```
              FR1-IMGT                CDR1-IMGT      FR2-IMGT      CDR2-IMGT                 FR3-IMGT                          CDR3-IMGT    FR4-IMGT
              (1-26)                  (27-38)        (39-55)       (56-65)                   (66-104)                          (105-117)    (118-128)
          A            B             BC        C       C'    C'C"      C"       D        E         F                  FG          G
        (1-15)        (16-26)        (27-38)  (39-46) (47-55) (56-65) (66-74) (75-84)  (85-96)   (97-104)           (105-117)   (118-128)
        -------->      -------->      ------>  ----->  ----->  ----->  ----->  ----->   ----->    ----->            ------->     ----------
        1     10 15 16   23 26 27      38 3941 46 47   55 56  65 66  74 75   84 85 89  96 97    104 105 11112 117 118      128
        |.........|..| |........|..| |........| |.|..| |.....| |.....| |.....| |.|..| |........| |.|......|      |.....||...| |.......|

8693 L  DIQMTQSPSTLSASV GDRVTITCSAS SRV.......GY MHWYQQKP GKAPKLLIY DT.......S KLASGVP.S RFSGSG..SG TEFTLTISSLQP DDFATYYC FQGSG....YPFT FGGGTKVEIK
                                                                                                                          ||

IGKV1-5*01   DIQMTQSPSTLSASV GDRVTITCRAS QSI......SSW LAWYQQKP GKAPKLLIY DA.......S SLESGVP.S RFSGSG..SG TEFTLTISSLQP DDFATYYC QQYNSYS
Homo sapiens                    S   SRV        GY MH                T         K A                                 F GSG
                                                                                                                          LT FGGGTKVEIK
                                                                                                                          F

                                                                                                                          IGKJ4*01
                                                                                                                          Homo sapiens
```

B CH1 and C-KAPPA

❷ Alignment with the closest gene and allele from the IMGT C domain directory: *Homo sapiens* (human)

```
          A        AB      B         BC      C       CD      D            DE          E      EF   F        FG          G
        (1-15)   (16-26)  (27-38)   (39-45) (77-84)                     (85-96)  (97-104) (105-117) (118-128)
        -------->  -------->         ------>  ------>                     -------->  ------>
        1      10 15 16   2326 27     38 3941 45     77      84        85  89   96 97   104 105      117 118
        87654321|.......|....|123|......|..| |........| |.|..|1234567|......|234567776543321|...|......|12|.......|    |.........|   |.........|

8693 H  ....ASTKGPSVFPLAPSSKSTS...GGTAALGCLVK DYFP..EPVT VSWNSGALTS....GVHTFPAVLQSS......GLYSLSSVVTVPSSSL...GTQTYIC NVNHKP..SNTKV DKRV......

IGHG1*03    ....ASTKGPSVFPLAPSSKSTS...GGTAALGCLVK DYFP..EPVT VSWNSGALTS....GVHTFPAVLQSS......GLYSLSSVVTVPSSSL...GTQTYIC NVNHKP..SNTKV DKRV
Homo sapiens
```

❷ Alignment with the closest gene and allele from the IMGT C domain directory: *Homo sapiens* (human)

```
          A        AB      B         BC      C       CD      D            DE          E      EF   F        FG          G
        (1-15)   (16-26)  (27-38)   (39-45) (77-84)                     (85-96)  (97-104) (105-117) (118-128)
        -------->  -------->         ------>  ------>                     -------->  ------>
        1      10 15 16   2326 27     38 3941 45     77      84        85  89   96 97   104 105      117 118
        87654321|.......|....|123|......|..| |........| |.|..|1234567|......|234567776543321|...|......|12|.......|    |.........|   |.........|

8693 L  ....RTVAAPSVFIFPPSDEQLK...SGTASVVCLLN NFYP..REAK VQWKVDNALQSG..NSQESVTEQDSKD.....STYSLSSTLTLSKADY..EKHKVYAC EVTHQG..LSSPV TKSFNRGEC.

IGKC*01     ....RTVAAPSVFIFPPSDEQLK...SGTASVVCLLN NFYP..REAK VQWKVDNALQSG..NSQESVTEQDSKD.....STYSLSSTLTLSKADY..EKHKVYAC EVTHQG..LSSPV TKSFNRGEC
Homo sapiens
```

FIGURE 2 **IMGT/DomainGapAlign alignments. A, VH and V-KAPPA. B, CH1 and C-KAPPA. The closest V-REGION and J-REGION identified at the amino acid level are aligned with the user sequence (here, motavizumab INN 8693, as example). The VH and V-KAPPA are identified as having 86.9% and 83% identity at the amino acid level with the *Homo sapiens* IGHV2-70*01 and IGKV1-5*01, respectively (% identity is shown in an upper section online). Amino acid differences are indicated below the V and J alignments. The FR-IMGT and CDR-IMGT, strands and loops are according to the IMGT unique numbering for V domain (28, 29, 30, 32). The CH1 and C-KAPPA are identified as having 100% identity at the amino acid level with the *H. sapiens* IGHG1*03 CH1 and IGKC*01, respectively. IMGT/DomainGapAlign displays the C-domain amino acid sequence of the user, with IMGT gaps and delimitations of the strands, turns, and loops, according to the IMGT unique numbering (31, 32). doi:10.1128/microbiolspec.AID-0001-2012.f2**

motavizumab is 100% identical to the IGKC*01 allele (Fig. 2B). IGKC*01 is one of the four IGKC alleles that correspond to a Km3 allele, characterized by an alanine (Ala) A45.1 ('.1' for the first position in the transverse CD strand) and a valine (Val) V101 (50).

The IMGT/DomainGapAlign results include tables with the characteristics of the AA changes (49) shown in strands, turns, and loops. The IMGT Collier de Perles of the analyzed C domain is also available with highlighted AA differences (in pink circles online) with the closest allele domain sequence.

ANTIBODY 3D STRUCTURES

IMGT/3Dstructure-DB Card

IMGT/3Dstructure-DB (26, 48) (http://www.imgt.org), the IMGT 3D structure database, is queried through a user-friendly interface and different displays for the results can be chosen from the database home page (48). Each entry in the database is detailed in an IMGT/3Dstructure-DB card that provides access to all sequence data related to that entry, and, in particular, for antibodies, the paired heavy and light chains, and for IG/antigen (Ag) complexes, the ligands (if peptides or proteins). IMGT uses the 'PDB code' (4 letters and/or numbers) as 'IMGT entry ID.' An additional letter separated by an underscore ('_') identifies the different chains in a 3D structure. For example, the 3ixt entry that corresponds to the 3D structure of an IG/antigen (Ag) complex (motavizumab Fab in complex with the antigen 'ligand' Fusion glycoprotein F1) comprises two crystallographic complexes (as indicated in the column CC with the colors red and blue), with for one of them (CC1, red), the following chains: 3ixt_H (VH-CH1) and 3ixt_L (L-KAPPA) for the IG Fab, and 3ixt_P for the antigen ('ligand'). Eight tabs are available at the top of each card: 'Chain details,' 'Contact analysis,' 'Paratope and epitope,' '3D visualization Jmol or QuickPDB,' 'Renumbered

IMGT file,' 'IMGT numbering comparison,' 'References and links,' and 'Printable card.'

IMGT/3Dstructure-DB Chain Details

The section 'Chain details' of the IMGT/3Dstructure-DB card comprises, for each chain, information first on the chain itself, then per domain.

1. The information for each chain includes:

   - 'Chain ID' (e.g., 3ixt_H),
   - 'Chain length' in amino acids (e.g., 225),
   - 'IMGT chain description' with the delimitations of the different domains (e.g., VH-CH1 = VH (1-120) [D1] + CH1 (121-210) [D2]),
   - 'Chain sequence' with delimitations of the regions and domains, highlighting of AA (in orange color) that are different from the closest genes and alleles, and links to *Sequence in FASTA format* and to *Sequence in IMGT format*.

2. The information for a V-DOMAIN, as an example, includes:

   - 'IMGT domain description' (e.g., VH (1-120) [D1]),
   - 'IMGT gene and allele name' with the percentage of identity for the V and a link to *Alignment details*
   - 'IMGT gene and allele name' with the percentage of identity for the J as well as other alleles giving the same percentage of identity), and a link to *Alignment details*,
   - '2D representation': links to *IMGT Collier de Perles on one layer* or *IMGT Collier de Perles on two layers,*
   - 'Contact analysis': a link to *Domain contacts (overview)*,
   - 'CDR-IMGT lengths' (e.g., [10.7.12]),
   - 'Sheet composition' (e.g., [A'BDE][A"CC'C "FG]),
   - the domain amino acid sequence with CDR-IMGT delimitations and highlighting of AA (in orange color) that are different from the closest V and J genes and alleles,
   - the link to *IMGT/DomainGapAlign results*.

IMGT/3Dstructure-DB Contact Analysis

The IMGT/3Dstructure-DB Contact analysis (26, 48) provides extensive information on the atom pair contacts between domains and/or chains and on the internal contacts in an IMGT/3Dstructure-DB entry. Atom pair contacts are obtained in IMGT/3Dstructure-DB by a local program in which atoms are considered to be in contact when no water molecule can take place between them and are characterized by their atom contact types (Noncovalent, Polar, Hydrogen bond, etc.) and their atom contact categories ([BB] Backbone/backbone, [SS] Side chain/side chain, etc.) (26, 48).

This information can be obtained at three different levels:

1. Domain contacts (overview),
2. Domain pair contacts ('DomPair') that provides information on the contacts between a pair of domains or between a domain and a ligand (e.g., between the VH domain of motavizumab (3ixt_H chain) and the ligand (3ixt_P chain) (Fig. 3A), or between the V-KAPPA domain of motavizumab (3ixt_L chain) and the ligand (3ixt_P chain) (Fig. 3B),
3. Residue pair contacts, or more precisely, IMGT Residue@Position (R@P) pair contacts.

R@P represents one of the major breakthroughs of the IMGT unique numbering for 3D structures. Indeed, in IMGT, any residue (amino acid) that belongs to an antibody domain (and more generally, any amino acid that belongs to a V or C domain of an IgSF protein, or to a G domain of a MhSF protein [32]) is characterized by its position in the domain. An R@P is defined by the IMGT position numbering, the residue name, the IMGT domain description, and the IMGT chain ID (e.g., 35 – ALA (A) – VH – 3ixt_H). Structural information and contacts for a given 'R@P' are provided in the IMGT Residue@Position card that includes general information (PDB file numbering, IMGT file numbering, residue full name and formula), and structural information 'IMGT LocalStructure@Position' (secondary structure, Phi and Psi angles [in degrees] and accessible surface area [ASA] [in square angstroms]). The IMGT Residue@Position cards can be accessed directly from the amino acid sequences of the IMGT/3Dstructure-DB card or from the IMGT Colliers de Perles, by clicking on one AA.

IMGT Paratope and Epitope

In an IG/Ag complex, the amino acids in contact at the interface between the IG and the Ag constitute the paratope on the IG surface, and the epitope on the Ag surface (Fig. 3C). In IMGT/3Dstructure-DB, the 'IMGT paratope and epitope' of IG/Ag complexes is determined automatically by combining contact analysis with an interaction scoring function and are described in a standardized way. Thus, the IG paratope of 3ixt (motavizumab Fab) (Fig. 3C) comprises amino acids of VH (3ixt_H chain) and of V-KAPPA (3ixt_L chain). Fifteen amino acids of the antibody, 8 from VH and 7 from V-KAPPA, form the paratope (Fig. 3C). Eight of the 8 positions belong to the VH CDR-IMGT [10.7.12] (A35 to the CDR1-IMGT; W58, D59, and K64 to the CDR2-IMGT; and I109, F110, N112, and F113 to the CDR3-IMGT). Seven of the 7 positions belong to the V-KAPPA CDR-IMGT [5.3.9] (G37 and Y38 to the CDR1-IMGT; D56 to the CDR2-IMGT; and G107, S108, G109, and Y114 to the CDR3-IMGT). These results emphasize the importance of using the IMGT unique numbering for standardized antibody analysis and confirm that the CDR-IMGT structural delimitations correspond to the V-domain interactions with the antigen.

The Ag epitope of 3ixt (Fig. 3C) comprises AA of the Fusion glycoprotein F1 (3ixt_P). Eleven amino acids form the Ag epitope. Each amino acid that belongs to the epitope is defined by its position in the chain in the 3D structure (if the AA is part of a V, C, or G domain, the position is given according to the IMGT unique numbering (32).

Clicking on a residue in 'Paratope details' or in 'Epitope details' (Fig. 3C) provides the

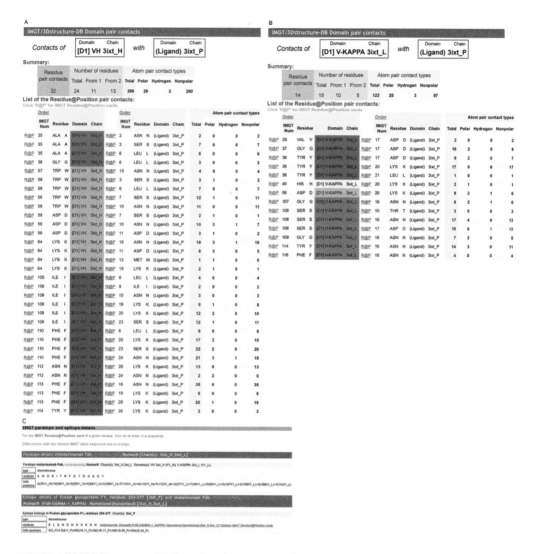

FIGURE 3 IMGT/3Dstructure-DB Domain pair contacts and IMGT paratope and epitope details. A, IMGT/3Dstructure-DB Domain pair contacts between the VH of motavizumab (3ixt_H) and the Fusion glycoprotein F1 (ligand) (3ixt_P). B, IMGT/3Dstructure-DB Domain pair contacts between the V-KAPPA of motavizumab (3ixt_L) and the Fusion glycoprotein F1 (ligand) (3ixt_P). 'Polar,' 'Hydrogen bonds,' and 'Nonpolar' were selected before display, in 'Atom contact types.' Amino acids belonging to the CDR1-IMGT, CDR2-IMGT, and CDR3-IMGT are colored online according to the IMGT color menu (red, orange, and purple, respectively, for VH; blue, green, and green-blue, respectively, for V-KAPPA). In this 3D structure, all but one amino acid that contact the antigen belong to the CDR-IMGT. Clicking on R@P gives access to the IMGT Residue@Position cards (26, 48). C, 'IMGT paratope and epitope details' of the IG/Ag complex '3ix't is shown. Each AA that belongs to the IG paratope is characterized by its position in the V domains according to the IMGT unique numbering (29, 30, 32). Thus, 'A (35V1_A)' means that the alanine (A) is at position 35 of the V domain 1 of 3ixt_A (VH). In the same way, 'G(107V1_B)' means that the glycine (G) is at position 107 of the V domain 1 of 3ixt_B (V-KAPPA). Each AA that belongs to the antigenic determinant (epitope) is characterized by its position (here, position in the chain, in the 3D structure). For example, 'S (3_C)' means that the serine (S) is at position 3 of the Fusion glycoprotein F1 ligand (3ixt_C), whereas 'SN (23-24_C)' means that the serine (S), asparagine (N) are at positions 23, 24. The 'IMGT paratope and epitope' analysis of the IG/Ag 3D structure (3ixt) is from IMGT/3Dstructure-DB (http://www.imgt.org). doi:10.1128/microbiolspec.AID-0001-2012.f3

R@P card for each AA that belongs to the paratope or epitope, respectively.

IMGT/StructuralQuery and IMGT/DomainSuperimpose

IMGT/DomainSuperimpose (3) (IMGT® Home page, http://www.imgt.org) allows one to superimpose the 3D structures of two domains from IMGT/3Dstructure-DB, and demonstrate that the same IMGT numbering is found at the same positions of the framework of the heavy and light chains and for the lower part of the CDR-IMGT loops of the two domains. IMGT/StructuralQuery (3) allows the retrieval the IMGT/3Dstructure-DB entries containing a V, C, or G domain, based on specific structural characteristics of the intramolecular interactions: phi and psi angles, accessible surface area, type of atom contacts, distance in angstroms between amino acids, R@P pair contacts, and, for the V domain, CDR-IMGT length or pattern.

IMGT/2Dstructure-DB AND IMGT/mAb-DB

In a further effort to bridge the gap between sequences and 3D structures, a new extension of IMGT/3Dstructure-DB, designated as IMGT/2Dstructure-DB, was created to describe and analyze amino acid sequences of paired chains of heavy and light chains of antibodies for which no 3D structures are available. These amino acid sequences are analyzed and managed with the IMGT criteria of standardized gene and allele nomenclature (classification), standardized labels (description), and IMGT unique numbering and IMGT Colliers de Perles (numerotation) (10). IMGT/2Dstructure-DB uses the IMGT/3Dstructure-DB informatics frame and interface that allows one to analyze, manage, and query antibodies as polymeric receptors made of several chains, in contrast to the IMGT/LIGM-DB sequence database that analyzes and manages IG sequences, individually. The current IMGT/2Dstructure-DB entries include amino acid sequences of the paired heavy and light chains of antibodies from WHO-INN (24, 25) and those from Kabat (annotated by IMGT and for which there are no available nucleotide sequences, the others already being in IMGT/LIGM-DB). IMGT/2Dstructure-DB entries also include the INN amino acid sequences of FPIA (suffix -cept) and those of CPCA with a Fc (for increased half-life) (prefix ef-).

Queries can be made on an individual entry, using the Entry ID (e.g., for an INN entry, the 4-number code, e.g., 8693) or the Molecule name (e.g., motavizumab). Search can be made on Entry type (e.g., 'INN'), and on criteria detailed in the IMGT/2Dstructure-DB Query page, http://www.imgt.org). In the results page, clicking on an IMGT entry ID gives access to the IMGT/2Dstructure-DB card (42). The IMGT/2Dstructure-DB card provides standardized IMGT information on chains and domains and IMGT Colliers de Perles on one or two layers, identical to that of an IMGT/3Dstructure-DB card; however, the information on experimental structural data (hydrogen bonds in IMGT Collier de Perles on two layers, Contact analysis) is only available in the corresponding IMGT/3Dstructure-DB card, if the antibodies have been crystallized (26, 48). For therapeutic antibodies, queries can be made from the IMGT/mAb-DB user-friendly interface (http://www.imgt.org) on search criteria, such as characteristics (conjugated, radiolabeled...), IG classes or subclasses for complete IG or format (Fab, scFv, etc.) for IG fragments, specificity (target name and species), clinical indication, development status, etc.

TOWARD TARGETED AND CUSTOMIZED THERAPEUTIC ANTIBODIES

IMGT provides antibody informatics with a standardized system for sequences and structures (6, 7), from amino acid characteristics at given positions (49), to IG gene and allele identification, and to 3D structures analysis (antibody/antigen contact analysis, paratope/

epitope description). Since its creation in 1989, and owing to a strong expertise and background in immunogenetics, IMGT has defined IG alleles and developed databases and tools and web resources for IG polymorphism, as demonstrated by IMGT/GENE-DB (18), IMGT Alignments of alleles and the correspondences between IGHG and IGKC genes and the C-domain Gm and Km allotypes (50). The extension of the IMGT unique numbering to the IgSF and to the MhSF proteins other than IG or TR has opened new perspectives for the standardized description of the polymorphism of the antigens (epitopes belonging to V, C, or G domains) and of the Fc receptors (FCGR of the IgSF, FCGRT of the MhSF) and for the characterization of their interactions (antibody/antigen, FcR/antibody). Given the importance of these interactions in the antibody specificity and affinity on the one hand and in the antibody pharmacokinetics/pharmacodynamics and half-life on the other hand, the IMGT integrated and standardized approach provides the genetic knowledge for allowing antibody informatics to answer the needs of targeted and customized therapy in the context of personalized medicine.

AVAILABILITY AND CITATION

Authors who use IMGT databases and tools are encouraged to cite this article and to quote the IMGT Home page (http://www.imgt.org). Online access to IMGT databases and tools is freely available for academics and under licenses and contracts for companies.

ACKNOWLEDGMENTS

I thank Gérard Lefranc for helpful discussions, Sophia Kossida and Souphatta Sasorith for reading the manuscript, Denis Moreno for the figures, and the IMGT team for its expertise and constant motivation. IMGT is a registered trademark of CNRS. IMGT is a member of the International Medical Informatics Association (IMIA). IMGT was funded in part by the BIOMED1 (BIOCT930038), Biotechnology BIOTECH2 (BIO4CT960037), 5th PCRDT Quality of Life and Management of Living Resources (QLG2-2000-01287), and 6th PCRDT Information Science and Technology (ImmunoGrid, FP6 IST-028069) programs of the European Union (EU), and by the Agence Nationale de la Recherche ANR (BIOSYS06_135457, FLAVORES). IMGT is currently supported by the Centre National de la Recherche Scientifique (CNRS), the Ministère de l'Enseignement Supérieur et de la Recherche (MESR), the Université Montpellier 2, the GIS IBiSA, the Région Languedoc-Roussillon (Grand Plateau Technique pour la Recherche [GPTR], GEPETOS), and the Labex MAbImprove (ANR-10-LABX-53). This work was granted access to the HPC resources of CINES under the allocations 2010-2014-036029 made by GENCI (Grand Equipement National de Calcul Intensif).

Conflicts of interest: I declares no conflicts.

CITATION

Lefranc M-P. 2014. Antibody informatics: IMGT, the International ImMunoGeneTics Information System. Microbiol Spectrum 2(2):AID-0001-2012.

REFERENCES

1. **Lefranc M-P, Lefranc G.** 2001. *The Immunoglobulin FactsBook.* Academic Press, London, United Kingdom.
2. **Lefranc M-P, Lefranc G.** 2001. *The T Cell Receptor FactsBook.* Academic Press, London, United Kingdom.
3. **Lefranc M-P, Giudicelli V, Ginestoux C, Jabado-Michaloud J, Folch G, Bellahcene F, Wu Y, Gemrot E, Brochet X, Lane J, Regnier L, Ehrenmann F, Lefranc G, Duroux P.** 2009. IMGT®, the international ImMunoGeneTics information system®. *Nucl Acids Res* 37:D1006–D1012.
4. **Giudicelli V, Lefranc M-P.** 1999. Ontology for immunogenetics: IMGT-ONTOLOGY. *Bioinformatics* 15:1047–1054.
5. **Lefranc M-P, Giudicelli V, Ginestoux C, Bosc N, Folch G, Guiraudou D, Jabado-Michaloud J,**

Magris S, Scaviner D, Thouvenin V, Combres K, Girod D, Jeanjean S, Protat C, Yousfi Monod M, Duprat E, Kaas Q, Pommié C, Chaume D, Lefranc G. 2004. IMGT-ONTOLOGY for immunogenetics and immunoinformatics. *In Silico Biol* **4**:17–29.

6. Lefranc M-P, Clément O, Kaas Q, Duprat E, Chastellan P, Coelho I, Combres K, Ginestoux C, Giudicelli V, Chaume D, Lefranc G. 2005. IMGT-Choreography for Immunogenetics and Immunoinformatics. *In SilicoBiol* **5**:45–60.

7. Lefranc M-P, Giudicelli V, Regnier L, Duroux P. 2008. IMGT®, a system and an ontology that bridge biological and computational spheres in bioinformatics. *Brief Bioinform* **9**:263–275.

8. Duroux P, Kaas Q, Brochet X, Lane J, Ginestoux C, Lefranc M-P, Giudicelli V. 2008. IMGT-Kaleidoscope, the formal IMGT-ONTOLOGY paradigm. *Biochimie* **90**:570–583.

9. Giudicelli V, Lefranc M-P. 2012. IMGT-ONTOLOGY 2012. *Front Genet* **3**:79. doi:10.3389/fgene.2012.00079.

10. Lefranc M-P. 2013. IMGT-ONTOLOGY, p 964–972. *In* Dubitzky W, Wolkenhauer O, Cho K, Yokota H (ed), *Encyclopedia of Systems Biology*, doi:10.1007/978-1-4419-9863-7. Springer Science+Business Media, LLC012, Rueil-Malmaison, France.

11. Lefranc M-P. 2011. From IMGT-ONTOLOGY CLASSIFICATION Axiom to IMGT standardized gene and allele nomenclature: for immunoglobulins (IG) and T cell receptors (TR). *Cold Spring Harb Protoc* **6**:627–632. pii: pdb.ip84. doi:10.1101/pdb.ip84.

12. Lefranc M-P. 2001. Nomenclature of the human immunoglobulin genes, p A.1P.1–A.1P.37. *In* Coligan JE, Bierer BE, Margulies DE, Shevach EM, Strober W (ed), *Current Protocols in Immunology*. John Wiley and Sons, Hoboken, NJ.

13. Lefranc M-P. 2001. Nomenclature of the human T cell receptor genes, p A.1O.1–A.1O.23. *In* Coligan JE, Bierer BE, Margulies DE, Shevach EM, Strober W (ed), *Current Protocols in Immunology*. John Wiley and Sons, Hoboken, NJ.

14. Wain HM, Bruford EA, Lovering RC, Lush MJ, Wright MW, Povey S. 2002. Guidelines for human gene nomenclature. *Genomics* **79**:464–470.

15. Bruford EA, Lush MJ, Wright MW, Sneddon TP, Povey S, Birney E. 2008. The HGNC Database in 2008: a resource for the human genome. *Nucl Acids Res* **36**:D445–D448.

16. Lefranc M-P. 2007. WHO-IUIS Nomenclature Subcommittee for immunoglobulins and T cell receptors report. *Immunogenetics* **59**:899–902.

17. Lefranc M-P. 2008. WHO-IUIS Nomenclature Subcommittee for immunoglobulins and T cell receptors report August 2007, 13th International Congress of Immunology, Rio de Janeiro, Brazil. *Dev Comp Immunol* **32**:461–463.

18. Giudicelli V, Chaume D, Lefranc M-P. 2005. IMGT/GENE-DB: a comprehensive database for human and mouse immunoglobulin and T cell receptor genes. *Nucl Acids Res* **33**:D256–D261.

19. Letovsky SI, Cottingham RW, Porter CJ, Li PW. 1998. GDB: the Human Genome Database. *Nucl Acids Res* **26**:94–99.

20. Maglott DR, Katz KS, Sicotte H, Pruitt KD. 2000. NCBI's LocusLink and RefSeq. *Nucl Acids Res* **28**:126–128.

21. Maglott D, Ostell J, Pruitt KD, Tatusova T. 2007. Entrez Gene: gene-centered information at NCBI. *Nucl Acids Res* **35**:D26–D31.

22. Stabenau A, McVicker G, Melsopp C, Proctor G, Clamp M, Birney E. 2004. The Ensembl core software libraries. *Genome Res* **14**:929–933.

23. Wilming LG, Gilbert JG, Howe K, Trevanion S, Hubbard T, Harrow JL. 2008. The vertebrate genome annotation (Vega) database. *Nucl Acids Res* **36**:D753–D760.

24. Lefranc M-P. 2011. Antibody nomenclature: from IMGT-ONTOLOGY to INN definition. *mAbs* **3**:1–2.

25. World Health Organization. 2011. General policies for monoclonal antibodies, p 8–10. *In International Nonproprietary Names (INN) for Biological and Biotechnological Substances, INN Working Document 05.179, Update 2011*. http://www.who.int/medicines/services/inn/en.

26. Ehrenmann F, Kaas Q, Lefranc M-P. 2010. IMGT/3Dstructure-DB and IMGT/DomainGapAlign: a database and a tool for immunoglobulins or antibodies, T cell receptors, MHC, IgSF and MhcSF. *Nucl Acids Res* **38**:D301–D307.

27. Poiron C, Wu Y, Ginestoux C, Ehrenmann F, Duroux P, Lefranc M-P. 2010. IMGT/mAb-DB: the IMGT® database for therapeutic monoclonal antibodies, poster 101. 11èmes Journées Ouvertes de Biologie, Informatique et Mathématiques (JOBIM), Montpellier, France, 7 to 9 September 2010.

28. Lefranc M-P. 1997. Unique database numbering system for immunogenetic analysis. *Immunol Today* **18**:509.

29. Lefranc M-P. 1999. The IMGT unique numbering for Immunoglobulins, T cell receptors and Ig-like domains. *The Immunologist* **7**:132–136.

30. Lefranc M-P, Pommié C, Ruiz M, Giudicelli V, Foulquier E, Truong L, Thouvenin-Contet V, Lefranc G. 2003. IMGT unique numbering for immunoglobulin and T cell receptor variable domains and Ig superfamily V-like domains. *Dev Comp Immunol* **27**:55–77.

31. Lefranc M-P, Pommié C, Kaas Q, Duprat E, Bosc N, Guiraudou D, Jean C, Ruiz M, Da Piedade I,

Rouard M, Foulquier E, Thouvenin V, Lefranc G. 2005. IMGT unique numbering for immuno-globulin and T cell receptor constant domains and Ig superfamily C-like domains. *Dev Comp Immunol* 29:185–203.

32. Lefranc M-P. 2011. IMGT Unique Numbering for the Variable (V), Constant (C), and Groove (G) Domains of IG, TR, MH, IgSF, and MhSF. *Cold Spring Harb Protoc* 6:633–642. pii: pdb.ip85. doi:10.1101/pdb.ip85.

33. Lefranc M-P, Duprat E, Kaas Q, Tranne M, Thiriot A, Lefranc G. 2005. IMGT unique numbering for MHC groove G-DOMAIN and MHC superfamily (MhcSF) G-LIKE-DOMAIN. *Dev Comp Immunol* 29:917–938.

34. Ruiz M, Lefranc M-P. 2002. IMGT gene identi-fication and Colliers de Perles of human immunoglobulins with known 3D structures. *Immunogenetics* 53:857–883.

35. Kaas Q, Lefranc M-P. 2007. IMGT Colliers de Perles: standardized sequence-structure repre-sentations of the IgSF and MhcSF superfamily domains. *Curr Bioinformatics* 2:21–30.

36. Kaas Q, Ehrenmann F, Lefranc M-P. 2007. IG, TR and IgSf, MHC and MhcSF: what do we learn from the IMGT Colliers de Perles? *Brief Funct Genomic Proteomic* 6:253–264.

37. Lefranc M-P. 2011. IMGT Collier de Perles for the Variable (V), Constant (C), and Groove (G) Domains of IG, TR, MH, IgSF, and MhSF. *Cold Spring Harb Protoc* 6:643–651. pii: pdb.ip86. doi:10.1101/pdb.ip86.

38. Ehrenmann F, Giudicelli V, Duroux P, Lefranc M-P. 2011. IMGT/Collier-de-Perles: IMGT Stan-dardized Representation of Domains (IG, TR, and IgSF Variable and Constant Domains, MH and MhSF Groove Domains). *Cold Spring Harb Protoc* 6:726–736. pii: pdb.prot5635. doi:10.1101/pdb. prot5635.

39. Lefranc M-P. 2004. IMGT, the international ImMunoGenetics information system®. *In* Lo BKC (ed), *Antibody Engineering: Methods and Protocols*, 2nd edition. Humana Press, Totowa, NJ. *Meth Mol Biol* 248:27–49.

40. Lefranc M-P. 2009. Antibody databases and tools: The IMGT® experience, p 91–114. *In* An Z (ed), *Therapeutic Monoclonal Antibodies: from Bench to Clinic*. John Wiley and Sons, Hoboken, NJ.

41. Ehrenmann F, Duroux P, Giudicelli V, Lefranc M-P. 2010. Standardized sequence and struc-ture analysis of antibody using IMGT®, p 11–31. *In* Kontermann R, Dübel S (ed), *Antibody Engi-neering*, vol **2**. Springer-Verlag, Heidelberg, Germany.

42. Lefranc MP, Ehrenmann F, Ginestoux C, Duroux P, Giudicelli V. 2012. Use of IMGT® databases and tools for antibody engineering and humanization. *In* Chames P (ed), *Antibody Engi-neering*. Humana Press, Springer, New York, NY. *Meth Mol Biol* 907:3–37.

43. Alamyar E, Giudicelli V, Shuo L, Duroux P, Lefranc M-P. 2012. IMGT/HighV-QUEST: the IMGT® web portal for immunoglobulin (IG) or antibody and T cell receptor (TR) analysis from NGS high throughput and deep sequencing. *Immunome Res* 8:26.

44. Giudicelli V, Brochet X, Lefranc M-P. 2011. IMGT/V-QUEST: IMGT Standardized Analysis of the Immunoglobulin (IG) and T Cell Receptor (TR) Nucleotide Sequences. *Cold Spring Harb Protoc* 6:695–715. pii: pdb.prot5633. doi:10.1101/ pdb.prot5633.

45. Giudicelli V, Lefranc M-P. 2011. IMGT/ JunctionAnalysis: IMGT Standardized Analysis of the V-J and V-D-J Junctions of the Rearranged Immunoglobulins (IG) and T Cell Receptors (TR). *Cold Spring Harb Protoc* 6:716–725. pii: pdb. prot5634. doi:10.1101/pdb.prot5634.

46. Alamyar E, Duroux P, Lefranc M-P, Giudicelli V. 2012. IMGT® tools for the nucleotide analysis of immunoglobulin (IG) and T cell receptor (TR) V-(D)-J repertoires, polymorphisms, and IG muta-tions: IMGT/V-QUEST and IMGT/HighV-QUEST for NGS. *In* Christiansen F, Tait B (ed), *Immunogenetics*. Humana Press, Springer, New York, NY. *Meth Mol Biol* 882:569–604.

47. Ehrenmann F, Lefranc M-P. 2011. IMGT/ DomainGapAlign: IMGT Standardized Analysis of Amino Acid Sequences of Variable, Constant, and Groove Domains (IG, TR, MH, IgSF, MhSF). *Cold Spring Harb Protoc* 6:737–749. pii: pdb. prot5636. doi:10.1101/pdb.prot5636.

48. Ehrenmann F, Lefranc M-P. 2011. IMGT/ 3Dstructure-DB: Querying the IMGT Database for 3D Structures in Immunology and Immuno-informatics (IG or Antibodies, TR, MH, RPI, and FPIA). *Cold Spring Harb Protoc* 6:750–761. pii: pdb.prot5637. doi:10.1101/pdb.prot5637.

49. Pommié C, Levadoux S, Sabatier R, Lefranc M-P. 2004. IMGT standardized criteria for statistical analysis of immunoglobulin V-REGION amino acid properties. *J Mol Recognit* 17:17–32.

50. Lefranc M-P, Lefranc G. 2012. Human Gm, Km and Am allotypes and their molecular character-ization: a remarkable demonstration of poly-morphism. *In* Christiansen F, Tait B (ed), *Immunogenetics*. Humana Press, Springer, New York, NY. *Meth Mol Biol* 882:635–680.

Probing Antibody-Antigen Interactions

22

GUOCHENG YANG,[1] STEFANIE N. VELGOS,[2] SHANTA P. BODDAPATI,[3] and MICHAEL R. SIERKS[1]

PROBING ANTIBODY-ANTIGEN INTERACTIONS

Antibodies bind antigens via noncovalent bonds, such as hydrogen bonds, ionic, hydrophobic, and Van der Waals forces, and their interactions depend strongly on the distance between two interacting molecules. While each individual bond is weak, the collective noncovalent bonds between the antibody and antigen can be strong when all the interacting molecules work together synergistically. Because there are a very large number of these interactions and the antigen and antibody are large, flexible, dynamic molecules, binding between an antibody and antigen is a very complex process. The binding interactions may also be time dependent, because formation of an antibody-antigen complex may involve a sequential series of interactions which induce conformational changes that generate some bonds while breaking others. Because of the dynamic and transient state of antibody-antigen interactions, measurements of the antibody-antigen interactions can be quite complicated and inconsistent, and the results may vary depending on the sample treatment conditions and technique utilized (1).

[1]Department of Chemical Engineering, Arizona State University, Tempe, AZ 85287-6006; [2]Mayo Clinic Arizona, Phoenix, AZ 85054; [3]Department of Biomedical Engineering, Oregon Health and Science University, Portland, OR 97239.
Antibodies for Infectious Diseases
Edited by James E. Crowe, Jr., Diana Boraschi, and Rino Rappuoli
© 2015 American Society for Microbiology, Washington, DC
doi:10.1128/microbiolspec.AID-0010-2013

Classical immunoassays such as radioimmunoassay (RIA) and enzyme-linked immunosorbent assay (ELISA) are widely used to determine the affinity and specificity of antibodies to their target antigens. These assays typically involve the immobilization of the antigen or antibody onto a solid support, followed by the introduction of labeled analyte at varying concentrations and the measurement of bound analyte to determine the binding constant (K_D) of the antibody. While these methods are widely utilized, there are some limitations in their application. For example, RIA and ELISA generally require large amounts of sample, chemical modification to the antigen or antibody for immobilization, and the need of a label. Consequently, modern immunochemical techniques, which include label-free detection, a single-molecule detection level, and a low sample volume system, have been developed to overcome these limitations and to complement the classical methods to study antibody-antigen interactions. Here, we will review three conceptually different techniques that can be used to study and quantify bulk and single-molecule-level antibody-antigen interactions: (i) surface plasmon resonance (SPR), a label-free method to measure both on and off rates of antibody-antigen interactions; (ii) fluorescence-activated cell sorting (FACS) that enables high-throughput screening of surface-bound proteins; and (iii) atomic force microscopy (AFM) that enables a molecular-level detection of individual antibody-antigen binding. These techniques differ from traditional immunoassays in that they do not require high sample volumes or concentrations, SPR and AFM do not require additional labeling, SPR provides real-time in situ detection of antibody-antigen interactions, and AFM can provide detailed structural information of the target antigen. These techniques expand the capabilities of classical immunoassays and are particularly useful when the quantity of antibody or antigen is limited, or when the purification process is tedious and difficult, or when the structure of the analytes is unstable or cannot be immobilized.

SPR: a Label-Free Detection System

SPR is an optical technique that offers real-time, label-free detection of binding interactions between the immobilized biomolecule and the free-flowing analyte. SPR measures changes in mass at the sensor surface as the analyte interacts with the immobilized biomolecule, and this increase in mass is proportional to the increase in refractive index (discussed later). A typical SPR instrument comprises three main components: (i) a microfluidic cartridge, (ii) a sensor chip, and (iii) an optical detection unit (Fig. 1A). The microfluidic assembly allows the analyte to pass over the sensor surface in a continuous and controlled flow, while maintaining a constant analyte concentration. The sensor chip is usually made of a glass support with a thin gold-sensing layer (2). The gold-sensing surface of the chip is in direct contact with a flow cell (the sample side), while the glass support is placed directly adjacent to a glass prism on the detector side (Fig. 1B). A light source, typically a light-emitting diode, emits a wedge of polarized light (3) onto the prism, which has the same refractive index as the glass substrate. The angle of incident from the light-emitting diode source is increased until the prism reflects light at or beyond the critical angle of the sensor surface such that total internal reflection (TIR) occurs (Fig. 1B).

TIR occurs when a light beam is propagated through two nonabsorbing media of different refractive indices (like glass-buffer or glass-air) (4). This reflected energy from the light beam excites the electrons of the gold atoms in the outer orbitals, thus causing the excited electrons to become delocalized and to form plasmons (4). The delocalized electrons (plasmons) resonate on the gold surface and emit evanescent waves, which propagate from the glass sensor chip (high refractive index) to

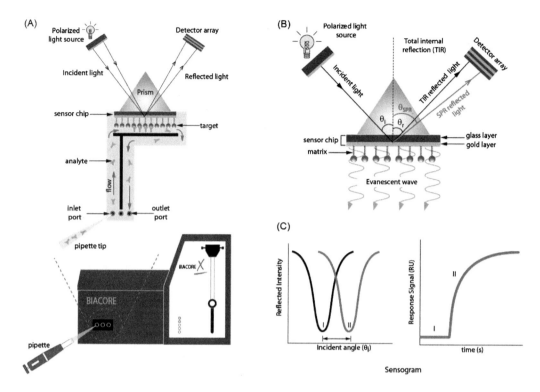

FIGURE 1 Schematic illustration of a BIAcore SPR instrument. (A) The BIAcore system contains three main elements crucial to its operation: the integrated microfluidic cartridge (IFC) (light gray L-shaped block), sensor chip, and optical detection unit. (B) A simplistic overview of how SPR works. (C) The transformation of the shift in incident angles to the response signal in an SPR sensogram. doi:10.1128/microbiolspec.AID-0010-2013.f1

the medium (low refractive index). The resonance energy transfer between the evanescent wave and the surface plasmons on the metal surface causes a decrease in the incident light intensity (3). TIR only occurs at a specific angle of the incident light reflection (5), and the SPR-reflected light angle depends on the refractive index of the medium close to the gold film surface (3). As mass accumulates at the sensor chip surface owing to biomolecular interactions, it causes a change in localized solute concentration, which corresponds to a change in the refractive index of the medium. This translates into a change in the SPR angle (5) and the SPR angle is often reported as resonance units (RUs) (Fig. 1C) (3). By monitoring the SPR signal, it is possible to quantify the interaction between

the target and analyte, to determine the kinetics of binding interactions (on and off rates), and to determine the concentrations of the amount of analyte in a sample (Fig. 2). Because the detection sensitivity of SPR mainly depends on the distance of the analyte from the sensor surface, although some electrostatic attraction or conformational changes may induce changes in SPR angles (6), SPR can detect virtually any interacting molecules regardless of their nature.

Several SPR experimental setups can be used to obtain data, including direct binding, surface competition, or inhibition-in-solution assays (7). For immobilization of antigen or antibody, a variety of different surface chemistries (e.g., dextran, carboxylation, and streptavidin coating) are available so that binding

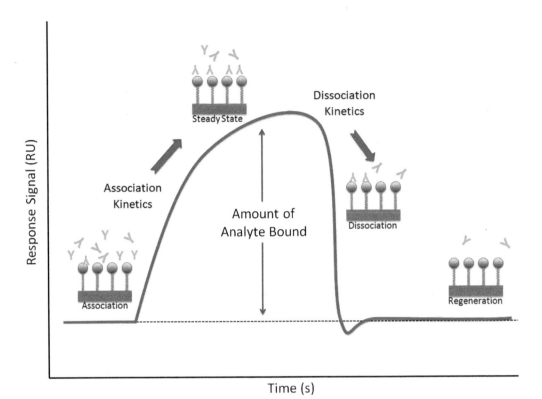

FIGURE 2 An SPR sensogram depicting the different stages of a binding event. After the target has been immobilized, a baseline RU is established by using only running buffer in the flow system. Upon injection of the analyte, the RU on the sensogram gradually increases, indicating that the system is in the association phase where the analyte binds to the target. It is important to note that some bound molecules have already begun to dissociate during analyte injection. The RU reaches saturation at steady state, where the associating and dissociating molecules are in equilibrium. Once the analyte injection is completed and is replaced by running buffer, the system is in the pure dissociation phase, which is marked by a decrease in RU. The sensor chip regeneration is performed, and baseline RU should be restored. doi:10.1128/microbiolspec.AID-0010-2013.f2

artifacts and high nonspecific binding can be avoided (8).

SPR has important benefits over conventional immunofluorescence or ELISA-type assays for studying interactions between immobilized biomolecules and a solution-phase analyte. SPR measurements are based on refractive index changes and do not require the need of a label or the need for a multistep protocol (9). Also, since SPR measurements are performed in real time instead of by using equilibrium endpoints, it provides useful thermodynamic and kinetic information of the system, including binding enthalpies and entropies, and the kinetic on and off rates. In

addition to antibody-antigen interactions, SPR has also been used to measure protein–peptide and protein-DNA interactions, cellular ligation, and DNA hybridization (9, 10).

FACS Offers High-Throughput Screening of Antibodies

FACS is an application of flow cytometry that uses fluorescently labeled reagents to detect antigens expressed on cells or other particles. This technique can be effectively used to determine antibody-antigen interactions. One major advantage of using FACS for studying antibody-antigen interactions is that the target antigen does not need to be modified or immobilized. In FACS, cells are first labeled directly or indirectly with fluorophore-conjugated antibodies. The labeled cell-antibody mixture is suspended in a stream of fluid, and the cells can then be sorted and analyzed individually. Laser light is directed onto the stream of cells and the scattering characteristics of the cells are used to analyze cell size, granularity, and expression of the antigen of interest on the cell surface (11). Thus, multiple antibodies can be used to simultaneously detect the expression of several antigens of interest on the cell surface (Fig. 3). Cells with desired characteristics can be collected for further growth and characterization.

Flow cytometry was first used to determine the equilibrium binding constant K_D for a recombinant single-chain antibody fragment (scFv) binding to the CD34 antigen (12). In this case, yeast cells expressing the scFv were conjugated with a labeled antibody and the antigen concentration was varied. The antigen-antibody binding can be quantified using flow cytometry by measuring the mean fluorescence intensity (MFI) for the antibody and antigen binding over a range of concentrations. The K_D can be calculated assuming MFI is directly proportional (fixed constant ratio) to the number of binding events, since both rates of binding and dissociation are equal at equilibrium (Eq. 1). With the use of single-site first-order binding kinetics, and assuming that the concentration of free scFv is much larger than the number of binding sites (12), the K_D and maximum fluorescence values (F_{max}) values can be obtained by using Eq. 1 and Eq. 2, respectively. Equation 2 is generally referred to as a Lineweaver-Burke plot. A similar approach was also used to quantify the K_D values of botulinum toxin specific antibodies using flow cytometry (13). FACS-based selection techniques were also used to select for scFv's against several proteins and phosphopeptides by using a nonimmune yeast surface display library where the scFv's were displayed on the yeast cell surface by genetically coupling the scFv gene to a yeast agglutinin receptor (14). K_D values of the scFv's calculated using FACS were similar to values obtained by using SPR (15).

$$K_D = \frac{k_{off}}{k_{on}} = \frac{[Ab][Ag]}{[Ab \cdot Ag]} \tag{1}$$

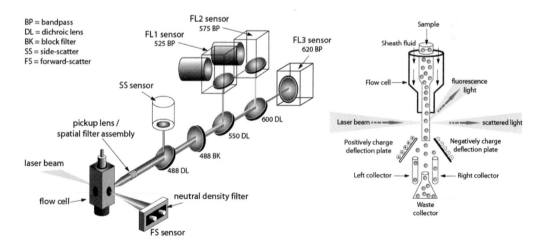

FIGURE 3 Schematic illustration of a FACS system. (A) A flow cytometer showing the light path, sensors, optics, and filters used (figure adapted from _Applied Microbiology and Biotechnology_ [11] with permission of with permission of Beckman-Coulter). (B) A simplified illustration of the principles of flow cytometry with the use of FACS. FL, fluorescent light. doi:10.1128/microbiolspec.AID-0010-2013.f3

where K_D = equilibrium binding constant,

k_{on} = association constant,
k_{off} = dissociation constant,
[Ab] = antibody concentration,
[Ag] = antigen concentration, and
[Ab·Ag] = antibody-antigen complex concentration

$$\frac{1}{F-F_b} = \frac{1}{F_{max}} + \left(\frac{K_D}{F_{max}}\right)\left(\frac{1}{[scFv]}\right) \tag{2}$$

where F_b = background fluorescence,
F_{max} = maximum fluorescence, and
[scFv] = concentration of scFv

FACS-based analysis can also be used to screen and select for antibodies from second-generation libraries containing mutations of a parent antibody (16, 17, 18). FACS selection was used to isolate higher-affinity variants from a library of clones generated from a parent anti-fluorescein 4-4-20 antibody (19). The dissociation of antigen from scFv follows a first-order kinetic model since the dissociation rate (k_{off}) depends on the amount of antigen bound to the surface-displayed scFv on the yeast (Eq. 3). A plot of the exponential decay of MFI with time enables calculation of the amount of bound antigen providing the system is initially saturated with excess antigen (Eq. 4). Antibody clones can be selected from the library based on k_{off} values, reducing the number of clones that need to be tested for further screening or characterization.

$$\frac{dF}{dt} = -k_{off}F \tag{3}$$

$$F_t = F_0 e^{-k_{off}t} \tag{4}$$

where F_t = MFI at time, t, and F_o = initial MFI.

FACS-based analysis of antigen-antibody binding is a convenient and reliable method. Because it does not need purified form of the protein, it can be used at the stage of selection and screening of antibodies. In addition, screening methods that use FACS analysis will be able to differentiate positive clones based on affinity. Unlike other selection methods that collect all positive binders for further rounds of amplification, high and low binders can be separately sorted for further amplification.

Single-Molecule Antigen-Antibody Detection Using AFM

The previous techniques describe methods that can be used to analyze bulk antigen-antibody interactions. However, sometimes it is beneficial to study single-molecule interactions. Antibody-antigen binding interactions are complex and dynamic processes, and proteins may have a multitude of variable conformations complicating or preventing bulk measurements. AFM is a powerful technique that can be used to measure single-molecule antibody-antigen interactions.

Three major techniques have been used to explore single molecular interactions: optical tweezers, magnetic tweezers, and AFM. Among them, optical tweezers and magnetic tweezers use either a laser optical trap or a magnetic force field to move a particle with molecules linked on it, while AFM uses a tiny stylus of a few nanometers in radius to directly probe and move the single molecule in three dimensions. An excellent review describing the different principles and instrumentation setups and discussing the resolution and other limitations is available (20). Although optical tweezer and magnetic tweezer techniques are considered to be noninvasive, they are not particularly well suited for measuring protein interactions because of their low pico-Newton measurement range (0.1 to 100 pN). AFM, however, can be effectively used to study interactions between molecules because it has a relatively large measurement range, is simple to operate, and has a unique ability to simultaneously image the sample and measure force interactions.

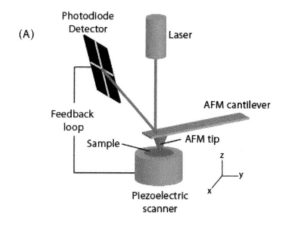

(A)

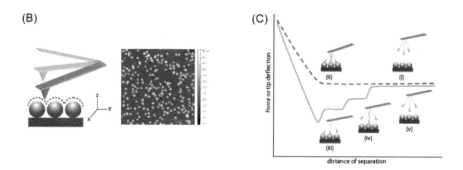

FIGURE 4 **Schematic illustration of an AFM. (A) A typical AFM setup comprises an AFM cantilever, a laser source, a photodetector, and a piezoelectric scanner. (B) AFM topographical imaging is acquired when the tip raster scans the sample surface in the X-Y direction, while the tip deflection is recorded in the Z direction. (C) AFM force-distance curve. The force plot is generated when the tip (i) approaches the surface (red dash line), (ii) contacts the surface and moves with the surface up to a preset point. In the retracting phase (green solid line), the tip retracts from the surface and experiences (iii) one or (iv) more bond-breaking events before completely dissociating from the surface and (v) returning to its original point. doi:10.1128/microbiolspec.AID-0010-2013.f4**

AFM was derived from scanning probe microscopy, which was invented by Binnig et al. in 1984 (21). AFM typically contains four main parts: (i) a tip attached to a flexible cantilever, (ii) a laser signal and a photodetector sensing the movement of the tip, (iii) a piezoelectric scanner controlling the X-Y-Z position of the sample, and (iv) a feedback loop controlling the movement of these three parts (Fig. 4). While the tip raster scans the sample surface, the laser beam is projected off the back of the cantilever onto the photodetector. The tip deflection caused by tip-sample interaction is reflected as a lateral or vertical shift of the laser spot on the photodetector. This shift is used to adjust the X-Y-Z extension of the scanner, to maintain the distance between the sample and the scanning tip at the prescribed set point value, which corresponds to the specific interaction force between the tip and sample. The X-Y-Z position of the sample generated from this process is recorded as the topography of the sample, also known as the height image. This primary imaging mode of AFM is also known as contact-mode AFM, in which the tip is in constant contact with the sample. To reduce interactions between the tip and sample, Hansma et al. invented a new way of oscillating a tip at a high frequency over the sample within a short distance, which is known as intermittent contact or tapping mode AFM (22).

AFM is able to produce high-resolution images of sample topography in aqueous/liquid environments with the use of minimal sample preparation and without the need to stain the sample. Images with nanometer resolution laterally and Angstrom resolution vertically can be readily obtained (23, 24, 25). In addition to generating high-resolution images, AFM is also particularly useful for measuring interaction forces between molecules. Since the tip on the cantilever is free to move above the sample surface, it can be modeled as a spring with a spring constant of k. According to Hooke's law, the force exerted between the tip and sample can be calculated from the deflection of the tip (Δz) multiplied by the spring constant k (Eq. 5). For any sudden change in the force interaction between the tip and surface due to the rupture of a bond or unfolding of a molecule, a sharp change in the force curve will be observed. Such special force curves will have multiple peaks or a sawtooth pattern, which is characteristic of nonspecific binding events.

$$F_{tip} = -k(\Delta z) \qquad (5)$$

where k = spring constant and Δz = tip deflection.

Most cantilevers and tips used for AFM imaging are made either of silicon nitride (Si_3N_4) or silicon (Si), which provides excellent mechanical elasticity. By fabricating the cantilevers in different geometric shapes and sizes, tips with different spring constants can be constructed. Selecting the cantilever with the right spring constant is critically important for performing protein interaction measurements. The smaller the spring constant, the more sensitive the cantilever is and the weaker force it can detect; on the other hand, the more

flexible the tip is, the more difficult it is to obtain good images. Contact mode imaging and noncontact mode imaging usually use cantilevers of different spring constants, and not all of them are suitable for force interaction studies because of sensitivity limits.

To prevent nonspecific binding interactions, the protein of interest can be attached onto the cantilever tip. Two common approaches are used, either esterification or silanization. In general, 3-aminophenyl-trimethoxysilane is used for silanization and ethanolamine is used for esterification (26). Both of these approaches add functional amine groups onto the end the tip. The amine groups are sequentially connected with glutaraldehyde, which can then be used to connect the target protein onto the tip. If needed, an extended polyethylene glycol linker can be added to allow more flexibility for the attached protein to minimize steric constraints.

AFM was initially used to study the binding interaction between streptavidin and biotin, one of the strongest protein/protein bonds known in nature. With the use of AFM, the force interaction between streptavidin and biotin was calculated to be ~0.35 nN (27) and between the essentially similar avidin and biotin to be ~0.16 nN (28). The difference in these two calculated values may result from the different experimental setups used where one protocol utilized a flat surface to immobilize the protein, and the other used curved agarose beads to minimize the potential for multiple binding events.

Nonspecific binding interactions are a problem in all antibody-antigen techniques, and this is equally true for single-molecule measurements using AFM. The use of nonreactive blocking agents and detergents to minimize nonspecific interactions has been extensively applied in traditional antibody-antigen assays such as ELISA. Similar approaches can be used for single molecule force spectroscopy to differentiate specific antibody-antigen interaction from nonspecific backgrounds as demonstrated on a ferritin and antiferritin system, by using bovine serum albumin and Tween 20 as unreactive proteins and detergents, respectively (29).

It is important to point out that single-molecule interaction forces as measured by AFM at a specific pulling rate represent a single point in a spectrum of binding strength. It is expected that different forces will be observed at different pulling rates. This principle was elegantly demonstrated by measuring the same streptavidin-biotin attractive forces with the use of a technique called surface biomembrane force probe (30). The biomembrane force probe is a single-molecule force apparatus, from which the interaction force is detected from the deformation of the vesicle or cell membrane with molecules attached. The measured bond strengths varied from 5 pN to 170 pN, depending on the rate at which the forces were applied. By analyzing the slope of the force versus the loading rate, it is possible to estimate the activation barriers of the interaction complex at a specific loading rate.

Similar experiments using AFM have also been performed to determine the binding force between the Fv fragments of antilysozyme and lysozyme (31). At a loading rate of 5,000 pN/s, multiples of characteristic unbinding force of ~50 pN were detected from 900 binding curves, which likely represents the rupture of a single Fv and lysozyme complex. As expected, the measured pulling force varied at different loading rates. It is interesting to note that the kinetic off-rate dissociation constant extrapolated at zero force is $\sim 1 \times 10^{-3}$ s^{-1}, which is in the same range as the value obtained using SPR ($\sim 3 \times 10^{-3}$ s^{-1}).

SELECTING ANTIBODIES WITH DIFFERENT SPECIFICITIES BY USING SPR, FACS, AND AFM

While the various techniques described above can be effectively used to measure and study antibody-antigen interactions, the same techniques can also be used to select for antibodies with target-specific binding properties. Anti-body-binding domains can be displayed on the surface of cells or virus particles, enabling the selection of displayed antibody fragments that have particular binding properties or that have improved affinity compared with a parent antibody. In the following section, we will briefly describe how the different aforementioned techniques can also be used to select for antibody fragments with improved binding characteristics.

SPR-Based Antibody Selection

SPR utilizes a microfluidic platform to first bind and then elute antibodies from antigens immobilized on the chip surface. This feature can also be utilized to select for higher binding variants of antibodies from a pool of antibodies. For example, in a study by Yuan et al., a library of higher binding variants of a parent antibody binding the protein β-amyloid (Aβ) were selected by using SPR (32). On average, antibody clones selected by SPR had fivefold better dissociation rates than clones selected by conventional means, and the best dissociation rate obtained with SPR was almost 10 times better than that obtained conventionally (32).

SPR technology has also been used to characterize binding epitopes of two different scFv's isolated against Aβ (33). While traditional immunoassays such as immunoblot, ELISA, and immunoprecipitations can be used for epitope mapping, SPR does not require a washing step to remove unbound material, which also makes it possible to characterize low-affinity and transient interactions (33). In this study by Liu et al., different peptide epitopes of Aβ (Aβ1-16, Aβ17-28, Aβ29-42) were immobilized to SPR substrates and different scFv's were injected over the chips. Binding specificity can be readily detected by the association curves (Fig. 5). The association (k_a) and dissociation (k_d) rate constants and the dissociation constants ($K_D = k_a/k_d$) for the entire AB peptide were also determined (Fig. 6) by fitting the data to a single binding site model. The higher affinity of H1v2 [$K_D = (2.47$

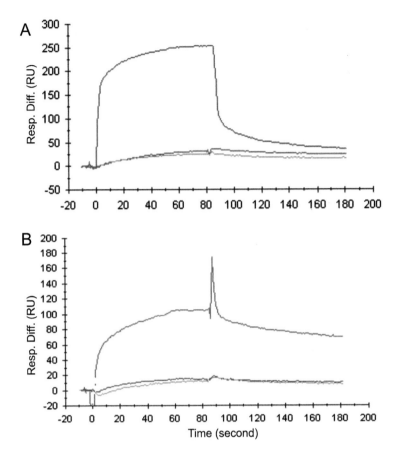

FIGURE 5 Association curves demonstrate that H1v2 binds AB17-28 (A) and C1 binds AB29-40 (B).
doi:10.1128/microbiolspec.AID-0010-2013.f5

$\pm 0.122) \times 10^{-7}$ M] compared with C1 [$K_D = 1.63 \pm 0.74) \times 10^{-6}$ M] is primarily due to differences in the association rate constant, k_a, rather than in the dissociation rate constant, k_d.

FACS-Based Antibody Selection

FACS can also be used to select for surface display antibodies with increased binding affinities. Proteins such as antibody fragment libraries can be displayed on the surface of yeast cells by fusing the antibody fragment to a yeast agglutinin receptor (14). Cells can be tagged with fluorescently labeled markers to identify the number of antibody fragments displayed and the number of antigen molecules bound (15). Cells can then be sorted to isolate cells expressing antibody fragments with high affinity for the given target antigen. By the use of this protocol, antibody fragments with high affinity against antigens, including epidermal growth factor receptor, hen egg lysozyme, and p-53 phosphopeptides were readily isolated (14). A schematic for the process of selection is shown in Fig. 7. The K_D values can be determined as described earlier. One of the major advantages of using flow cytometry-based techniques is the ability to distinguish between binders with high and low affinities. Negative selection steps can also be included in the selection process to facilitate isolation of antibody fragments with specific binding properties. For example, an scFv that selectively inhibited only one side of

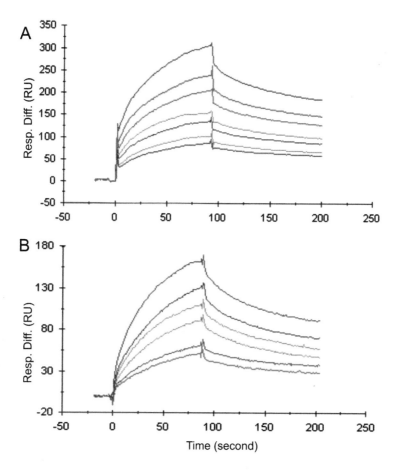

FIGURE 6 Association (k_a) and dissociation (k_d) rate constants and dissociation constants ($K_D = k_a/k_d$) of H1v2 (A) and C1 (B) to monomeric AB1-40. doi:10.1128/microbiolspec.AID-0010-2013.f6

a target proteolytic cleavage site on the amyloid precursor protein was isolated by first eliminating all cells that bound to a highly immunogenic site on one side of the cleavage site corresponding to the amino terminus of the Aβ protein implicated in Alzheimer's disease (34). Monitoring the panning process by using flow cytometry ensured that the negative selection successfully eliminated cells binding the nondesired antigen. Other panning techniques can be used to evaluate the individual clones for antigen binding. FACS enables the panning process to be monitored in real time, greatly facilitating the efficient selection of desired antibody fragments.

AFM-Based Antibody Selection

Since individual protein-binding events can be monitored by AFM, this provides a powerful tool to facilitate the isolation of antibody fragments with very selective binding specificities. For example, antibodies that recognize specific protein variants or morphologies can have important implications for studying, diagnosing and treating different diseases. We developed an AFM-based biopanning protocol that utilizes the nanoscale imaging capability of the AFM and the diversity of phage display antibody libraries to isolate antibody fragments with very specific binding properties (35) (Fig. 8). With the use of this AFM-based method, antibody fragments against selected protein

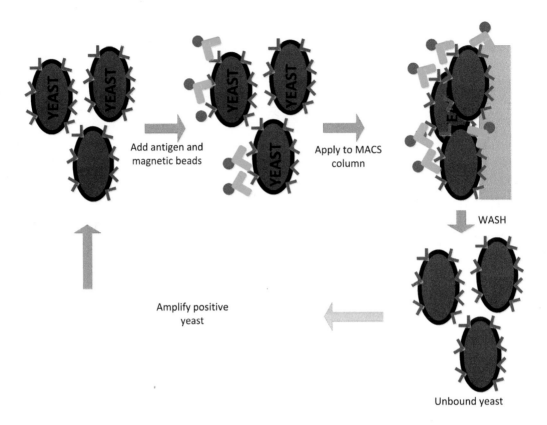

Add antigen and
magnetic beads

Apply to MACS
column

WASH

Unbound yeast

Amplify positive
yeast

FIGURE 7 Illustration of magnetic bead-based (MACS) biopanning. Yeast cells expressing antibody fragments (scFv's) are grown in medium containing galactose to induce expression and incubated with biotinylated antigen and streptavidin or neutravidin magnetic beads. Yeast cells are loaded into a magnetic column, and those expressing antigen-binding scFv's are retained. After multiple washes, bound yeast cells can be plunged out and the process can be repeated several times to enrich for antigen binders. doi:10.1128/microbiolspec.AID-0010-2013.f7

morphology targets can be used with high efficiency with the use of minimal sample volumes and without the need to modify or label the antigen.

In AFM biopanning, the target antigen is first immobilized on mica and then imaged by using AFM to confirm that the desired antigen morphology is present. A phage library is then added to the antigen-coated mica to select for the phage clones that have the strongest affinity to that particular protein morphology (Fig. 9). AFM is used to monitor each step of the biopanning process, including binding, washing, and elution, greatly increasing the efficiency of the panning process and ensuring that a high percentage of recovered clones have the desired binding specificity. With the

use of this AFM-based biopanning technique, antibody fragments with specificity for a variety of target protein morphologies were isolated, including different oligomeric and fibrillar forms of α-synuclein (36, 37) and Aβ (38, 39, 40).

Most antibody selection methods require significant amounts of purified antigen target for selection and screening and involve several rounds of amplification to enrich the number of positive clones present in the eluted mixture. However, many biologically important antigen targets are either scant in availability, difficult to purify, or may be unstable. In order to isolate antibodies to such antigens, a more direct method would be to directly "fish" out the desired antibodies. By the use of the AFM cantilever as the "fishing pole," a single-phage

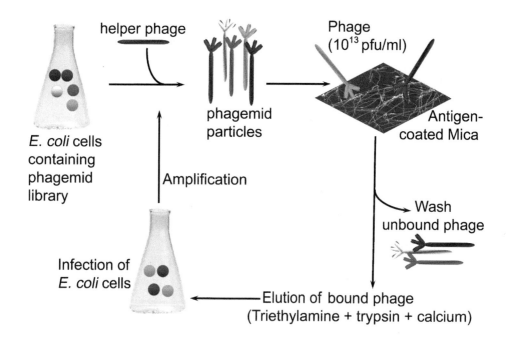

FIGURE 8 Overview of the AFM-biopanning process. The target antigen is first adsorbed on the mica surface, and the selection of phage is performed by using multiple rounds of biopanning. Any unbound phage is subsequently washed and removed, and bound phages are eluted from the mica surface. The eluted phages are then amplified, purified, and used for subsequent rounds of panning. doi:10.1128/ microbiolspec.AID-0010-2013.f8

recovery technique using AFM was developed based on the principles of the AFM biopanning technology (41). An image of the target protein-scFv complex is first acquired to determine the presence of a desired target protein-phage. Once the protein-scFv complex of interest is determined, the AFM tip is positioned over the target and the applied force is increased in order to "pick up" the phage-displaying scFv bound to the target protein. The DNA of the scFv can be recovered and amplified from the single-phage molecule on the AFM tip by using PCR. The advantages of this AFM single-phage recovery technology include (i) selection for morphology-specific scFv's from a mixture of different antigens, (ii) detection and recovery of antibodies of transiently stable protein morphologies, and (iii) recovery of antibodies from different regions of the same protein aggregate, e.g., the sides, ends, or along the axis of a fibril. With the ability to screen, select, and recover antibodies on one platform by using minimal amounts of target protein, this AFM technology is very useful to generate affinity reagents to a variety of target protein morphologies of interest that may be difficult to isolate by conventional methods such as ELISA. This protocol enables endless possibilities to detect the presence of various transient intermediate protein structures that occur in vivo and that may be involved in various human diseases.

SUMMARY

Antibody-antigen binding is a complex and dynamic process driven by various noncovalent forces including hydrogen bond, van der Waals, ionic, and hydrophobic interactions. Since both antigen and antibody are flexible molecules that are constantly moving, the different forces between the antibody and antigen are also

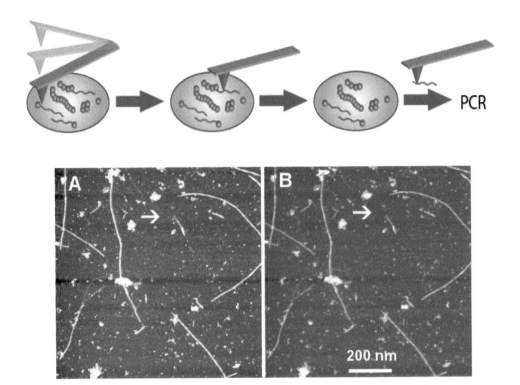

FIGURE 9 Single-phage recovery using AFM. (Top) Phage DNA recovery on the AFM tip using PCR. (Bottom) AFM image of the sample before (A) and after (B) phage "pickup." doi:10.1128/microbiolspec.AID-0010-2013.f9

constantly changing during binding and unbinding events to accommodate for the changes to the structure of each molecule. Therefore, it is crucial to understand and determine the thermodynamic properties of antibody-antigen interactions, such as the equilibrium binding (K_D), association (k_{on}), and dissociation rate (k_{off}) constants, in order to elucidate the affinity and specificity of an antibody to its target antigen. Traditional immunoassays such as RIA and ELISA have long been used to determine the steady-state equilibrium interactions between an antibody and antigen and are excellent techniques for large-volume, high-throughput screening of antibodies against an array of antigens. However, these techniques are not suitable for more intricate analysis such as a precise characterization of an antibody-antigen interaction, the determination of antibody specificity for rare and unstable antigens, or for a low-volume–high-throughput screening of antibody libraries.

Here, we present three additional techniques, SPR, FACS, and AFM, that can also be used to characterize antibody-antigen interactions. Each technique has unique detection methods and provides some advantages over traditional immunoassays. SPR offers a real-time, label-free detection system by measuring the changes in refractive index of the sensor chip surface. This allows for continuous monitoring of the kinetic profile between an immobilized agent and free-flowing analyte, and thermodynamic constants can be easily obtained from the SPR sensograms. In addition, different sensor surface chemistries are available for antigen or antibody immobilization, which increases the overall number and variety of targets that can be analyzed. FACS utilizes fluorescently labeled antibodies for characterization of binding events on cell surfaces in order to sort and count cells that have the desired properties. Additionally, the use of multiple labeled antibodies is possible in

FACS, which allows for the simultaneous analysis of multiple targets on a single cell. Because thousands of particles per second can be easily counted and sorted by using FACS, this technique is very efficient for drug or antibody screening. Finally, AFM provides a high-sensitivity detection method to detect antibody-antigen interactions without the need of a label. Individual molecular forces between an antibody and antigen can be elucidated by using the AFM, as well as the folding and unfolding of a biomolecule by varying the loading rates. In addition to force measurements, the intricate structures or morphologies of biomolecules can be obtained by using the AFM with high resolution. These capabilities can facilitate more precise antibody selection methods against different target protein morphologies.

The demand for antibodies with higher affinity and specificity is increasingly important for both diagnostic and therapeutic applications to eliminate nonspecific and off-target interactions. In order to design and synthesize the next-generation set of antibodies, analytical methods are needed to characterize, screen, sort, select, and determine the binding kinetics of the antibodies against an array of antigens. The techniques discussed in this article are among some of the modern analytical tools that can be used to study antibody-antigen interactions. They are good alternatives or complementary techniques to the classical immunoassays in providing a fast, label-free, low-volume, high-throughput screening of antibodies with high specificity and a molecular level of detection resolution.

ACKNOWLEDGMENT

Conflicts of interest: We disclose no conflicts.

CITATION

Yang G, Velgos SN, Boddapati SP, Sierks MR. 2014. Probing antibody-antigen interactions. Microbiol Spectrum 2(1):AID-0010-2013

REFERENCES

1. **Reverberi R, Reverberi L.** 2007. Factors affecting the antigen-antibody reaction. *Blood Transfus* **5:**227–240.
2. **Ritzefeld M, Sewald N.** 2012. Real-time analysis of specific protein-DNA Interactions with surface plasmon resonance. *J Amino Acids* **2012:** 816032.
3. **Zhu G, Yang B, Jennings RN.** 2000. Quantitation of basic fibroblast growth factor by immunoassay using BIAcore 2000. *J Pharm Biomed Anal* **24:**281–290.
4. **Jonsson U, Fägerstam L, Ivarsson B, Johnsson B, Karlsson R, Lundh K, Löfås S, Persson B, Roos H, Ronnberg I, et al.** 1991. Real-time biospecific interaction analysis using surface plasmon resonance and a sensor chip technology. *Biotechniques* **11:**620–627.
5. **Guo X.** 2012. Surface plasmon resonance based biosensor technique: a review. *J Biophotonics* **5:** 483–501.
6. **Mannen T, Yamaguchi S, Honda J, Sugimoto S, Kitayama A, Nagamune T.** 2001. Observation of charge state and conformational change in immobilized protein using surface plasmon resonance sensor. *Anal Biochem* **293:**185–193.
7. **Karlsson R, Kullman-Magnusson M, Hamalainen MD, Remaeus A, Andersson K, Borg P, Gyzander E, Deinum J.** 2000. Biosensor analysis of drug-target interactions: direct and competitive binding assays for investigation of interactions between thrombin and thrombin inhibitors. *Anal Biochem* **278:**1–13.
8. **Kruger R, Kuhn W, Müller T, Woitalla D, Graeber M, Kösel S, Przuntek H, Epplen JT, Schöls L, Riess O.** 1998. Ala30Pro mutation in the gene encoding alpha-synuclein in Parkinson's disease. *Nat Genet* **18:**106–108.
9. **Daghestani HN, Day BW.** 2010. Theory and applications of surface plasmon resonance, resonant mirror, resonant waveguide grating, and dual polarization interferometry biosensors. *Sensors (Basel)* **10:**9630–9646.
10. **Boozer C, Kim G, Cong S, Guan H, Londergan T.** 2006. Looking towards label-free biomolecular interaction analysis in a high-throughput format: a review of new surface plasmon resonance technologies. *Curr Opin Biotechnol* **17:**400–405.
11. **Rieseberg M, Kasper C, Reardon KF, Scheper T.** 2001. Flow cytometry in biotechnology. *Appl Microbiol Biotechnol* **56:**350–360.
12. **Benedict CA, MacKrell AJ, Anderson WF.** 1997. Determination of the binding affinity of an anti-CD34 single-chain antibody using a novel, flow cytometry based assay. *J Immunol Methods* **201:** 223–231.

13. **Lou J, Geren I, Garcia-Rodriguez C, Forsyth CM, Wen W, Knopp K, Brown J, Smith T, Smith LA, Marks JD.** 2010. Affinity maturation of human botulinum neurotoxin antibodies by light chain shuffling via yeast mating. *Protein Eng Des Sel* **23:**311–319.

14. **Feldhaus MJ, Siegel RW, Opresko LK, Coleman JR, Feldhaus JM, Yeung YA, Cochran JR, Heinzelman P, Colby D, Swers J, Graff C, Wiley HS, Wittrup KD.** 2003. Flow-cytometric isolation of human antibodies from a nonimmune *Saccharomyces cerevisiae* surface display library. *Nat Biotechnol* **21:**163–170.

15. **Chao G, Lau WL, Hackel BJ, Sazinsky SL, Lippow SM, Wittrup KD.** 2006. Isolating and engineering human antibodies using yeast surface display. *Nat Protoc* **1:**755–768.

16. **Li B, Zhao L, Guo H, Wang C, Zhang X, Wu L, Chen L, Tong Q, Qian W, Wang H, Guo Y.** 2009. Characterization of a rituximab variant with potent antitumor activity against rituximab-resistant B-cell lymphoma. *Blood* **114:**5007–5015.

17. **Geuijen CA, Clijsters-van der Horst M, Cox F, Rood PM, Throsby M, Jongeneelen MA, Backus HH, van Deventer E, Kruisbeek AM, Goudsmit J, de Kruif J.** 2005. Affinity ranking of antibodies using flow cytometry: application in antibody phage display-based target discovery. *J Immunol Methods* **302:**68–77.

18. **Daugherty PS, Chen G, Olsen MJ, Iverson BL, Georgiou G.** 1998. Antibody affinity maturation using bacterial surface display. *Protein Eng* **11:**825–832.

19. **Boder ET, Midelfort KS, Wittrup KD.** 2000. Directed evolution of antibody fragments with monovalent femtomolar antigen-binding affinity. *Proc Natl Acad Sci USA* **97:**10701–10705.

20. **Neuman KC, Nagy A.** 2008. Single-molecule force spectroscopy: optical tweezers, magnetic tweezers and atomic force microscopy. *Nature Methods* **5:**491–505.

21. **Binnig G, Rohrer H, Gerber C, Weibel E.** 1982. Surface studies by scanning tunneling microscopy. *Phys Rev Lett* **49:**57–61.

22. **Hansma PK, Cleveland JP, Radmacher M, Walters DA, Hillner PE, Bezanilla M, Fritz M, Vie D, Hansma HG, Prater CB, Massie J, Fukunaga L, Gurley J, Elings V.** 1994. Tapping mode atomic-force microscopy in liquids. *Appl Phys Lett* **64:**1738–1740.

23. **Matsko N.** 2007. Atomic force microscopy applied to study macromolecular content of embedded biological material. *Ultramicroscopy* **107:**95–105.

24. **Melling M, Hochmeister S, Blumer R, Schilcher K, Mostler S, Behnam M, Wilde J, Karimian-Teherani D.** 2001. Atomic force microscopy imaging of the human trigeminal ganglion. *Neuroimage* **14:**1348–1352.

25. **Nag K, Munro JG, Hearn SA, Rasmusson J, Petersen NO, Possmayer F.** 1999. Correlated atomic force and transmission electron microscopy of nanotubular structures in pulmonary surfactant. *J Struct Biol* **126:**1–15.

26. **Ebner A, Hinterdorfer P, Gruber HJ.** 2007. Comparison of different aminofunctionalization strategies for attachment of single antibodies to AFM cantilevers. *Ultramicroscopy* **107:**922–927.

27. **Lee GU, Kidwell DA, Colton RJ.** 1994. Sensing discrete streptavidin-biotin interactions with atomic force microscopy. *Langmuir* **10:**354–357.

28. **Florin EL, Moy VT, Gaub HE.** 1994. Adhesion forces between individual ligand-receptor pairs. *Science* **264:**415–417.

29. **Wakayama J, Sekiguchi H, Akanuma S, Ohtani T, Sugiyama S.** 2008. Methods for reducing nonspecific interaction in antibody-antigen assay via atomic force microscopy. *Anal Biochem* **380:**51–58.

30. **Merkel R, Nassoy P, Leung A, Ritchie K, Evans E.** 1999. Energy landscapes of receptor-ligand bonds explored with dynamic force spectroscopy. *Nature* **397:**50–53.

31. **Berquand A, Xia N, Castner DG, Clare BH, Abbott NL, Dupres V, Adriaensen Y, Dufrene YF.** 2005. Antigen binding forces of single antilysozyme Fv fragments explored by atomic force microscopy. *Langmuir* **21:**5517–5523.

32. **Yuan B, Schulz P, Liu R, Sierks MR.** 2006. Improved affinity selection using phage display technology and off-rate based selection. *Electron J Biotechnol* **9:**171–175.

33. **Liu R, Yuan B, Emadi S, Zameer A, Schulz P, McAllister C, Lyubchenko Y, Goud G, Sierks MR.** 2004. Single chain variable fragments against beta-amyloid (Abeta) can inhibit Abeta aggregation and prevent abeta-induced neurotoxicity. *Biochemistry* **43:**6959–6967.

34. **Boddapati S, Levites Y, Sierks MR.** 2011. Inhibiting β-secretase activity in Alzheimer's disease cell models with single-chain antibodies specifically targeting APP. *J Mol Biol* **405:**436–447.

35. **Barkhordarian H, Emadi S, Schulz P, Sierks MR.** 2006. Isolating recombinant antibodies against specific protein morphologies using atomic force microscopy and phage display technologies. *Protein Eng Des Sel* **19:**497–502.

36. **Emadi S, Barkhordarian H, Wang MS, Schulz P, Sierks MR.** 2007. Isolation of a human single chain antibody fragment against oligomeric alpha-synuclein that inhibits aggregation and prevents alpha-synuclein-induced toxicity. *J Mol Biol* **368:**1132–1144.

37. **Emadi S, Kasturirangan S, Wang MS, Schulz P, Sierks MR.** 2009. Detecting morphologically distinct oligomeric forms of alpha-synuclein. *J Biol Chem* **284:**11048–11058.

38. **Zameer A, Kasturirangan S, Emadi S, Nimmagadda SV, Sierks MR.** 2008. Anti-oligomeric Abeta single-chain variable domain antibody blocks Abeta-induced toxicity against human neuroblastoma cells. *J Mol Biol* **384:**917–928.

39. **Kasturirangan S, Li L, Emadi S, Boddapati S, Schulz P, Sierks M.** 2012. Nanobody specific for oligomeric β-amyloid stabilizes nontoxic form. *Neurobiol Aging* **33:**1320–1328.

40. **Marcus WD, Wang H, Lindsay SM, Sierks MR.** 2008. Characterization of an antibody scFv that recognizes fibrillar insulin and beta-amyloid using atomic force microscopy. *Nanomedicine* **4:**1–7.

41. **Lyubchenko Y, Gall A, Shlyakhtenko L, Harrington R, Jacobs B, Oden P, Lindsay S.** 1992. Atomic force microscopy imaging of double stranded DNA and RNA. *J Biomol Struct Dyn* **10:** 589–606.

Radiolabeled Antibodies for Therapy of Infectious Diseases

23

EKATERINA DADACHOVA[1,2] and ARTURO CASADEVALL[2,3]

INTRODUCTION

There is a growing need for alternatives to conventional antibiotics for the treatment of infectious diseases. The number of bacterial pathogens that are resistant even to the most powerful antibiotics is growing each year. HIV remains an incurable disease more than 30 years since its identification. Since 1979 there has been a >200% increase in the annual number of cases of invasive fungal infections in the United States. To exacerbate these problems, the number of patients who cannot fight infections because of impaired immunity is growing and includes HIV patients, patients who have been through cancer chemotherapy, and organ transplant recipients.

Radioimmunotherapy (RIT) is based on the interaction between the pair of antigen and antibody to carry cytocidal amounts of ionizing radiation to the vicinity of specific cellular targets. Currently, RIT is clinically utilized in the treatment of primary, refractory, and recurrent non-Hodgkin lymphoma with the radiolabeled monoclonal antibodies (mAbs) Zevalin and Bexxar, and it offers several significant advantages over naked antibody strategies: (i) RIT delivers lethal radiation, such that it does not merely interfere with a single cellular pathway but leads to physical destruction of targeted cells via radiation-induced

[1]Department of Radiology; [2]Department of Microbiology and Immunology; [3]Department of Medicine, Albert Einstein College of Medicine of Yeshiva University, Bronx, NY 10461.
Antibodies for Infectious Diseases
Edited by James E. Crowe, Jr., Diana Boraschi, and Rino Rappuoli
© 2015 American Society for Microbiology, Washington, DC
doi:10.1128/microbiolspec.AID-0023-2014

apoptosis/autophagy/necrosis; (ii) RIT is not subject to drug resistance mechanisms such as efflux through drug efflux pumps in malignant cells; (iii) the effectiveness of RIT does not depend on the immunological status of the host; (iv) RIT has the potential to reduce the number of doses used to combat infections with standard therapies from weeks or months to a single or limited number of doses of RIT.

A decade ago we suggested the use of RIT for the treatment of the fungal pathogen *Cryptococcus neoformans* (1). Since then we have evaluated the suitability of this approach to treating fungal infections for its efficacy and safety as well as expanded it to treating infections due to bacteria and viruses (Fig. 1). Here we provide a brief overview of the preclinical development of RIT for infectious diseases.

FUNGAL INFECTIONS

We started with the investigation of RIT potency against *C. neoformans* fungal infection (1).

C. neoformans results in life-threatening meningoencephalitis, which affects people with a compromised immune system and is responsible for higher mortality among individuals with AIDS in sub-Saharan Africa than tuberculosis (2). The availability of good animal models and well-characterized mAbs to *C. neoformans* antigens provided an impetus to use this pathogen for investigating RIT for infections. Importantly, immunotherapy in patients with *C. neoformans* with the capsule polysaccharide-binding antibody 18B7 has already been evaluated clinically (3). Therapeutic studies employed AJ/Cr mice infected systemically with *C. neoformans*. A/JCr mice succumb to the systemic infection with *C. neoformans*, most likely because of the partial complement deficiency (4). The survival of mice treated with radiolabeled *C. neoformans*–specific mAb 18B7 was significantly longer than the survival of mice treated with irrelevant labeled IgG1 or phosphate-buffered saline. We utilized a radiolabeled irrelevant mAb (^{213}Bi- or ^{188}Re-IgG$_1$ MOPC21) to take

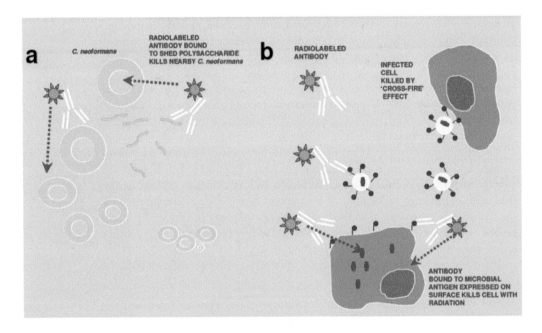

FIGURE 1 Mechanisms of RIT efficacy against infections. (a) Direct targeting of microbial cells with the radiolabeled organism-specific antibodies. (b) Killing of virally infected host cells by targeting viral antigens expressed on the surface of infected cells. doi:10.1128/microbiolspec.AID-0023-2014.f1

into account the possibility of the radiolabeled IgG binding to Fc receptors on phagocytic cells present at the infected site, which might lead to nonspecific killing of some *C. neoformans* cells. Interestingly, treatment with 100 μCi ^{213}Bi-18B7 resulted in 60% of mice in the ^{213}Bi group surviving on day 75 post-therapy ($P < 0.05$). In the ^{188}Re group 40% and 20% of animals were alive after treatment with 100 ($P < 0.005$) and 50 ($P < 0.05$) μCi ^{188}Re-18B7, respectively. In contrast, mice in control groups died from *C. neoformans* infection on days 35 to 40 (Fig. 2a). Administration of RIT resulted in significant reduction of fungal burden in lungs and brains of mice with *C. neoformans* 48 h after RIT administration when compared to control groups. No difference in the percentage decrease of the fungal burden in the lungs was observed between the groups that received 50 and 100 μCi ^{188}Re-18B7. In contrast, the administration of 200 μCi ^{188}Re-18B7 led to pronounced reduction in lung CFUs when compared to the lower activities ($P < 0.05$). We concluded that giving a radiolabeled antibody to fungal polysaccharide to infected mice led to the prolongation in survival and reduction in organ fungal burden.

Subsequently we investigated whether RIT was effective in a different mouse model—immunocompetent C57BL6 mice—and whether it would be effective in the setting of more established cryptococcal infection. RIT kills the microorganisms primarily by targeted cytocidal radiation, so it was paramount to establish its presumed independence from the immune status of the host. Additionally, showing that RIT can be efficacious in the setting of the established infections accompanied by the high fungal load would be useful for its future translation into the clinic. For this purpose C57BL6 mice were infected intravenously (i.v.) via the tail vein with 10^6 *C. neoformans* cells and were left either untreated or treated intraperitoneally (i.p.) with 100 μCi ^{213}Bi-18B7 24 h postinfection, 100 μCi ^{188}Re-18B7 24 h postinfection, or 100 μCi ^{188}Re-18B7 48 h postinfection (5). Administration of ^{188}Re-18B7 mAb 24 h post-

infection resulted in one log reduction in the lung CFUs ($P = 0.04$), while no reduction in CFUs was observed in the brains ($P = 0.07$) (Fig. 2b). Treatment with ^{213}Bi-18B7 mAb 24 h postinfection completely killed fungal cells in the lungs and the brains (the plating assay sensitivity was 50 CFUs) (Fig. 2b), which agreed with the results of Gomon methenamine silver (GMS) staining. Interestingly, for established infection at 48 h, ^{188}Re-18B7 mAb efficiently decreased CFUs in the lungs ($P = 0.03$) and also notably decreased the number of fungal cells in the brains of treated mice ($P = 0.02$) (Fig. 2b). The latter observation might stem from the increased permeability of the blood-brain barrier caused by the presence of infection, which results in facilitating the entrance of the radiolabeled antibody into the brain (6). We concluded from this study that RIT demonstrated efficacy in both early and established infection in immunocompetent C57BL6 mice. In our previous work we showed RIT efficacy in complement-deficient AJ/Cr mice. The results are consistent with and supportive of the presumed RIT independence of the status of the host's immune system. Such a finding is encouraging for the treatment of opportunistic infections in cancer and organ transplant patients.

As a part of our effort to demonstrate the value of RIT as an anti-infective strategy, we compared its efficacy with amphotericin B, which is one of the major antifungal drugs (7). AJ/Cr mice were infected i.v. with 3×10^5 melanized or nonmelanized *C. neoformans* cells. Twenty-four hours after infection the mice were given i.p. either 100 μCi ^{213}Bi-18B7 or amphotericin in its deoxycholate form at 1 μg/g body weight at 24, 48, and 72 h, were given both treatments, or were left untreated. Mouse survival was observed for 60 days. The lungs and brains were analyzed at 60 days postinfection. This analysis demonstrated that treatment with amphotericin did not significantly decrease lung and brain CFUs in either nonmelanized or melanized *C. neoformans* groups (Fig. 2c) ($P > 0.05$). RIT administration resulted in noted decreases in fungal burden in comparison with the untreated controls and

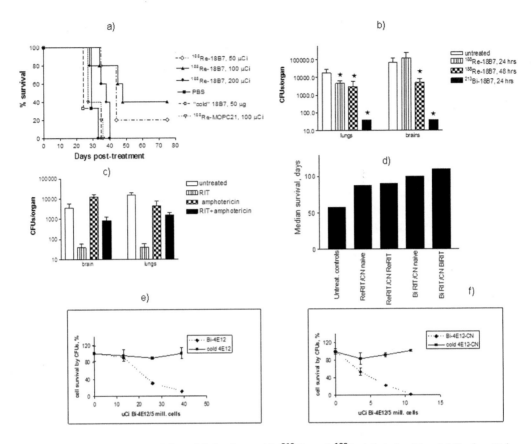

FIGURE 2 RIT of experimental fungal infections with ^{213}Bi- and ^{188}Re-labeled mAbs. (a) Kaplan-Meier survival curves for A/JCr mice infected i.v. with 10^5 *C. neoformans* cells 24 h prior to treatment with 50 to 200 μCi ^{188}Re-labeled mAbs. Animals injected with phosphate-buffered saline or 50 μg cold 18B7 served as controls. (b) RIT of C57BL6 mice infected i.v. with 10^6 *C. neoformans* cells: CFUs in the brains and the lungs of RIT-treated and control mice. Mice were treated i.p. with either 100 μCi ^{213}Bi-18B7 24 h postinfection, 100 μCi ^{188}Re-18B7 24 h postinfection, or 100 μCi ^{188}Re-18B7 48 h postinfection or were left untreated and sacrificed 75 days posttreatment. The detection limit of the method was 50 CFUs. No CFUs were found in the brains and lungs of mice treated with 100 μCi ^{213}Bi-18B7, which are presented in the graph as 40 CFUs/organ. The asterisks show the groups in which the CFUs were significantly different from the untreated controls. (c) Comparison of RIT and amphotericin B efficacy toward melanized *C. neoformans in vivo*. CFUs in the lungs and brains of mice infected with melanized *C. neoformans*. AJ/Cr mice were infected i.v. with 3×10^5 *C. neoformans* cells and were given either 100 μCi ^{213}Bi-18B7 RIT or amphotericin B at 1 μg/g body weight on days 1, 2, and 3 postinfection or combined treatment or left untreated. The detection limit of the method was 50 CFUs. No CFUs were found in the brains and lungs of mice infected with melanized *C. neoformans* cells and treated with RIT, which are presented in the graph as 40 CFUs/organ. (d) Median survival of AJ/Cr mice infected i.v. with 5×10^4 *C. neoformans* and treated 24 h later with 150 μCi ^{188}Re-18B7 or 125 μCi ^{213}Bi-18B7 mAb. CN$_{naïve}$ cells from ATCC; CN$_{Re\ RIT}$, cells recovered from mice treated with ^{188}Re-18B7 mAb; CN$_{Bi\ RIT}$, cells recovered from mice treated with ^{213}Bi-18B7 mAb; Re RIT/CN$_{naïve}$, mice infected with CN$_{naïve}$ and treated with ^{188}Re-18B7; Bi RIT/CN$_{naïve}$, mice infected with CN$_{naïve}$ and treated with ^{213}Bi-18B7; Re RIT/CN$_{Re\ RIT}$, mice infected with CN$_{Re\ RIT}$ and treated with ^{188}Re-18B7; Bi RIT/CN$_{Bi\ RIT}$, mice infected with CN$_{Bi\ RIT}$ and treated with ^{213}Bi-18B7. (e, f) RIT with ^{213}Bi-4E12 antibody to Hsp60: (e) RIT of *C. albicans*; (f) RIT of *C. neoformans*. Each experiment was performed three times, and the results shown are from one typical experiment. The CFUs for each antibody dose were plated in triplicate. doi:10.1128/microbiolspec.AID-0023-2014.f2

the amphotericin-treated mice ($P \ll 0.05$). Of note, the fungus was practically cleared from the brains of the RIT-treated nonmelanized *C. neoformans* group (sensitivity of the detection was 50 CFUs), while in the melanized *C. neoformans* group RIT was capable of practically clearing the infection from both brain and lungs. Our most important result was the observation of the RIT efficacy in reducing fungal burden in lungs and brains when compared to the high 1-μg/g dose of amphotericin, when the majority of mice treated with RIT were able to almost completely clear the infection. The explanation of the inability of amphotericin to decrease the fungal burden in the organs of partially complement-deficient AJ/Cr mice 3 days posttreatment was provided by the subsequent amphotericin study showing a trend toward a decrease in CFUs in brains and lungs that manifested itself only on day 14 of treatment with amphotericin B (7).

Our results are in accordance with the published data showing that amphotericin was able to produce only a 1 to 1.5 log reduction in CFUs in immunocompetent mice such as CD-1 and BALB/c, and all mice succumbed to *C. neoformans* infection around day 24 (8, 9). Our results also agree with the clinical reports that show that a short course of amphotericin was not able to sterilize cerebrospinal fluid or blood of patients and that correlated the rate of sterilization with patient survival (10). Our observations underline the advantages of RIT, which has pronounced antimicrobial effects *in vivo* after just one injection, compared to long and often ineffective treatments with amphotericin, which has long-lasting side effects.

Despite radiation being a weak mutagen, the belief that even low doses of ionizing radiation are able to create potentially dangerous cellular mutants persists within the scientific community and the lay public alike. To evaluate the possibility that RIT might select for the radiation resistance in *C. neoformans* cells *in vivo*, AJ/Cr mice were infected with *C. neoformans* cells recovered from mice treated previously with ^{188}Re-18B7 mAb (CN$_{Re-RIT}$),

with ^{213}Bi-18B7 mAb (CN$_{Bi-RIT}$), or with the RIT-naïve *C. neoformans* cells (CN$_{naïve}$) (11). We treated *C. neoformans*-infected mice with 150 μCi ^{188}Re-18B7 or 125 μCi ^{213}Bi-18B7 24 h after i.v. infection and then observed the mice for survival and weight loss. The number of deaths in mice infected with CN$_{Re-RIT}$ or CN$_{Bi-RIT}$ was similar to that in mice infected with CN$_{naïve}$ ($P > 0.05$) (Fig. 2d). Mice given ^{213}Bi-18B7 mAb survived longer ($P = 0.04$) than those given ^{188}Re-18B7 (Fig. 2d), most likely due to the higher killing power of ^{213}Bi-emitted alpha particles when compared to ^{188}Re-emitted beta particles. In general, the interaction of fungal cells with particulate radiation resulted in the loss of the cells' ability to divide (1, 12), which could provide an explanation for the nonemergence of radiation-resistant phenotypes post-RIT. The residual cells that replicated post-RIT were probably shielded from the antibodies that received radiation from a biofilm, an abscess, or a host cell.

Finally, in an effort to develop broader antifungal therapy that did not rely on pathogen-specific mAbs, we investigated the targeting of antigens shared by major invasive fungal infection-causing fungi (pan-fungal antigens) to deliver RIT without the need for specific mycological diagnosis or concerns about drug resistance. We explored the possibility of targeting common cell-wall-associated antigens, which also happen to be the dominate virulence factors for these fungal pathogens. The majority of fungal cells, in both yeast and hyphal forms, display beta-glucans on their cell surface. Cassone and colleagues generated a mAb to beta-glucans in *Candida albicans, C. neoformans,* and *Aspergillus fumigatus* in animal models (13–15). Heat shock protein 60 (Hsp60) is a major regulator of virulence in *Histoplasma capsulatum*, and mAbs directed to this protein are protective in murine histoplasmosis (16). We established that a mAb to *H. capsulatum* Hsp60 also bound other pathogenic fungal species but did not react with human Hsp60 (16). Melanin is present in the cell wall of diverse human fungal pathogens, and a mAb 6D2 to fungal melanin was shown to bind *C. neoformans, H. capsulatum, Aspergillus* spp., *C. albicans, Scytalidium dimidiatum, Sporothrix schenckii, Paracoccidioides brasiliensis, Coccidioides posadassi,* and *Blastomyces dermatitidis* (17). To explore the feasibility of using RIT to target these pan-antigens we utilized mAbs 4E12, an IgG2a to fungal HSP60; 2G8, an IgG 2b to beta-(1,3)-glucan; and 6D2, an IgM to melanin, and radiolabeled them with ^{213}Bi (18). *C. neoformans* and *C. albicans* were used to evaluate the cytocidal effects of these radiolabeled mAbs. ^{213}Bi-labeled mAbs to HSP60 (Fig. 2e,f) and to the beta-(1,3)-glucan each decreased the viability of both fungi in the 80 to 100% range. The ^{213}Bi-6D2 mAb to melanin eliminated 50% of *C. neoformans* cells but did not kill *C. albicans*. Treatment with unlabeled mAbs and with radiolabeled isotype-matching control mAbs resulted in no killing. These results point to the possibility of developing RIT against fungal pathogens by targeting shared fungal antigens. This approach could be utilized against fungal infections for which current therapies are not working well.

BACTERIAL INFECTIONS

Streptococcus pneumoniae, an important cause of community-acquired pneumonia, meningitis, and bacteremia, was selected for evaluating the feasibility of RIT against bacterial diseases (19). A human mAb D11 that binds to pneumococcal capsular polysaccharide 8 (PPS 8) was chosen as a delivery vehicle for RIT and was radiolabeled with a short-range alpha-emitter, ^{213}Bi. The RIT administration resulted in a higher percentage of mice surviving in the ^{213}Bi-D11-treated group compared to the untreated group ($P < 0.01$) (Fig. 3a). In contrast, giving mice 5 μg unlabeled D11 mAb did not lead to the prolongation in survival in comparison to untreated mice ($P > 0.05$). Radiolabeled irrelevant IgM also did not show any therapeutic results ($P > 0.05$) and, in contrast, fewer mice survived its administration when compared to the untreated group. A possible

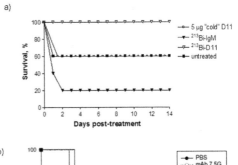

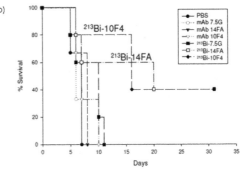

FIGURE 3 **RIT of bacterial infections. (a) *S. pneumoniae*, ^{213}Bi-labeled mAbs in C57BL/6 mice. Mice were infected i.p. with 1,000 organisms 1 h before treatment with mAbs. (b) RIT of *B. anthracis* Sterne infection with ^{213}Bi-labeled mAbs. Mice were infected 1 h prior to labeled-mAb treatment. Survival experiment was repeated three times with similar results. Controls include unlabeled mAbs given in the same amounts (15 μg) as radiolabeled mAbs.**
doi:10.1128/microbiolspec.AID-0023-2014.f3

explanation could be the absence of a target for the irrelevant radiolabeled mAb to bind to, which resulted in an excessive dose of radiation to the blood-rich dose-limiting organs such as bone marrow. Mice in control groups died from bacteremia on days 1 to 3, while 87 to 100% of mice given 80 μCi ^{213}Bi-D11 survived. Measuring CFUs in the blood of the RIT-treated mice demonstrated that they were not bacteremic at 3, 6, and 10 h posttreatment or on days 3 and 14. RIT with radiolabeled D11 did not cause any weight loss in treated animals. In summary, this proof of principle study was the first to demonstrate the ability of RIT to treat experimental bacterial infection.

Later we investigated RIT for experimental *Bacillus anthracis* infection. *B. anthracis* is a potential agent for bioterrorism and biological weapons, which underscores the necessity for additional, different mode of action therapies for anthrax (20). The surface expression of toxins on bacterial cells was demonstrated by indirect immunofluorescence experiments with mAbs to protective antigen (7.5G γ2b and 10F4 γ1) and lethal factor (mAb 14FA γ2b). Scatchard analysis of mAbs binding to the bacterial surface demonstrated high binding constants and multiple binding sites on the surface of bacteria, which provided the impetus for RIT studies. The mAbs to the toxins were radiolabeled with either ^{188}Re or ^{213}Bi for investigating the microbicidal potential of RIT. ^{213}Bi-labeled mAbs were more efficient *in vitro* than ^{188}Re-labeled mAbs in killing *B. anthracis* Sterne bacterial cells. Giving i.p. ^{213}Bi-labeled mAbs 10F4 and 14FA to A/JCr mice lethally infected with *B. anthracis* cells significantly prolonged their survival (Fig. 3b). Our results point to RIT's utility in treating experimental anthrax infection with mAbs targeting *B. anthracis* tri-partite toxin components and suggest that toxigenic bacteria may be targeted with radiolabeled mAbs to its toxins.

Finally, we recently investigated the potential of RIT against germinating *B. anthracis* spores (21). *B. anthracis* spores are covered by an impenetrable two-layered exosporium, which is composed of a basal layer and an external hair-like nap. The nap consists of filaments, which in turn are composed of trimers of a collagen-like glycoprotein BclA. BclA is considered to be an immunodominant antigen on the spore surface. The antibodies to BclA are highly specific and can specifically identify *B. anthracis* spores among the spores produced by other *Bacillus* species. We investigated whether EA2-1 mAb to BclA armed with ^{213}Bi would be capable of sterilizing *B. anthracis* spores. We chose an alpha-emitter ^{213}Bi for this study, as this radionuclide was successfully used in our previous research on RIT for bacterial pathogens such as *S. pneumoniae* and *B. anthracis*.

First, we confirmed the previous reports that the spores were completely resistant to the external gamma radiation. Our initial RIT experiments demonstrated that dormant spores were not killed by ^{213}Bi -EA2-1 mAb either. Only when the dose of ^{213}Bi-EA2-1 mAb reached 300 μCi was the significant spore killing observed. However, this killing was not mAb-specific, as the isotype control mAb labeled with 300 μCi ^{213}Bi showed the same results. Our next step was to examine the effects of RIT on the germinating versus dormant spores. The reasoning for that was that the spores become pathogenic in a host when they start germinating and dividing, which leads to the development of anthrax disease. In addition, it is known from classical radiobiology that dividing cells are much more susceptible to ionizing radiation damage than cells that are not dividing. Thus, the germinating spores might present a better target for RIT. The experiments showed that 75 and 150 μCi ^{213}Bi-EA2-1 killed significant numbers of germinating spores, while the matching activities of the isotype matching control mAb did not. We concluded from this study that while dormant spores are resistant to both external radiation and RIT, the germinating spores are RIT-susceptible, and this line of study should be investigated further, possibly in animal models.

HIV

The HIV epidemic remains a major worldwide health problem. Highly active antiretroviral therapy (HAART), a combination of drugs that inhibits enzymes essential for HIV replication, can decrease the viremia to almost undetectable levels and decrease the likelihood of opportunistic infections in the majority of patients. As a result, patients on HAART now survive for decades. However, HAART regimens are complex and require lifelong use, and many have significant long-term side effects such as metabolic syndrome, cardiotoxicity, etc. A replication-competent virus that "hides" in latently infected cells serves as a source of viremia that emerges rapidly after the discontinuation of HAART. A modality that specifically targets and eliminates HIV-infected cells in patients on HAART could be a major contributor toward the eradication of persistent HIV cellular reservoirs. We hypothesized that RIT could be able to kill virally infected cells. RIT for viral diseases would target viral antigens on infected cells and consequently would provide a completely different approach for treating HIV.

Initially, we studied the efficacy of RIT against HIV infection in SCID mice using an HIV envelope-specific human mAb 246-D to gp41 that we radiolabeled with ^{213}Bi or ^{188}Re (22). For these experiments human peripheral blood mononuclear cells (hPBMCs) were infected with HIV-1$_{JR-CSF}$ and injected intrasplenically into SCID mice, and radiolabeled mAbs were given i.p. 1 h later. The mice were sacrificed 72 h after RIT, and the presence of the residual HIV-infected cells was established by quantitative coculture (23). This time interval was chosen to provide enough time for the ^{188}Re-radiolabel (its physical half-life is 16.9 h) on the mAb to deliver a lethal cytotoxic dose to the infected cells. Adminis-

tration of ^{188}Re-armed 246-D mAb before or after intrasplenic injection with HIV-infected hPBMCs significantly decreased the numbers of HIV-infected cells in mice (Fig. 4a). Similar results were obtained with ^{213}Bi-246-D (Fig. 4a). In contrast, control SCID mice that received equivalent amounts of "cold" mAb 246-D or a radiolabeled isotype-matched control mAb showed no reduction in the average number of infected cells detected in their spleens. These results established the feasibility of using RIT to specifically target and eliminate HIV-infected hPBMCs *in vivo* and provided a first experimental proof for the concept of fighting viral infections by targeting virally infected cells with the radioactively armed mAbs to viral antigens. We anticipate that the same approach could be useful for treatment of other chronic viral infections, e.g., hepatitis C (24).

It should be noted that the antibodies used in RIT do not neutralize the virus and consequently are not expected to exert selective pressure on the virus. Only the epitopes on the

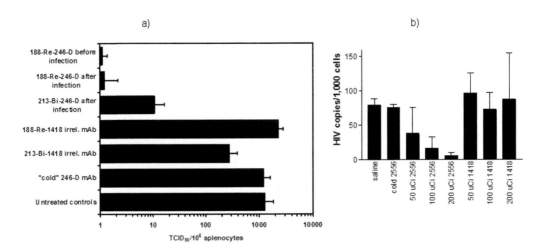

FIGURE 4 **RIT of SCID mice injected intrasplenically with JR-CSF HIV-infected human PBMCs and treated with** ^{188}**Re- and** ^{213}**Bi-labeled human anti-gp41 mAbs 246-D (a) or 2556 (b). (a) Limiting coculture results for 246-D mAb. Mice received either 20 µg cold anti-gp41 mAb 246-D, 100 µCi (20 µg)** ^{213}**Bi-1418 or 80 µCi (20 µg)** ^{188}**Re-1418 as isotype-matching controls, 80 µCi (20 µg)** ^{188}**Re-246-D, or 100 µCi (20 µg)** ^{213}**Bi-246-D i.p. 1 h after injection of PBMCs. In some experiments mice were given 80 µCi (20 µg)** ^{188}**Re-246-D i.p. 1 h prior to injection of HIV-infected PBMCs. (b) PCR data for RIT with 50, 100, and 200 µCi** ^{213}**Bi-2556 mAb. The cold 2556, untreated mice, and matching activities of the irrelevant 1418 mAb were used as controls.**
doi:10.1128/microbiolspec.AID-0023-2014.f4

viral proteins that are conserved throughout all HIV strains and clades, which is consistent with their role in the maintenance of envelope protein structure, are chosen as targets for RIT. As a result, even in case of a mutation, such epitopes will probably be present on mutated viral particles and, as a result, on HIV-infected cells. In this regard RIT has certain advantages over immunotoxins to eradicate infected cells. In immunotoxins a mAb is conjugated to immunogenic toxin and thus can elicit an immune response, while in RIT no responses to radiolabeled human mAbs have been observed. RIT is a highly versatile modality due to the availability of the radionuclides with various emissions and decay schemes. Recently we identified a human mAb 2556 as a superb reagent for the development of an RIT-based HIV elimination strategy (25). mAb 2556 is a human mAb to a conserved domain of HIV gp41 glycoprotein and was able to outperform the endogenous antibodies in HIV-positive serum for binding to gp41. This latter quality is very important because it means that the antibody target site is not likely to be obscured by endogenous antibodies produced by infected individuals.

To investigate the feasibility of killing HIV-infected cells with radiolabeled 2556 mAb *in vivo* we used two HIV mouse models—a splenic model (22) and the Mosier model (26). As in the previous study (22), human mAb 1418 (IgG1) to parvovirus B19 (27) was used as an irrelevant isotype-matched control. As in our previous study, HIV-infected hPBMCs were given intrasplenically to SCID mice. After 1.5 h, these mice were given a single injection of [213]Bi-2556 or control mAbs. The radioactivity doses were 50, 100, and 200 μCi per animal (1 mg of mAb 2556/kg body weight). Three days following treatment, the mice were sacrificed, their spleens were harvested, and the viral load was determined by real-time PCR for HIV-1 DNA. The results demonstrated that [213]Bi-2556 killed HIV-infected hPBMCs much more effectively than isotype-matching control mAb armed with the same amounts of radioactivity or cold mAb 2556 (Fig. 4b). To

investigate the potential bone marrow toxicity of RIT, the peripheral blood of treated mice was analyzed for platelet counts. A drop in platelet numbers would be evidence of an undesirable effect of the radiolabeled mAb on the bone marrow, indicating hematologic toxicity (28). There was no difference in platelet counts between RIT-treated and control mice, consistent with no significant acute hematologic toxicity.

Subsequently [213]Bi-2556 was further evaluated in the SCID mouse model described by Mosier (26). The Mosier model involves i.p. implantation of hPBMCs into SCID mice, resulting in activation of T cells, thus providing a cellular population easily infected by HIV and mimicking the widespread lymphocyte activation observed in chronic HIV infection. HIV infection of hu-PBL SCID mice led to the loss of CD4+ T cells, as also seen as a result of HIV infection in human hosts. The Mosier model has been broadly utilized in evaluating the efficacy of antiviral drugs (29, 30). Similar to the splenic model, RIT led to a several log reduction in viral load in groups treated with 25, 50, and 100 μCi [213]Bi-2556 relative to controls (*P* < 0.05). These results are encouraging for further development of RIT as a backbone strategy for HIV eradication. We are currently planning a pilot clinical trial of RIT in HIV-infected patients on HAART.

CONCLUSIONS

The foreign nature of microbial cells results in their display of antigens that are not found anywhere in the human body, making RIT for infectious diseases more specific than RIT for cancer, since tumor-associated antigens are also sometimes found on normal tissues. As a consequence, the specificity of RIT for infections at least theoretically should be much more pronounced than in cancer, given higher selectivity and specificity for target cells. This exquisite specificity will lead to precise targeting, which in turn should translate into a highly efficacious treatment not accompanied by side effects. Additionally, the technology for linking radionuclides to mAbs is well established, so the lessons learned in the development of RIT in oncology could be readily applied to infectious diseases. Also, U.S. hospitals that are now regularly using RIT to treat cancer patients are fully equipped for initiating infectious disease RIT since the two use the same approach and differ only in the type of antibody used. An added bonus that would occur with some isotopes is the possibility for imaging patients receiving RIT to ascertain the targeting of radiolabeled mAbs to tissue and the anatomical extent of infection. We believe a combination of need together with the presence of a mature technology means that the time is ripe for deploying RIT into the clinic to combat infectious diseases.

ACKNOWLEDGMENTS

E. Dadachova was supported by the National Institute of Allergy and Infectious Disease (NIAID) grant AI60507 and by the Bill and Melinda Gates Foundation Grand Exploration Grant. A. Casadevall was supported by NIAID grants AI033142 and AI033774.

Conflicts of interest: We declare no conflicts.

CITATION

Dadachova E, Casadevall A. 2014. Radiolabeled antibodies for therapy of infectious diseases. Microbiol Spectrum 2(6):AID-0023-2014.

REFERENCES

1. **Dadachova E, Nakouzi A, Bryan R, Casadevall A.** 2003. Ionizing radiation delivered by specific antibody is therapeutic against a fungal infection. *Proc Natl Acad Sci USA* **100:**10942–10947.

2. **Park BJ, Wannemuehler KA, Marston BJ, Govender N, Pappas PG, Chiller TM.** 2009. Estimation of the current global burden of cryptococcal meningitis among persons living with HIV/AIDS. *AIDS* **23:**525–530.

3. **Larsen RA, Pappas PG, Perfect J, Aberg JA, Casadevall A, Cloud GA, James R, Filler S, Dismukes WE.** 2005. Phase I evaluation of the safety and pharmacokinetics of murine-derived anticryptococcal antibody 18B7 in subjects with treated cryptococcal meningitis. *Antimicrob Agents Chemother* **49:**952–958.

4. **Rhodes JC, Wicker LS, Urba WJ.** 1980. Genetic control of susceptibility to *Cryptococcus neoformans* in mice. *Infect Immun* **29:**494–499.

5. **Jiang Z, Bryan RA, Morgenstern A, Bruchertseifer F, Casadevall A, Dadachova E.** 2012. Treatment of early and established *Cryptococcus neoformans* infection with radiolabeled antibodies in immunocompetent mice. *Antimicrob Agents Chemother* **56:**552–554.

6. **Pai MP, Sakoglu U, Peterson SL, Lyons CR, Sood R.** 2009. Characterization of BBB permeability in a preclinical model of cryptococcal meningoencephalitis using magnetic resonance imaging. *J Cereb Blood Flow Metab* **29:**545–553.

7. **Bryan RA, Jiang Z, Howell RC, Morgenstern A, Bruchertseifer F, Casadevall A, Dadachova E.** 2010. Radioimmunotherapy is more effective than antifungal treatment in experimental cryptococcal infection. *J Infect Dis* **202:**633–637.

8. **Clemons KV, Stevens DA.** 1998. Comparison of fungizone, Amphotec, AmBisome, and Abelcet for treatment of systemic murine cryptococcosis. *Antimicrob Agents Chemother* **42:**899–902.

9. **Kakeya H, Miyazaki Y, Senda H, Senda H, Kobayashi T, Seki M, Izumikawa K, Yamamoto Y, Yanagihara K, Tashiro T, Kohno S.** 2008. Efficacy of SPK-843, a novel polyene antifungal, in a murine model of systemic cryptococcosis. *Antimicrob Agents Chemother* **52:**1871–1872.

10. **Bicanic T, Muzoora C, Brouwer AE, Brouwer AE, Meintjes G, Longley N, Taseera K, Rebe K, Loyse A, Jarvis J, Bekker LG, Wood R, Limmathurotsakul D, Chierakul W, Stepniewska K, White NJ, Jaffar S, Harrison TS.** 2009. Independent association between rate of clearance of infection and clinical outcome of HIV-associated cryptococcal meningitis: analysis of a combined cohort of 262 patients. *Clin Infect Dis* **49:**702–709.

11. **Bryan RA, Jiang Z, Huang X, Morgenstern A, Bruchertseifer F, Sellers R, Casadevall A, Dadachova E.** 2009. Radioimmunotherapy is effective against a high infection burden of *Cryptococcus neoformans* in mice and does not select for radiation-resistant phenotypes in cryptococcal cells. *Antimicrob Agents Chemother* **53:**1679–1682.

12. **Bryan RA, Huang X, Morgenstern A, Bruchertseifer F, Casadevall A, Dadachova E.** 2008. Radio-fungicidal effects of external gamma radiation and antibody-targeted beta and alpha radiation on *Cryptococcus neoformans. Antimicrob Agents Chemother* **52:**2232–2235.

13. **Torosantucci A, Chiani P, Bromuro C, De Bernardis F, Palma AS, Liu Y, Mignogna G, Maras B, Colone M, Stringaro A, Zamboni S, Feizi T, Cassone A.** 2009. Protection by anti-beta-glucan antibodies is associated with restricted beta-1,3 glucan binding specificity and inhibition of fungal growth and adherence. *PLoS One* **4:** e5392. doi:10.1371/journal.pone.0005392.

14. **Rachini A, Pietrella D, Lupo P, Torosantucci A, Chiani P, Bromuro C, Proietti C, Bistoni F, Cassone A, Vecchiarelli A.** 2007. An anti-beta-glucan monoclonal antibody inhibits growth and capsule formation of *Cryptococcus neoformans in vitro* and exerts therapeutic, anticryptococcal activity *in vivo*. *Infect Immun* **75:**5085–5094.

15. **Torosantucci A, Bromuro C, Chiani P, De Bernardis F, Berti F, Galli C, Norelli F, Bellucci C, Polonelli L, Costantino P, Rappuoli R, Cassone A.** 2005. A novel glyco-conjugate vaccine against fungal pathogens. *J Exp Med* **202:**597–606.

16. **Guimaraes AJ, Frases S, Gomez FJ, Zancope-Oliveira RM, Nosanchuk JD.** 2009. Monoclonal antibodies to heat shock protein 60 alter the pathogenesis of *Histoplasma capsulatum*. *Infect Immun* **77:**1357–1367.

17. **Nosanchuk JD, Casadevall A.** 2006. Impact of melanin on microbial virulence and clinical resistance to antimicrobial compounds. *Antimicrob Agents Chemother* **50:**3519–3528.

18. **Bryan RA, Guimaraes AJ, Hopcraft S, Jiang Z, Bonilla K, Morgenstern A, Bruchertseifer F, Del Poeta M, Torosantucci A, Cassone A, Nosanchuk JD, Casadevall A, Dadachova E.** 2012. Towards developing a universal treatment for fungal disease using radioimmunotherapy targeting common fungal antigens. *Mycopathologia* **73:**463–471.

19. **Dadachova E, Burns T, Bryan RA, Apostolidis C, Brechbiel MW, Nosanchuk JD, Casadevall A, Pirofski L.** 2004. Feasibility of radioimmunotherapy of experimental pneumococcal infection. *Antimicrob Agents Chemother* **48:**1624–1629.

20. **Rivera J, Nakouzi AS, Morgenstern A, Bruchertseifer F, Dadachova E, Casadevall A.** 2009. Radiolabeled antibodies to *Bacillus anthracis* toxins are bactericidal and partially therapeutic in experimental murine anthrax. *Antimicrob Agents Chemother* **53:**4860–4868.

21. **Rivera J, Morgenstern A, Bruchertseifer F, Kearney JF, Turnbough CL Jr, Dadachova E, Casadevall A.** 2014. Microbicidal power of alpha radiation in sterilizing germinating *Bacillus anthracis* spores. *Antimicrob Agents Chemother* **58:**1813–1815.

22. **Dadachova E, Patel MC, Toussi S, Apostolidis C, Morgenstern A, Brechbiel MW, Gorny MK, Zolla-Pazner S, Casadevall A, Goldstein H.** 2006. Targeted killing of virally infected cells by radiolabeled antibodies to viral proteins. *PLoS Med* **3:**e427. doi:10.1371/journal.pmed.0030427.

23. **Ho DD, Moudgil T, Alam M.** 1989. Quantitation of human immunodeficiency virus type 1 in the blood of infected persons. *N Engl J Med* **321:**1621–1625.

24. **Casadevall A, Goldstein H, Dadachova E.** 2007. Targeting viruses-harboring host cells with radiolabeled antibodies. *Expert Opin Biol Ther* **7:**595–597.

25. **Dadachova E, Kitchen SG, Bristol G, Baldwin GC, Revskaya E, Empig C, Thornton GB, Gorny MK, Zolla-Pazner S, Casadevall A.** 2012. Pre-clinical evaluation of a 213Bi-labeled 2556 antibody to HIV-1 gp41 glycoprotein in HIV-1 mouse models as a reagent for HIV eradication. *PLoS One* **7:**e31866. doi:10.1371/journal.pone.0031866.

26. **Mosier DE.** 1996. Viral pathogenesis in hu-PBL-SCID mice. *Sem Immunol* **8:**255–262.

27. **Gigler A, Dorsch S, Hemauer A, Williams C, Kim S.** 1999. Generation of neutralizing human monoclonal antibodies against parvovirus B19 proteins. *J Virol* **73:**1974–1979.

28. **Milenic DE, Brady ED, Brechbiel MW.** 2004. Antibody-targeted radiation cancer therapy. *Nat Rev Drug Discov* **3:**488–499.

29. **Uckun FM, Rajamohan F, Pendergrass S, Ozer Z, Waurzyniak B, Mao C.** 2003. Structure-based design and engineering of a nontoxic recombinant pokeweed antiviral protein with potent-anti-human immunodeficiency virus activity. *Antimicrob Agents Chemother* **47:**1052–1061.

30. **Uckun FM, Qazi S, Pendergrass S, Lisowski E, Waurzyniak B, Chen CL, Venkatachalam TK.** 2002. *In vivo* toxicity, pharmacokinetics, and anti-human immunodeficiency virus activity of stavudine-5'-(p-bromophenyl methoxyalaninyl phosphate) stampidine in mice. *Antimicrob Agents Chemother* **46:**3428–3436.

ALTERNATE SYSTEMS
FOR EXPRESSION

Plant-Derived Monoclonal Antibodies for Prevention and Treatment of Infectious Disease

24

ANDREW HIATT,[1] KEVIN J. WHALEY,[1] and LARRY ZEITLIN[1]

INTRODUCTION

Production and evaluation of monoclonal antibodies (MAbs) produced in plants to combat infectious diseases (IDs) has been ongoing for almost 20 years (1). With the recent FDA approval of the first plant-derived biologic (2), development of rapid manufacturing technology (3), and the capability of producing MAbs with homogenous mammalian glycosylation (4), a wave of infectious disease (and other) MAbs that are plant-derived are expected to enter clinical trials in the next several years. This review is intended to summarize the results of research on plant-derived MAbs to infectious pathogens that have completed animal or clinical studies.

PRODUCTION OF MAbs IN PLANTS

Rationale for Manufacturing ID MAbs in Plants

There are a number of advantageous characteristics of plant systems for production of anti-infective antibodies. One in particular has to do with the ease with which complex, multicomponent isotypes can be assembled (1, 5). The

[1]Mapp Biopharmaceutical, Inc., San Diego, CA 92121.
Antibodies for Infectious Diseases
Edited by James E. Crowe, Jr., Diana Boraschi, and Rino Rappuoli
© 2015 American Society for Microbiology, Washington, DC
doi:10.1128/microbiolspec.AID-0004-2012

most structurally complex type of antibody, a secretory immunoglobulin A (sIgA) consisting of four different chains, can be assembled in plants to produce functional, protease-resistant antibody molecules appropriate for use in environments where other types of antibodies are not found (e.g., the gastrointestinal tract) (1). Since mucosal surfaces are often the site of entry of infectious pathogens (6), the technology that can provide an appropriate type of antibody isotype for that environment could be uniquely suited for combating infectious diseases. Moreover, the use of antibodies at mucosal surfaces emphasizes preventive strategies that would deny entry to pathogens, rather than postexposure or therapeutic strategies. Preventive applications of antibodies inherently require a much larger scale of production due to a requirement for repeated dosing. Because preventive strategies ordinarily involve larger populations, an appropriate unit cost for a preventative antibody can be achieved at a sufficiently large production scale (7, 8). The ability to scale up production without incurring excessive capital requirements or a change in production methods is a hallmark of production in plants (7).

Transgenic Technologies for Plant-Based MAb Production

The first technology that was employed to express an antibody in a plant involved the transfer of recombinant selectable vectors into small pieces of leaf ("leaf discs") (9) by use of *Agrobacterium tumefaciens* infection as the transformation vehicle (1, 5). The early results of plant expression of a MAb to an infectious pathogen (1) demonstrated a number of principles about the variety of MAb isotypes that can be produced in plants as well as the characteristics and localization of those antibodies within the plant leaf (1). Early experiments exploring the capabilities of plants for expressing, assembling, and secreting complex immunoglobulins used a

plant transformation technology that was almost entirely based on regeneration of plants from infected plant cells carrying the antibody-encoding cDNAs (5). Infection was accomplished using engineered *Agrobacterium* that could selectively deliver the immunoglobulin-encoding DNAs to the plant cell nucleus (9). This process of creating fertile transgenic plants suffered from the significant period of time required for regeneration (~1 year) but did benefit from the ability to cross-pollinate the resulting plants to derive progeny that produced a desired combination of immunoglobulin chains (1, 5). In the first set of transgenic experiments, plants expressing IgG(γ) or Ig(κ) chains were cross-pollinated to produce progeny expressing assembled antibody (5). These IgGs possessed the same specificity when compared to the original mammalian cell-derived MAb. In subsequent experiments, the IgG constant region was replaced with a hybrid constant region consisting of both IgG and IgA components (1). When these hybrid heavy chain plants were crossed with plants expressing kappa, J chain, and secretory component, an assembled sIgA was produced. Microscopic examination of antibody accumulation showed that specific cell types, predominantly bundle sheath cells, were responsible for the relatively high level of sIgA accumulation in these plants.

Overall, the results demonstrated that a variety of immunoglobulin isotypes could be expressed in plants to yield complex, functional antibodies and that multiple immunoglobulin chains could be assembled into antibodies by stepwise cross-pollination of plants containing immunoglobulin genes. Moreover, the use of a hybrid constant region could result in assembly and high-level production of a class of antibody that is not ordinarily observed from mammalian cell culture. Perhaps due to their inherent biochemical stability, the hybrid sIgA accumulated in these plants to levels that are not ordinarily observed in transgenics (~5% of extractable protein).

Transient Technologies for Plant-Based MAb Production

Recent plant-based manufacturing techniques have been aimed at deriving a higher level of expression and, importantly, a short time frame to generate MAb. One commercially viable technique, referred to as "magnifection," involves transient expression of the MAb wherein the infection of the cell is accomplished after introducing several pro-vectors into *Agrobacterium tumefaciens* that can deliver noncompeting viral components (derived from tobacco mosaic virus and potato virus X) as well as the MAb genes to plant cells (3, 10). In this sense, *Agrobacterium* is the vehicle for primary infection of the plant, whereas the ultimately recombined, functional viral replicon provides cell-to-cell spread, amplification, and high expression (Fig. 1). The technology appears to be the most rapid path from genes to full-length, assembled MAb, i.e., 14 days from gene delivery to purified MAb (10). The manufacturing technology can easily accommodate hundreds of grams per month for preclinical and clinical studies as well as commercial scale (7, 8). Because antibody drug development has evolved into a highly iterative process where sequential modifica-

tions are introduced into candidate molecules and evaluated for changes in efficacy, the shortened time frame to multi-gram-level production may accelerate this process greatly.

Technologies for Controlling MAb N Glycosylation

Recently, transgenic technology has been used to generate plants that yield MAbs with homogenous N glycosylation patterns (4) (Fig. 2). Specifically, using RNA interference technology, *Nicotiana benthamiana* plants have been generated that have dramatically reduced xylosyl or fucosyl transferase enzymatic activities (ΔXF) (11). Antibodies expressed in this transgenic plant contain a single dominant N-glycan species consisting of biantennary N-glycans with terminal *N*-acetylglucosamine on both branches (GnGn) that shows significantly enhanced binding to FcγRIIIa, as has been observed with other nonfucosylated MAbs derived from other sources (11). A plant-derived anti-human immunodeficiency virus (anti-HIV) antibody produced in these plants was the first example of using glycoengineering to improve the antiviral activity of a MAb (11).

Introduction of the β-1,4-galactosyl transferase gene into this ΔXF plant background resulted in a fully galactosylated and relatively homogeneous N-glycosylation. These MAbs (11) consisted of two broadly neutralizing anti-HIV MAbs (2G12, 4E10) and displayed improved virus neutralization potency when compared with other glycoforms produced in plants and in CHO cells.

The final sugar addition in many mammalian glycans is sialylation (12). Terminal α-2,6-sialic acid is an important mediator of diverse biological activities. In particular, sialylation appears to play a crucial role in the efficacy of intravenous immunoglobulin for autoimmune diseases (13, 14, 15). Plants do not make sialic acid; however, the entire biosynthetic pathway for antibody sialylation has been incorporated into ΔXF *Nicotiana* plants (12). IgG antibodies expressed in the sialo-engineered plants have a

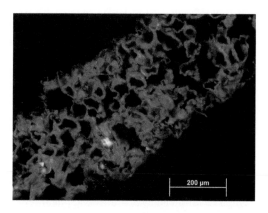

FIGURE 1 **Fluorescent immunocytochemistry of a *N. benthamiana* leaf 7 days after magnifection. Tissue was stained with Cy3-labeled anti-human IgG. Image courtesy of Jeffrey Pudney, Boston University Medical College. doi:10.1128/microbiolspec.AID-0004-2012.f1**

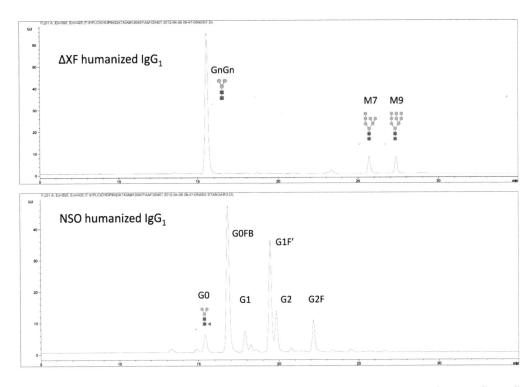

FIGURE 2 **N glycosylation of a humanized IgG1 produced in ΔXF *N. benthamiana* and mammalian cell culture (NS0 cells) as determined by 2-AA glycan analysis. doi:10.1128/microbiolspec.AID-0004-2012.f2**

significant percentage of molecules with α-2,6-sialic acid termini that can exceed the percentage observed in intravenous immunoglobulin.

In sum, the glycoengineering that has been accomplished to date has provided a variety of glycoforms with either enhanced biological activity (e.g., antiviral) or fully human glycans.

PLANT-DERIVED MAbs AGAINST ID TARGETS

To date, a variety of plant-produced MAbs have been described. The focus here is on MAbs that have been tested for efficacy in animals or humans (Table 1).

Dental Caries MAbs

Clinical evaluation of the plant-produced Guy's 13 sIgA/G has been performed (16). In

an initial trial, patients received 9 days of chlorhexidine treatment to eliminate *Streptococcus mutans* from their oral cavities followed by two treatments per week for 3 weeks with Guy's 13 sIgA/G, saline, or control antibody. Patients treated with the plant-derived Guy's 13 had no recolonization with *S. mutans* ($n = 4$), whereas patients treated with saline ($n = 4$) or control antibody ($n = 3$) were all recolonized. All treatments in this study were performed in a dental clinic. In a subsequent trial testing home treatment, 56 eligible adults had 9 days of treatment with chlorhexidine and were randomized equally to a group receiving 0, 2, 4, or 6 topical applications of plant-produced Guy's 13 followed by 6, 4, 2, or 0 applications of placebo, respectively, over a 3-week period. After 6 months, there were no significant differences in *S. mutans* levels by number of applications, relative to placebo. No adverse effects were observed during the study, and it

TABLE 1 **In vivo studies with plant-derived MAbs against ID targets**

Pathogen	MAb descriptor	Expression host	Test model	Efficacy	P	Comments (reference)[a]
Anthrax	Receptor-human Fc fusion	*N. benthamiana*	Rabbit	100%	<0.05	2 mg/kg delivered 1 h after 100 LD_{50} inhalation challenge (69)
	Aglycosylated human IgG1	*N. benthamiana*	Mouse	100%	<0.01	8 mg/kg delivered to mice prior to i.p. challenge with 20 LD_{50}; 5 mg/kg delivered to macaques prior to 500 LD_{50} aerosol challenge (68)
			Macaque	100%	<0.05	
C. perfringens ETX	Chimeric IgG1	*N. benthamiana*	Mouse	100%	<0.001	0.8 mg/kg delivered prior to i.v. challenge (Uzal and Zeitlin, unpublished)
Ebola virus	Humanized IgG1	*N. benthamiana*	Mouse	100%	<0.01	2 mg/kg delivered prior to i.p. challenge with 30,000 LD_{50} (21)
	3-MAb IgG1 cocktail	*N. benthamiana*	Macaque	67 – 100%	<0.05	50 mg/kg delivered 1 h to 2 days after 1,000 LD_{50} i.m. challenge (26)
HSV	Humanized IgG1	Soybean	Mouse	100%	<0.001	0.5 mg/ml delivered vaginally prior to 10 LD_{50} vaginal challenge (27)
Rabies	Human IgG	*N. tabacum*	Hamster	100%	<0.01	3 IU of MAb 4 h after intracerebral challenge with 3×10^5 LD_{50} (36)
RSV	Humanized IgG1	*N. benthamiana*	Cotton rat	>10[2b]	<0.001	5 mg/kg delivered prior to i.n. challenge of 2×10^4 PFU (Zeitlin et al., submitted)
SEB	Chimeric IgG1	*N. benthamiana*	Mouse	100%	<0.001	0.4 mg/kg delivered prior to i.p. challenge with 5 LD_{50} (Roy and Zeitlin, unpublished)
S. mutans	Murine SIgA/G	*N. tabacum*	Human	100%	<0.05	2–5 mg/kg prevented natural recolonization over the 3-mo course of study (18)
WNV	Humanized IgG1	*N. benthamiana*	Mouse	80–90%	<0.001	1–5 mg/kg delivered 2 days post-footpad challenge with 5–10 LD_{50} (54)

[a]LD_{50}, 50% lethal dose; i.p., intraperitoneal; i.v., intravenous; i.m., intramuscular; i.n., intranasal.
[b]Reduction in viral lung titer.

was concluded that plant-produced Guy's 13 is safe but not effective at the frequency, concentration, and number of applications used in that study. However, subsequent clinical evaluation did define the effective parameters of administration. CaroRx, the commercial name for the plant-produced Guy's 13 anti-caries MAb product, is intended for regular oral topical preventative administration. New clinical trials have indicated that this treatment can effectively eliminate decay-causing bacteria for up to 2 years (16, 17, 18, 19). CaroRx has demonstrated efficacy and safety in a phase 2 clinical trial (www.planetbiotechnology.com/products.html) (20).

Ebola Virus MAbs

Recent outbreaks in central Africa and concerns about weaponization highlight the lack of any vaccine or treatment for Ebola virus infection. A recent study focused on the role of antibody glycosylation in the development of an immunoprotectant for Ebola virus revealed potential advantages of plant production of MAbs against infectious pathogens (21). An anti-Ebola glycoprotein (GP) MAb was produced in ΔXF *Nicotiana* plants, resulting in MAb with a highly homogenous distribution of N-glycoforms (90% GnGn) and lacking potentially immunogenic plant-specific β1,2 xylose and core α1,3 fucose. The MAb, h-13F6, recognizes the heavily glycosylated mucin-like domain of GP. h-13F6 does not neutralize in vitro, as assessed by inhibition of plaque formation, even in the presence of complement (21), suggesting an important role for Fc-mediated effector functions in in vivo protection. The plant-derived h-13F6 was compared with h-13F6 produced in CHO cells in a lethal mouse Ebola virus challenge model. The plant-derived h-13F6 carrying N-glycans lacking fucose showed threefold-superior potency to h-13F6 with typical CHO glycosylation patterns (21). Elimination of core fucose has been shown to dramatically improve antibody-dependent cellular cytotoxicity (ADCC) activity in vitro and in vivo through improved affinity for FcγRIII (22, 23, 24, 25). Indeed, affinity analyses of the plant- and CHO-derived h-13F6 confirmed that elimination of core fucose from h-13F6 resulted in an improved affinity for FcγRIII. In total, these results suggested that ADCC is an important mechanism of protection by this MAb. Further studies have now been performed showing that a cocktail of 3 *Nicotiana*-derived anti-Ebola GP MAbs (including h-13F6) can protect rhesus macaques from lethal challenge: 100% survival was observed when the MAbs were administered an hour after challenge and 67% survival when delivered 1 or 2 days postchallenge (26). This study demonstrated a greater therapeutic window as well as reduced viral burden and level of disease compared to other therapeutics in development (26).

HSV and HIV MAbs: Preventing Sexual Transmission

The earliest in vivo comparison study of a plant-produced and a cell culture-produced MAb involved a humanized anti-herpes simplex virus (anti-HSV) glycoprotein B antibody made in soybeans compared to the same MAb expressed in mammalian cell culture of Sp2/0 cells (27). The comparative assays included diffusion and stability in mucus as well as prevention of vaginal transmission of genital herpes in the mouse. No significant difference was observed in these assays, and vaginal delivery of 10 μg of either MAb provided 100% protection against vaginal challenge with HSV type 2 (27). A microbicide containing a cocktail of HSV and HIV MAbs is currently being evaluated for efficacy in the simian HIV nonhuman primate model and is expected to enter a clinical safety trial in 2014 (K. Whaley and F. Villinger, personal communication).

A number of broadly neutralizing HIV MAbs have been produced in plants and evaluated on the basis of binding ability as well as structure (28, 29, 30, 31). For example, one of the broadly neutralizing MAbs, 2G12, has been produced in transgenic maize plants (29), and the HIV neutralization capability of the antibody is equal to or superior to that of the same antibody produced in CHO cells. 2G12 has also been transiently produced in the ΔXF *Nicotiana* line and was found to contain a relatively homogeneous N-glycan species without detectable xylose or α-1,3-fucose residues (4). In general, plant-derived 2G12 was indistinguishable from CHO-derived 2G12 with respect to electrophoretic properties as well as functional properties (i.e., antigen binding and HIV neutralization activity). In some cases, plant-produced HIV MAbs appear to have enhanced potency compared to CHO-produced MAbs. Fully galactosylated 4E10 (another broadly neutralizing MAb) and 2G12 were reported to be severalfold higher in neutralization potency than CHO-produced MAbs (11). In addition, sialylated 2G12 exhibits in vitro HIV neutralization potency similar to that of other glycoforms derived from plants and CHO cells (12). Other plant expression systems have been used to produce these MAbs as well: 4E10 has been produced in a transgenic tobacco rhizosection system (31), and a fusion protein of the broadly neutralizing HIV MAb b12 and cyanovirin produced in transgenic tobacco increased HIV potency compared to b12 or cyanovirin alone (32).

Rabies Virus MAbs

Since more than 10 million people annually receive rabies virus postexposure prophylaxis in the form of equine antirabies immunoglobulin or human antirabies immunoglobulin (HRIG), together with rabies vaccine (33), there is a worldwide shortage of these immunoglobulins. The limited supply and the additional risk of adverse reactions associated with equine antirabies immunoglobulin have spurred the search for new MAbs. In addition, the high cost of HRIG has been a significant impediment in providing postexposure prophylaxis against rabies (34). To address these limitations, transgenic plants have been used as an efficient production system for the expression of functional therapeutic antirabies MAbs (35). In the first report of systemic administration of a plant-derived MAb to provide immunoprotection, a human anti-rabies MAb was purified from transgenic tobacco plants and characterized structurally and for its effectiveness in vivo (36). The plant-derived MAb was compared with an equivalent human MAb expressed in murine-human hybridoma cell lines (37, 38) and/or commercial HRIG for neutralization activity, protein stability, N-glycan processing, and the efficacy of rabies virus postexposure prophylaxis in exposed animals. The plant-derived MAb was as effective at neutralizing the activity of the rabies virus as the mammalian-derived antibody or HRIG. Due to the incorporation of an endoplasmic retention signal on the MAb heavy chain (to increase accumulation), the plant-derived MAb contained mainly oligomannose type N-glycans (90%) and had no potentially antigenic $\alpha(1,3)$-linked fucose residues. The plant-derived MAb had a shorter serum half-life than mammalian cell-derived MAb but was as efficient as HRIG for postexposure prophylaxis against rabies

virus in hamsters, indicating that differences in N-glycosylation do not affect the efficacy of the antibody in this model (38).

RSV MAbs

Synagis is the only MAb approved by the FDA for an ID indication and currently generates sales of greater than $1 billion/year. Although Synagis is an effective drug for respiratory syncytial virus (RSV) immunoprophylaxis in at-risk neonates, ongoing analyses on the pharmacoeconomics suggest that Synagis may not be cost-effective in actual use, nor even when its use is restricted very tightly to its labeled population (39, 40, 41, 42, 43, 44). A less expensive RSV MAb could improve the pharmacoeconomics in neonates and open up additional markets; RSV is a significant cause of morbidity and mortality in the elderly as well as in hematopoietic stem cell transplant patients. Several RSV-neutralizing MAbs have been produced in *Nicotiana* using magnifection and have been tested in the cotton rat model of protective efficacy (80). Synagis and the identical amino acid sequence expressed in *Nicotiana* were superior to other candidate MAbs and were essentially indistinguishable in terms of affinity, neutralization, and in vivo protection, providing greater than 100-fold reduction in viral lung titer when dosed at 5 mg/kg of body weight. The data also suggested that the *Nicotiana*-derived MAb was more potent therapeutically than Synagis, raising the possibility that enhanced ADCC conferred by the ΔXF *Nicotiana* N-glycans may be responsible for improved efficacy in an established RSV infection (80).

WNV MAbs

West Nile virus (WNV) has in the past been responsible for outbreaks of mild illness in regions of Africa, the Middle East, Asia, and Australia. In the 1990s, however, the epidemiology of infection changed and new outbreaks in Eastern Europe were associated with higher rates of severe neurological disease (45). In 1999, WNV entered North America, and since then, WNV has spread to all 48 of the lower United States as well as to parts of Canada, Mexico, the Caribbean, and South America. Because of the increased range, the number of human cases has continued to rise: in the United States between 1999 and 2008, 28,961 cases that reached clinical attention were confirmed and associated with 1,131 deaths (46). The lack of effective and specific antiviral treatment for infection by WNV or other flaviviruses (47) has prompted the search for highly specific therapies, including MAbs. Although small-molecule antiviral agents have been described with activity against WNV in vitro, efficacy in vivo has been limited (48). A humanized murine MAb (Hu–E16) that binds to a highly conserved epitope on domain III (DIII) of the WNV envelope (E) protein has been described (49). This MAb blocks viral fusion at low concentrations (50, 51) and has therapeutic activity in rodents even after WNV has entered the central nervous system (52, 53). Magnifection has been used to produce high levels of the Hu-E16 MAb, which retained neutralizing activity and significant pre- and postexposure therapeutic activity in mice (54). The therapeutic activity was virtually equivalent to that observed with mammalian cell culture-derived Hu-E16 with 80 to 90% survival when delivered 2 or 4 days postchallenge (54).

MAbs to Bacterial Toxins

Anthrax MAbs

Anthrax toxin-specific antibodies have previously been shown to provide passive protection against an anthrax challenge (55, 56, 57, 58). These antibodies, generally against protective antigen, protect rats, guinea pigs, rabbits, and nonhuman primates when administered within a time frame of several hours before or after the exposure to inhalation anthrax (59, 60, 61, 62, 63, 64, 65, 66, 67, 68). A transgenic *Nicotiana*-derived nonglycosylated MAb directed against protective antigen has been evaluated (68). This antibody neutralized

anthrax lethal toxin activity in vitro and protected mice from lethal intraperitoneal challenge with spores. The nonglycosylated MAb possessed superior efficacy (100% protection) against an aerosol challenge compared with the glycosylated form (40%) after a single 5-mg/kg of body weight intravenous administration in nonhuman primates. This was attributed to the shortened half-life observed with the glycosylated MAb. In general, the data demonstrate that the absence of N-linked glycans does not affect the ability of this MAb to protect animals against a lethal spore challenge. The results also demonstrate that plant production is an appropriate technology for generating nonglycosylated MAbs and could be useful in meeting the production challenge involved in the treatment of inhalation anthrax in humans. An additional plant-derived immunotherapeutic utilized a recombinant fusion protein comprised of a fusion of a human receptor for anthrax toxins (capillary morphogenesis protein 2 [CMG2]) and the Fc of human IgG1, for long-circulating half-life and immune effector cell interaction (69). CMG2-Fc, purified from tobacco plants, fully protected rabbits against a lethal challenge with *Bacillus anthracis* spores at a dose of 2 mg/kg of body weight administered at the time of challenge. Treatment with CMG2-Fc did not interfere with the development of the animals' own immunity to anthrax, as treated animals that survived an initial challenge also survived a rechallenge 30 days later (69).

Clostridium Perfringens ETX

Potential aggressors have shown interest in the biological weapons potential of *C. perfringens*, and the UN Special Commission identified it as having been developed and potentially weaponized in Iraq (70, 71). Epsilon toxin (ETX) is the most potent of the *C. perfringens* toxins, with a mouse intravenous lethal dose of 100 ng per kg of body weight (72). A previously identified mouse MAb, 4D7, with potent neutralizing activity (73) was chimerized with human constant regions and produced in the magnifection system. This

MAb demonstrated 100% prophylactic and postexposure efficacy against challenge (F. Uzal and L. Zeitlin, unpublished data).

SEB

Staphylococcal enterotoxin B (SEB) is an extremely potent enterotoxin involved in a large proportion of cases of toxic shock syndrome as well as a very significant mediator of staphylococcal food poisoning (74, 75, 76). Because of its extreme potency, current interest in SEB relates to its potential for use as a biowarfare or bioterrorism agent. There are currently no therapeutic options available for SEB exposure. SEB MAb production in the magnifection system resulted in very high levels of MAb accumulation (77). A human-mouse chimeric MAb against SEB has now been shown to provide 100% protection in mouse lethal aerosol and systemic challenge models (C. Roy, L. Zeitlin, et al., unpublished data).

Plant-Produced MAbs for Purification of ID Antigens

MAbs specific for particular ID antigens have also been produced in plants to facilitate large-scale purification of the antigen for use as a vaccine. For example, a recombinant antibody specific for the HBsAg was purified from transgenic *Nicotiana tabacum* plants to test its ability to immunopurify a yeast rHBsAg to be putatively used as a vaccine in humans. The purification system was mainly based on recombinant protein A expanded bed adsorption chromatography, which has been widely used for MAb purification (78, 79). In this chromatography, a strong interaction among the protein A and Fc fragments of the antibodies is normally produced, allowing high recovery and purity. Additionally, its main advantage is the capacity to be introduced as a primary recovery operation to handle unclarified materials, yielding a combination of clarification, concentration, and adsorptive purification in a single step. Further preclinical evaluation has demonstrated that the MAb readily interacts with cell surface HBsAgs and displays complement-dependent cytotoxicity in a manner that was similar to anti-HBs human immunoglobulins used clinically. This product is now being used in Cuba in the manufacturing of HBsAg for active immunization.

CONCLUSION

Since the early days of plant expression of antibodies (5), research into the application of the technology for preventing or treating infectious pathogens has resulted in established clinical efficacy in one case and fundamental proof of concept in others. In addition, the ability of plants to readily assemble antibodies that are appropriate for applications involving mucosal and topical surfaces derives from the various ways that different antibody components can be assembled as well as the fidelity of the endomembrane system of plants in efficiently assembling and secreting antibody molecules. Further, the ability to manufacture MAb with specific mammalian N-glycosylation patterns allows for customization of biological activity. Now that a plant-derived biologic has found regulatory acceptance, the path to approval of novel antibody anti-infectives derived from plants should be straightforward. Whereas it remains to be seen the extent to which plant-derived antibody products will enjoy benefit of scale, the promise of a production system that can provide novel anti-infectives at low cost to a large market continues to drive research in the field.

ACKNOWLEDGMENT

We declare a conflict of interest: L.Z. and K.J.W. are co-owners of Mapp Biopharmaceutical, Inc.

CITATION

Hiatt A, Whaley KJ, Zeitlin L. 2014. Plant-derived monoclonal antibodies for prevention and treatment of infectious disease. Microbiol Spectrum 2(1):AID-0004-2012.

REFERENCES

1. Ma JK, Hiatt A, Hein M, Vine ND, Wang F, Stabila P, van Dolleweerd C, Mostov K, Lehner T. 1995. Generation and assembly of secretory antibodies in plants. *Science* **268:**716–719.

2. Aviezer D, Brill-Almon E, Shaaltiel Y, Hashmueli S, Bartfeld D, Mizrachi S, Liberman Y, Freeman A, Zimran A, Galun E. 2009. A plant-derived recombinant human glucocerebrosidase enzyme—a preclinical and phase I investigation. *PLoS One* **4:**e4792–e4796.

3. Giritch A, Marillonnet S, Engler C, van Eldik G, Botterman J, Klimyuk V, Gleba Y. 2006. Rapid high-yield expression of full-size IgG antibodies in plants co-infected with noncompeting viral vectors. *Proc Natl Acad Sci USA* **103:**14701–14706.

4. Strasser R, Stadlmann J, Schahs M, Stiegler G, Quendler H, Mach L. 2008. Generation of glycoengineered *Nicotiana benthamiana* for the production of monoclonal antibodies with a homogeneous human-like N-glycan structure. *Plant Biotech J* **6:**392–402.

5. Hiatt A, Cafferkey R, Bowdish K. 1989. Production of antibodies in transgenic plants. *Nature* **342:** 76–78.

6. Bemark M, Boysen P, Lycke NY. 2012. Induction of gut IgA production through T cell-dependent and T cell-independent pathways. *Ann N Y Acad Sci* **1247:**97–116.

7. Pogue GP, Vojdani F, Palmer KE, Hiatt E, Hume S, Phelps J, Long L, Bohorova N, Kim D, Pauly M, Velasco J, Whaley K, Zeitlin L, Garger SJ, White E, Bai Y, Haydon H, Bratcher B. 2010. Production of pharmaceutical-grade recombinant aprotinin and a monoclonal antibody product using plant-based transient expression systems. *Plant Biotechnol J* **8:**638–654.

8. Klimyuk V, Pogue G, Herz S, Butler J, Haydon H. 2012. Production of recombinant antigens and antibodies in *Nicotiana benthamiana* using 'magnifection' technology: GMP-compliant facilities for small- and large-scale manufacturing. *Curr Top Microbiol Immunol* doi:10.1007/82_2012_212. [Epub ahead of print.]

9. Horsch RB, Fraley RT, Rogers SG, Sanders PR, Lloyd A, Hoffmann N. 1984. Inheritance of functional foreign genes in plants. *Science* **223:** 496–498.

10. Hiatt A, and Pauly M. 2006. Monoclonal antibodies from plants: a new speed record. *Proc Natl Acad Sci USA* **103:**14645–14646.

11. Strasser R, Castilho A, Stadlmann J, Kunert R, Quendler H, Gattinger P. 2009. Improved virus neutralization by plant-produced anti-HIV antibodies with a homogeneous beta1,4-galactosylated N-glycan profile. *J Biol Chem* **284:**20479–20485.

12. Castilho A, Strasser R, Stadlmann J, Grass J, Jez J, Gattinger P, Kunert R, Quendler H, Pabst M, Leonard R, Altmann F, Steinkellner H. 2010. In planta protein sialylation through overexpression of the respective mammalian pathway. *J Biol Chem* **285:**15923–15930.

13. Jefferis R. 2005. Glycosylation of recombinant antibody therapeutics. *Biotechnol Prog* **21:**11–16.

14. Nimmerjahn F, Ravetch JV. 2008. Anti-inflammatory actions of intravenous immuno-globulin. *Annu Rev Immunol* **26:**513–533.

15. Anthony RM, Wermeling F, Ravetch JV. 2012. Novel roles for the IgG Fc glycan. *Ann NY Acad Sci* **1253:**170–180.

16. Ma JK, Hikmat BY, Wycoff K, Vine ND, Chargelegue D, Yu L, Hein MB, Lehner T. 1998. Characterization of a recombinant plant monoclonal secretory antibody and preventive immunotherapy in humans. *Nat Med* **4:**601–606.

17. Ma JK, and Lehner T. 1990. Prevention of colonization of *Streptococcus mutans* by topical application of monoclonal antibodies in human subjects. *Arch Oral Biol* **35:**115–122.

18. Ma JK, Hunjan M, Smith R, Lehner T. 1989. Specificity of monoclonal antibodies in local passive immunization against *Streptococcus mutans*. *Clin Exp Immunol* **77:**331–337.

19. Weintraub JA, Hilton JF, White JM, Hoover CI, Wycoff KL, Yu L, Larrick JW, Featherstone JD. 2005. Clinical trial of a plant-derived antibody on re-colonization of mutans streptococci. *Caries Res* **39:**241–250.

20. De Muynck B, Navarre C, Boutry M. 2010. Production of antibodies in plants: status after twenty years. *Plant Biotechnol J* **8:**529–563.

21. Zeitlin L, Pettitt J, Scully C, Bohorova N, Kim D, Pauly M, Hiatt A, Ngo L, Steinkellner H, Whaley KJ, Olinger GG. 2011. Enhanced potency of a fucose-free monoclonal antibody being developed as an Ebola virus immunoprotectant. *Proc Natl Acad Sci USA* **108:**20690–20694.

22. Niwa R, Shoji-Hosaka E, Sakurada M, Shinkawa T, Uchida K, Nakamura K, Matsushima K, Ueda R, Hanai N, Shitara K. 2004. Defucosylated chimeric anti-CC chemokine receptor 4 IgG1 with enhanced antibody-dependent cellular cytotoxicity shows potent therapeutic activity to T-cell leukemia and lymphoma. *Cancer Res* **64:** 2127–2133.

23. Cox KM, Sterling JD, Regan JT, Gasdaska JR, Frantz KK, Peele CG, Black A, Passmore D, Moldovan-Loomis C, Srinivasan M, Cuison S, Cardarelli PM, Dickey LF. 2006. Glycan optimization of a human monoclonal antibody in the aquatic plant *Lemna minor*. *Nat Biotechnol* **24:** 1591–1597.

24. Umaña P, Jean-Mairet J, Moudry R, Amstutz H, Bailey JE. 1999. Engineered glycoforms of an antineuroblastoma IgG1 with optimized antibody-dependent cellular cytotoxic activity. *Nat Biotechnol* **17:**176–180.

25. Junttila TT, Parsons K, Olsson C, Lu Y, Xin Y, Theriault J, Crocker L, Pabonan O, Baginski T, Meng G, Totpal K, Kelley RF, Sliwkowski MX. 2010. Superior in vivo efficacy of afucosylated trastuzumab in the treatment of HER2-amplified breast cancer. *Cancer Res* **70:**4481–4489.

26. Olinger GG, Pettitt JD, Kim DH, Working C, Bohorov O, Bratcher B, Hiatt E, Hume SD, Johnson AK, Morton J, Pauly MH, Whaley KJ, Lear CM, Biggins JE, Scully C, Hensley LE, Zeitlin L. 2012. Delayed treatment of Ebola virus infection with plant-derived monoclonal antibodies provides protection in rhesus macaques. *Proc Natl Acad Sci USA* doi:10.1073/pnas.1213709109.

27. Zeitlin L, Olmsted SS, Moench TR, Co MS, Martinell BJ, Paradkar VM, Russell DR, Queen C, Cone RA, Whaley KJ. 1998. A humanized monoclonal antibody produced in transgenic plants for immunoprotection of the vagina against genital herpes. *Nat Biotechnol* **16:**1361–1364.

28. Forthal DN, Gach JS, Landucci G, Jez J, Strasser R, Kunert R, Steinkellner H. 2010. Fc-glycosylation influences Fcγ receptor binding and cell-mediated anti-HIV activity of monoclonal antibody 2G12. *J Immunol* **185:**6876–6882.

29. Rademacher T, Sack M, Arcalis E, Stadlmann J, Balzer S, Altmann F. 2008. Recombinant antibody 2G12 produced in maize endosperm efficiently neutralizes HIV-1 and contains predominantly single GlcNAc N-glycans. *Plant Biotech J* **6:**189–201.

30. Ramessar K, Rademacher T, Sack M, Stadlmann J, Platis D, Stiegler G. 2008. Cost-effective production of a vaginal protein microbicide to prevent HIV transmission. *Proc Natl Acad Sci USA* **105:**3727–3732.

31. Drake PMW, Barbi T, Sexton A, McGowan E, Stadlmann J, Navarre C. 2009. Development of rhizosecretion as a production system for recombinant proteins from hydroponic cultivated tobacco. *FASEB J* **23:**3581–3589.

32. Sexton A, Harman S, Shattock RJ, Ma JK. 2009. Design, expression and characterization of a multivalent, combination HIV microbicide. *FASEB J* **23:**3590–3600.

33. Anonymous. 2002. Rabies vaccines. *Wkly Epidemiol Rec* **77:**109–120.

34. Wilde H, Tipkong P, Khawplod P. 1999. Economic issues in postexposure rabies treatment. *J Travel Med* **6:**238–242.

35. Daniell H, Streatfield SJ, Wycoff K. 2001. Medical molecular farming: production of antibodies, biopharmaceuticals and edible vaccines in plants. *Trends Plant Sci* **6:**219–226.

36. Ko K, Tekoah Y, Rudd PM, Harvey DJ, Dwek RA, Spitsin S, Hanlon CA, Rupprecht C, Dietzschold B, Golovkin M, Koprowski H. 2003. Function and glycosylation of plant-derived antiviral monoclonal antibody. *Proc Natl Acad Sci USA* **100:**8013–8018.

37. Dietzschold B, Gore M, Casali P, Ueki Y, Rupprecht CE, Notkins AL, Koprowski H. 1990. Biological characterization of human monoclonal antibodies to rabies virus. *J Virol* **6:**3087–3090.

38. Prosniak M, Faber M, Hanlon CA, Rupprecht CE, Hooper DC, Dietzschold B. 2003. Development of a cocktail of recombinant-expressed human rabies virus-neutralizing monoclonal antibodies for postexposure prophylaxis of rabies. *J Infect Dis* **188:**53–56.

39. Joffe S, Ray GT, Escobar GJ, Black SB, Lieu TA. 1999. Cost-effectiveness of respiratory syncytial virus prophylaxis among preterm infants. *Pediatrics* **104**(3 Pt 1):419–427.

40. Lofland JH, O'Connor JP, Chatterton ML, Moxey ED, Paddock LE, Nash DB, Desai SA. 2000. Palivizumab for respiratory syncytial virus prophylaxis in high-risk infants: a cost-effectiveness analysis. *Clin Ther* **22:**1357–1369.

41. Numa A. 2000. Outcome of respiratory syncytial virus infection and a cost-benefit analysis of prophylaxis. *J Paediatr Child Health* **36:**422–427.

42. Barton LL, Grant KL, Lemen RJ. 2001. Respiratory syncytial virus immune globulin: decisions and costs. *Pediatr Pulmonol* **32:**20–28.

43. Vogel A, McKinlay M, Ashton T, Lennon D, Harding J, Pinnock R, Graham D, Grimwood K, Pattemore P, Schousboe M. 2002. Cost-effectiveness of palivizumab in New Zealand. *J Paediatr Child Health* **38:**352–357.

44. Roeckl-Wiedmann I, Liese JG, Grill E, Fischer B, Carr D, Belohradsky BH. 2003. Economic evaluation of possible prevention of RSV-related hospitalizations in premature infants in Germany. *Eur J Pediatr* **162:**237–244.

45. Hubalek Z, Halouzka J. 1999. West Nile fever—a reemerging mosquito-borne viral disease in Europe. *Emerg Infect Dis* **5:**643–650.

46. Diamond MS. 2009. Progress on the development of therapeutics against West Nile virus. *Antivir Res* **83:**214–227.

47. Furuta Y, Takahashi K, Shiraki K, Sakamoto K, Smee DF, Barnard DL, Gowen BB, Julander JG, Morrey JD. 2009. T-705 (favipiravir) and related compounds: novel broad-spectrum inhibitors of RNA viral infections. *Antivir Res* **82:**95–102.

48. Morrey JD, Taro BS, Siddharthan V, Wang H, Smee DF, Christensen AJ, Furuta Y. 2008.

Efficacy of orally administered T-705 pyrazine analog on lethal West Nile virus infection in rodents. *Antivir Res* **80**:377–379.

49. **Oliphant T, Engle M, Nybakken GE, Doane C, Johnson S, Huang L, Gorlatov S, Mehlhop E, Marri A, Chung KM, Ebel GD, Kramer LD, Fremont DH, Diamond MS.** 2005. Development of a humanized monoclonal antibody with therapeutic potential against West Nile virus. *Nat Med* **11**:522–530.

50. **Pierson TC, Xu Q, Nelson S, Oliphant T, Nybakken GE, Fremont DH, Diamond MS.** 2007. The stoichiometry of antibody-mediated neutralization and enhancement of West Nile virus infection. *Cell Host Microbe* **1**:135–145.

51. **Thompson BS, Moesker B, Smit JM, Wilschut J, Diamond MS, Fremont DH.** 2009. A therapeutic antibody against West Nile virus neutralizes infection by blocking fusion within endosomes. *PLoS Pathog* **5**:e1000453.

52. **Morrey JD, Siddharthan V, Olsen AL, Roper GY, Wang H, Baldwin TJ, Koenig S, Johnson S, Nordstrom JL, Diamond MS.** 2006. Humanized monoclonal antibody against West Nile virus envelope protein administered after neuronal infection protects against lethal encephalitis in hamsters. *J Infect Dis* **194**:1300–1308.

53. **Samuel MA, Wang H, Siddharthan V, Morrey JD, Diamond MS.** 2007. Axonal transport mediates West Nile virus entry into the central nervous system and induces acute flaccid paralysis. *Proc Natl Acad Sci USA* **104**:17140–17145.

54. **Lai H, Engle M, Fuchs A, Keller T, Johnson S, Gorlatov S, Diamond MS, Chen Q.** 2010. Monoclonal antibody produced in plants efficiently treats West Nile virus infection in mice. *Proc Natl Acad Sci USA* **107**:2419–2424.

55. **Beedham RJ, Turnbull PC, Williamson ED.** 2001. Passive transfer of protection against Bacillus anthracis infection in a murine model. *Vaccine* **19**:4409–4416.

56. **Henderson J, Bauly JM, Ashford DA, Oliver SC, Hawes CR, Lazarus CM, Venis MA, Napier RM.** 1997. Retention of maize auxin-binding protein in the endoplasmic reticulum: quantifying escape and the role of auxin. *Planta* **202**:313–323.

57. **Little SF, Leppla SH, Cora E.** 1988. Production and characterization of monoclonal antibodies to the protective antigen component of *Bacillus anthracis* toxin. *Infect Immun* **56**:1807–1813.

58. **Pitt ML, Little SF, Ivins BE, Fellows P, Barth J, Hewetson J.** 2001. In vitro correlate of immunity in a rabbit model of inhalational anthrax. *Vaccine* **19**:4768–4773.

59. **Beebe LE, Zhong J, Clagett M, Babin M, Ou Y, Roschke V.** 2003. Protection against inhalation anthrax induced lethality by a human monoclonal antibody to protective antigen in rabbits and cynomolgus monkeys, abstr. 3836. *Progr Abstr 43rd Intersci Conf Antimicrob Agents Chemother*, Chicago, IL.

60. **Beebe LE, Babin M, Barnewall R, Zhong J, Choi G.** 2004. Post-exposure therapeutic potential of PAMAb in an inhalation model of anthrax in New Zealand White rabbits (NZW), abstr. 167G. *Abstr 2004 Am Soc Microbiol Biodefense Res Meet*, Baltimore, MD.

61. **Mabry R, Rani M, Geiger R, Hubbard GB, Carrion R Jr, Brasky K, Patterson JL, Georgiou G, Iverson BL.** 2005. Passive protection against anthrax by using a high-affinity antitoxin antibody fragment lacking an Fc region. *Infect Immun* **73**:8362–8368.

62. **Mohamed N, Clagett M, Li J, Jones S, Pincus S, D'Alia G, Nardone L, Babin M, Spitalny G, Casey L.** 2005. A high-affinity monoclonal antibody to anthrax protective antigen passively protects rabbits before and after aerosolized *Bacillus anthracis* spore challenge. *Infect Immun* **73**:795–802.

63. **Peterson JW, Comer JE, Noffsinger DM, Wenglikowski A, Walberg KG, Chatuev BM.** 2006. Human monoclonal anti-protective antigen antibody completely protects rabbits and is synergistic with ciprofloxacin in protecting mice and guinea pigs against inhalation anthrax. *Infect Immun* **74**:1016–1024.

64. **Peterson JW, Comer JE, Baze WB, Noffsinger DM, Wenglikowski A, Walberg KG.** 2007. Human monoclonal antibody AVP-21D9 to protective antigen reduces dissemination of the *Bacillus anthracis* Ames strain from the lungs in a rabbit model. *Infect Immun* **75**:3414–3424.

65. **Sawada-Hirai R, Jiang I, Wang F, Sun SM, Nedellec R, Ruther P.** 2004. Human anti-anthrax protective antigen neutralizing monoclonal antibodies derived from donors vaccinated with anthrax vaccine adsorbed. *J Immune Based Ther Vaccines* **2**:5.

66. **Vitale L, Blanset D, Lowy I, O'Neill T, Goldstein J, Little SF.** 2006. Prophylaxis and therapy of inhalational anthrax by a novel monoclonal antibody to protective antigen that mimics vaccine-induced immunity. *Infect Immun* **74**:5840–5847.

67. **Wild MA, Kumor K, Nolan MJ, Lockman H, Bowdish KS.** 2007. A human antibody against anthrax protective antigen protects rabbits from lethal infection with aerosolized spores. *Hum Antibodies* **16**:99–105.

68. **Mett V, Chichester JA, Stewart ML, Musiychuk K, Bi H, Reifsnyder CJ, Hull AK, Albrecht MT, Goldman S, Baillie LW, Yusibov V.** 2011. A nonglycosylated, plant-produced human monoclonal antibody against anthrax protective antigen

protects mice and non-human primates from B. anthracis spore challenge. *Hum Vaccin* **7**(Suppl): 183–190.

69. **Wycoff KL, Belle A, Deppe D, Schaefer L, Maclean JM, Haase S, Trilling AK, Liu S, Leppla SH, Geren IN, Pawlik J, Peterson JW.** 2011. Recombinant anthrax toxin receptor-Fc fusion proteins produced in plants protect rabbits against inhalational anthrax. *Antimicrob Agents Chemother* **55**:132–139.

70. **Bowmann E.** 1998. *Iraqi Chemical and Biological Weapons Capabilities*, p 1–5. Congressional Research Service, Washington, DC.

71. **Cordesman RA.** 1998. *UNSCOM Main Achievements*, p 67–71. United Nations Special Commission (UNSCOM), New York, NY.

72. **Gill DM.** 1982. Bacterial toxins: a table of lethal amounts. *Microbiol Rev* **46**:86–94.

73. **Hauer PJ, Clough NE.** 1999. Development of monoclonal antibodies suitable for use in antigen quantification potency tests for clostridial veterinary vaccines. *Dev Biol Stand* **101**:85–94.

74. **Burnett JC, Henchal EA, Schmaljohn AL, Bavari S.** 2005. The evolving field of biodefence: therapeutic developments and diagnostics. *Nat Rev Drug Discov* **4**:281–297.

75. **Schlievert PM.** 1993. Role of superantigens in human disease. *J Infect Dis* **167**:997–1002.

76. **Schlievert PM.** 1986. Staphylococcal enterotoxin B and toxic-shock syndrome toxin-1 are significantly associated with non-menstrual TSS. *Lancet* **i**:1149–1150.

77. **Karauzum H, Chen G, Abaandou L, Mahmoudieh M, Boroun AR, Shulenin S, Devi VS, Stavale E, Warfield KL, Zeitlin L, Roy CJ, Sidhu SS, Aman MJ.** 2012. Synthetic human monoclonal antibodies toward staphylococcal enterotoxin B (SEB) protective against toxic shock syndrome. *J Biol Chem* **287**:25203–25215.

78. **Valdés R, Reyes B, Alvarez T, García J, Montero JA, Figueroa A, Gómez L, Padilla S, Geada D, Abrahantes MC, Dorta L, Fernández D, Mendoza O, Ramirez N, Rodriguez M, Pujol M, Borroto C, Brito J.** 2003. Hepatitis B surface antigen immunopurification using a plant-derived specific antibody produced in large scale. *Biochem Biophys Res Commun* **310**:742–747.

79. **Blank GS, Zapata G, Fahrner R, Milton M, Yedinak C, Knudsen H, Schmelzer C.** 2001. Expanded bed adsorption in the purification of monoclonal antibodies: a comparison of process alternatives. *Bioseparation* **10**:65–71.

80. **Zeitlin L, Bohorov O, Bohorova N, Hiatt A, Kim Do H, Pauly MH, Velasco J, Whaley KJ, Barnard DL, Bates JT, Crowe JE Jr, Piedra PA, Gilbert BE.** 2013. Prophylactic and therapeutic testing of *Nicotiana*-derived RSV-neutralizing human monoclonal antibodies in the cotton rat model. *mAbs* **5**(2):263–269. doi:10.4161/mabs. 23281. Epub Feb 8 2013.

Vector-Mediated *In Vivo* Antibody Expression

25

BRUCE C. SCHNEPP[1] and PHILIP R. JOHNSON[1]

INTRODUCTION

The holy grail of human immunodeficiency virus (HIV) vaccine development is an immunogen that elicits antibodies that neutralize field strains of the virus. In recent years, we have gained tremendous insights into the structure and function of the HIV envelope glycoprotein, but limited progress has been made in designing such immunogens. These sobering observations underscore the tremendous hurdles that must be overcome to develop an effective HIV vaccine (1, 2, 3, 4, 5). Foremost among these hurdles is the inability to induce antibodies that neutralize a wide array of HIV field isolates. Such antibodies are rare, and, until recently, only a handful of these antibodies had been isolated (6, 7, 8, 9). Over the past few years, a much larger number of HIV antibodies have been identified that have a much broader range of neutralization and are orders of magnitude more potent than the previously identified group (10, 11, 12, 13). These antibodies were isolated from the high-throughput screening of sera from HIV-1-infected individuals and categorized as "elite neutralizers" based on their neutralization breadth and potency (14). Extensive sequence analysis of these potent, broadly neutralizing antibodies revealed that high levels of somatic mutations were involved to generate the mature antibody (11). Furthermore, the maturation may have involved repeated rounds of antibody selection through HIV antigen interaction, a process that may

[1]The Children's Hospital of Philadelphia, Abramson Research Center, Philadelphia, PA 19104.
Antibodies for Infectious Diseases
Edited by James E. Crowe, Jr., Diana Boraschi, and Rino Rappuoli
© 2015 American Society for Microbiology, Washington, DC
doi:10.1128/microbiolspec.AID-0016-2014

not be possible to duplicate from a traditional HIV protein subunit or viral vector vaccine.

Given the obstacles required to generate this class of broadly neutralizing antibodies by current vaccine strategies, one option is to deliver these antibodies by passive immunization. Passive immunization schemes using neutralizing antibodies have protected monkeys from simian-human immunodeficiency virus (SHIV) challenge infections (15, 16, 17, 18, 19, 20). Unfortunately, an injection of antibodies every few weeks is neither practical nor cost-effective as a large-scale human vaccine approach. The vector-mediated gene transfer vaccine strategy eliminates the problems with passive antibody transfer and uses a viral vector to deliver the potent, broadly neutralizing antibodies directly to muscle by *gene* transfer. In this scheme, the antibody gene of choice is packaged into an adeno-associated virus (AAV) vector, which is then delivered by direct intramuscular injection. Thereafter, antibody molecules are endogenously synthesized in myofibers and passively distributed to the circulatory system (21). In a proof-of-concept experiment in a large animal model, rhesus monkeys were injected with AAV vectors expressing monkey antibodies able to neutralize simian immunodeficiency virus (SIV) (22). The neutralizing antibodies were detected in the serum for over 6 years following a single intramuscular injection. Furthermore, monkeys were protected from infection and the development of AIDS following challenge with virulent SIV.

The concept of immunoprophylaxis by gene transfer is significant in that it can rapidly move existing and newly discovered molecules that block HIV infection into the clinic. In fact, the development of molecules that inhibit all steps in HIV entry could create a multilayered blockade against HIV infection and provide a shortcut to an HIV vaccine. These molecules could be directed at any or all points of HIV entry including (i) gp120 binding to CD4, (ii) gp120 binding to CCR5, and (iii) membrane fusion. This concept need not be limited to HIV. In fact, the general strategy of "immunoprophylaxis by antibody gene transfer" can be applied to other difficult vaccine targets like hepatitis C virus, malaria, respiratory syncytial virus, and tuberculosis.

IMPORTANCE OF HIV-NEUTRALIZING ANTIBODIES

The need for a vaccine is still great, with approximately 35 million people currently infected with HIV, and more than 2 million new adult infections every year. Two earlier vaccine approaches, each targeting a different arm of the immune response, were evaluated in large efficacy trials. Both approaches failed to protect vaccine recipients from infection, and neither diminished viral replication after infection (23, 24, 25, 26). The more recent RV144 trial in Thailand using a canarypox virus expressing HIV proteins in conjunction with a gp120 subunit showed moderate efficacy (31%), indicating that protection may be achievable with the right immunogen (27). Detailed analyses of the RV144 study results revealed two significant correlations with infection among vaccine recipients. The presence of IgG antibodies against V1V2 Env may have contributed to protection against HIV-1 infection, whereas high levels of Env-specific IgA antibodies correlated inversely with infection (28). Very recently, the HVTN 505 trial was stopped for futility. The HVTN 505 trial showed no difference in HIV-1 infections between those recipients who received the vaccine and those receiving placebo (29). Vaccine recipients did generate IgG antibodies to Env; however, the majority were nonneutralizing with low reactivity to the V1V2 antigen (29).

The observations from these clinical trials, that neutralizing antibodies may be essential for an effective vaccine, is reinforced by the large number of new, highly potent broadly neutralizing antibodies (bNAbs) that have been identified by using improved screening and sequencing techniques. These new antibodies were isolated by high-throughput screening of sera from healthy HIV-1-infected individuals categorized as "elite neutralizers" based on their neutralization breadth and potency (10, 11, 12, 13, 14, 30, 31, 32, 33). Detailed analyses of these antibodies indicated they are approximately 10- to 100-fold more potent and have an increased breadth compared with the original 4 isolates (6, 7, 8, 9). Furthermore, this new class of antibodies can neutralize HIV-1 through binding to a variety of envelope domains including the CD4 binding site (VRC01, NIH45-46, and PGV04) (13, 31, 34), glycan-containing regions in the variable loops (PG9, PG16, PGT121, and PGT128)(11, 12), and the membrane-proximal external region (MPER) on gp41 (10E8) (30).

Epitope mapping of these new, potent antibodies has invigorated the vaccine field by providing precise regions to target when designing new protein or subunit vaccine antigens to induce bNAbs (35). However, even with this new wealth of information at hand, generating bNAbs with improved, redesigned antigens may still prove to be problematic. Extensive sequence analysis of these potent broadly neutralizing antibodies reveal that high levels of somatic mutations (as much as 30%) can occur in the generation of the mature antibody (11, 13, 31, 33, 36). Furthermore, the maturation may have involved repeated rounds of antibody selection through HIV antigen interaction. In light of this, several groups have developed novel immunogens, such as glycopeptides or computation-derived multimerized nanoparticles, that are designed to induce bNAbs (37, 38). These immunogens can bind to both mature bNAbs as well as the receptors of their germline (naïve) B cells, which can trigger the activation and maturation process required to produce a bNAb.

Passive immunization using neutralizing monoclonal antibodies has protected monkeys from SHIV challenge infections (15, 16, 17, 18, 19, 20, 39). In a recent study by Moldt et al. (39), they showed that passively administered PGT121 can mediate sterilizing immunity against SHIV in monkeys at serum concentrations that were significantly lower than those observed in previous studies (as low as 1.8 μg/ml). While this study demonstrated the potential for passive immunization with the new class of bNAbs, unfortunately, an injection of antibodies every few weeks is not practical or cost-effective as a large-scale human prophylactic vaccine approach. Given these difficulties, we developed a second option: isolate the representative antibody gene and use gene transfer technology to endow a target host with the gene. In this way, the antibody gene directs endogenous expression of the antibody molecule, and the host (in theory) will now have the antibody in its circulation. Thus, after a single injection, the muscle now serves as a depot to synthesize the bNAbs that are passively distributed to the circulatory system (Fig. 1). The host is now armed with a potent bNAb against HIV-1 that effectively bypasses the adaptive immune system. This is in contrast to the traditional idea of passive immunization whereby the purified antibodies are injected intravenously into the host to provide protection from infection. However, because of the antibody half-life, the levels decline, requiring repeated injections. The obvious advantage is that antibody gene transfer engenders the host with long-term antibody persistence from a single injection due to endogenous antibody expression.

HIV-NEUTRALIZING ANTIBODIES AS A VACCINE

While induction of bNAbs by various next-generation immunization strategies holds promise, the question remains as to the best use of the human monoclonal antibodies that have already been isolated and characterized. One obvious option is passive immunization.

VECTOR EXPRESSION SYSTEMS FOR ANTIBODY GENE TRANSFER

Our chosen vector to deliver the antibody gene is the recombinant adeno-associated virus (rAAV) vector, which is derived from wild-type AAV. AAV is a *Dependovirus* with a 4.7-kb single-strand DNA genome that contains only two genes (*rep* and *cap*) flanked by inverted

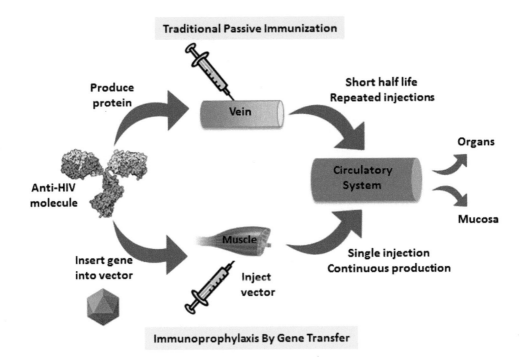

FIGURE 1 **Immunoprophylaxis by antibody gene transfer. Passive immunization involves intravenous delivery of purified antibodies to engender the host with short-lived immunity in serum and mucosa. In contrast, vector-mediated antibody gene transfer uses a viral vector to deliver the antibody *gene* to the host via intramuscular injection. The antibody is produced endogenously in the muscle and secreted into the circulatory system and mucosa providing long-term protection from infection. (Reprinted from reference 72 [Schnepp BC, Johnson PR. 2014. Adeno-associated virus delivery of broadly neutralizing antibodies. *Curr Opin HIV AIDS* 9:205–256] with permission.) doi:10.1128/microbiolspec.AID-0016-2014.f1**

terminal repeats (ITRs). AAV natural infection is common and has not been associated with any disease. Multiple AAV serotypes have been identified with different transduction efficiencies in different tissues, offering flexibility for gene transfer targets such as muscle or liver (40). rAAV vectors have an established record of high-efficiency gene transfer in a variety of model systems (41, 42). Following injection, the rAAV vector genome can form stable nonintegrating circular episomes that can persist in nondividing cells (43, 44, 45). Because of these features, rAAV vectors have become popular gene delivery vehicles for use in clinical studies for the treatment of diseases such as alpha1-antitrypsin deficiency, cystic fibrosis, hemophilia B, Leber's congenital amaurosis, lipoprotein lipase (LPL) deficiency, Parkinson's disease, and muscular dystrophy (46).

rAAV gene transfer vectors are devoid of the endogenous *rep* and *cap* genes, and consist of the antibody gene expression cassette flanked by the AAV ITRs (Fig. 2). The ITRs (145 bp each), which are necessary for rAAV vector genome replication and packaging, are the only part of the AAV genome present in the rAAV vectors. One method for antibody expression utilizes a two-promoter system whereby the heavy- and light-chain genes are transcribed independently by using two different promoters and polyadenylation signals within the same rAAV vector genome (Fig. 2) (47). Another method uses a single promoter for expression of both the heavy and light chains, which are separated by the foot-and-mouth-disease virus (FMDV) 2A peptide, which undergoes self-cleavage to produce separate heavy- and light-chain proteins

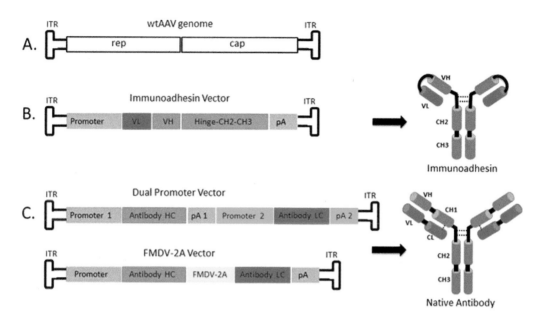

FIGURE 2 rAAV vectors for antibody gene transfer. (A) The wild-type AAV (wtAAV) genome consists of the *rep* and *cap* genes flanked by inverted terminal repeats (ITRs). For rAAV vectors, the *rep* and *cap* genes are removed and replaced by an antibody expression cassette flanked by ITRs, which are necessary for rAAV vector genome replication and packaging. (B) Immunoadhesins contain the antibody variable domains (VL, variable light; VH, variable heavy) usually joined by a flexible protein linker. The variable domains are connected to the hinge and constant heavy-chain domains (CH2 and CH3). The immunoadhesins can form dimers through disulfide bonding in the hinge region. (C) Full antibodies can be expressed by using either a dual promoter or single-promoter system. For dual promoter expression, the antibody heavy and light chains are each expressed separately from their own promoter. For the single promoter system, the heavy and light chains are expressed as a single polypeptide separated by the foot-and-mouth-disease virus 2A peptide (FMDV-2A). The FMDV-2A peptide can undergo self-cleavage to give rise to separate heavy and light chains. doi:10.1128/microbiolspec.AID-0016-2014.f2

(Fig. 2) (48). The advantage of this system is that the heavy and light chains can potentially be expressed in a 1:1 ratio using a single promoter, which may translate to more efficient expression. However, a potential disadvantage is that the FMDV-2A peptide is derived from a viral sequence and may be immunogenic in the host causing immune clearance of cells expressing the antibody.

Another option is to create an immunoadhesin version of the neutralizing antibody. Immunoadhesins are chimeric, antibody-like molecules that combine the functional domain of a binding protein like a scFv or CD4 extracellular domains 1 and 2 (D1D2) with an immunoglobulin constant domain (49) (Fig. 2), and have been shown to be effective in disease models including HIV, SIV, and influenza (22, 50, 51). A typical immunoadhesin lacks the

constant light-chain domain and the constant heavy-chain domain 1 (CH1); however, it can be expressed as a single polypeptide from a single promoter, and forms dimers through disulfide bonding in the hinge region. While immunoadhesins have many attractive features such as efficient expression/secretion *in vivo*, they also have some drawbacks. Immunoadhesins may not exhibit the same neutralization breadth and potency as the native antibody. While we have seen cases where a specific immunoadhesin functions identically to its native antibody counterpart, we have also seen an immunoadhesin become 10-fold less potent at neutralizing HIV-1 (unpublished observation). Thus, immunoadhesins must be fully characterized and compared with the native antibody from which they were derived before consideration as a vaccine. Another drawback to using immunoadhesins is possible immunogenicity. Immunoadhesins are not naturally occurring proteins and may contain amino acid linkers connecting the variable domains (Fig. 2), which could trigger an immune response leading to the loss of expression. However, it should be noted that Enbrel (etanercept), an immunoadhesin consisting of the tumor necrosis factor receptor fused to IgG1-Fc, was well tolerated in patients for long-term treatment (10 years) of rheumatoid arthritis (52).

PROOF-OF-CONCEPT STUDIES IN ANIMAL MODELS

We first developed the concept of using antibody gene transfer in 2002 (47). Because of the significant obstacles that confronted both active and passive immunization strategies, we began to explore an alternate strategy to generate serum antibodies that neutralize primary isolates of HIV-1. At that time, only a few monoclonal antibodies existed (6, 7, 8, 9). We chose to express IgG1b12 to test the feasibility of antibody gene transfer using rAAV vectors. To generate the IgG1b12 expression construct, the IgG1b12 heavy and light chains were expressed independently in the same rAAV vector using the dual-promoter system. The resulting vector was injected into the quadriceps muscles of immunodeficient mice (to avoid immune responses to human IgG). IgG1b12 was expressed in mouse muscle (confirmed by histochemical staining), and biologically active antibody was found in sera for over 6 months (47). Characteristic biologic activity was determined by HIV neutralization assays against IgG1b12 sensitive/resistant viruses. This study provided the first evidence that: (i) rAAV vectors transferred antibody genes to muscle; (ii) myofibers produced antibodies; (iii) antibodies were distributed to the circulation; and (iv) such antibodies were biologically active.

While these initial findings supported the hypothesis that antibody gene transfer to the muscle can produce systemic levels of HIV-neutralizing activity without the need for an active humoral response, it was difficult to determine if this activity would translate to protection from a challenge infection. Therefore, our next goal was to test our hypothesis in a macaque challenge model, but we were faced with the problem that the human antibody IgGb12 was viewed as foreign in a macaque, triggering an immune response that lead to the elimination of IgG1b12 expression. We then turned to using rhesus-derived antibodies by taking advantage of native macaque SIV gp120-specific Fab molecular clones that had been derived directly from SIV-infected macaques (53). When designing the antibody gene transfer vectors, we chose to express the Fabs as immunoadhesins, which in pilot experiments in mice were superior to single-chain (scFv) or whole-antibody (IgG) molecules with respect to steady-state serum concentrations (unpublished data).

For the macaque experiments, we constructed immunoadhesins derived from two different SIV Fab fragments (4L6 and 5L7), as well as a third immunoadhesin containing the rhesus CD4 D1D2, which was modeled after CD4-Ig fusion proteins (54). All of the constructs neutralized *in vitro* the proposed SIV challenge stock (SIVmac316), indicating that the immunoadhesins were functioning like the original Fab clones (22). The 3 immunoadhesins were injected into 3 monkeys each (for 9 total), followed by an intravenous SIV challenge 4 weeks later, including 6 naïve controls. Immunoadhesin expression levels were as high as 190 μg/ml at the time of challenge (4 weeks postinjection) and peaked around 6 months with levels reaching 400 μg/ml in some animals (22). Overall, 6 of the 9 monkeys receiving the immunoadhesins were completely protected after challenge, while all 6 naïve controls became infected. Analysis of the 3 monkeys from the immunoadhesin group that became infected revealed that these specific animals had developed an immune response to the immunoadhesin by 3 weeks postinjection, suggesting a correlation between an immune response to the immunoadhesin and failure to protect from infection. We have performed longitudinal studies of the protected monkeys, which are now over 6 years postinjection. Immunoadhesin levels dropped to a stable level of approximately 20 μg/ml, which has persisted for over the past 4 years. The monkeys have remained negative for SIV infection and have not developed an immune response to the immunoadhesins (unpublished observation). Thus, this crucial study was instrumental in proving the concept of vector-mediated gene transfer as a viable HIV vaccine.

More recently, other investigators performed rAAV vector-mediated gene transfer expression/challenge studies, which they called vectored immunoprophylaxis (VIP) (55). They expressed the native, full antibodies of 2G12, IgG1b12, 2F5, 4E10, and VRC01 using the single-promoter FMDV-2A system. Following intramuscular rAAV injection in mice, antibody expression levels greater than 100 μg/ml were observed for at least 12 months. Using a humanized mouse model, they further showed that these rAAV vectors provided protection following HIV challenge, with antibody serum levels as low as 8.3 μg/ml (antibody VRC01). These encouraging results reinforce the efficacy of the antibody gene transfer approach, especially when potent antibodies such as VRC01 are used. Taken together, these murine and primate studies show that vector-mediated antibody gene transfer can bypass the adaptive immune response and engender the host with antibodies that provide protection from infection. Furthermore, antibody expression can persist several years following a single injection, suggesting that long-term protection is possible.

ANTIBODY GENE TRANSFER FOR HIV-POSITIVE INDIVIDUALS

While antibody gene transfer shows great promise for providing protection from HIV infection, one obvious question is whether this strategy can also be used for antibody therapy in HIV-positive individuals. To answer the question, HIV-infected humanized mice received an intravenous injection of a rAAV (serotype 8)

vector expressing bNAb 10-1074 (56), which targets the base of the V3 stem of gp120 (57). These mice maintained a high level of antibody 10-1074 expression of around 200 μg/ml for the entire length of the 67-day observation period. During this time, 6 of the 7 mice in the group were able to control HIV plasma viral loads, whereas 1 mouse exhibited viral escape. As seen with escape mutants from passive immunization studies (56, 58), sequence analysis of the gp120 of these escape viruses revealed mutations in the 10-1074 binding site that conferred resistance to the antibody. It remains to be seen if simultaneously administering rAAV vectors expressing multiple bNAbs could dramatically reduce or even possibly eliminate the generation of escape mutants. Furthermore, long-term studies will be required to see if escape mutants could arise over time, even in the presence of multiple antibodies. These results in humanized mice suggest that using vector-mediated gene transfer to deliver bNAbs to HIV-infected individuals could be a viable option, possibly even used in conjunction with standard antiretroviral therapy (ART). An overriding theme is that multiple bNAbs would be required to provide the selective pressure to avoid viral escape mutants. Multiple antibodies could target different gp120 domains such as the exterior loops, CD4 binding site, and MPER. Furthermore, multiple antibodies could be used that target different stages of viral entry including CD4 binding, CCR5 binding, and membrane fusion. Of course, this strategy of the simultaneous use of multiple antibodies against multiple viral targets or stages of entry could also be applicable in a prophylactic vaccine approach for maximum efficacy.

ANTIBODY GENE TRANSFER FOR RESPIRATORY TRACT INFECTIONS

The use of vector-mediated antibody gene transfer has not been limited to just HIV (Table 1). Respiratory syncytial virus (RSV) is a major cause of severe respiratory infection in high-risk populations (such as infants) for

TABLE 1 Vector-mediated antibody gene transfer studies

Application	Antibody	Reference
HIV vaccine	SIV immunoadhesins, 4E10, 2G12, 2F5, b12, VRC01, PG9[a]	Lewis 2002 (47), Johnson 2009 (22), Balazs 2012 (55)
HIV therapy	10-1074	Horwitz 2013 (56)
RSV vaccine	Palivizumab	Skaricic 2008 (59)
Influenza vaccine	FI6, F10, CR6261	Limberis 2013 (61), Balazs 2013 (62)
Drug addiction	NIC9D9, GNC92H2	Hicks 2012 (65), Rosenberg 2012 (66)
Cancer therapy	DC101	Fang 2005 (48)

[a]The first clinical trial using rAAV vector-mediated PG9 antibody gene transfer began in 2014 as a result of collaboration between The Children's Hospital of Philadelphia, The International AIDS Vaccine Initiative, and the Division of AIDS (DAIDS) in the National Institute of Allergy and Infectious Diseases.

which a vaccine is not yet available. Currently, the only way to prevent infection is through the passive administration of anti-RSV antibodies, such as palivizumab (also known as Synagis, manufactured by MedImmune). This antibody can be administered intramuscularly once each month during the RSV season (winter and spring) to prevent RSV infection. While this treatment is effective, it is costly and limited to high-risk individuals, which are attributes that make it a prime candidate for antibody gene transfer. Instead of repeated monthly injections of the purified antibody, the antibody could be endogenously expressed from a single injection using antibody gene transfer and provide a constant level of protective anti-RSV antibodies in the host.

The study used different vector systems to deliver antibodies against RSV infection (59). They compared the expression and efficacy of a mouse version of palivizumab in a mouse model system when delivered by either a rAAV vector (serotype rh.10) or adenovirus (Ad) vector. Adenovirus vectors have the capacity for high-level gene transfer with rapid and robust transgene expression. However, Ad vectors are highly immunogenic, and transduced cells

are quickly cleared by the immune system, resulting in the rapid loss of transgene expression. In contrast, rAAV vectors have very low immunogenicity and can give rise to long-term gene (antibody) expression for potentially the life of the individual. The Ad-palivizumab vector was administered intravenously, with palivizumab detected in the lungs by day 3 postadministration. Following an intranasal RSV challenge 7 days postadministration, the mice showed >5-fold decrease in RSV titers in the lung compared with control animals. Long-term antibody expression and challenge studies were done using the rAAVrh.10-palivizumab vector via intrapleural administration. Palivizumab was detected in the serum of these animals by 8 weeks postadministration that started to peak by week 20. These rAAVrh.10-palivizumab mice were intranasally challenged with RSV at 7 and 21 weeks' postadministration. They showed 14.3-fold and 10.6-fold lower numbers of RSV PFU in the lungs, indicating that protection against RSV infection can be sustained at least 21 weeks postdelivery of an rAAV vector.

Antibody gene transfer studies using rAAV vectors have also been done to prevent influenza. Although traditional vaccination strategies for influenza are quite effective, they may not be adequate for a possible zoonotic strain that could lead to a pandemic (such as the 2009 H1N1). In this case, the time needed to develop a traditional vaccine may not be rapid enough. The rationale is that vector-mediated antibody gene transfer could quickly deliver a bNAb that is effective against multiple strains of influenza that would provide protection against a pandemic. One study looked at delivering the bNAb antibody FI6 (60) as an immunoadhesin using rAAV serotype 9 via intranasal delivery in mice and ferrets (51). FI6 immunoadhesin expression was detected in the nasal and lung lavage fluids of mice 14 days after vector administration at concentrations ranging from 0.5 to 2.0 μg/ml. Animals challenged as early as 3 days after rAAV9-FI6 administration could be protected. Furthermore, this strategy was able to protect both mice and ferrets from the exposure of lethal doses of various clinical isolates of H5N1 and H1N1. An additional study (61) also demonstrated that rAAV9-FI6 administration showed partial efficacy in mice challenged with the newly emergent avian H7N9, which is believed to be transmitted from poultry to humans.

A separate study used a similar strategy but with intramuscular administration of the rAAV antibody vector in mice (62). They expressed antibodies F10 (63) and CR6261 (64) in an rAAV serotype 8 vector by using the FMDV-2A expression system. Antibody expression levels in the serum reached 200 µg/ml at 5 weeks after intramuscular injection, with levels still around 10 µg/ml out to at least 11 months after a single injection. These treated mice were protected from diverse strains of H1N1 influenza when challenged at either of these time points (5 weeks and 11 months), demonstrating once again the incredible potential for this strategy as a vaccine. The results from both the intranasal (51) and intramuscular (62) routes of vector administration reinforce the flexibility of vector-mediated gene transfer and provide important proof-of-concept studies that could lead to translation into humans.

ANTIBODY GENE TRANSFER FOR DRUG ADDICTION

Perhaps a less conventional use of vector-mediated antibody gene transfer is a potential role in the treatment of drug/substance addiction. Antibodies exist that can bind to these substances in the blood and prevent their transfer to the brain, which leads to their addictive properties. Antibody therapy for addiction would require routine, costly injections, which once again makes this a prime candidate for antibody gene transfer. NIC9D9 is an antinicotine antibody that was delivered intravenously (targeting the liver) to mice by using a rAAVrh.10 vector (65). NIC9D9 antibody was detected in the serum for the length of the 18-week study. Following intravenous nicotine delivery, the rAAV-NIC9D9 mice had

83% of the nicotine bound to the NIC9D9 antibody in serum, which drastically reduced the amount of serum delivered to the brain. Furthermore, these mice had reduced cardiovascular effects compared with control animals. These results indicate that this strategy may hold promise as an effective preventative therapy for nicotine addiction.

Along the same line, GNC92H2 is a mouse monoclonal antibody with high affinity for cocaine. This antibody was also delivered to mice by using the rAAVrh.10 vector via intravenous injection (66). GNC92H2 was detected in the serum for the entire duration of the 24-week study. The GNC92H2 antibody was able to sequester intravenously administered cocaine in the blood, thereby protecting the brain from the effects of cocaine. Furthermore, these mice showed suppressed cocaine-induced hyperactivity derived from weekly cocaine exposure (12 to 17 weeks after rAAVrh.10 vector administration). These findings offer an alternative intervention to cocaine addiction therapy. High-affinity cocaine antibodies could be maintained long term in the serum following a single administration. This strategy could be coupled with traditional behavioral therapies for a combined approach for the treatment of cocaine addiction.

ANTIBODY GENE TRANSFER FOR CANCER

The vector-mediated antibody gene transfer strategy can be expanded for use in noninfectious disease applications where antibodies still play a critical role, such as cancer treatment. In a study by Fang et al. (48), they examined the efficacy of an antitumor antibody to reduce tumor growth in a mouse model system. They used an rAAV8 vector that expressed antibody DC101 by the FMDV-2A system. Antibody DC101 is an antiangiogenic monoclonal antibody that targets vascular endothelial cell growth factor receptor-2 (VEGFR2). Mice given an intravenous injection of rAAV8-DC101 could express high levels (>1 mg/ml) of the antibody in the serum for the length of the 5-month monitoring period. Mice receiving this rAAV vector exhibited shrinkage of tumors and prolonged survival time compared with untreated control animals. These encouraging results set the stage for combining antibody gene transfer technology with the ever increasing number of antibody-based therapies for cancers that include such antibodies as Herceptin and Avastin (Genentech), to name a few.

DRAWBACKS OF rAAV ANTIBODY GENE TRANSFER

Essentially any therapeutic or immunoprophylactic protein can be expressed by using rAAV vector gene transfer, as long as it fits within the vector packaging limit. However, one must be careful that the expressed protein is not immunogenic in the host. However, this is also the same concern for all exogenously (passively) administered proteins, including monoclonal antibodies and other biologics. Most, if not all, of the 25 monoclonal antibodies that have been approved as therapeutics have exhibited some level of immunogenicity (67, 68). Several factors may contribute to immunogenicity including antibody structure, dosing regimen, and the recipient's genetic background. Also, it remains to be determined if an antibody that was endogenously expressed in the host via gene transfer will be more or less immunogenic than when passively administered as an exogenously produced protein. The big question is what effect would an immune response to the transgene have in the host? In the simplest scenario, as was seen in the nonhuman primate studies (22), the appearance of anti-antibody responses would limit the vaccine efficiency through loss of transgene expression, with no adverse events observed. Ultimately, at this stage, it is difficult to predict with any certainty which, if any, of the candidates would be immunogenic, and what the consequences would be. Human clinical trials will be the best predictor.

Perhaps of greater concern is the risk that the antibody will bind off-target causing an unanticipated adverse event. Preclinical testing, such as passive administration and Good Laboratory Practice (GLP) human tissue binding studies, can help avert most of these issues. However, if off-target effects occur *in vivo*, there is currently no efficient method to stop antibody gene expression. As the data shows from animal models, antibodies are expressed for potentially the life of the host following a single intramuscular administration. A few studies have attempted to regulate gene expression from rAAV gene transfer vectors in mice and monkeys (69, 70, 71), but these schemes are transient and require continuous exogenous drug administration to maintain a constant level of gene expression. Clearly, identifying an efficient method to permanently eliminate antibody gene expression in the host is a top priority if rAAV vector-mediated antibody gene transfer is to become applicable for wide-scale use.

ACKNOWLEDGMENT

Conflicts of interest: We declare no conflicts.

CITATION

Schnepp BC, Johnson PR. 2014. Vector-mediated *in vivo* antibody expression. Microbiol Spectrum 2(4):AID-0016-2014.

REFERENCES

1. **Desrosiers R.** 2004. Prospects for an AIDS vaccine. *Nat Med* **10:**221–223.
2. **Fauci AS, Johnston MI, Dieffenbach CW, Burton DR, Hammer SM, Hoxie JA, Martin M, Overbaugh J, Watkins DI, Mahmoud A, Greene WC.** 2008. HIV vaccine research: the way forward. *Science* **321:**530–532.
3. **Morgan C, Marthas M, Miller C, Duerr A, Cheng-Mayer C, Desrosiers R, Flores J, Haigwood N, Hu SL, Johnson RP, Lifson J, Montefiori D, Moore J, Robert-Guroff M, Robinson H, Self S, Corey L.** 2008. The use of nonhuman primate models in HIV vaccine development. *PLoS Med* **5:**e173. doi:10.1371/journal.pmed.0050173.

4. **Walker B, Burton D.** 2008. Toward an AIDS vaccine. *Science* **320:**760–764.

5. **Watkins DI.** 2008. Basic HIV Vaccine development. *Top HIV Med* **16:**7–8.

6. **Burton DR, Pyati J, Koduri R, Sharp SJ, Thornton GB, Parren PW, Sawyer LS, Hendry RM, Dunlop N, Nara PL, et al.** 1994. Efficient neutralization of primary isolates of HIV-1 by a recombinant human monoclonal antibody. *Science* **266:**1024–1027.

7. **Muster T, Steindl F, Purtscher M, Trkola A, Klima A, Himmler G, Ruker F, Katinger H.** 1993. A conserved neutralizing epitope on gp41 of human immunodeficiency virus type 1. *J Virol* **67:**6642–6647.

8. **Trkola A, Purtscher M, Muster T, Ballaun C, Buchacher A, Sullivan N, Srinivasan K, Sodroski J, Moore JP, Katinger H.** 1996. Human monoclonal antibody 2G12 defines a distinctive neutralization epitope on the gp120 glycoprotein of human immunodeficiency virus type 1. *J Virol* **70:**1100–1108.

9. **Zwick MB, Labrijn AF, Wang M, Spenlehauer C, Saphire EO, Binley JM, Moore JP, Stiegler G, Katinger H, Burton DR, Parren PW.** 2001. Broadly neutralizing antibodies targeted to the membrane-proximal external region of human immunodeficiency virus type 1 glycoprotein gp41. *J Virol* **75:**10892–10905.

10. **Burton DR, Poignard P, Stanfield RL, Wilson IA.** 2012. Broadly neutralizing antibodies present new prospects to counter highly antigenically diverse viruses. *Science* **337:**183–186.

11. **Walker LM, Huber M, Doores KJ, Falkowska E, Pejchal R, Julien JP, Wang SK, Ramos A, Chan-Hui PY, Moyle M, Mitcham JL, Hammond PW, Olsen OA, Phung P, Fling S, Wong CH, Phogat S, Wrin T, Simek MD, Koff WC, Wilson IA, Burton DR, Poignard P.** 2011. Broad neutralization coverage of HIV by multiple highly potent antibodies. *Nature* **477:**466–470.

12. **Walker LM, Phogat SK, Chan-Hui PY, Wagner D, Phung P, Goss JL, Wrin T, Simek MD, Fling S, Mitcham JL, Lehrman JK, Priddy FH, Olsen OA, Frey SM, Hammond PW, Kaminsky S, Zamb T, Moyle M, Koff WC, Poignard P, Burton DR.** 2009. Broad and potent neutralizing antibodies from an African donor reveal a new HIV-1 vaccine target. *Science* **326:**285–289.

13. **Wu X, Yang ZY, Li Y, Hogerkorp CM, Schief WR, Seaman MS, Zhou T, Schmidt SD, Wu L, Xu L, Longo NS, McKee K, O'Dell S, Louder MK, Wycuff DL, Feng Y, Nason M, Doria-Rose N, Connors M, Kwong PD, Roederer M, Wyatt RT, Nabel GJ, Mascola JR.** 2010. Rational design of envelope identifies broadly neutralizing human monoclonal antibodies to HIV-1. *Science* **329:**856–861.

14. **Simek MD, Rida W, Priddy FH, Pung P, Carrow E, Laufer DS, Lehrman JK, Boaz M, Tarragona-Fiol T, Miiro G, Birungi J, Pozniak A, McPhee DA, Manigart O, Karita E, Inwoley A, Jaoko W, Dehovitz J, Bekker LG, Pitisuttithum P, Paris R, Walker LM, Poignard P, Wrin T, Fast PE, Burton DR, Koff WC.** 2009. Human immunodeficiency virus type 1 elite neutralizers: individuals with broad and potent neutralizing activity identified by using a high-throughput neutralization assay together with an analytical selection algorithm. *J Virol* **83:**7337–7348.

15. **Baba TW, Liska V, Hofmann-Lehmann R, Vlasak J, Xu W, Ayehunie S, Cavacini LA, Posner MR, Katinger H, Stiegler G, Bernacky BJ, Rizvi TA, Schmidt R, Hill LR, Keeling ME, Lu Y, Wright JE, Chou TC, Ruprecht RM.** 2000. Human neutralizing monoclonal antibodies of the IgG1 subtype protect against mucosal simian-human immunodeficiency virus infection. *Nat Med* **6:**200–206.

16. **Mascola JR, Stiegler G, VanCott TC, Katinger H, Carpenter CB, Hanson CE, Beary H, Hayes D, Frankel SS, Birx DL, Lewis MG.** 2000. Protection of macaques against vaginal transmission of a pathogenic HIV-1/SIV chimeric virus by passive infusion of neutralizing antibodies. *Nat Med* **6:**207–210.

17. **Parren PW, Marx PA, Hessell AJ, Luckay A, Harouse J, Cheng-Mayer C, Moore J, Burton DR.** 2001. Antibody protects macaques against vaginal challenge with a pathogenic R5 simian/human immunodeficiency virus at serum levels giving complete neutralization in vitro. *J Virol* **75:**8340–8347.

18. **Hessell AJ, Poignard P, Hunter M, Hangartner L, Tehrani DM, Bleeker WK, Parren PW, Marx PA, Burton DR.** 2009. Effective, low-titer antibody protection against low-dose repeated mucosal SHIV challenge in macaques. *Nat Med* **15:**951–954.

19. **Hessell AJ, Rakasz EG, Poignard P, Hangartner L, Landucci G, Forthal DN, Koff WC, Watkins DI, Burton DR.** 2009. Broadly neutralizing human anti-HIV antibody 2G12 is effective in protection against mucosal SHIV challenge even at low serum neutralizing titers. *PLoS Pathog* **5:**e1000433. doi:10.1371/journal.ppat.1000433.

20. **Willey R, Nason MC, Nishimura Y, Follmann DA, Martin MA.** 2010. Neutralizing antibody titers conferring protection to macaques from a simian/human immunodeficiency virus challenge using the TZM-bl assay. *AIDS Res Hum Retroviruses* **26:**89–98.

21. **Berkhout B, Sanders RW.** 2012. Gene therapy as a vaccine for HIV-1. *Expert Opin Biol Ther* **12:**1315–1321.

22. **Johnson PR, Schnepp BC, Zhang J, Connell MJ, Greene SM, Yuste E, Desrosiers RC, Clark KR.** 2009. Vector-mediated gene transfer engenders long-lived neutralizing activity and protection against SIV infection in monkeys. *Nat Med* **15:** 901–906.

23. **Buchbinder SP, Mehrotra DV, Duerr A, Fitzgerald DW, Mogg R, Li D, Gilbert PB, Lama JR, Marmor M, Del Rio C, McElrath MJ, Casimiro DR, Gottesdiener KM, Chodakewitz JA, Corey L, Robertson MN.** 2008. Efficacy assessment of a cell-mediated immunity HIV-1 vaccine (the Step Study): a double-blind, randomised, placebo-controlled, test-of-concept trial. *Lancet* **372:**1881–1893.

24. **Flynn NM, Forthal DN, Harro CD, Judson FN, Mayer KH, Para MF.** 2005. Placebo-controlled phase 3 trial of a recombinant glycoprotein 120 vaccine to prevent HIV-1 infection. *J Infect Dis* **191:**654–665.

25. **McElrath MJ, De Rosa SC, Moodie Z, Dubey S, Kierstead L, Janes H, Defawe OD, Carter DK, Hural J, Akondy R, Buchbinder SP, Robertson MN, Mehrotra DV, Self SG, Corey L, Shiver JW, Casimiro DR.** 2008. HIV-1 vaccine-induced immunity in the test-of-concept Step Study: a case-cohort analysis. *Lancet* **372:**1894–1905.

26. **Pitisuttithum P, Gilbert P, Gurwith M, Heyward W, Martin M, van Griensven F, Hu D, Tappero JW, Choopanya K.** 2006. Randomized, double-blind, placebo-controlled efficacy trial of a bivalent recombinant glycoprotein 120 HIV-1 vaccine among injection drug users in Bangkok, Thailand. *J Infect Dis* **194:**1661–1671.

27. **Rerks-Ngarm S, Pitisuttithum P, Nitayaphan S, Kaewkungwal J, Chiu J, Paris R, Premsri N, Namwat C, de Souza M, Adams E, Benenson M, Gurunathan S, Tartaglia J, McNeil JG, Francis DP, Stablein D, Birx DL, Chunsuttiwat S, Khamboonruang C, Thongcharoen P, Robb ML, Michael NL, Kunasol P, Kim JH.** 2009. Vaccination with ALVAC and AIDSVAX to prevent HIV-1 infection in Thailand. *N Engl J Med* **361:**2209–2220.

28. **Haynes BF, Gilbert PB, McElrath MJ, Zolla-Pazner S, Tomaras GD, Alam SM, Evans DT, Montefiori DC, Karnasuta C, Sutthent R, Liao HX, DeVico AL, Lewis GK, Williams C, Pinter A, Fong Y, Janes H, DeCamp A, Huang Y, Rao M, Billings E, Karasavvas N, Robb ML, Nauy V, de Souza MS, Paris R, Ferrari G, Bailer RT, Soderberg KA, Andrews C, Berman PW, Frahm N, De Rosa SC, Alpert MD, Yates NL, Shen X, Koup RA, Pitisuttithum P, Kaewkungwal J, Nitayaphan S, Rerks-Ngarm S, Michael NL, Kim JH.** 2012. Immune-correlates analysis of an HIV-1 vaccine efficacy trial. *N Engl J Med* **366:** 1275–1286.

29. **Hammer SM, Sobieszczyk ME, Janes H, Karuna ST, Mulligan MJ, Grove D, Koblin BA, Buchbinder SP, Keefer MC, Tomaras GD, Frahm N, Hural J, Anude C, Graham BS, Enama ME, Adams E, DeJesus E, Novak RM, Frank I, Bentley C, Ramirez S, Fu R, Koup RA, Mascola JR, Nabel GJ, Montefiori DC, Kublin J, McElrath MJ, Corey L, Gilbert PB.** 2013. Efficacy trial of a DNA/rAd5 HIV-1 preventive vaccine. *N Engl J Med* **369:**2083–2092.

30. **Huang J, Ofek G, Laub L, Louder MK, Doria-Rose NA, Longo NS, Imamichi H, Bailer RT, Chakrabarti B, Sharma SK, Alam SM, Wang T, Yang Y, Zhang B, Migueles SA, Wyatt R, Haynes BF, Kwong PD, Mascola JR, Connors M.** 2012. Broad and potent neutralization of HIV-1 by a gp41-specific human antibody. *Nature* **491:** 406–412.

31. **Scheid JF, Mouquet H, Ueberheide B, Diskin R, Klein F, Oliveira TY, Pietzsch J, Fenyo D, Abadir A, Velinzon K, Hurley A, Myung S, Boulad F, Poignard P, Burton DR, Pereyra F, Ho DD, Walker BD, Seaman MS, Bjorkman PJ, Chait BT, Nussenzweig MC.** 2011. Sequence and structural convergence of broad and potent HIV antibodies that mimic CD4 binding. *Science* **333:**1633–1637.

32. **Zhou T, Georgiev I, Wu X, Yang ZY, Dai K, Finzi A, Kwon YD, Scheid JF, Shi W, Xu L, Yang Y, Zhu J, Nussenzweig MC, Sodroski J, Shapiro L, Nabel GJ, Mascola JR, Kwong PD.** 2010. Structural basis for broad and potent neutralization of HIV-1 by antibody VRC01. *Science* **329:**811–817.

33. **Bonsignori M, Hwang KK, Chen X, Tsao CY, Morris L, Gray E, Marshall DJ, Crump JA, Kapiga SH, Sam NE, Sinangil F, Pancera M, Yongping Y, Zhang B, Zhu J, Kwong PD, O'Dell S, Mascola JR, Wu L, Nabel GJ, Phogat S, Seaman MS, Whitesides JF, Moody MA, Kelsoe G, Yang X, Sodroski J, Shaw GM, Montefiori DC, Kepler TB, Tomaras GD, Alam SM, Liao HX, Haynes BF.** 2011. Analysis of a clonal lineage of HIV-1 envelope V2/V3 conformational epitope-specific broadly neutralizing antibodies and their inferred unmutated common ancestors. *J Virol* **85:**9998–10009.

34. **Falkowska E, Ramos A, Feng Y, Zhou T, Moquin S, Walker LM, Wu X, Seaman MS, Wrin T, Kwong PD, Wyatt RT, Mascola JR, Poignard P, Burton DR.** 2012. PGV04, an HIV-1 gp120 CD4 binding site antibody, is broad and potent in neutralization but does not induce conformational changes characteristic of CD4. *J Virol* **86:**4394–4403.

35. **Kwong PD, Mascola JR, Nabel GJ.** 2013. Broadly neutralizing antibodies and the search for an HIV-1 vaccine: the end of the beginning. *Nat Rev Immunol* **13**:693–701.

36. **Zhou T, Zhu J, Wu X, Moquin S, Zhang B, Acharya P, Georgiev IS, Altae-Tran HR, Chuang GY, Joyce MG, Do Kwon Y, Longo NS, Louder MK, Luongo T, McKee K, Schramm CA, Skinner J, Yang Y, Yang Z, Zhang Z, Zheng A, Bonsignori M, Haynes BF, Scheid JF, Nussenzweig MC, Simek M, Burton DR, Koff WC, Mullikin JC, Connors M, Shapiro L, Nabel GJ, Mascola JR, Kwong PD.** 2013. Multidonor analysis reveals structural elements, genetic determinants, and maturation pathway for HIV-1 neutralization by VRC01-class antibodies. *Immunity* **39**:245–258.

37. **Alam SM, Dennison SM, Aussedat B, Vohra Y, Park PK, Fernandez-Tejada A, Stewart S, Jaeger FH, Anasti K, Blinn JH, Kepler TB, Bonsignori M, Liao HX, Sodroski JG, Danishefsky SJ, Haynes BF.** 2013. Recognition of synthetic glycopeptides by HIV-1 broadly neutralizing antibodies and their unmutated ancestors. *Proc Natl Acad Sci USA* **110**:18214–18219.

38. **Jardine J, Julien JP, Menis S, Ota T, Kalyuzhniy O, McGuire A, Sok D, Huang PS, MacPherson S, Jones M, Nieusma T, Mathison J, Baker D, Ward AB, Burton DR, Stamatatos L, Nemazee D, Wilson IA, Schief WR.** 2013. Rational HIV immunogen design to target specific germline B cell receptors. *Science* **340**:711–716.

39. **Moldt B, Rakasz EG, Schultz N, Chan-Hui PY, Swiderek K, Weisgrau KL, Piaskowski SM, Bergman Z, Watkins DI, Poignard P, Burton DR.** 2012. Highly potent HIV-specific antibody neutralization in vitro translates into effective protection against mucosal SHIV challenge in vivo. *Proc Natl Acad Sci USA* **109**:18921–18925.

40. **Asokan A.** 2010. Reengineered AAV vectors: old dog, new tricks. *Discov Med* **9**:399–403.

41. **Coura Rdos S, Nardi NB.** 2007. The state of the art of adeno-associated virus-based vectors in gene therapy. *Virol J* **4**:99. doi:10.1186/1743-422X-4-99

42. **Daya S, Berns KI.** 2008. Gene therapy using adeno-associated virus vectors. *Clin Microbiol Rev* **21**:583–593.

43. **Nowrouzi A, Penaud-Budloo M, Kaeppel C, Appelt U, Le Guiner C, Moullier P, von Kalle C, Snyder RO, Schmidt M.** 2012. Integration frequency and intermolecular recombination of rAAV vectors in non-human primate skeletal muscle and liver. *Mol Ther* **20**:1177–1186.

44. **Penaud-Budloo M, Le Guiner C, Nowrouzi A, Toromanoff A, Cherel Y, Chenuaud P, Schmidt M, von Kalle C, Rolling F, Moullier P, Snyder RO.** 2008. Adeno-associated virus vector genomes persist as episomal chromatin in primate muscle. *J Virol* **82**:7875–7885.

45. **Schnepp BC, Clark KR, Klemanski DL, Pacak CA, Johnson PR.** 2003. Genetic fate of recombinant adeno-associated virus vector genomes in muscle. *J Virol* **77**:3495–3504.

46. **Aalbers CJ, Tak PP, Vervoordeldonk MJ.** 2011. Advancements in adeno-associated viral gene therapy approaches: exploring a new horizon. *F1000 Med Rep* **3**:17. doi:10.3410/M3-17.

47. **Lewis AD, Chen R, Montefiori DC, Johnson PR, Clark KR.** 2002. Generation of neutralizing activity against human immunodeficiency virus type 1 in serum by antibody gene transfer. *J Virol* **76**:8769–8775.

48. **Fang JM, Qian JJ, Yi SY, Harding TC, Tu GH, VanRoey M, Jooss K.** 2005. Stable antibody expression at therapeutic levels using the 2A peptide. *Nat Biotechnol* **23**:584–590.

49. **Ashkenazi A, Chamow SM.** 1997. Immunoadhesins as research tools and therapeutic agents. *Curr Opin Immunol* **9**:195–200.

50. **Capon DJ, Chamow SM, Mordenti J, Marsters SA, Gregory T, Mitsuya H, Byrn RA, Lucas C, Wurm FM, Groopman JE, Broder S, Smith DH.** 1989. Designing CD4 immunoadhesins for AIDS therapy. *Nature* **337**:525–531.

51. **Limberis MP, Adam VS, Wong G, Gren J, Kobasa D, Ross TM, Kobinger GP, Tretiakova A, Wilson JM.** 2013. Intranasal antibody gene transfer in mice and ferrets elicits broad protection against pandemic influenza. *Sci Transl Med* **5**:187ra172. doi:10.1126/scitranslmed.3006299

52. **Weinblatt ME, Bathon JM, Kremer JM, Fleischmann RM, Schiff MH, Martin RW, Baumgartner SW, Park GS, Mancini EL, Genovese MC.** 2011. Safety and efficacy of etanercept beyond 10 years of therapy in North American patients with early and longstanding rheumatoid arthritis. *Arthritis Care Res (Hoboken)* **63**:373–382.

53. **Johnson WE, Sanford H, Schwall L, Burton DR, Parren PW, Robinson JE, Desrosiers RC.** 2003. Assorted mutations in the envelope gene of simian immunodeficiency virus lead to loss of neutralization resistance against antibodies representing a broad spectrum of specificities. *J Virol* **77**:9993–10003.

54. **Allaway GP, Ryder AM, Beaudry GA, Maddon PJ.** 1993. Synergistic inhibition of HIV-1 envelope-mediated cell fusion by CD4-based molecules in combination with antibodies to gp120 or gp41. *AIDS Res Hum Retroviruses* **9**:581–587.

55. **Balazs AB, Chen J, Hong CM, Rao DS, Yang L, Baltimore D.** 2012. Antibody-based protection against HIV infection by vectored immunoprophylaxis. *Nature* **481**:81–84.

56. **Horwitz JA, Halper-Stromberg A, Mouquet H, Gitlin AD, Tretiakova A, Eisenreich TR, Malbec M, Gravemann S, Billerbeck E, Dorner M, Buning H, Schwartz O, Knops E, Kaiser R, Seaman MS, Wilson JM, Rice CM, Ploss A, Bjorkman PJ, Klein F, Nussenzweig MC.** 2013. HIV-1 suppression and durable control by combining single broadly neutralizing antibodies and antiretroviral drugs in humanized mice. *Proc Natl Acad Sci USA* **110:**16538–16543.

57. **Mouquet H, Scharf L, Euler Z, Liu Y, Eden C, Scheid JF, Halper-Stromberg A, Gnanapragasam PN, Spencer DI, Seaman MS, Schuitemaker H, Feizi T, Nussenzweig MC, Bjorkman PJ.** 2012. Complex-type N-glycan recognition by potent broadly neutralizing HIV antibodies. *Proc Natl Acad Sci USA* **109:**E3268–E3277.

58. **Klein F, Halper-Stromberg A, Horwitz JA, Gruell H, Scheid JF, Bournazos S, Mouquet H, Spatz LA, Diskin R, Abadir A, Zang T, Dorner M, Billerbeck E, Labitt RN, Gaebler C, Marcovecchio PM, Incesu RB, Eisenreich TR, Bieniasz PD, Seaman MS, Bjorkman PJ, Ravetch JV, Ploss A, Nussenzweig MC.** 2012. HIV therapy by a combination of broadly neutralizing antibodies in humanized mice. *Nature* **492:**118–122.

59. **Skaricic D, Traube C, De B, Joh J, Boyer J, Crystal RG, Worgall S.** 2008. Genetic delivery of an anti-RSV antibody to protect against pulmonary infection with RSV. *Virology* **378:**79–85.

60. **Corti D, Voss J, Gamblin SJ, Codoni G, Macagno A, Jarrossay D, Vachieri SG, Pinna D, Minola A, Vanzetta F, Silacci C, Fernandez-Rodriguez BM, Agatic G, Bianchi S, Giacchetto-Sasselli I, Calder L, Sallusto F, Collins P, Haire LF, Temperton N, Langedijk JP, Skehel JJ, Lanzavecchia A.** 2011. A neutralizing antibody selected from plasma cells that binds to group 1 and group 2 influenza A hemagglutinins. *Science* **333:**850–856.

61. **Limberis MP, Racine T, Kobasa D, Li Y, Gao GF, Kobinger G, Wilson JM.** 2013. Vectored expression of a broadly neutralizing antibody (FI6) in mouse airway provides partial protection against a new avian influenza A (H7N9) virus. *Clin Vaccine Immunol* **20:**1836–1837.

62. **Balazs AB, Bloom JD, Hong CM, Rao DS, Baltimore D.** 2013. Broad protection against influenza infection by vectored immunoprophylaxis in mice. *Nat Biotechnol* **31:**647–652.

63. **Sui J, Hwang WC, Perez S, Wei G, Aird D, Chen LM, Santelli E, Stec B, Cadwell G, Ali M, Wan H, Murakami A, Yammanuru A, Han T, Cox NJ, Bankston LA, Donis RO, Liddington RC, Marasco WA.** 2009. Structural and functional bases for broad-spectrum neutralization of avian and human influenza A viruses. *Nat Struct Mol Biol* **16:**265–273.

64. **Throsby M, van den Brink E, Jongeneelen M, Poon LL, Alard P, Cornelissen L, Bakker A, Cox F, van Deventer E, Guan Y, Cinatl J, ter Meulen J, Lasters I, Carsetti R, Peiris M, de Kruif J, Goudsmit J.** 2008. Heterosubtypic neutralizing monoclonal antibodies cross-protective against H5N1 and H1N1 recovered from human IgM+ memory B cells. *PLoS One* **3:**e3942. doi:10.1371/journal.pone.0003942

65. **Hicks MJ, Rosenberg JB, De BP, Pagovich OE, Young CN, Qiu JP, Kaminsky SM, Hackett NR, Worgall S, Janda KD, Davisson RL, Crystal RG.** 2012. AAV-directed persistent expression of a gene encoding anti-nicotine antibody for smoking cessation. *Sci Transl Med* **4:**140ra187. doi:10.1126/scitranslmed.3003611

66. **Rosenberg JB, Hicks MJ, De BP, Pagovich O, Frenk E, Janda KD, Wee S, Koob GF, Hackett NR, Kaminsky SM, Worgall S, Tignor N, Mezey JG, Crystal RG.** 2012. AAVrh.10-mediated expression of an anti-cocaine antibody mediates persistent passive immunization that suppresses cocaine-induced behavior. *Hum Gene Ther* **23:**451–459.

67. **Keizer RJ, Huitema AD, Schellens JH, Beijnen JH.** 2010. Clinical pharmacokinetics of therapeutic monoclonal antibodies. *Clin Pharmacokinet* **49:**493–507.

68. **Kessler M, Goldsmith D, Schellekens H.** 2006. Immunogenicity of biopharmaceuticals. *Nephrol Dial Transplant* **21**(Suppl 5)**:**9–12.

69. **Fang J, Yi S, Simmons A, Tu GH, Nguyen M, Harding TC, VanRoey M, Jooss K.** 2007. An antibody delivery system for regulated expression of therapeutic levels of monoclonal antibodies in vivo. *Mol Ther* **15:**1153–1159.

70. **Rivera VM, Gao GP, Grant RL, Schnell MA, Zoltick PW, Rozamus LW, Clackson T, Wilson JM.** 2005. Long-term pharmacologically regulated expression of erythropoietin in primates following AAV-mediated gene transfer. *Blood* **105:**1424–1430.

71. **Nguyen M, Huan-Tu G, Gonzalez-Edick M, Rivera VM, Clackson T, Jooss KU, Harding TC.** 2007. Rapamycin-regulated control of anti-angiogenic tumor therapy following rAAV-mediated gene transfer. *Mol Ther* **15:**912–920.

72. **Schnepp BC, Johnson PR.** 2014. Adeno-associated virus delivery of broadly neutralizing antibodies. *Curr Opin HIV AIDS* **9:**205–256.

Index